Lifestyle Psychiatry

Lifestyle Medicine is a practice which adopts evidence-based lifestyle interventions as a primary modality to prevent, treat, and reverse chronic diseases. The six main pillars of this specialty include physical activity, nutrition, stress resilience, cessation or risk reduction of substance use, quality sleep, and connectivity. *Lifestyle Psychiatry: Through the Lens of Behavioral Medicine* is grounded in the same pillars, drawing upon theories, methods, and empirical findings from health psychology and behavioral medicine.

Lifestyle Psychiatry is a rapidly emerging area within healthcare informed by rigorous research within the social and biological sciences, public health, and medicine. A volume in the *Lifestyle Medicine* series, this book uses a comprehensive biopsychosocial approach to prevent and treat psychiatric disorders and promote mental and physical well-being through evidenced-based lifestyle interventions.

Features:

- Draws upon theories, methods, and empirical findings from health psychology and behavioral medicine.
- Provides evidence-based research on the bi-directionality of mental and physical health.
- Addresses fundamental neuroscience concepts and applies them to practical aspects of lifestyle practices, mental health, and brain health.

Appropriate for clinicians, primary care physicians, and those practicing in specialized areas, the information in this book provides users with practical tools to help explain, prevent, and treat psychiatric disorders and associated maladaptive health behaviors in patients.

Lifestyle Medicine

Series Editor: *James M. Rippe, Professor of Medicine,*
University of Massachusetts Medical School

Led by James M. Rippe, MD, founder of the Rippe Lifestyle Institute, this series is directed to a broad range of researchers and professionals consisting of topical books with clinical applications in nutrition and health, physical activity, obesity management, and applicable subjects in lifestyle medicine.

For more information, please visit: www.routledge.com/Lifestyle-Medicine/book-series/CRCLM

Lifestyle Psychiatry
Through the Lens of Behavioral Medicine

Edited by

Gia Merlo, MD, MBA, MEd
NYU Rory Meyers College of Nursing, New York, NY
NYU Grossman School of Medicine, New York, NY

Christopher P. Fagundes, PhD
Department of Psychological Sciences
Rice University, Houston, TX

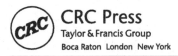

CRC Press
Taylor & Francis Group
Boca Raton London New York

CRC Press is an imprint of the
Taylor & Francis Group, an **informa** business

Designed cover image: Shutterstock

First edition published 2024
by CRC Press
2385 NW Executive Center Drive, Suite 320, Boca Raton FL 33431

and by CRC Press
4 Park Square, Milton Park, Abingdon, Oxon, OX14 4RN

CRC Press is an imprint of Taylor & Francis Group, LLC

ISBN: 978-1-032-23099-3 (hbk)
ISBN: 978-1-032-23097-9 (pbk)
ISBN: 978-1-003-27567-1 (ebk)

DOI: 10.1201/b22810

Typeset in Times
by KnowledgeWorks Global Ltd.

Contents

SECTION I   Theoretical Frameworks

SECTION II   Biopsychosocial Processes: Basic Concepts and Disease Implications

SECTION III   Risk and Protective Lifestyle Factors for Mental Health and Psychological Well-Being

SECTION IV Physical and Mental Health Conditions

SECTION V *Specific Populations*

About the Editors

Gia Merlo, MD, MBA, MEd is a clinical professor of nursing and senior advisor on wellness, a clinical professor of psychiatry at the NYU Grossman School of Medicine, and a fellow of the American College of Lifestyle Medicine. She recently published a textbook *Lifestyle Nursing* (Taylor & Francis/CRC Press, August 2022) that expands Lifestyle Medicine (an evidence-based approach in preventing, treating, and oftentimes, reversing chronic diseases) to nursing. Her first book, *Principles of Medical Professionalism* (Oxford University Press, 2021), stresses the importance of physician wellness, the need to address the social determinants of health, as well as the need to address chronic diseases with prevention. Merlo is the associate editor of the *American Journal of Lifestyle Medicine*. She is a contributing author of the American College of Lifestyle Medicine's (ACLM) curriculum *Lifestyle Medicine 101* and of the board review course, *Foundations to Lifestyle Medicine*. Merlo is a part of the Psychiatry Faculty Group Practice at NYU Grossman School of Medicine and sees patients at NYU Langone Health Psychiatry. She completed her Master of Education in Health Professions at Johns Hopkins University School of Education in August 2022 and is currently an Adjunct Faculty at Johns Hopkins helping students in the program complete their capstone projects. She is chair of the Mental and Behavioral Health Member Interest Group of the ACLM and founding chair of the American Psychiatric Association Lifestyle Psychiatry Caucus. She has been involved in clinician care and medical education for nearly 30 years in professional development and mental health, particularly for healthcare professionals.

Christopher P. Fagundes, PhD is a health psychologist and tenured professor in the Department of Psychological Sciences at Rice University. He uses theories and methods from clinical, social, and developmental psychology to examine how interpersonal relationships, loss, and trauma impact the molecular and cellular processes associated with diseases of older adulthood in diverse populations (e.g., cardiovascular disease, stroke, age-related cognitive decline, Alzheimer's disease & related dementias). He also develops and tests mechanism-focused interventions that target behavioral, psychological, and interpersonal processes underlying quality of life, age-related cognitive decline, and diseases of older adulthood. His grant portfolio includes longitudinal studies and clinical trials, which aim to improve the health and well-being of dementia family caregivers, cognitively impaired older adults, and recent widow(er)s. Over the last half-decade, he has been awarded over 10 million dollars in funding for his research (mainly from the National Institutes of Health). He has authored over 130 publications and is on the editorial board for *Psychological Science* and *Psychoneuroendocrinology*. He has been the primary mentor on several National Institutes of Health training fellowships. Dr. Fagundes is an elected fellow of the Academy of Behavioral Medicine Research, the leading honorary organization for scientists working at the interface of behavior and medicine.

Contributors

Liana Abascal, PhD, MPH
Alliant International University
San Diego, California

Leo Alexander III, PhD
School of Labor and Employment
    Relations and Department of
    Psychology
University of Illinois
Urbana-Champaign, Illinois

Joanne Angosta, PhD
Department of Psychology
University of Houston
Houston, Texas

Daniel Argueta, BA
Department of Psychological
    Sciences
Rice University
Houston, Texas

Mirna L. Arroyo-Miranda, DrPH JD
Department of Psychology
University of Houston
Houston, Texas

Gabrielle Bachtel, BS
Lake Erie College of Osteopathic
    Medicine
Bradenton, Florida

Martha A. Belury, PhD, RDN
The Ohio State University
Columbus, Ohio

Jennifer Braim, BS
University of Pittsburgh
School of Medicine
Pittsburgh, Pennsylvania

Ryan Linn Brown, PhD
Department of Psychiatry and
    Behavioral Sciences
University of California
San Francisco, California

Jolanta Burke, CPsychol, PhD
Royal College of Surgeons
Dublin, Ireland

Kari R. Campbell, MS
University of Pittsburgh Medical
    Center
Pittsburgh, Pennsylvania

Steven E. Carlson, MS
Department of Psychology
University of Utah
Salt Lake City, Utah

Allison J. Carroll, PhD
Department of Psychiatry and
    Behavioral Sciences
Northwestern University Feinberg
    School of Medicine
Chicago, Illinois

Vanika Chawla, MD, FRCPC
Department of Psychiatry & Behavioral
    Sciences
Stanford University School of Medicine
Palo Alto, California

Diana A. Chirinos, PhD
Department of Preventive
    Medicine
Northwestern University Feinberg
    School of Medicine
Chicago, Illinois

Dorothy T. Chiu, PhD
University of California, Berkeley &
Osher Center for Integrative Health
University of California
San Francisco, California

Lauren E. Chu, BA
Department of Biobehavioral Health
The Pennsylvania State University
State College, Pennsylvania

Matthew R. Cribbet, PhD
Department of Psychology
The University of Alabama
Tuscaloosa, Alabama

Jenny M. Cundiff, PhD
Department of Psychology
University of Alabama
Tuscaloosa, Alabama

Kristin M. Davis, PhD
Department of Biobehavioral Health
The Pennsylvania State University
State College, Pennsylvania

Marcel A. de Dios, MS, PhD
Health Research Institute
University of Houston
Houston, Texas

Andrea N. Decker, MA
Department of Psychology
The University of Alabama
Tuscaloosa, Alabama

Bryan T. Denny, PhD
Department of Psychological Sciences
Rice University
Houston, Texas

Lisa M. Diamond, PhD
Department of Psychology
University of Utah
Salt Lake City, Utah

Eva E. Dicker, MA
Department of Psychological
 Sciences
Rice University
Houston, Texas

Emma Dotson, DNP, AGPCNP-BC
Swedish Center for Healthy Aging
Swedish Neuroscience Institute
Seattle, Washington

Dawn M. Eichen, PhD
Department of Pediatrics
University of California
San Diego, California

Elissa Epel, PhD
Department of Psychiatry and
 Behavioral Sciences
University of California
San Francisco, California

Christopher P. Fagundes, PhD
Department of Psychological
 Sciences
Rice University
Houston, Texas

Robert D. Faulk, MA
Department of Psychology
University of Alabama
Tuscaloosa, Alabama

Lorena A. Ferguson, MA
Department of Psychological
 Sciences
Rice University
Houston, Texas

Heather Freeman, PsyD, E-RYT 500
Department of Psychiatry & Behavioral
 Sciences
Stanford University School of
 Medicine
Palo Alto, California

Christopher G. Engeland, PhD
The Pennsylvania State University
University Park, Pennsylvania

Joshua M. Garcia, BS
Department of Psychology
University of Houston
Houston, Texas

Luz M. Garcini, PhD, MPH
Department of Psychological Sciences
Rice University
Houston, Texas

Lorra Garey, PhD
Department of Psychology
University of Houston
Houston, Texas

Michelle T. Garza, MS
Center for Research to Advance
    Community Health
University of Texas at San Antonio
San Antonio, Texas

Pauline N. Goodson, BA
Department of Psychological Sciences
Rice University
Houston, Texas

Kaivalya Gudooru, BS
Center for Research to Advance
    Community Health
University of Texas at San Antonio
San Antonio, Texas

Emily A. Halvorson, MA
Department of Psychology
The University of Alabama
Tuscaloosa, Alabama

Elissa J. Hamlat, PhD
Department of Psychiatry and
    Behavioral Sciences
University of California
San Francisco, California

Charles F. Hodgman, MS
Department of Health and Human
    Performance
University of Houston
Houston, Texas

Nancy Isenberg, MD, MPH, FAAN
Medical Director, Swedish Center
    for Healthy Aging/Women's Brain
    Health Program
Swedish Neuroscience Institute
Seattle, Washington

Cramer J. Kallem, MA
University of Pittsburgh School of
    Medicine
Pittsburgh, Pennsylvania

Brooke Y. Kauffman, PhD
Department of Psychology
University of Houston
Houston, Texas

Joshua Landvatter, MA
Department of Psychology and Health
    Psychology Program
University of Utah
Salt Lake City, Utah

Emily C. LaVoy, PhD
Department of Health and Human
    Performance
University of Houston
Houston, Texas

Stephanie L. Leal, PhD
Department of Psychological Sciences
Rice University
Houston, Texas

Liana Lianov, MD, MPH
Royal College of Surgeons
Dublin, Ireland

Andrea P. Ochoa Lopez, MA
Department of Psychology
University of Houston
Houston, Texas

Richard B. Lopez, PhD
Department of Psychological &
    Cognitive Sciences
Worcester Polytechnic Institute
Worcester, Massachusetts

Annelise A. Madison, MA
The Ohio State University
Columbus, Ohio

Maryam S. Makowski, PhD
Department of Psychiatry & Behavioral
    Sciences
Stanford University School of
    Medicine
Palo Alto, California

Francisco D. Marquez, ScM, MA
Department of Psychology
The University of Alabama
Tuscaloosa, Alabama

Michelle N. Martinez, MA
Department of Psychology
University of Houston
Houston, Texas

Megan Marumoto, MD
Psychiatrist
Kailua, Hawaii
New York, New York

Luis D. Medina, PhD
Department of Psychology
University of Houston
Houston, Texas

Gia Merlo, MD, MBA, MEd
Department of Psychiatry
NYU Grossman School of Medicine
New York, New York
NYU Rory Meyers College of Nursing
New York, New York

Emma Moughan, BA
Department of Psychological &
    Cognitive Sciences
Worcester Polytechnic Institute
Worcester, Massachusetts

Kyle W. Murdock, PhD
Department of Biobehavioral
    Health
The Pennsylvania State
    University
State College, Pennsylvania

Douglas L. Noordsy, MD
Director of Lifestyle Psychiatry
Department of Psychiatry & Behavioral
    Sciences
Stanford University School of Medicine
Palo Alto, California

Jensine Paoletti, PhD
Rice University
Houston, Texas

Julia Starkovsky, MA
Department of Psychiatry and
    Behavioral Sciences
Northwestern University Feinberg
    School of Medicine
Chicago, Illinois

Jennifer L. Steel, PhD
University of Pittsburgh
School of Medicine
Pittsburgh, Pennsylvania

Steven G. Sugden, MD, MPH
Huntsman Mental Health Institute
University of Utah Spencer Fox Eccles
    School of Medicine
Salt Lake City, Utah

Tracey Tacana, BS
Department of Psychology and Health
    Psychology Program
University of Utah
Salt Lake City, Utah

Emily K. Tillman, MS, MSW
University of Pittsburgh Medical Center
Pittsburgh, Pennsylvania

A. Janet Tomiyama, PhD
Department of Psychology
University of California
Los Angeles, California

Autena Torbati, PhD
VA Palo Alto Health Care System
Palo Alto, California

Bert N. Uchino, PhD
Department of Psychology and Health
   Psychology Program
University of Utah
Salt Lake City, Utah

Alyssa M. Vela, PhD
Department of Surgery, Division of
   Cardiac Surgery
Northwestern University Feinberg
   School of Medicine
Chicago, Illinois

Ivanova Veras-de Jesús, BA
Department of Psychological Sciences
Rice University
Houston, Texas

Wendi Waits, MD
Psychiatrist
Kailua, Hawaii

Morgann West, BA
Department of Psychiatry and
   Behavioral Sciences
Northwestern University Feinberg
   School of Medicine
Chicago, Illinois

Paula G. Williams, PhD
Department of Psychology
University of Utah
Salt Lake City, Utah

Molly A. Wright, BS
The Pennsylvania State University
University Park, Pennsylvania

Lydia Wu-Chung, MA
Department of Psychological
   Sciences
Rice University
Houston, Texas

Allison Young, MD
Psychiatrist
Palm Beach Gardens, Florida

Anthony Zannas, PhD
Department of Psychiatry
University of North Carolina
Chapel Hill, North Carolina

Khadija Ziauddin, MBBS, MPH
Department of Psychological
   Sciences
Rice University
Houston, Texas

Michael J. Zvolensky, PhD
Department of Psychology
University of Houston
Houston, Texas

Foreword

It is a great pleasure to write the Foreword to this important book. *Lifestyle Psychiatry: Through the Lens of Behavioral Medicine*, edited by Drs. Gia Merlo and Christopher P. Fagundes, stands as the latest volume in the *Lifestyle Medicine Series* for which I am honored to serve as the Series Editor.

Drs. Merlo and Fagundes start from the fundamental insight that a bi-directional relationship exists between mental and physical health. Mental health guides the processes of physical health, and in turn, physical health undergirds the processes of mental health. Launching from this bidirectional platform, the editors and their contributors then leap into the area of behavioral medicine. They underscore the salient point that both mental and physical health are fostered and driven by daily habits and actions. Linking these three areas of research and practical application provides fundamental new insights into the human condition. This synthesis is both profound and long overdue.

Understanding the intrinsic links between mind and body and how they underpin human behavior and health is complicated but necessary. The journey to understand these interrelationships will fundamentally change the way we think about, and conduct research in, human behavior and both physical and mental health in the future. The field of exploring how lifestyle habits and actions impact both physical and mental health is a journey worth exploring. We could not have better guides than Drs. Merlo and Fagundes to inform this path.

The emerging area of lifestyle psychiatry, which combines the exploration of psychology, psychiatry, and behavioral medicine, represents one of the most exciting new areas in healthcare to emerge in the past decade. As the editors of this volume point out, however, this new field is subject to the danger of devolving into silos since it involves combining the expertise, backgrounds, and point of view of three separate groups of professionals. Drs. Merlo and Fagundes, aided by the group of high-level chapter authors they have selected, do a magnificent job of bridging these potentially disparate disciplines into a compelling and evidence-based book.

Lifestyle Psychiatry: Through the Lens of Behavioral Medicine is divided into two broad conceptual frameworks. The first half of the book elucidates the processes of neuroscience to provide the theoretical basis for how the brain guides behavior. This foundation then leads to the second area where these fundamental neuroscience concepts are applied to practical issues related to lifestyle habits and practices. The book concludes with an important section applying these insights to specific populations.

I particularly enjoyed how the authors blended solid evidence-based information on psychiatry and neurobiology with practical applications of how these fundamental understandings have the potential to motivate behavior change.

Behavior change is the holy grail of lifestyle medicine and should be the central focus of many aspects of mainstream medicine. For this reason, in all four editions of my *Lifestyle Medicine* academic textbook, I devoted a large section to behavioral medicine. The editors of the current book take the next step and provide solid evidence-based neurobiology and psychiatric concepts to further articulate and underpin how behavior occurs and how it can be changed.

As a cardiologist, I have been interested in brain health and its relationship to heart health for many years. In fact, in the most recent volume I have written in the *Lifestyle Medicine Series* entitled *"Integrating Lifestyle Medicine and Cardiovascular Health and Disease Prevention,"* I devoted three chapters to issues related to mental health, cognition, and brain health. The concept of brain health came into focus for me with the recent publication from the American Heart Association (AHA) and American Stroke Association (ASA) entitled *"Defining Optimal Brain Health in Adults: A Presidential Advisory from the American Heart Association/American Stroke Association."* This seminal work defined optimal brain health as "an optimal capacity to function adaptively in the environment." The Presidential Advisory goes on to state that "a healthy brain is essential for living a longer and fuller life. Brain health enables thought, planned action, and emotional connections that affect the daily lives and progress of individuals, families, and communities. Sustaining brain over the course of a lifetime is important to allow one to maximize one's overall ability and independence."

As recommended in the AHA/ASA document, brain health can be optimally preserved by following the framework developed by the American Heart Association entitled "Life's Simple 7" which is a summary of recommendations for managing blood pressure, controlling cholesterol, reducing blood sugar, becoming more physically active, improving nutrition, losing weight if necessary, and stopping smoking as mechanisms to preserve both heart health and brain health. (This rubric has subsequently been modified by the addition of a recommendation for healthy sleep, turning the mantra into "Life's Essential 8" further connecting heart health and brain health).

Brain health and mental health are intimately linked together and inextricably tied to behavior which is a concept that provides the intellectual foundation for the current book. I particularly enjoyed the seamless way the editors and their contributors stitched together the fundamentals of neuroscience into practical applications for the pillars of lifestyle medicine. These include physical activity, nutrition, stress, substance abuse, and healthy sleep.

I had the honor of naming the field of "lifestyle medicine" with the first edition of my multi-authored academic textbook in this area published in 1999. The 4th edition of my *Lifestyle Medicine* book will be published in 2024. The *Lifestyle Medicine Series* has been designed to expand and deepen the concept of lifestyle medicine and further tie the field to robust evidence. We have published seven books in the Lifestyle Medicine Series, with six more coming in the next two years. The books already published in the Lifestyle Medicine series include such topics as physical activity, obesity management, women's health, behavioral counseling, integrating lifestyle medicine into diabetes and pre-diabetes care, and linking lifestyle medicine to cardiovascular health and disease prevention.

In the next two years, additional books will include ones on lifestyle medicine and family practice, and geriatrics. In all instances, I have challenged the editors to bridge their underlying academic discipline to the robust evidence that now exists in the area of lifestyle medicine. This task has been beautifully accomplished in the current book edited by Merlo and Fagundes.

All of this brings me back to this important book *Lifestyle Psychiatry: Through the Lens of Behavioral Medicine*. I believe that the approach taken in this volume represents the future of lifestyle medicine. Just as the editors state in their Preface, "Lifestyle medicine is a field that addresses chronic diseases through prevention, treatment and in many cases reversal through lifestyle interventions. Lifestyle psychiatry, mental health, and brain health are central to every aspect of lifestyle medicine." I could not agree more!

The editors and contributors to this volume have done a masterful job of bridging the gap between neuroscience and its practical application to behaviors in our daily lives. This is the essence of lifestyle medicine and the cornerstone for the bidirectional relationship between mental health and physical health. The beneficiaries of this important synthesis will be not only practitioners in psychiatry, psychology, and behavioral medicine, but in the final analysis, the lives of all of the patients that they touch.

James M. Rippe, MD
Founder and Director, Rippe Lifestyle Institute
Professor of Medicine, UMass Chan Medical School

Preface

Lifestyle Psychiatry: Through the Lens of Behavioral Medicine

Having a psychiatrist and a psychologist co-edit a book focused on preventing and managing mental and physical health may seem odd to some readers — especially those working in settings where mental health providers do not interface with other health care providers clinically. This book represents the end product of a multi-year partnership between a clinically-oriented psychiatrist and a research-oriented psychologist who share the same fundamental assumption: positive health behaviors and emotional well-being provide the foundation for good physical health. The idea to collaborate on this project came from a phone call between Merlo and Fagundes that started as a casual phone conversation about each other's current research interests and career directions. One of us had just published a book on Lifestyle Medicine (Merlo), and the other was formulating a new Ph.D. program in health psychology at Rice University (Fagundes). A discussion about the similarities and differences between Lifestyle Medicine and Health Psychology ensued; we noticed considerable overlap. Both fields maintain that good health can be obtained by practicing positive health behaviors and maintaining psychological health. In addition, both disciplines are built on a research foundation that values empirically supported interventions. The differences we identified in subsequent conversations related to the clinical-research divide. Lifestyle Medicine articles seemed more clinically oriented than health psychology articles, emphasizing practical applications. Health psychology articles generally required a background in research and psychological theory to extract the key points. It became apparent throughout our collaboration that these disciplines reflected our own biases for this book. Rather than posing a barrier, we think one of this book's significant strengths comes from this difference. Having a professor who maintains a sizeable National Institutes of Health (NIH)-funded research lab co-edit a book on Lifestyle Psychiatry with a clinical professor with an active psychiatry practice helped ensure the book included high-quality research that is accessible and translatable.

At many institutions, psychiatrists and other mental health providers still work in silos, until called upon to address a potential psychiatric patient. The roots of this healthcare model stem from a time when the medical community viewed mental and physical health as independent entities, and acute disorders were the primary cause of morbidity and mortality. Yet, for those born in the latter half of the 20th century, chronic illnesses have replaced acute disorders as the primary cause of morbidity and mortality. Unlike acute illnesses, chronic diseases take decades to develop and are primarily caused and managed by psychological, behavioral, and social factors.

Because chronic illnesses are governed by psychosocial factors, a background in psychological theory, mental health, and empirically supported health behavior change interventions is critical for almost all providers. For example, there are now well-established evidenced-based lifestyle interventions that reliably elicit behavior change and improve emotional and social well-being. Unfortunately, most providers lack the knowledge base to deliver these interventions. Asking healthcare professionals from non-mental health disciplines to learn and stay abreast of the current state of the science in psychology and psychiatry by sifting through the vast array of studies and reviews, often filled with jargon, is unreasonable. The field of Lifestyle Psychiatry represents a disciplinary solution to this issue.

Lifestyle Medicine is a field that addresses chronic diseases through prevention, treatment, and in many cases reversal, through lifestyle interventions. Lifestyle psychiatry, mental health, and brain health are central to every aspect of lifestyle medicine. With a focus on good mental health and behavior change, the field uses empirically supported interventions to target health behaviors and well-being. In the same way, lifestyle medicine tackles the roots of medical conditions; transdiagnostic considerations of mental well-being allow us to address the underlying processes that shape our minds. The American Heart Association recently updated its essentials to include psychological well-being, which falls within mental health providers' expertise and scope of practice. By presenting the material through a research lens that is accessible and translatable, we hope this book will help break down the silos and unite the different fields of study within lifestyle psychiatry.

Lifestyle Psychiatry is practiced in several hospitals nationwide, including Harvard, Stanford, and NYU, and by a handful of practitioners. NIH-funded studies on core topics within Lifestyle Medicine are currently being run at hundreds of research institutions. The silos in the field of Lifestyle Psychiatry are real. Disciplinary separation, intellectual distance within lifestyle psychiatry, and the divide between research and practice hinder its growth and impact. This book aims to break down these barriers to collaborative and communicative efforts within the lifestyle psychiatry sphere. We also aim to present an integrative approach to the clinical applications of lifestyle interventions with a behavioral medicine lens that is strongly grounded in research.

The Australasian Psychiatry Guidelines were amended in 2019 to include lifestyle interventions as first-line treatments for patients with mild to moderate mood disorders and mild anxiety disorders. This book is intended to assist and educate students and residents in psychiatry residency programs and clerkships at medical schools. In the absence of adequate training in lifestyle interventions in mental health and brain health, budding clinicians rely exclusively upon medications and psychotherapy as their first lines of treatment. However, over 80% of chronic diseases can be addressed by lifestyle interventions. The bi-directionality between mental and physical health is significant and well-established in the literature. It is also important to note that over 50% of patients with psychiatric disorders prefer treatment from their primary care physicians. Therefore, this book may also serve as a resource for clinicians in the primary care setting. Marrying the concepts of psychology, psychiatry, and traditional medicine serves to help our patients as whole beings. The fractionation of healthcare creates artificial boundaries between disciplines that can be confusing and fail to account for this bidirectionality of well-being. Lifestyle Psychiatry aims to acknowledge the connections between stress, the immune response, mood, and various medical conditions, to alleviate the suffering and improve the outcomes of our patients.

Lifestyle Psychiatry has been emerging as a discipline for a decade in Australasia. Doug Noordsy cemented this concept in the literature through his edition of *Lifestyle Psychiatry*, published by American Psychiatric Association press in 2019. Noordsy has generously contributed a chapter to our text, and our book aims to add new dimensions to the constructs proposed in his volume.

Neither of us expected how much change and growth we would experience with each other and from our contributing authors over the last few years. Indeed, we have embraced our differences with curiosity and a passion for learning. Through this collaborative piece, we have broadened our perspectives, expanded our knowledge, challenged our assumptions, and overcome obstacles to accomplish more than we could have individually achieved. We sincerely hope this volume reflects this translational growth and helps the reader embrace such a process in their own practice and research.

Gia Merlo, MD
Christopher P. Fagundes, PhD

Acknowledgments

Many colleagues, students, friends, and family members have contributed to the success of bringing this book to life. We owe an enormous gratitude to them. In particular, we are exceedingly grateful for the contributing authors who generously contributed their expertise.

We thank Kristi English for organizing the receipt and review of each chapter and ensuring tasks were completed promptly and in an organized manner. Her contribution to the book's organization cannot be understated. In addition, we want to express our gratitude to Daniel Argueta, who worked tirelessly to ensure that final drafts were formatted and edited appropriately. His dedication to this project was invaluable. We wish to acknowledge Marzieh Majd for initiating contact with each chapter author during the initial stages of the project.

Dr. James Rippe, who has single-handedly moved lifestyle medicine forward with his vision for the *American Journal of Lifestyle Medicine*, groundbreaking books on lifestyle medicine, and now the lifestyle medicine series of books has been and continues to be a shining light in the field of lifestyle medicine. His patience and good judgment are invaluable and deeply appreciated.

The team at Taylor and Francis, especially Randy Brehm, Senior Editor, are such a pleasure to work with. Tom Connelly provided much-needed support to see this process through to completion.

Without our families' support and encouragement, nothing would be possible. Dr. Fagundes would like to thank Katherine, Madeleine, and Juliette Fagundes for their patience, love, and support during each stage of the book's development. In addition, he thanks Randy, Marty, Suzi, Matthew, Jacob, Nancy, and Charlie for their love and support.

Gia Merlo especially would like to thank her family and friends who have shown such love and kindness throughout the process, especially Monisha, Wayne, and Torin Lewis.

Section I

Theoretical Frameworks

Section 1

Theoretical Frameworks

1 Introduction to Lifestyle Psychiatry

Gia Merlo, MD, MBA, MEd and
Christopher P. Fagundes, PhD

KEY POINTS

- Lifestyle psychiatry is an emerging interventional field that targets health behavior change and patient well-being.
- The burgeoning field of lifestyle medicine aims to facilitate the treatment, management, and prevention of lifestyle-related conditions through evidence-based lifestyle interventions.
- Lifestyle medicine adopts a transdiagnostic approach that uses the biopsychosocial model of health to combine evidence-based and cost-effective lifestyle interventions that can be personalized to individual needs in conjunction with pharmacological and surgical interventions to provide well-rounded patient care.

1.1 CHRONIC ILLNESSES AND LIFESTYLE: PSYCHIATRY'S ROLE

Perhaps the most dramatic change in medicine over the past century is that chronic illnesses have supplanted acute infectious disease as the primary cause of morbidity and mortality. As a result, there has been a profound transition in predominant health problems from acute ailments to chronic illnesses in recent decades. Chronic diseases, such as cardiovascular disease, stroke, diabetes, and cancer, are currently the leading causes of mortality in the United States and many other developed countries.[1] Medical advancements and improvements within the healthcare system have led to increased life expectancies across the globe.[2] However, a longer lifespan increases the potential for chronic disease onset and progression. The worldwide crisis of increasing chronic disease prevalence has significant consequences for individuals, families, communities, and entire societies.[3] This phenomenon is driven by various factors, including, but not limited to, lifestyle behaviors such as physical inactivity, unhealthy diets, and risky substance use (e.g., tobacco, alcohol), as well as aging populations and environmental factors.[4] Chronic diseases can lead to disability, reduced quality of life, increased healthcare costs, and premature death. Individuals with chronic diseases often require ongoing medical care and support, which can be costly and significantly burden healthcare systems.[4] Addressing the chronic disease crisis requires a comprehensive transdiagnostic approach that includes prevention, early detection, and effective management of chronic diseases. Most chronic diseases can be prevented, managed, or treated with health-promoting lifestyle habits.[5] Therefore, efforts within the public health space must promote healthy lifestyle behaviors and access to affordable healthcare while finding ways to improve the healthcare system's capacity to manage chronic diseases effectively.

Mental health is the cornerstone for health and well-being. The mission of the emerging field of lifestyle medicine is to facilitate the treatment, management, and prevention of lifestyle-related conditions through evidence-based lifestyle interventions. Lifestyle medicine practitioners work with patients to develop personalized lifestyle plans that focus on the six pillars of lifestyle medicine, as well as educate patients on the importance of making healthy lifestyle choices. A growing body of evidence indicates the neurobiological pathways between lifestyle factors and mental health.[6] The current chronic disease crisis is intrinsically interconnected with the ongoing mental health crisis. Data suggest that one-third of individuals with a physical health condition are also affected by a mental health condition.[7] One in eight people worldwide were living with a mental disorder in 2019. The first year of the COVID-19 pandemic alone resulted in an increase in mental disorders, such as anxiety and major depressive disorders, by almost 30%.[8] Recent epidemiological data reveal that mental illness and lifestyle factors are leading causes of the global burden of disease.[9]

Mental health has been a public health concern for centuries. Historically, mental illness was often stigmatized and misunderstood. The concept of mental health is increasingly recognized as a critical component of overall health and well-being with significant efforts being made to increase access to mental health care and to reduce the stigma associated with mental illness. Organizations such as the World Health Organization (WHO) have been involved in mental health since their inception. Mental health was included as part of the WHO's constitution to promote health and prevent disease as early as the mid-20th century: "Health is a state of complete physical, mental, and social well-being and not merely the absence of disease or infirmity."[10] Addressing both the global chronic disease and mental health crises will require a transdiagnostic approach that considers symptomatology, social determinants of health, and individual lifestyle factors that each have a significant impact on health outcomes. It is impossible to adequately address overall health without considering all components of the biopsychosocial model of health. Lifestyle psychiatry is a burgeoning empirically-supported interventional field that targets health behavior change and patient well-being.

Wellness is defined as positive health that exemplifies quality of life and well-being.[11] Mental health is characterized by emotional well-being, health-supporting behavioral adjustment, freedom from anxiety, and the capacity to establish close connections while managing life stressors.[12] Brain health, as defined by the WHO, fosters optimal brain development, cognitive health, and well-being throughout the lifespan.[13] Wellness, mental health, and brain health are impacted by well-being, a state of relationship contentment with low levels of distress, overall good physical and mental health, and good quality of life.[12]. Six pillars of lifestyle medicine address and promote overall well-being: whole-food, plant-predominant eating patterns; physical activity; stress management; risky substance harm reduction; positive social connectivity; and restorative sleep.[14]

1.2   TRANSDIAGNOSTIC APPROACH TO HEALTHCARE

The field of lifestyle medicine adopts a biopsychosocial model of health. One of the key benefits of a transdiagnostic approach is that it identifies standard underlying processes that contribute to different causes of suboptimal mental health, brain health, physical health, and overall well-being.[15] For example, many mental health disorders, such as anxiety, depression, and substance abuse, share common cognitive processes, such as negative thinking patterns and difficulties regulating emotions. A transdiagnostic approach may provide more effective and efficient treatment for a wide range of health problems by targeting the underlying processes rather than treating the symptoms of specific diagnoses.[16] The field of lifestyle psychiatry, and lifestyle medicine more broadly, is well suited to adopt a transdiagnostic approach because strategies for successful health behavior change are similar regardless of the lifestyle pillar one is changing. By providing patients with a set of skills to target core processes underlying behavior change and relapse prevention, practitioners can target multiple lifestyle pillars simultaneously rather than sequentially.

A transdiagnostic approach can also be particularly crucial concerning the improvement of mental health and brain health because it can allow for a more personalized and individualized treatment approach to well-being. Clinicians can tailor treatment plans and lifestyle interventions to each patient's specific needs and challenges through a biopsychosocial lens and, thus, produce more effective health outcomes and improved brain health and mental health.[17-21] Healthcare professionals can use lifestyle medicine to help individuals achieve optimal health, manage chronic diseases more effectively, and reduce the burden of chronic disease on society.

1.3   SOCIAL DETERMINANTS OF HEALTH

Contextual factors like the social environment represent critical links to mental and physical health. Social determinants of health are the economic, social, and environmental conditions in which people live, work, and play. A large body of research shows that income, education, race/ethnicity, health literacy, language differences, discrimination, and other factors related to socioeconomic position (SEP) are potent determinants of health. These social determinants govern lifestyle behaviors and access to quality health care through several mechanisms described throughout this book. For example, SEP, an indicator of family income and social position, shapes one's immediate living environment, which in turn, impacts access to safe areas to engage in physical activity. These gaps in health outcomes related to SEP are due to a multitude of factors, including limited access to healthcare services, education, and resources; unhealthy lifestyle behaviors, exposure to environmental toxins, and chronic stress.[22-28] People with lower SEP are more likely to experience poorer physical health outcomes, such as chronic conditions like obesity, heart disease, and diabetes, and have a higher risk of premature mortality.[29] Lower SEP is also associated with a higher risk of mental health disorders such as depression, anxiety, and substance abuse.[22,23] People with lower SEP may experience chronic stress, leading to brain structure and function changes and increasing the risk of mental illness.[30,31] SEP can also impact brain health. Research has shown that individuals with lower SEP have a higher risk of cognitive decline, dementia, and other age-related brain disorders.[32,33] Addressing social and economic inequalities and inequities can improve health outcomes and promote well-being across diverse patient populations.

1.4 PERSONALITY AND INDIVIDUAL FACTORS

Personality and individual factors can significantly impact health and well-being.[34] There are several taxonomies for conceptualizing individual personality differences inspired by different theoretical traditions.[35] Developed within the trait theory tradition, the five-factor model has been particularly useful for understanding the relationship between personality traits and physical health outcomes.[35] It is also reliably associated with certain health behaviors and physiological reactivity profiles. Personality traits such as optimism and resilience can help individuals cope with stress, positively affecting their well-being. Personality traits such as neuroticism and extraversion have been linked to mental health issues such as anxiety and depression, which can negatively impact well-being.[36] [37] Some personality traits may be linked to genetic predispositions that can affect health outcomes. For instance, some studies suggest that individuals with certain personality traits may be more susceptible to heart disease.[38] Individual factors such as motivation, self-efficacy, and self-control can affect an individual's health behaviors, such as exercise, diet, and substance use.[39–42] For example, individuals with higher levels of self-efficacy may be more likely to engage in healthy behaviors. Individual factors such as social skills and social support can influence an individual's ability to form and maintain relationships, thereby positively affecting mental health and well-being.[43] Personality and individual factors are crucial determinants of health and well-being. Personality may be particularly useful for clinicians when prescribing personalized lifestyle interventions. However, it is important to note that the five-factor structure strength lies in its ability to describe *which* personality characteristics are associated with health outcomes. Yet, other theoretical perspectives are more adept at explaining *how* individual differences respond to their social environment in ways that impact physical health (e.g., social-cognitive tradition, circumplex of personality metatraits, interpersonal circumplex).[34] Accordingly, when developing tailored lifestyle interventions, it may be prudent for intervention developers to take into account multiple theoretical perspectives.

Personality frequently feeds directly into individuals' abilities and/or tendencies for emotional regulation, which is also a critical factor in maintaining optimal mental, brain, and physical health.[44,45] Emotional regulation refers to the ability to manage and respond to emotions in a healthy and adaptable way.[46,47] Poor emotional regulation has been linked to various mental health issues, such as anxiety, depression, and borderline personality disorder.[48–54] Individuals who struggle with emotional regulation may experience intense and overwhelming emotions, which can lead to negative thoughts, behaviors, and coping strategies.[54–56] Chronic stress, which can result from poor emotional regulation, has been linked to various health issues.[57] Poor emotional regulation can also lead to unhealthy lifestyle behaviors such as overeating, substance use, and a sedentary lifestyle, which can negatively impact well-being.[58–60] Effective emotional regulation has been linked to positive mental health outcomes such as improved mood, reduced anxiety, and increased resilience. It can also lead to health-promoting lifestyle behaviors such as regular exercise, a balanced diet, and good sleep hygiene. Brain health can also be promoted through effective emotional regulation through stress reduction and neuroprotection from structural and functional changes associated with chronic stress in the emotional regulation centers of the brain.[61–64] Developing effective emotional regulation strategies can help individuals better manage their emotions, improve their overall well-being, and reap the full benefits of medical interventions and treatment.

1.5 COGNITIVE AND BEHAVIORAL APPROACHES

Cognitive and behavioral approaches to lifestyle medicine are essential to mental health and brain health because they address the interplay between behavior, cognition, and emotion, critical factors in overall health and well-being.[65,66] Cognitive and behavioral intervention approaches effectively treat a range of mental health disorders, such as anxiety, depression, and post-traumatic stress disorder.[15,67–69] These approaches involve identifying and changing negative thoughts and behaviors that contribute to developing and maintaining disorders and thoughts and behaviors that may contribute to unhealthy lifestyle choices.[65,68] For example, cognitive behavioral therapy may involve helping an individual identify and challenge negative thoughts about exercise or healthy eating. Therefore, cognitive and behavioral approaches can allow individuals to develop and maintain healthier lifestyle habits supporting brain health and cognitive functioning. Better health outcomes and improved quality of life can be achieved by addressing the interactions between behavior, cognition, and emotions in lifestyle medicine.[70]

1.6 POSITIVE PSYCHOLOGY

Applying positive psychology constructs can contribute to promoting and maintaining mental health through lifestyle medicine.[71] Positive psychology and lifestyle medicine emphasize the importance of adopting healthy lifestyle behaviors and promoting positive psychological well-being.[72–78] Positive psychology focuses on understanding and promoting positive emotions, attitudes, and behaviors, such as gratitude, optimism, resilience, and mindfulness. It recognizes the importance of positive emotions and their impact on physical health, mental health, brain health, and well-being. Positive psychology interventions, such as meditation and gratitude protocols, have been shown to improve health outcomes, such as reducing symptoms of depression and anxiety.[79] Lifestyle medicine and positive psychology recognize that a holistic approach to health includes positive psychological well-being and lifestyle interventions that have a powerful impact on overall well-being and quality of life.[80–83]

1.7 BIOPSYCHOSOCIAL MODEL OF HEALTH

Aside from the cognitive-behavioral and positive psychology-based view of lifestyle medicine, the biopsychosocial model is an approach to health and illness that addresses the biological, psychological, and social factors that influence a person's overall well-being.[84] Biological factors include genetic predisposition, health behaviors, and physiological processes. Psychological factors refer to a person's mental and emotional state. Social factors include social support and connectivity, socioeconomic status, and cultural factors. There have been significant advancements in health neuroscience research over the past few decades, including neuroimaging techniques, an understanding of the brain-body connection, and neuroplasticity.[85-88] Neurotransmitters, brain circuits, and hormones are all part of the neurobiological system that affects mental health and brain health, underlies the function and structure of the nervous system, and regulates mood, behavior, and cognition.[89-92] Imbalances in neurobiological factors, including those related to genetics, the environment, and lifestyle habits, can lead to mental health disorders such as depression, anxiety, bipolar disorder, and schizophrenia.[89,90,93-95] Neurobiological factors can influence the autonomic nervous system, which modulates bodily functions such as heart rate, digestion, and respiratory rate. Stress and other emotional factors can lead to dysregulation of the autonomic nervous system, resulting in physical manifestations and increased risk of chronic diseases.[96-98] Understanding neurobiological factors can help healthcare practitioners discern the underlying causes of various health conditions and develop more effective treatments. Importantly, the biopsychosocial perspective is best utilized in lifestyle psychiatry when adopted in conjunction with other perspectives from positive psychology, personality psychology, and cognitive-behavioral theory.

1.8 AGE-RELATED DISEASES

Healthcare professionals can address the complex interplay between age-related diseases and their causative and associative factors through a biopsychosocial approach to lifestyle medicine. For example, a treatment plan for an individual with dementia may include medication to address biological factors, counseling to address psychological factors, and social activities and support to address social factors. Alzheimer's disease and related dementias (ADRDs) are a group of disorders that can be influenced by a wide range of biological, psychological, and social factors.[99-101] Healthcare practitioners need to understand the biological factors associated with ADRDs to properly diagnose the condition and consider treatments to slow its progression.[102] However, all factors related to ADRDs must be considered in a holistic manner to provide more comprehensive and effective care for individuals with ADRDs. ADRDs can cause significant psychological distress for both individuals with the condition and their caregivers.[103] Understanding the psychological impact of ADRDs can help providers provide appropriate support and interventions to improve quality of life for everyone involved in the treatment plan.[104] ADRDs can also impact an individual's social relationships and ability to participate in activities they enjoy.[105,106] Understanding social factors such as access to support systems, caregiving resources, and community engagement can help healthcare professionals develop care plans tailored to an individual's needs and preferences.

1.9 BRAIN HEALTH

In addition to purely cognitive and behavioral focused approaches to address psychopathology, the development of advanced neuroimaging techniques such as functional magnetic resonance imaging (fMRI) has allowed researchers to investigate and target cognitive, emotional, and thought processes in specific regions of the brain. Neurofeedback and neuroimaging can detect brain structural changes associated with Alzheimer's disease, major depressive disorder, and bipolar disorder.[107] A growing body of evidence demonstrates that the brain and body are intimately connected and that mental and emotional states can significantly impact physical health outcomes.[108–111] Mental disorder symptom severity exists on a spectrum. Expanding on the connection between mental health, brain health, and physical health can allow healthcare professionals to individualize and target lifestyle medicine techniques and interventions more efficiently and specifically. Current scientific limitations have given rise to the BrainHealth index, which measures whole brain health (cognition, social functioning, well-being, and real-life functions).[112] In conjunction with genetic and epigenetic considerations, the BrainHealth index may allow for earlier diagnoses and interventions. Early detection advances in health neuroscience have provided new insights and contributed to a better understanding of the neural basis of health and disease, which may help inform and adapt lifestyle treatments and interventions.[107,113]

1.10 TELOMERE AND IMAGING

Neuroimaging technologies are constantly evolving, as is the understanding of neurobiology's utility in medicine. Emerging research has suggested a link between mental health and cellular aging.[114–116] Telomeres are the protective caps at the ends of chromosomes that shorten with each cell division, leading to cellular aging and eventual cell death.[117] Telomere shortening has been associated with several age-related diseases, including cardiovascular disease, diabetes, and cancer.[118–120] Studies have found that individuals with mental health disorders, such as depression and anxiety, may have shorter telomeres than individuals without these disorders.[121–124] Additionally, individuals who experience chronic stress, which is often associated with mental health disorders, have also been found to exhibit shorter telomeres.[125] Stress linked to mental health disorders and chronic stress can activate the body's stress response system, leading to increased inflammation and oxidative stress, which can cause telomere shortening.[126]

Chronic activation of the stress response system can also cause damage to DNA and other cellular structures, contributing to cellular aging.[126] Inflammaging refers to a state of chronic, low-grade inflammation that results from the aging process.[127,128] It is a complex phenomenon that involves a variety of different biological processes and molecular pathways. Some factors contributing to inflammation include changes in the composition of the gut microbiome, increased oxidative stress, and a decline in immune function.[129,130] Growing evidence suggests that inflammaging may be linked to mental and brain health outcomes. Lifestyle medicine has been shown to disrupt the proinflammatory cycle of cellular stress in some biological pathways.[131] Therefore, researchers can develop lifestyle strategies for promoting healthy aging and preventing age-related cognitive decline and mental health problems by better understanding the underlying mechanisms of inflammaging and its effects on the brain.

1.11 HEALTH NEUROSCIENCE

Health neuroscience research has provided a mechanistic neurobiological understanding of lifestyle factors that govern mental and brain health. Health neuroscience
is a transdisciplinary field that focuses on understanding the neural basis of health and
disease. It integrates neuroscience, psychology, and clinical medicine principles to
investigate the relationship between the brain, behavior, and health outcomes. Reward
processing, regulating, and valuation are all critical processes in the brain that influence lifestyle behaviors and overall well-being.[132,133] The brain's reward system is a
complex neural network that regulates responses to pleasurable stimuli, such as food
and social interactions. Humans are naturally motivated to engage in activities that
the brain finds rewarding. For example, the pleasure of eating certain foods can lead
to overeating, contributing to weight gain and other health problems.[134] The brain's
reward system can be a powerful motivator for positive lifestyle behaviors. However,
improper regulation or impairment of the reward system in the brain can lead to
unhealthy behavior patterns and difficulty regulating behavior and making healthy
lifestyle choices. The prefrontal cortex, a brain region involved in decision-making
and self-control, regulates the brain's reward system.[132,135–137] Inhibitory mechanisms
governed by the prefrontal cortex can facilitate health-promoting decision-making
and resistance to unhealthy temptations.[132] Valuation refers to the brain's process of
assigning value to different stimuli and experiences.[132] Humans have an innate priority for activity and experiences that are perceived as valuable.[132,138,139] Therefore, the
valuation process plays a critical role in shaping lifestyle behaviors. For example,
if high value is placed on work and career success, an individual may neglect other
important aspects of a healthy lifestyle, including relationships and stress-reducing
leisure activities. Healthcare providers can use this knowledge to optimize their
patient's brain function and healthy lifestyle habits. Engaging in activities perceived
as rewarding in moderation can improve self-control and decision-making skills.[140]
Patients must be encouraged to consistently re-evaluate personal values to ensure that
they align with their overall well-being goals and the physical, mental, and emotional
symptoms that are being managed in their treatment plan.

1.12 PILLARS OF LIFESTYLE MEDICINE

Lifestyle medicine is based on six pillars that have been identified as key components for the maintenance of optimal health and the prevention of chronic diseases,
including restorative sleep, physical activity, nutrition, positive connectivity, risky
substance harm reduction, and stress management. Clinicians with psychiatric and
psychological training can clearly see how their expertise transcends all the pillars
of lifestyle medicine. The lifestyle medicine clinician, especially those practicing
lifestyle psychiatry, will be well served in educating patients around what they can
do to address these six pillars that all have emerging evidence-based data.

1.12.1 SLEEP

Lack of sleep has been linked to various mental health problems, including depression, anxiety, and mood disorders.[141,142] Sleep is essential for a properly functioning

autonomic, neuroendocrine, and immune system. Poor sleep has been linked to an increased risk of obesity, diabetes, cardiovascular disease, and other chronic health conditions.[143] Sleep is also critical for brain health, including cognitive functioning, memory consolidation, and learning. The brain consolidates memories and processes information essential for optimal brain functioning during sleep.[144] Chronic sleep deprivation can lead to cognitive impairment, memory loss, and other neurological problems.[145] Sleeping well each night can improve mood, increase energy levels, boost the immune system, and optimize brain functioning. Healthcare providers must address good sleep hygiene practices with patients to maintain optimal mental, brain, and physical health.

Those with unhealthy sleep patterns are at risk for stress-related disorders, mental health disorders, obesity, cancer, type 2 diabetes, and cardiovascular-related morbidity and mortality.[143,146] Insufficient sleep dysregulates the autonomic nervous system, diurnal cortisol patterns, and the synthesis of proteins.[147,148] Individuals with disrupted circadian rhythms are at a higher risk for breast cancer, DNA damage, dysregulated cytokine production balance, cancer, psychological stress, and depression.[149–151] Humans need less sleep to maintain health as they age. Although there is some individual-level variability, adults generally require 7 to 8 hours of sleep daily to avoid an increased risk of poor health outcomes.[152]

For individuals who struggle to achieve good sleep hygiene, cognitive behavioral therapy for insomnia (CBT-I) is a highly effective treatment option that can provide long-lasting patient benefits. CBT-I typically involves a combination of techniques designed to help patients change their sleep-related thoughts and behaviors. CBT-I has been shown to improve the quality of sleep for patients.[153,154] Patients undergoing CBT-I can fall asleep faster, stay asleep longer, and feel more rested and refreshed. Many people with insomnia use sleeping pills to help them sleep. Sleep-inducing medications can be habit-forming and have adverse side effects.[155] CBT-I can reduce the need for medication to induce sleep, which can help patients avoid these risks. The benefits of CBT-I are often long-lasting, whereas medications can provide short-term relief.[156] CBT-I teaches patients techniques that can be used across the lifespan to improve sleep. Insomnia can contribute to mental health issues like anxiety and depression.[157,158] CBT-I can help to improve mental health by enhancing sleep quality. Healthcare practitioners can work with patients to identify specific factors contributing to their insomnia and develop a treatment plan addressing them. Therefore, CBT-I is another lifestyle intervention that can be tailored to each patient's individual needs.

1.12.2 Physical Activity

In addition to sleep, exercise is an essential and effective component of a healthy lifestyle and should be addressed by all healthcare professionals. Adults should have 150 minutes of moderate-intensity exercise or 75 minutes of vigorous aerobic physical activity per week.[159] Children and adolescents require 60 minutes a day of moderate or vigorous exercise.[159]

Exercise has been shown to have numerous mental health benefits, including reduced symptoms of depression and anxiety, improved mood, and increased self-esteem.[160–162] Exercise can also help reduce stress, improve cognitive functioning, and promote better sleep, all of which can improve mental health.[160,163] Incorporating regular exercise into one's daily routine is essential for maintaining good physical health and reducing the risk of chronic health conditions. Moreover, data has demonstrated that exercise promotes the growth of new brain cells, reduces the risk of age-related cognitive decline, and improves brain function in people with neurological disorders such as Alzheimer's disease and Parkinson's disease.[160,162,163]

Physical activity is a significant risk factor for over 30 chronic diseases. Those who meet the current guidelines for physical activity lower their risk of all-cause morbidity and mortality by almost 20%.[164] Physical inactivity is associated with cancer, cardiovascular disease, type 2 diabetes, the onset and progression of cognitive decline and mental illness, and some forms of dementia.[165] In addition to its impact on physical health, physical activity also reduces the risk for mental health disorders. In a recent meta-analysis that included 49 prospective studies, those considered physical activity were 17% less likely to develop major depression than those not.[166]

1.12.3   NUTRITION: WHOLE-FOOD, PLANT-PREDOMINANT EATING PATTERN

Lifestyle medicine recommends a whole, primarily plant-based diet with fruits, vegetables, whole grains, legumes, nuts, and seeds. The field of lifestyle medicine encourages healthcare professionals to encourage their patients to maintain a diet low in red and processed meats, refined grains, sugar, and other saturated and trans-fat sources. Saturated fat raises blood levels of total cholesterol, triglycerides, and low-density lipoproteins (LDL), contributing to heart disease, stroke, and other vascular-related disorders.[167] Indeed, there is growing evidence that it significantly contributes to some forms of dementia.[168] Likewise, sugar intake, even in moderate amounts, promotes a similar lipid pattern and is associated with heart disease, stroke, and type 2 diabetes.[167] The Mediterranean diet and Dietary Approaches to Stop Hypertension (DASH) diet are evidence-based eating pattern recommendations that promote overall well-being.[169] Postprandial triglycerides and proinflammatory cytokine production, predictors of cardiovascular-related disease mortality associated with the Western diet, can be diminished by exercise, sleep quality, and changes in diet to follow lifestyle medicine guidelines.[170,171] The brain-gut-microbiota (BGM) system also affects brain and mental health. The gut microbiota interacts with the brain via the vagus nerve, the hypothalamic-pituitary-adrenal axis, the immune response, the intestinal epithelium, and the blood-brain barrier. Increasing evidence shows that depression and other mental health disorders impact the composition of the gut microbiome bi-directionally. When the gut microbiome is imbalanced (called dysbiosis), there is an increased appearance of pathology associated with the BGM.[172-179] Adherence to a whole food, plant-predominant eating pattern can promote diversity of gut microbiota, positively affecting mental and brain health via the BGM.

1.12.4   POSITIVE CONNECTIVITY

Social connection has been linked to depression, anxiety, and other mental health problems.[180] Studies have found that people with strong social connections are less likely to experience symptoms of mental illness and are more resilient in the face of stress. Social connection is also associated with physical health outcomes,[181] such as cardiovascular disease, cancer, type 2 diabetes, stroke, and some forms of dementia. The reasons for this are multifaceted. First, people with strong social connections are likelier to engage in healthy behaviors. They are less likely to smoke, drink alcohol excessively, or engage in unhealthy behaviors. Social connections are also critical for regulating the stress-response system; those with low levels of social connection have higher blood pressure, poorer cellular immune function, and an overactive proinflammatory state.

1.12.5 HARMFUL SUBSTANCE RISK REDUCTION

Tobacco and alcohol use are associated with DNA damage, cancer, and other chronic diseases.[182,183] The use of illicit drugs and abuse of prescription drugs have led to a rise in age-adjusted drug overdose rates each year since 2000 except for 2017.[184] Stress and depression are among the most significant risk factors for substance abuse.[185-188] Incorporating exercise and strong social connectedness can lower addiction risk.[189-191] Substance abuse can lead to addiction, a chronic relapsing condition characterized by compulsive substance-seeking behaviors and use despite harmful consequences. Substance abuse can lead to various mental health problems, including depression, anxiety, mood disorders, and psychotic disorders. It can also worsen existing mental health problems and make them more challenging to treat. Addiction can significantly impact all areas of a person's life, including relationships, work, and health. Early intervention can help to prevent further harm and improve overall health outcomes.

1.12.6 STRESS MANAGEMENT

Psychological stress can directly dysregulate physiological processes associated with premature aging, morbidity, and mortality. Stress also significantly impacts lifestyle choices, often leading to unhealthy habits and behaviors. Those experiencing stress are more likely to consume foods high in sugar, fat, and calories, rather than healthier options.[192] Weight gain and poor nutrition independently predict risk for disease and premature mortality.[193] Stress can trigger emotional eating. Emotional eating is an unhealthy coping mechanism for difficult emotions or life events that can lead to overeating, binge-eating, and cravings for high-calorie, high-fat, or sugary foods.[194] Stress can also disrupt normal eating patterns and lead to skipping meals or irregular eating, affecting metabolism, energy levels, and overall health. Metabolic health may be improved with interventions that improve stress and diet.[192,195,196]

1.13 BURNOUT

Burnout is a state of emotional, physical, and mental exhaustion caused by prolonged and excessive stress that can significantly affect well-being.[197] As a specific type of chronic stressor, burnout can lead to various physical health problems, such as chronic fatigue, and increase the risk of developing chronic illnesses such as hypertension, cardiovascular disease, and diabetes. Burnout can also contribute to various mental health problems, such as depression, anxiety, and mood disorders. Individuals with burnout can experience feelings of hopelessness, detachment, and loss of motivation.[198] Chronic burnout is associated with reduced emotion regulation, executive function, and attention.[199–202] Recognizing and addressing the signs of burnout, as well as taking steps to manage stress and prevent burnout, are important considerations in the field of lifestyle medicine.

1.14 CLINICAL APPLICATIONS

Lifestyle psychiatry can be part of a comprehensive treatment approach to promote overall health and well-being in individuals with psychotic disorders. A healthy diet that is rich in nutrients and regular exercise can help to improve the symptoms of psychotic disorders.[203–207] Healthcare professionals can work with patients to develop exercise plans that are safe and effective for their specific needs. Sleep disruptions worsen symptoms of psychotic disorders. Providers can work with patients to develop healthy sleep habits and address any problems contributing to their symptoms. Stress can also exacerbate symptoms of psychotic disorders. Therefore, effective stress management strategies can be an important part of treatment.[208–210] Strategies to reduce or eliminate substance use should be explored with patients with psychotic disorders, as substance use can worsen symptoms of psychotic disorders.

Physicians are encouraged to take "lifestyle medicine vital signs" as a means of comprehensive patient care. Addressing, preventing, and treating mental health conditions with lifestyle medicine techniques is accessible and affordable. Healthcare providers must use evidence-based strategies to ensure that their efforts to improve patient outcomes through lifestyle interventions are well-received, encouraging, and effective and promote the patient-provider connection.

REFERENCES

1. Armstrong GL, Conn LA, Pinner RW. Trends in infectious disease mortality in the United States during the 20th century. *JAMA*. 1999;281:61–66. doi:10.1001/jama. 281.1.61
2. Woolf SH, Schoomaker H. Life expectancy and mortality rates in the United States, 1959–2017. *JAMA*. 2019;322:1996–2016. doi:10.1001/jama.2019.16932
3. McGinnis JM, Williams-Russo P, Knickman JR. The case for more active policy attention to health promotion. *Health Affairs (Millwood)*. 2002;21:78–93. doi:10.1377/hlthaff.21.2.78
4. Schroeder SA. Shattuck lecture. We can do better–improving the health of the American people. *The New England Journal of Medicine*. 2007;357:1221–1228. doi:10.1056/NEJMsa073350
5. Rippe JM. *Lifestyle Medicine*. Taylor & Francis; 2019.
6. Firth J, Solmi M, Wootton RE, Vancampfort D, Schuch FB, Hoare E, *et al*. A meta-review of 'lifestyle psychiatry': The role of exercise, smoking, diet and sleep in the prevention and treatment of mental disorders. *World Psychiatry*. 2020;19:360–380. doi:10.1002/wps.20773
7. *Chronic Illness and Mental Health: Recognizing and Treating Depression*. National Institute of Mental Health (NIMH). n.d. URL: https://www.nimh.nih.gov/health/publications/chronic-illness-mental-health (Accessed 24 April 2023).

8. *Mental disorders.* n.d. URL: https://www.who.int/news-room/fact-sheets/detail/mental-disorders (Accessed 24 April 2023).
9. Global, regional, and national burden of 12 mental disorders in 204 countries and territories, 1990–2019: A systematic analysis for the global burden of disease study 2019. *The Lancet Psychiatry.* 2022;9:137–150. doi:10.1016/S2215-0366(21)00395-3.
10. Constitution of the World Health Organization. *American Journal of Public Health and the Nation's Health.* 1946;36:1315–1323. doi:10.2105/ajph.36.11.1315
11. Corbin CB, Pangrazi RP. *Toward a Uniform Definition of Wellness: A Commentary.* President's Council on Physical Fitness and Sports, 200 Independence Avenue, S; 2001.
12. *APA Dictionary of Psychology.* n.d. URL: https://dictionary.apa.org/ (Accessed 24 April 2023).
13. *Brain Health.* n.d. URL: https://www.who.int/health-topics/brain-health (Accessed 24 April 2023).
14. Pere D. Building physician competency in lifestyle medicine: A model for health improvement. *American Journal of Preventive Medicine.* 2017;52:260–261. doi:10.1016/j.amepre.2016.11.001
15. Dozois D, Seeds P, Collins K. Transdiagnostic approaches to the prevention of depression and anxiety. *Journal of Cognitive Psychotherapy.* 2009;23:44–59. doi:10.1891/0889-8391.23.1.44
16. Barlow DH, Allen LB, Choate ML. Toward a unified treatment for emotional disorders - republished article. *Behavior Therapy.* 2016;47:838–853. doi:10.1016/j.beth.2016.11.005
17. Minich DM, Bland JS. Personalized lifestyle medicine: Relevance for nutrition and lifestyle recommendations. *ScientificWorldJournal.* 2013;2013:129841. doi:10.1155/2013/129841
18. Ozomaro U, Wahlestedt C, Nemeroff CB. Personalized medicine in psychiatry: Problems and promises. *BMC Medicine.* 2013;11:132. doi:10.1186/1741-7015-11-132
19. Gutner CA, Galovski T, Bovin MJ, Schnurr PP. Emergence of transdiagnostic treatments for PTSD and posttraumatic distress. *Current Psychiatry Reports.* 2016;18:95. doi:10.1007/s11920-016-0734-x
20. Bolton P, Lee C, Haroz EE, Murray L, Dorsey S, Robinson C, *et al.* A transdiagnostic community-based mental health treatment for comorbid disorders: Development and outcomes of a randomized controlled trial among Burmese refugees in Thailand. *PLOS Medicine.* 2014;11:e1001757. doi:10.1371/journal.pmed.1001757
21. McQuaid RJ. Transdiagnostic biomarker approaches to mental health disorders: Consideration of symptom complexity, comorbidity and context. *Brain, Behavior, and Immunity – Health.* 2021;16:100303. doi:10.1016/j.bbih.2021.100303
22. Alegría M, NeMoyer A, Falgas I, Wang Y, Alvarez K. Social determinants of mental health: Where we are and where we need to go. *Current Psychiatry Reports.* 2018;20:95. doi:10.1007/s11920-018-0969-9
23. Bhugra D, Moussaoui D, Craig TJ, eds. *Oxford Textbook of Social Psychiatry.* Oxford, New York: Oxford University Press; 2022.
24. Fisher M, Baum F. The social determinants of mental health: Implications for research and health promotion. *Australian and New Zealand Journal of Psychiatry.* 2010;44:1057–63. doi:10.3109/00048674.2010.509311
25. Kyle T, Dunn JR. Effects of housing circumstances on health, quality of life and health-care use for people with severe mental illness: A review. *Health & Social Care in the Community.* 2008;16:1–15. doi:10.1111/j.1365-2524.2007.00723.x
26. Martin MS, Maddocks E, Chen Y, Gilman SE, Colman I. Food insecurity and mental illness: Disproportionate impacts in the context of perceived stress and social isolation. *Public Health.* 2016;132:86–91. doi:10.1016/j.puhe.2015.11.014

27. Compton MT, Shim R. This issue: The social determinants of mental health. *Psychiatric Annals.* 2014;44:17–20. doi:10.3928/00485713-20140108-03

28. Silver E, Mulvey EP, Swanson JW. Neighborhood structural characteristics and mental disorder: Faris and Dunham revisited. *Social Science & Medicine.* 2002;55:1457–1470. doi:10.1016/s0277-9536(01)00266-0

29. Stringhini S, Berkman L, Dugravot A, Ferrie JE, Marmot M, Kivimaki M, et al. Socioeconomic status, structural and functional measures of social support, and mortality: The British Whitehall II Cohort Study, 1985–2009. *American Journal of Epidemiology.* 2012;175:1275–1283. doi:10.1093/aje/kwr461

30. Dennis E, Manza P, Volkow ND. Socioeconomic status, BMI, and brain development in children. *Translational Psychiatry.* 2022;12:33. doi:10.1038/s41398-022-01779-3

31. Shaked D, Millman ZB, Moody DLB, Rosenberger WF, Shao H, Katzel LI, et al. Sociodemographic disparities in corticolimbic structures. *PLoS One.* 2019;14:e0216338. doi:10.1371/journal.pone.0216338

32. Cha H, Farina MP, Hayward MD. Socioeconomic status across the life course and dementia-status life expectancy among older Americans. *SSM Population Health.* 2021;15:100921. doi:10.1016/j.ssmph.2021.100921

33. Deckers K, Cadar D, van Boxtel MPJ, Verhey FRJ, Steptoe A, Köhler S. Modifiable risk factors explain socioeconomic inequalities in dementia risk: Evidence from a population-based prospective cohort study. *Journal of Alzheimer's Disease.* 2019; 71:549–57. doi:10.3233/JAD-190541

34. Smith TW. Toward a more systematic, cumulative, and applicable science of personality and health: Lessons from type D personality. *Psychosomatic Medicine.* 2011;73:528–532. doi:10.1097/PSY.0b013e31822e095e

35. Eysenck HJ. Trait theories of personality. *Companion Encyclopedia of Psychology.* Routledge; 1994.

36. Widiger TA, Sellbom M, Chmielewski M, Clark LA, DeYoung CG, Kotov R, et al. Personality in a hierarchical model of psychopathology. *Clinical Psychological Science.* 2019;7:77–92. doi:10.1177/2167702618797105

37. Brandes CM, Tackett JL. Contextualizing neuroticism in the hierarchical taxonomy of psychopathology. 2019. doi:10.31234/osf.io/23jm5

38. Smith TW, Williams PG, Segerstrom SC. Personality and physical health. *APA Handbook of Personality and Social Psychology, Volume 4: Personality Processes and Individual Differences.* Washington, DC, US: American Psychological Association; 2015:639–661.

39. Bauman AE, Reis RS, Sallis JF, Wells JC, Loos RJF, Martin BW, et al. Correlates of physical activity: Why are some people physically active and others not? *Lancet* 2012;380:258–71. doi:10.1016/S0140-6736(12)60735-1

40. Ahn J, Kim I. The effect of autonomy and self-control on changes in healthy lifestyles of inactive college students through regular exercise. *International Journal of Environmental Research and Public Health.* 2022;19:10727. doi:10.3390/ijerph191710727

41. Yang C, Zhou Y, Cao Q, Xia M, An J. The relationship between self-control and self-efficacy among patients with substance use disorders: Resilience and self-esteem as mediators. *Frontiers in Psychiatry.* 2019;10:388. doi:10.3389/fpsyt.2019.00388

42. Nezami BT, Lang W, Jakicic JM, Davis KK, Polzien K, Rickman AD, et al. The effect of self-efficacy on behavior and weight in a behavioral weight loss intervention. *Health Psychology.* 2016. doi:10.1037/hea0000378

43. Hughes ME, Waite LJ. Marital biography and health at mid-life. *Journal of Health and Social Behavior.* 2009;50:344–358.

44. Lopez RB, Denny BT. Negative affect mediates the relationship between use of emotion regulation strategies and general health in college-aged students. *Personality and Individual Differences.* 2019;151. doi:10.1016/j.paid.2019.109529

45. DeSteno D, Gross JJ, Kubzansky L. Affective science and health: The importance of emotion and emotion regulation. *Health Psychology.* 2013;32:474–486. doi:10.1037/a0030259

46. Gross JJ. The emerging field of emotion regulation: An integrative review. *Review of General Psychology.* 1998;2:271–299.

47. Gross JJ. The extended process model of emotion regulation: Elaborations, applications, and future directions. *Psychological Inquiry.* 2015;26:130–137. doi:10.1080/1047840X.2015.989751

48. Skodol AE, Gunderson JG, Pfohl B, Widiger TA, Livesley WJ, Siever LJ. The borderline diagnosis I: Psychopathology, comorbidity, and personality structure. *Biological Psychiatry.* 2002;51:936–950. doi:10.1016/s0006-3223(02)01324-0

49. Tomko RL, Trull TJ, Wood PK, Sher KJ. Characteristics of borderline personality disorder in a community sample: Comorbidity, treatment utilization, and general functioning. *Journal of Personality Disorders.* 2014;28:734–750. doi:10.1521/pedi_2012_26_093

50. Carpenter RW, Trull TJ. Components of emotion dysregulation in borderline personality disorder: A review. *Current Psychiatry Reports.* 2013;15:335. doi:10.1007/s11920-012-0335-2

51. Houben M, Claes L, Sleuwaegen E, Berens A, Vansteelandt K. Emotional reactivity to appraisals in patients with a borderline personality disorder: A daily life study. *Borderline Personality Disorder and Emotion Dysregulation.* 2018;5:18. doi:10.1186/s40479-018-0095-7

52. Bradley B, DeFife JA, Guarnaccia C, Phifer J, Fani N, Ressler KJ, *et al.* Emotion dysregulation and negative affect: Association with psychiatric symptoms. *The Journal of Clinical Psychiatry.* 2011;72:685–91. doi:10.4088/JCP.10m06409blu

53. Hofmann SG, Sawyer AT, Fang A, Asnaani A. Emotion dysregulation model of mood and anxiety disorders. *Depression and Anxiety.* 2012;29:409–416. doi:10.1002/da.21888

54. Espejo EP, Hammen C, Brennan PA. Elevated appraisals of the negative impact of naturally occurring life events: A risk factor for depressive and anxiety disorders. *Journal of Abnormal Child Psychology.* 2012;40:303–315. doi:10.1007/s10802-011-9552-0

55. Gómez de La Cuesta G, Schweizer S, Diehle J, Young J, Meiser-Stedman R. The relationship between maladaptive appraisals and posttraumatic stress disorder: A meta-analysis. *European Journal of Psychotraumatology.* 2019;10:1620084. doi:10.1080/20008198.2019.1620084

56. Kelly RE, Dodd AL, Mansell W. "When my moods drive upward there is nothing I can do about it": A review of extreme appraisals of internal states and the bipolar spectrum. *Frontiers in Psychology.* 2017;8:1235. doi:10.3389/fpsyg.2017.01235

57. Zahniser E, Conley CS. Interactions of emotion regulation and perceived stress in predicting emerging adults' subsequent internalizing symptoms. *Motivation and Emotion.* 2018;42:763–773. doi:10.1007/s11031-018-9696-0

58. Munsch S, Meyer AH, Quartier V, Wilhelm FH. Binge eating in binge eating disorder: A breakdown of emotion regulatory process? *Psychiatry Research.* 2012;195:118–124. doi:10.1016/j.psychres.2011.07.016.

59. Harrison A, Genders R, Davies H, Treasure J, Tchanturia K. Experimental measurement of the regulation of anger and aggression in women with anorexia nervosa. *Clinical Psychology & Psychotherapy.* 2011;18:445–452. doi:10.1002/cpp.726

60. Szasz PL, Szentagotai A, Hofmann SG. Effects of emotion regulation strategies on smoking craving, attentional bias, and task persistence. *Behaviour Research and Therapy.* 2012;50:333–340. doi:10.1016/j.brat.2012.02.010

61. Compare A, Zarbo C, Shonin E, Van Gordon W, Marconi C. Emotional regulation and depression: A potential mediator between heart and mind. *Cardiovascular Psychiatry and Neurology.* 2014;2014:324374. doi:10.1155/2014/324374

62. Kraiss JT, Ten Klooster PM, Moskowitz JT, Bohlmeijer ET. The relationship between emotion regulation and well-being in patients with mental disorders: A meta-analysis. *Comprehensive Psychiatry.* 2020;102:152189. doi:10.1016/j.comppsych. 2020.152189

63. Suzuki H, Botteron KN, Luby JL, Belden AC, Gaffrey MS, Babb CM, et al. Structural-functional correlations between hippocampal volume and cortico-limbic emotional responses in depressed children. *Cognitive, Affective, & Behavioral Neuroscience.* 2013;13:135–151. doi:10.3758/s13415-012-0121-y

64. Weissman DG, Rodman AM, Rosen ML, Kasparek S, Mayes M, Sheridan MA, et al. Contributions of emotion regulation and brain structure and function to adolescent internalizing problems and stress vulnerability during the COVID-19 pandemic: A longitudinal study. *Biological Psychiatry: Global Open Science.* 2021;1:272–282. doi:10. 1016/j.bpsgos.2021.06.001

65. Gonzalez-Prendes AA, Resko S, Cassady CM. *2. Cognitive - Behavioral Therapy. 2. Cognitive - Behavioral Therapy.* Columbia University Press; 2019:20–66.

66. *eTextbook: A History of Modern Psychology, 11th Edition - 9780357694589 - Cengage.* n.d. URL: https://www.cengage.com/c/a-history-of-modern-psychology-11e-schultz/ 9780357694589 (Accessed 24 April 2023).

67. Loerinc AG, Meuret AE, Twohig MP, Rosenfield D, Bluett EJ, Craske MG. Response rates for CBT for anxiety disorders: Need for standardized criteria. *Clinical Psychology Review.* 2015;42:72–82. doi:10.1016/j.cpr.2015.08.004

68. Dobson KS, Backs-Dermott BJ, Dozois DJA. Cognitive and cognitive behavioral therapies.In: *Handbook of Psychological Change: Psychotherapy Processes & Practices for the 21st Century.* Hoboken, NJ, US: John Wiley & Sons, Inc.; 2000:409–28.

69. Hofmann SG, Asnaani A, Vonk IJ, Sawyer AT, Fang A. The efficacy of cognitive behavioral therapy: A review of meta-analyses. *Cognitive Therapy and Research.* 2012;36:427–440.

70. Reavell J, Hopkinson M, Clarkesmith D, Lane DA. Effectiveness of cognitive behavioral therapy for depression and anxiety in patients with cardiovascular disease: A systematic review and meta-analysis. *Psychosomatic Medicine.* 2018;80:742–753. doi:10.1097/PSY.0000000000000626

71. Seligman MEP. Positive health. *Journal of Applied Psychology.* 2008;57:3–18. doi:10. 1111/j.1464-0597.2008.00351.x

72. Bolier L, Haverman M, Westerhof GJ, Riper H, Smit F, Bohlmeijer E. Positive psychology interventions: A meta-analysis of randomized controlled studies. *BMC Public Health.* 2013;13:119. doi:10.1186/1471-2458-13-119

73. Chakhssi F, Kraiss JT, Sommers-Spijkerman M, Bohlmeijer ET. The effect of positive psychology interventions on well-being and distress in clinical samples with psychiatric or somatic disorders: A systematic review and meta-analysis. *BMC Psychiatry.* 2018;18:211. doi:10.1186/s12888-018-1739-2

74. Hendriks T, Schotanus-Dijkstra M, Hassankhan A, de Jong J, Bohlmeijer E. The efficacy of multi-component positive psychology interventions: A systematic review and meta-analysis of randomized controlled trials. *Journal of Happiness Studies.* 2020;21:357–390. doi:10.1007/s10902-019-00082-1

75. van Agteren J, Iasiello M, Lo L, Bartholomaeus J, Kopsaftis Z, Carey M, *et al.* A systematic review and meta-analysis of psychological interventions to improve mental wellbeing. *Nature Human Behaviour.* 2021;5:631–652. doi:10.1038/s41562-021-01093-w

76. White CA, Uttl B, Holder MD. Meta-analyses of positive psychology interventions: The effects are much smaller than previously reported. *PLoS One.* 2019;14:e0216588. doi:10.1371/journal.pone.0216588

77. Van Cappellen P, Rice EL, Catalino LI, Fredrickson BL. Positive affective processes underlie positive health behaviour change. *Psychology & Health.* 2018;33:77–97. doi: 10.1080/08870446.2017.1320798

Introduction to Lifestyle Psychiatry **19**

78. Fredrickson BL. Chapter one - positive emotions broaden and build. In: Devine P, Plant A, eds. *Advances in Experimental Social Psychology*, vol. 47. Academic Press; 2013:1–53.
79. Lianov LS, Fredrickson BL, Barron C, Krishnaswami J, Wallace A. Positive psychology in lifestyle medicine and health care: Strategies for implementation. *American Journal of Lifestyle Medicine*. 2019;13:480–486. doi:10.1177/1559827619838992
80. Diener E. New findings and future directions for subjective well-being research. *American Psychologist*. 2012;67:590–597. doi:10.1037/a0029541
81. Huppert FA, So TTC. Flourishing across Europe: Application of a new conceptual framework for defining well-being. *Social Indicators Research*. 2013;110:837–861. doi:10.1007/s11205-011-9966-7
82. Ryff CD. Psychological well-being revisited: Advances in the science and practice of eudaimonia. *Psychotherapy and Psychosomatics*. 2014;83:10–28. doi:10.1159/000353263
83. Seligman M *Flourish*. 2012.
84. Engel GL. The need for A new medical model: A challenge for biomedicine. *Science*. 1977;196:129–136.
85. Tardif CL, Gauthier CJ, Steele CJ, Bazin P-L, Schäfer A, Schaefer A, *et al*. Advanced MRI techniques to improve our understanding of experience-induced neuroplasticity. *Neuroimage*. 2016;131:55–72. doi:10.1016/j.neuroimage.2015.08.047
86. Cope TE, Weil RS, Düzel E, Dickerson BC, Rowe JB. Advances in neuroimaging to support translational medicine in dementia. *Journal of Neurology, Neurosurgery and Psychiatry*. 2021;92:263–270. doi:10.1136/jnnp-2019-322402
87. St. Marie R, Talebkhah KS. Neurological evidence of a mind-body connection: mindfulness and pain control. *American Journal of Psychiatry Residents' Journal*. 2018;13:2–5. doi:10.1176/appi.ajp-rj.2018.130401
88. Power BD, Nguyen T, Hayhow B, Looi J. Neuroimaging in psychiatry: An update on neuroimaging in the clinical setting. *Australas Psychiatry*. 2016;24:157–163. doi:10.1177/1039856215618525
89. Philip NS, Carpenter LL, Tyrka AR, Price LH. Nicotinic acetylcholine receptors and depression: A review of the preclinical and clinical literature. *Psychopharmacology (Berl)*. 2010;212:1–12. doi:10.1007/s00213-010-1932-6
90. Nutt DJ. Relationship of neurotransmitters to the symptoms of major depressive disorder. *The Journal of Clinical Psychiatry*. 2008;69(Suppl E1):4–7.
91. George MS, Ketter TA, Post RM. Prefrontal cortex dysfunction in clinical depression. *Depression*. 1994;2:59–72. doi:10.1002/depr.3050020202
92. Bremner JD, Vythilingam M, Vermetten E, Nazeer A, Adil J, Khan S, et al. Reduced volume of orbitofrontal cortex in major depression. *Biological Psychiatry*. 2002;51:273–279. doi:10.1016/s0006-3223(01)01336-1
93. Serafini G. Neuroplasticity and major depression, the role of modern antidepressant drugs. *World Journal of Psychiatry*. 2012;2:49–57. doi:10.5498/wjp.v2.i3.49
94. Majd M, Saunders EFH, Engeland CG. Inflammation and the dimensions of depression: A review. *Frontiers in Neuroendocrinology*. 2020;56:100800. doi:10.1016/j.yfrne.2019.100800.
95. Kalin NH. The critical relationship between anxiety and depression. *The American Journal of Psychiatry*. 2020;177:365–367. doi:10.1176/appi.ajp.2020.20030305
96. Denny BT, Ochsner KN. Behavioral effects of longitudinal training in cognitive reappraisal. *Emotion*. 2014;14:425–433. doi:10.1037/a0035276
97. Johansson L, Guo X, Waern M, Ostling S, Gustafson D, Bengtsson C, *et al*. Midlife psychological stress and risk of dementia: A 35-year longitudinal population study. *Brain*. 2010;133:2217–2224. doi:10.1093/brain/awq116
98. Kivipelto M, Mangialasche F, Ngandu T. Lifestyle interventions to prevent cognitive impairment, dementia and Alzheimer disease. *Nature Reviews Neurology*. 2018; 14:653–666. doi:10.1038/s41582-018-0070-3

99. Seshadri S, Wolf PA, Beiser A, Au R, McNulty K, White R, *et al.* Lifetime risk of dementia and Alzheimer's disease. The impact of mortality on risk estimates in the Framingham study. *Neurology.* 1997;49:1498–1504. doi:10.1212/wnl.49.6.1498

100. Dilworth-Anderson P, Hendrie HC, Manly JJ, Khachaturian AS, Fazio S, Social, Behavioral and Diversity Research Workgroup of the Alzheimer's Association. Diagnosis and assessment of Alzheimer's disease in diverse populations. *Alzheimer's & Dementia.* 2008;4:305–309. doi:10.1016/j.jalz.2008.03.001

101. *Racial and Ethnic Disparities in Alzheimer's Disease: A Literature Review.* ASPE. n.d. URL: https://aspe.hhs.gov/reports/racial-ethnic-disparities-alzheimers-disease-literature-review-0 (Accessed 24 April 2023).

102. Arenaza-Urquijo EM, Vemuri P. Resistance vs resilience to Alzheimer disease: Clarifying terminology for preclinical studies. *Neurology.* 2018;90:695–703. doi:10. 1212/WNL.0000000000005303

103. Brodaty H, Donkin M. Family caregivers of people with dementia. *Dialogues in Clinical Neuroscience.* 2009;11:217–228.

104. Ashworth RM. Looking ahead to a future with Alzheimer's disease: Coping with the unknown. *Ageing & Society.* 2020;40:1647–1668. doi:10.1017/S0144686X19000151

105. Fratiglioni L, Paillard-Borg S, Winblad B. An active and socially integrated life-style in late life might protect against dementia. *Lancet Neurology.* 2004;3:343–353. doi:10.1016/S1474-4422(04)00767-7

106. Pillai JA, Verghese J. Social networks and their role in preventing dementia. *Indian Journal of Psychiatry.* 2009;51:S22–S28.

107. Jack CR, Petersen RC, Xu Y, O'Brien PC, Smith GE, Ivnik RJ, et al. Rates of hippo-campal atrophy correlate with change in clinical status in aging and AD. *Neurology.* 2000;**55**:484–489. doi:10.1212/wnl.55.4.484

108. Clapp M, Aurora N, Herrera L, Bhatia M, Wilen E, Wakefield S. Gut microbiota's effect on mental health: The gut-brain axis. *Clinics and Practice.* 2017;7:987. doi:10.4081/cp.2017.987

109. Panza F, Frisardi V, Capurso C, D'Introno A, Colacicco AM, Imbimbo BP, et al. Late-life depression, mild cognitive impairment, and dementia: Possible con-tinuum? *The American Journal of Geriatric Psychiatry.* 2010;18:98–116. doi:10.1097/ JGP.0b013e3181b0fa13

110. Huey ED, Lee S, Cheran G, Grafman J, Devanand DP, Alzheimer's Disease Neuroimaging Initiative. Brain regions involved in arousal and reward processing are associated with apathy in Alzheimer's disease and frontotemporal dementia. *Journal of Alzheimer's Disease.* 2017;55:551–558. doi:10.3233/JAD-160107

111. Shimoda K, Kimura M, Yokota M, Okubo Y. Comparison of regional gray matter volume abnormalities in Alzheimer's disease and late life depression with hippocam-pal atrophy using VSRAD analysis: A voxel-based morphometry study. *Psychiatry Research.* 2015;232:71–75. doi:10.1016/j.pscychresns.2015.01.018

112. Chapman SB, Fratantoni JM, Robertson IH, D'Esposito M, Ling GSF, Zientz J, et al. A Novel BrainHealth index prototype improved by telehealth-delivered train-ing during COVID-19. *Frontiers in Public Health.* 2021;9:641754. doi:10.3389/ fpubh.2021.641754

113. Butters MA, Young JB, Lopez O, Aizenstein HJ, Mulsant BH, Reynolds CF, et al. Pathways linking late-life depression to persistent cognitive impairment and dementia. *Dialogues in Clinical Neuroscience.* 2008;10:345–357. doi:10.31887/DCNS.2008.10.3/ mabutters

114. Byers AL, Yaffe K. Depression and risk of developing dementia. *Nature Reviews Neurology.* 2011;**7**:323–331. doi:10.1038/nrneurol.2011.60

115. Han X, Hou C, Yang H, Chen W, Ying Z, Hu Y, et al. Disease trajectories and mortality among individuals diagnosed with depression: A community-based cohort study in UK biobank. *Molecular Psychiatry.* 2021;26:6736–6746. doi:10.1038/s41380-021-01170-6

116. Sariaslan A, Sharpe M, Larsson H, Wolf A, Lichtenstein P, Fazel S. Psychiatric comorbidity and risk of premature mortality and suicide among those with chronic respiratory diseases, cardiovascular diseases, and diabetes in Sweden: A nationwide matched cohort study of over 1 million patients and their unaffected siblings. *PLoS Medicine.* 2022;19:e1003864. doi:10.1371/journal.pmed.1003864

117. Gilson E, Londoño-Vallejo A. Telomere length profiles in humans: All ends are not equal. *Cell Cycle.* 2007;6:2486–2494. doi:10.4161/cc.6.20.4798

118. Haycock PC, Heydon EE, Kaptoge S, Butterworth AS, Thompson A, Willeit P. Leucocyte telomere length and risk of cardiovascular disease: Systematic review and meta-analysis. *BMJ.* 2014;349:g4227. doi:10.1136/bmj.g4227

119. Ma H, Zhou Z, Wei S, Liu Z, Pooley KA, Dunning AM, *et al.* Shortened telomere length is associated with increased risk of cancer: A meta-analysis. *PLoS One.* 2011;6:e20466. doi:10.1371/journal.pone.0020466

120. Wang Q, Zhan Y, Pedersen NL, Fang F, Hägg S. Telomere length and all-cause mortality: A meta-analysis. *Ageing Research Reviews.* 2018;48:11–20. doi:10.1016/j.arr.2018.09.002

121. Darrow SM, Verhoeven JE, Révész D, Lindqvist D, Penninx BWJH, Delucchi KL, et al. The association between psychiatric disorders and telomere length: A meta-analysis involving 14,827 persons. *Psychosomatic Medicine.* 2016;78:776–787. doi:10.1097/PSY.0000000000000356

122. Pousa PA, Souza RM, Melo PHM, Correa BHM, Mendonça TSC, Simões-E-Silva AC, et al. Telomere shortening and psychiatric disorders: A systematic review. *Cells.* 2021;10:1423. doi:10.3390/cells10061423

123. Verhoeven JE, Révész D, Epel ES, Lin J, Wolkowitz OM, Penninx BWJH. Major depressive disorder and accelerated cellular aging: Results from a large psychiatric cohort study. *Molecular Psychiatry.* 2014;19:895–901. doi:10.1038/mp.2013.151

124. Wolkowitz O, Reus V, Mellon S. Of sound mind and body: Depression, disease, and accelerated aging. *Dialogues in Clinical Neuroscience.* 2011;13:25–39. doi:10.31887/DCNS.2011.13.1/owolkowitz

125. Epel ES, Blackburn EH, Lin J, Dhabhar FS, Adler NE, Morrow JD, *et al.* Accelerated telomere shortening in response to life stress. *Proceedings of the National Academy of Sciences of the United States of America.* 2004;101:17312–17315. doi:10.1073/pnas.0407162101

126. Lin J, Epel E. Stress and telomere shortening: Insights from cellular mechanisms. *Ageing Research Reviews.* 2022;73:101507. doi:10.1016/j.arr.2021.101507

127. Furman D, Campisi J, Verdin E, Carrera-Bastos P, Targ S, Franceschi C, et al. Chronic inflammation in the etiology of disease across the life span. *Nature Medicine.* 2019;25:1822–1832. doi:10.1038/s41591-019-0675-0

128. Kotas ME, Medzhitov R. Homeostasis, inflammation, and disease susceptibility. *Cell.* 2015;160:816–827. doi:10.1016/j.cell.2015.02.010

129. Cohen S, Janicki-Deverts D, Doyle WJ, Miller GE, Frank E, Rabin BS, et al. Chronic stress, glucocorticoid receptor resistance, inflammation, and disease risk. *PNAS.* 2012;109:5995–5999. doi:10.1073/pnas.1118355109

130. Franceschi C, Garagnani P, Parini P, Giuliani C, Santoro A. Inflammaging: A new immune-metabolic viewpoint for age-related diseases. *Nature Reviews Endocrinology.* 2018;14:576–590. doi:10.1038/s41574-018-0059-4

131. Dossett ML, Fricchione GL, Benson H. A new era for mind–body medicine. *The New England Journal of Medicine.* 2020;382:1390–1391. doi:10.1056/NEJMp1917461

132. Lopez R, Cruz-Vespa I. The brain bases of regulation of eating behaviors: The role of reward, executive control, and valuation processes, and new paths to propel the field forward. *Current Opinion in Behavioral Sciences.* 2022;48:101214. doi:10.1016/j.cobeha.2022.101214

133. Johnson H. Neuroscience in social work practice and education. *Journal of Social Work Practice in the Addictions*. 2001;1:81–102. doi:10.1300/J160v01n03_06
134. Kringelbach ML, O'Doherty J, Rolls ET, Andrews C. Activation of the human orbito-frontal cortex to a liquid food stimulus is correlated with its subjective pleasantness. *Cerebral Cortex*. 2003;13:1064–1071. doi:10.1093/cercor/13.10.1064
135. Enax L, Hu Y, Trautner P, Weber B. Nutrition labels influence value computation of food products in the ventromedial prefrontal cortex. *Obesity (Silver Spring)*. 2015;23: 786–792. doi:10.1002/oby.21027
136. Gearhardt AN, Yokum S, Stice E, Harris JL, Brownell KD. Relation of obesity to neural activation in response to food commercials. *Social Cognitive and Affective Neuroscience*. 2014;9:932–938. doi:10.1093/scan/nst059
137. Whelan ME, Morgan PS, Sherar LB, Orme MW, Esliger DW. Can functional magnetic resonance imaging studies help with the optimization of health messaging for lifestyle behavior change? A systematic review. *Preventive Medicine*. 2017;99:185–196. doi:10.1016/j.ypmed.2017.02.004
138. Rangel A, Camerer C, Montague PR. A framework for studying the neurobiology of value-based decision making. *Nature Reviews Neuroscience*. 2008;9:545–556. doi:10.1038/nrn2357
139. Brosch T, Sander D. Neurocognitive mechanisms underlying value-based decision-making: From core values to economic value. *Frontiers in Human Neuroscience*. 2013;7:398. doi:10.3389/fnhum.2013.00398
140. Kelley NJ, Finley AJ, Schmeichel BJ. After-effects of self-control: The reward responsivity hypothesis. *Cognitive, Affective, & Behavioral Neuroscience*. 2019;19:600–618. doi:10.3758/s13415-019-00694-3
141. Clement-Carbonell V, Portilla-Tamarit I, Rubio-Aparicio M, Madrid-Valero JJ. Sleep quality, mental and physical health: A differential relationship. *International Journal of Environmental Research and Public Health*. 2021;18:460. doi:10.3390/ijerph18020460
142. Magee JC, Carmin CN. The relationship between sleep and anxiety in older adults. *Current Psychiatry Reports*. 2010;12:13–19. doi:10.1007/s11920-009-0087-9
143. Grandner Ma. Addressing sleep disturbances: An opportunity to prevent cardiometabolic disease? *International Review of Psychiatry*. 2014;26:155–176. doi:10.3109/09540261.2014.911148
144. Rasch B, Born J. About Sleep's role in memory. *Physiological Reviews*. 2013;93: 681–766. doi:10.1152/physrev.00032.2012
145. Bishir M, Bhat A, Essa MM, Ekpo O, Ihunwo AO, Veeraraghavan VP, et al. Sleep deprivation and neurological disorders. *BioMed Research International*. 2020;2020:5764017. doi:10.1155/2020/5764017
146. Chattu VK, Manzar MD, Kumary S, Burman D, Spence DW, Pandi-Perumal SR. The global problem of insufficient sleep and its serious public health implications. *Healthcare (Basel)*. 2018;7:1. doi:10.3390/healthcare7010001
147. Morris CJ, Aeschbach D, Scheer FAJL. Circadian system, sleep and endocrinology. *Molecular and Cellular Endocrinology*. 2012;349:91–104. doi:10.1016/j.mce.2011.09.003
148. Sequeira VCC, Bandeira PM, Azevedo JCM. Heart rate variability in adults with obstructive sleep apnea: A systematic review. *Sleep Science*. 2019;12:214–221. doi:10.5935/1984-0063.20190082
149. Dimitrov S, Lange T, Tieken S, Fehm HL, Born J. Sleep associated regulation of t helper 1/t helper 2 cytokine balance in humans. *Brain, Behavior, and Immunity*. 2004; 18:341–348. doi:10.1016/j.bbi.2003.08.004
150. Barragán R, Ortega-Azorín C, Sorlí JV, Asensio EM, Coltell O, St-Onge M-P, et al. Effect of physical activity, smoking, and sleep on telomere length: A systematic review

of observational and intervention studies. *Journal of Clinical Medicine.* 2021;11:76. doi:10.3390/jcm11010076

151. Mogavero MP, DelRosso LM, Fanfulla F, Bruni O, Ferri R. Sleep disorders and cancer: State of the art and future perspectives. *Sleep Medicine Reviews.* 2021;56:101409. doi:10.1016/j.smrv.2020.101409.

152. Chaput J-P, Dutil C, Sampasa-Kanyinga H. Sleeping hours: What is the ideal number and how does age impact this? *Nature and Science of Sleep.* 2018;10:421–430. doi:10.2147/NSS.S163071

153. Koffel EA, Koffel JB, Gehrman PR. A meta-analysis of group cognitive behavioral therapy for insomnia. *Sleep Medicine Reviews.* 2015;19:6–16. doi:10.1016/j.smrv.2014. 05.001

154. Trauer JM, Qian MY, Doyle JS, Rajaratnam SMW, Cunnington D. Cognitive behavioral therapy for chronic insomnia: A systematic review and meta-analysis. *Annals of Internal Medicine.* 2015;163:191–204. doi:10.7326/M14-2841

155. Mellman TA. Sleep and anxiety disorders. *Sleep Medicine Clinics.* 2008;3:261–268. doi:10.1016/j.jsmc.2008.01.010

156. Morin CM, Benca R. Chronic insomnia. *Lancet.* 2012;379:1129–1141. doi:10.1016/ S0140-6736(11)60750-2

157. Fang H, Tu S, Sheng J, Shao A. Depression in sleep disturbance: A review on a bidirectional relationship, mechanisms and treatment. *Journal of Cellular and Molecular Medicine.* 2019;23:2324–2332. doi:10.1111/jcmm.14170

158. Ohayon MM, Caulet M, Lemoine P. Comorbidity of mental and insomnia disorders in the general population. *Comprehensive Psychiatry.* 1998;39:185–197. doi:10.1016/ s0010-440x(98)90059-1

159. U.S. Department of Health and Human Services. *Physical Activity Guidelines for Americans, 2nd edition - Healthy People 2030 | health.gov.* https://Health.Gov/ Paguidelines/Second-Edition/Pdf/Physical_Activity_Guidelines_2nd_edition.Pdf. n.d. URL: https://health.gov/healthypeople/tools-action/browse-evidence-based-resources/ physical-activity-guidelines-americans-2nd-edition (Accessed 30 August 2022).

160. Falkai P, Schmitt A, Rosenbeiger CP, Maurus I, Hattenkofer L, Hasan A, *et al.* Aerobic exercise in severe mental illness: Requirements from the perspective of sports medicine. *Eur Archives of Psychiatry and Clinical Neuroscience.* 2022;272:643–677. doi:10.1007/s00406-021-01360-x

161. Chen Z, Lan W, Yang G, Li Y, Ji X, Chen L, et al. Exercise intervention in treatment of neuropsychological diseases: A review. *Frontiers in Psychology.* 2020;11:569206. doi:10.3389/fpsyg.2020.569206

162. Caponnetto P, Casu M, Amato M, Cocuzza D, Galofaro V, La, Morella A, *et al.* The effects of physical exercise on mental health: From cognitive improvements to risk of addiction. *International Journal of Environmental Research and Public Health.* 2021;18:13384. doi:10.3390/ijerph182413384

163. Pedersen BK, Saltin B. Exercise as medicine – Evidence for prescribing exercise as therapy in 26 different chronic diseases. *Scandinavian Journal of Medicine & Science in Sports.* 2015;25:1–72. doi:10.1111/sms.12581

164. Lee DH, Rezende LFM, Joh H-K, Keum N, Ferrari G, Rey-Lopez JP, et al. Long-term leisure-time physical activity intensity and all-cause and cause-specific mortality: A prospective cohort of US adults. *Circulation.* 2022;146:523–534. doi:10.1161/ CIRCULATIONAHA.121.058162

165. Knight JA. Physical inactivity: Associated diseases and disorders. *Annals of Clinical & Laboratory Science.* 2012;42:320–337.

166. Schuch FB, Vancampfort D, Firth J, Rosenbaum S, Ward PB, Silva ES, et al. Physical activity and incident depression: A meta-analysis of prospective cohort studies. *The American Journal of Psychiatry.* 2018;175:631–648. doi:10.1176/appi.ajp.2018.17111194

167. DiNicolantonio JJ, Lucan SC, O'Keefe JH. The evidence for saturated fat and for sugar related to coronary heart disease. *Progress in Cardiovascular Diseases*. 2016; 58:464–472. doi:10.1016/j.pcad.2015.11.006

168. Zhu R-Z, Chen M-Q, Zhang Z-W, Wu T-Y, Zhao W-H. Dietary fatty acids and risk for Alzheimer's disease, dementia, and mild cognitive impairment: A prospective cohort meta-analysis. *Nutrition*. 2021;90:111355. doi:10.1016/j.nut.2021.111355

169. Liu X, Morris MC, Dhana K, Ventrelle J, Johnson K, Bishop L, *et al*. Mediterranean-DASH intervention for neurodegenerative delay (MIND) study: Rationale, design and baseline characteristics of a randomized control trial of the MIND diet on cognitive decline. *Contemporary Clinical Trials*. 2021;102:106270. doi:10.1016/j.cct.2021.106270

170. Mora S, Rifai N, Buring JE, Ridker PM. Fasting compared with nonfasting lipids and apolipoproteins for predicting incident cardiovascular events. *Circulation*. 2008; 118:993–1001. doi:10.1161/CIRCULATIONAHA.108.777334

171. Stalenhoef AF, de Graaf J. Association of fasting and nonfasting serum triglycerides with cardiovascular disease and the role of remnant-like lipoproteins and small dense LDL. *Current Opinion in Lipidology*. 2008;19:355–361. doi:10.1097/MOL.0b013e328304b63c

172. Cekanaviciute E, Yoo BB, Runia TF, Debelius JW, Singh S, Nelson CA, *et al*. Gut bacteria from multiple sclerosis patients modulate human t cells and exacerbate symptoms in mouse models. *Proceedings of the National Academy of Sciences of the United States*. 2017;114:10713–10718. doi:10.1073/pnas.1711235114

173. Sampson TR, Debelius JW, Thron T, Janssen S, Shastri GG, Ilhan ZE, *et al*. Gut Microbiota regulate motor deficits and neuroinflammation in a model of Parkinson's disease. *Cell*. 2016;167:1469–1480.e12. doi:10.1016/j.cell.2016.11.018

174. Senthong V, Wang Z, Li XS, Fan Y, Wu Y, Tang WHW, *et al*. Intestinal Microbiota-generated metabolite trimethylamine-n-oxide and 5-year mortality risk in stable coronary artery disease: The contributory role of intestinal microbiota in a COURAGE-like patient cohort. *Journal of the American Heart Association*. 2016;5:e002816. doi:10.1161/JAHA.115.002816

175. Li J, Zhao F, Wang Y, Chen J, Tao J, Tian G, *et al*. Gut microbiota dysbiosis contributes to the development of hypertension. *Microbiome*. 2017;5:14. doi:10.1186/s40168-016-0222-x

176. Carding S, Verbeke K, Vipond DT, Corfe BM, Owen LJ. Dysbiosis of the gut microbiota in disease. *Microbial Ecology in Health and Disease*. 2015;26. doi:10.3402/mehd.v26.26191

177. Fond G, Boukouaci W, Chevalier G, Regnault A, Eberl G, Hamdani N, *et al*. The 'psychomicrobiotic': Targeting microbiota in major psychiatric disorders: A systematic review. *Pathologie Biologie (Paris)*. 2015;63:35–42. doi:10.1016/j.patbio.2014.10.003

178. Tai N, Wong FS, Wen L. The role of gut microbiota in the development of type 1, type 2 diabetes mellitus and obesity. *Reviews in Endocrine and Metabolic Disorders*. 2015;16:55–65. doi:10.1007/s11154-015-9309-0

179. Dunlop AL, Mulle JG, Ferranti EP, Edwards S, Dunn AB, Corwin EJ. The maternal microbiome and pregnancy outcomes that impact infant health: A review. *Advances in Neonatal Care*. 2015;15:377–385. doi:10.1097/ANC.0000000000000218

180. Gariépy G, Honkaniemi H, Quesnel-Vallée A. Social support and protection from depression: Systematic review of current findings in Western countries. *British Journal of Psychiatry*. 2016;209:284–293. doi:10.1192/bjp.bp.115.169094

181. Holt-Lunstad J. Why social relationships are important for physical health: A systems approach to understanding and modifying risk and protection. *Annual Review of Psychology*. 2018;69:437–458. doi:10.1146/annurev-psych-122216-011902

182. *Alcohol*. n.d. URL: https://www.who.int/news-room/fact-sheets/detail/alcohol (Accessed 24 April 2023).

183. CDCTobaccoFree. *Health Effects of Cigarette Smoking*. Centers for Disease Control and Prevention. 2022. URL: https://www.cdc.gov/tobacco/data_statistics/fact_sheets/ health_effects/effects_cig_smoking/index.htm (Accessed 24 April 2023).
184. Hedegaard H, Miniño AM, Spencer MR, Warner M. Drug Overdose Deaths in the United States, 1999–2020. NCHS Data Brief, No 428. Hyattsville, MD: National Center for Health Statistics; 2021. doi:10.15620/cdc:112340
185. National Institutes of Health. *Alcohol Alert Number 85* n.d. 2013.
186. Lawless MH, Harrison KA, Grandits GA, Eberly LE, Allen SS. Perceived stress and smoking-related behaviors and symptomatology in male and female smokers. *Addictive Behaviors*. 2015;51:80–3. doi:10.1016/j.addbeh.2015.07.011
187. Hajek P, Taylor T, McRobbie H. The effect of stopping smoking on perceived stress levels. *Addiction*. 2010;105:1466–71. doi:10.1111/j.1360-0443.2010.02979.x
188. Stein RJ, Pyle SA, Haddock CK, Poston WSC, Bray R, Williams J. Reported stress and its relationship to tobacco use among U.S. military personnel. *Military Medicine*. 2008;173:271–7. doi:10.7205/milmed.173.3.271
189. Thayer JF, Lane RD. A model of neurovisceral integration in emotion regulation and dysregulation. *Journal of Affective Disorders*. 2000;61:201–16. doi:10.1016/S0165-0327(00)00338-4
190. Ralevski E, Petrakis I, Altemus M. Heart rate variability in alcohol use: A review. *Pharmacology Biochemistry and Behavior*. 2019;176:83–92. doi:10.1016/j.pbb.2018. 12.003
191. Mannes ZL, Burrell LE, Bryant VE, Dunne EM, Hearn LE, Whitehead NE. Loneliness and substance use: The influence of gender among HIV+ Black/African American adults 50+. *AIDS Care*. 2016;28:598–602. doi:10.1080/09540121.2015.1120269
192. Tomiyama AJ. Stress and obesity. *Annual Review of Psychology*. 2019;70:703–718. doi:10.1146/annurev-psych-010418-102936
193. Letois F, Mura T, Scali J, Gutierrez L-A, Feart C, Berr C. Nutrition and mortality in the elderly over 10 years of follow-up: The three-city study. *British Journal of Nutrition*. 2016;116:882–889. doi:10.1017/S000711451600266X
194. Gibson EL. The psychobiology of comfort eating: Implications for neuropharmacological interventions. *Behavioural Pharmacology*. 2012;23:442–460. doi:10.1097/FBP. 0b013e328357bd4e
195. Epel ES, Crosswell AD, Mayer SE, Prather AA, Slavich GM, Puterman E, et al. More than a feeling: A unified view of stress measurement for population science. *Frontiers in Neuroendocrinology*. 2018;49:146–169. doi:10.1016/j.yfrne.2018.03.001
196. Dickerson SS, Kemeny ME. Acute stressors and cortisol responses: A theoretical integration and synthesis of laboratory research. *Psychological Bulletin*. 2004;130: 355–391. doi:10.1037/0033-2909.130.3.355.
197. Nabizadeh-Gharghozar Z, Adib-Hajbaghery M, Bolandianbafghi S. Nurses' job burnout: A hybrid concept analysis. *Journal of Caring Sciences*. 2020;9:154–161. doi:10. 34172/jcs.2020.023
198. Schaufeli W, Enzmann D. *The Burnout Companion to Study and Practice: A Critical Analysis*. CRC Press. 1998.
199. Maslach C, Jackson SE. The measurement of experienced burnout. *Journal of Organizational Behavior*. 1981;2:99–113. doi:10.1002/job.4030020205
200. *ICD - ICD-10 - International Classification of Diseases, Tenth Revision*. 2021. URL: https://www.cdc.gov/nchs/icd/icd10.htm (Accessed 24 April 2023).
201. Golembiewski RT, Munzenrider RF. Phases of burnout, modes and social support: Contributions to explaining differences in physical symptoms. *Journal of Managerial Issues*. 1990;2:176–183
202. Gryskiewicz N, Buttner EH. Testing the robustness of the progressive phase burnout model for a sample of entrepreneurs. *Educational and Psychological Measurement*. 1992;52:747–751. doi:10.1177/0013164492052003025

203. Li Y, Lv M-R, Wei Y-J, Sun L, Zhang J-X, Zhang H-G, *et al*. Dietary patterns and depression risk: A meta-analysis. *Psychiatry Research*. 2017;253:373–382. doi:10.1016/j.psychres.2017.04.020
204. Vancampfort D, Vansteelandt K, Scheewe T, Probst M, Knapen J, De Herdt A, *et al*. Yoga in schizophrenia: A systematic review of randomised controlled trials. *Acta Psychiatrica Scandinavica*. 2012;126:12–20. doi:10.1111/j.1600-0447.2012.01865.x
205. Balasubramaniam M, Telles S, Doraiswamy PM. Yoga on our minds: A systematic review of yoga for neuropsychiatric disorders. *Frontiers in Psychiatry*. 2013;3:117. doi:10.3389/fpsyt.2012.00117
206. Ho PA, Dahle DN, Noordsy DL. Why do people with schizophrenia exercise? A mixed methods analysis among community dwelling regular exercisers. *Frontiers in Psychiatry*. 2018;9:596. doi:10.3389/fpsyt.2018.00596.
207. Firth J, Marx W, Dash S, Carney R, Teasdale SB, Solmi M, et al. The effects of dietary improvement on symptoms of depression and anxiety: A meta-analysis of randomized controlled trials. *Psychosomatic Medicine*. 2019;81:265–280. doi:10.1097/PSY.0000000000000673
208. Pascoe MC, Bauer IE. A systematic review of randomised control trials on the effects of yoga on stress measures and mood. *Journal of Psychiatric Research*. 2015;68:270–282. doi:10.1016/j.jpsychires.2015.07.013
209. Mehta UM, Gangadhar BN. Yoga: Balancing the excitation-inhibition equilibrium in psychiatric disorders. *Progress in Brain Research*. 2019;244:387–413. doi:10.1016/bs.pbr.2018.10.024
210. Govindaraj R, Naik SS, Mehta UM, Sharma M, Varambally S, Gangadhar BN. Yoga therapy for social cognition in schizophrenia: An experimental medicine-based randomized controlled trial. *Asian Journal of Psychiatry*. 2021;62:102731. doi:10.1016/j.ajp.2021.102731

2 Transdiagnostic Processes

Brooke Y. Kauffman, PhD, Lorra Garey, PhD, and Michael J. Zvolensky, PhD

KEY POINTS

- The majority of health care money in the United States is spent on the treatment and management of chronic illnesses.
- The underlying cause of emotional and physical symptoms and disorders may be underpinned by a smaller set of affective-related transdiagnostic vulnerability processes.
- Better understanding and targeting transdiagnostic risk factors for anxiety and lifestyle behaviors can be a highly efficient clinical strategy for reducing the impact of disease on society.

2.1 DISEASE PREVENTION WITHIN THE CONTEXT OF ANXIETY

The majority of health care money spent in the United States (US) is focused on the treatment and management of chronic diseases.[1] The best pooled estimates suggest that up to 50% of chronic disease is preventable through modifying behavioral risk factors (i.e., lifestyle behaviors),[2] including tobacco use, physical inactivity, poor diet, sleep impairment, and substance use.[3] Importantly, many of the common behavioral risk factors for chronic disease share overlapping mechanisms (i.e., transdiagnostic processes) related to the interpretation, management, and regulation of negative mood experiences. Thus, intervening in disease mechanisms that contribute to an increased likelihood of engaging in health risk behavior can potentially impact lifestyle behaviors (singularly or simultaneously) and reduce both the prevalence and severity of chronic disease in the US and other regions of the world.

Anxiety symptoms and disorders contribute to chronic disease prevalence and severity.[4] The prevalence of anxiety symptoms and disorders among persons with physical disturbances (e.g., gastrointestinal symptoms) and conditions (e.g., inflammatory bowel disease) is estimated to be at least two to five times the rate observed in the general population.[5-8] Indeed, research has illustrated anxiety symptoms and disorders are strongly associated with poor physical health symptoms and disease of all major bodily systems (e.g., cardiovascular, respiratory, gastrointestinal, skeletal, hormonal).[9] Notably, the co-occurrence of more severe anxiety among persons with physical symptoms and conditions is associated with greater severity of illness.[10,11]

DOI: 10.1201/b22810-3

2.2   CLINICAL FRAMEWORK FOR UNDERSTANDING DISEASE VULNERABILITY PROCESSES

Identifying vulnerabilities for chronic disease onset and progression provides intervention targets for disease prevention. A *risk factor* is a variable that is related to and temporally precedes a disease/disorder.[12] These factors can predispose, precipitate, or perpetuate disease. *Causal risk factors* reflect variables that, when present or aggravated, produce systematic change that results in the development or progression of a disease.[12] *Proxy risk factors* are variables that are related to disease assessment, but this association is due to the proxy risk factor's relationship with another causal risk factor.[13] Thus, a proxy risk factor may "mark" risk, but not explain such risk. See Table 2.1 for examples.

TABLE 2.1
Risk Factor Definitions

Label	Definition	Example
Risk Factor	A variable that is related to and temporarily precedes a disease/disorder	An increase in plaque formation in blood vessels may precede the development of cardiac disease.
Maintenance Factor	A factor which reflects a variable that predicts the persistence of an existing outcome over time among individuals already demonstrating the outcome	For an individual with cardiac disease, a maintenance factor could be consistent high blood pressure.
Risk Factor Types		
Causal Risk Factors	Variables that, when modified in some way, produce systematic change (increase or decrease) in a dependent variable	Increasing cigarettes smoked per day may increase the risk of developing cardiac disease.
Proxy Risk Factor	Variables that are related to an outcome of interest, but this association is due to the relationship with another causal risk factor	Low socioeconomic status may "mark" a risk but not explain or account for systematic change in developing cardiac disease.
Risk Factor Subtypes (e.g., Malleability)		
Causal/Proxy: Fixed Marker	In terms of influencing an outcome variable, a fixed marker is a factor that cannot be changed	A person's genetics attribute to a predisposition for cardiac disease.
Causal/Proxy: Variable Risk Factor	In terms of influencing an outcome variable, a risk factor is able to be manipulated or changed	Engaging in a greater amount of sedentary behavior, whether this effort is directly influential or not (causal or proxy), may increase risk of developing cardiac disease.

Both causal and proxy risk factors often are categorized based on whether they are *malleable*. When a risk factor cannot be changed, it can be classified as a *fixed marker*, whereas when it can be changed, it can be classified as a *variable risk factor*.[14] A central task of developing efficacious prevention programs for disease involves efforts to isolate whether an identified variable is a fixed marker or a variable risk factor.[14] Both fixed markers and variable risk factors may be important for identifying vulnerable individuals, but only variable risk factors will be the ultimate target of the intervention. It also is important to note that a risk factor may be contrasted with a *maintenance factor*. A maintenance factor reflects a variable that predicts the persistence of an existing outcome over time among individuals already demonstrating the outcome;[15] a risk factor may also function as a maintenance factor. Therefore, an important component of disease prevention research is to explicate not only singular risk main effects but also how such factors interact with one another in the pathogenesis of disease. For this reason, it is necessary to understand moderators (variables that influence the association between a specific risk factor and disease) and mediators (variables that explain the relations between a risk factor and disease) that serve to qualify a relationship between a given risk factor and an outcome of interest.[16] It also is possible that a common or shared variable, such as a transdiagnostic cognitive vulnerability factor, may potentiate the development of *both* a given risk factor and an outcome.

2.3 TRANSDIAGNOSTIC PSYCHOLOGICAL VULNERABILITY PROCESSES

The underlying cause of emotional and physical symptoms and disorders may be a smaller set of affective-related transdiagnostic vulnerability processes that serve to initiate the process of disease development and progression (see Figure 2.1).[17]

Transdiagnostic vulnerability factors can be conceptualized as "causal, variable, and maintaining factors" within the risk factor framework.[12] A key aspect of

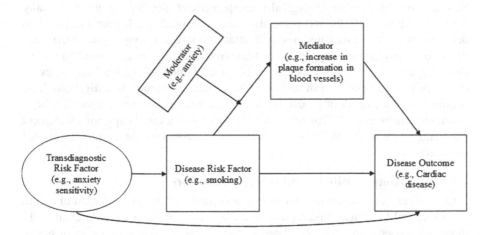

FIGURE 2.1   Transdiagnostic psychological vulnerability processes: pathways to disease development and progression.

transdiagnostic models of vulnerability is that they seek to identify fundamental processes underlying *multiple*, usually comorbid, psychopathologies and disease comorbidities.[18] We consider transdiagnostic emotional vulnerabilities as core processes that reflect one's characteristic *response* to emotion stimuli and states that subsequently contribute to physical health outcomes. Hence, transdiagnostic emotional vulnerabilities are conceptually independent of emotional symptoms like anxiety, depression, or stress, but may influence the latency and severity of these symptoms. This framework has informed a robust theoretical model based on the presumption that transdiagnostic conceptualization is particularly relevant to understanding the function of anxiety-related processes that underlie lifestyle or health behavior change within disease prevention.

2.4 TRANSDIAGNOSTIC PSYCHOLOGICAL FACTORS FOR ANXIETY AND LIFESTYLE BEHAVIORS

2.4.1 ANXIETY SENSITIVITY

Anxiety sensitivity is a relatively stable, but malleable factor[19] defined as the extent to which individuals believe anxiety and anxiety-related sensations (e.g., racing heart) have harmful personal consequences.[20,21] The global anxiety sensitivity construct encompasses lower-order fears of physical, mental, and publicly observable experiences.[22] According to expectancy theory, anxiety sensitivity serves to amplify anxious and fearful responses to evocative stimuli.[23] Theoretically, individuals higher in anxiety sensitivity are more likely to be frightened by harmless heart palpitations because they believe these sensations will lead to cardiac arrest or other feared outcomes, whereas individuals lower in anxiety sensitivity do not fear these sensations because they believe them to be benign.

2.4.1.1 Anxiety Sensitivity: Anxiety and Mood Disturbance Indicator

Research on the psychopathological consequences of anxiety sensitivity initially focused on panic attacks and panic disorder,[20] although work over the past two decades has extended such findings to illustrate anxiety sensitivity's role in the etiology of other psychopathology (e.g., Posttraumatic Stress Disorder, Major Depressive Disorder, etc.).[24–28] Such effects are not better explained by the tendency to experience negative affect or trait anxiety.[25] Moreover, numerous investigations have documented the impact of modifying anxiety sensitivity to enhance mood-related treatment outcomes.[29–31] That is, anxiety sensitivity is a chief explanatory element (mechanism) in treatment gains for intervention programs for certain emotional disorders.

2.4.1.2 Anxiety Sensitivity and Lifestyle Behaviors

There is evidence that anxiety sensitivity is involved in the exacerbation of health processes and behaviors, and represents a core mechanism in lifestyle change. To illustrate, anxiety sensitivity is related to clinical facets of a wide range of health conditions, such as chronic pain, gastrointestinal conditions, asthma, and vestibular pathology.[32–35] Although the precise pathways between anxiety sensitivity and health problems are complex, researchers have proposed specific pathways in which anxiety sensitivity may increase risk for chronic health problems, including through the avoidance of healthy behaviors (e.g., exercise avoidance) and engagement in unhealthy behaviors (e.g., emotional eating, substance use).[35] Thus, in regard to preventable causes of disease that are impacted by lifestyle behaviors, it is important to consider the role of anxiety sensitivity in this context.

2.4.2 DISTRESS TOLERANCE

Distress tolerance is defined as the perceived or objective ability to withstand negative or aversive conditions.[36] Distress tolerance can manifest in the perceived ability to tolerate distress as indicated typically by self-report methodologies or the objective ability to tolerate aversive experiences as indicated from behavioral tasks (e.g., cold pressor task).[36] The global distress tolerance construct consists of five domains, including tolerance to the following: (1) uncertainty, (2) ambiguity, (3) frustration, (4) negative emotional states, and (5) physical sensations.[36] Distress tolerance, although relatively stable, is also malleable.[36,37] Theoretically, individuals with low tolerance for distress are more likely to engage in escape/avoidance behaviors as a means to manage aversive conditions or states rather than adaptively cope with such experiences.[38]

2.4.2.1 Distress Tolerance: Anxiety and Mood Disturbance Indicator

Extant work has implicated low distress tolerance as a risk factor for psychopathology[36,39] and increased severity of negative mood symptoms.[40] Notably, distress tolerance is thought to be related, although distinct from, other psychological vulnerability factors (e.g., anxiety sensitivity, emotion regulation).[39,41] Indeed, within intervention research, distress tolerance is frequently isolated as a mechanism of change in the relationship between psychosocial treatment and improved psychopathology outcomes.[42,43]

2.4.2.2 Distress Tolerance and Lifestyle Behaviors

Existing research suggests distress tolerance may play a key role in guiding health behavior decisions.[44-46] Individuals with lower distress tolerance may engage in maladaptive coping strategies in an effort to escape or avoid negative internal states.[38] Consequently, these individuals may be at risk for the onset or maintenance of chronic disease as a result of affectively motivated lifestyle choices. In line with this perspective, low tolerance for distress has been consistently related to behaviors associated with chronic disease, such as smoking,[46] disordered eating behaviors (e.g., binge eating),[47] and alcohol misuse.[48]

2.4.3 EMOTION REGULATION

Emotion regulation involves observing, understanding, and evaluating one's emotions to subsequently utilize strategies to regulate emotional and behavioral responses.[49] Emotion regulation processes include five components: (1) influencing the exposure to a situation, (2) changing an aspect of the situation, (3) influencing which portions of the situation are perceived, (4) cognitive restructuring of the situation presented, and (5) directly changing the emotion-related behavior.[50] Theoretically, individuals who have difficulties regulating emotions may be more likely to engage in maladaptive coping mechanisms in response to aversive states.[51]

2.4.3.1 Emotion Regulation: Anxiety and Mood Disturbance Indicator

Difficulties regulating emotions are implicated in the etiology and maintenance of psychopathology.[52,53] Notably, these relations have been demonstrated across a variety of psychiatric conditions (e.g., anxiety and depressive disorders).[54,55] Extant interventions aimed at improving emotion regulation have demonstrated large effects in psychopathology symptom outcomes (e.g., panic, social anxiety, depression) suggesting emotion regulation as a putative mechanism of change.[56]

2.4.3.2 Emotion Regulation and Lifestyle Behaviors

Empirical evidence has highlighted the role of emotion regulation in contributing to maladaptive lifestyle choices.[57] For example, greater difficulties regulating emotions have been linked to many unhealthy behaviors associated with chronic disease, including substance use[57] and emotional eating.[58] An individual may be at greater risk for chronic disease due to an inability to access adaptive strategies to regulate distress.[59] For example, an individual with difficulties regulating emotions may be more apt to utilize maladaptive coping strategies (e.g., smoking, eating)[57,58] as a means of regulation thereby increasing the risk for chronic disease (e.g., cardiovascular disease).[59] Thus, emotion regulation may play a key role in promoting positive health-related changes among individuals engaging in unhealthy lifestyle behaviors.

2.5 SUMMARY

Although the treatment and management of chronic illnesses is a major public health concern, many of these illnesses can be prevented by modifying lifestyle behaviors (e.g., substance use, physical inactivity). Notably, individuals with chronic illness evidence significantly elevated rates of anxiety symptoms and clinical disorders compared to the general population, and such comorbidity impairs changing these lifestyle behaviors (e.g., diet, sleep, drug use). Better understanding and targeting transdiagnostic risk factors for anxiety and lifestyle behaviors can be a highly efficient clinical strategy for reducing the impact of disease on society. Although the present chapter focused on anxiety sensitivity, distress tolerance, and emotion regulation, these models can span across a wide range of other transdiagnostic psychological factors (e.g., experiential avoidance).

REFERENCES

1. Keehan SP, Poisal JA, Cuckler GA, et al. National health expenditure projections, 2015–25: Economy, prices, and aging expected to shape spending and enrollment. *Health Affairs*. 2016. doi:10.1377/hlthaff. 2016.0459
2. McGinnis M, Williams-Russo O, Knickman J. The case for more active policy attention to health promotion. *Health Affairs (Millwood)*. 2002;21:78–93.

3. Schroeder SA. We can do better—Improving the health of the American people. *New England Journal of Medicine.* 2007;357(12):1221–1228.
4. Bhattacharya R, Shen C, Sambamoorthi U. Excess risk of chronic physical conditions associated with depression and anxiety. *BMC Psychiatry.* 2014;14(1):10.
5. Mussell M, Kroenke K, Spitzer RL, Williams JBW, Herzog W, Löwe B. Gastrointestinal symptoms in primary care: Prevalence and association with depression and anxiety. *Journal of Psychosomatic Research.* 2008;64(6):605–612.
6. Neuendorf R, Harding A, Stello N, Hanes D, Wahbeh H. Depression and anxiety in patients with inflammatory bowel disease: A systematic review. *Journal of Psychosomatic Research.* 2016;87:70–80.
7. Thompson WG, Irvine EJ, Pare P, Ferrazzi S, Rance L. Functional gastrointestinal disorders in Canada: First population-based survey using Rome II criteria with suggestions for improving the questionnaire. *Digestive Diseases and Sciences.* 2002;47(1):225–235.
8. Roy-Byrne PP, Davidson KW, Kessler RC, et al. Anxiety disorders and comorbid medical illness. *General hospital Psychiatry.* 2008;30(3):208–225.
9. Zvolensky MJ, Smits JA. *Anxiety in Health Behaviors and Physical Illness.* Springer Science & Business Media; 2007.
10. Fiest KM, Bernstein CN, Walker JR, et al. Systematic review of interventions for depression and anxiety in persons with inflammatory bowel disease. *BMC Research Notes.* 2016;9:404.
11. Mittermaier C, Dejaco C, Waldhoer T, et al. Impact of depressive mood on relapse in patients with inflammatory bowel disease: A prospective 18-month follow-up study. *Psychosomatic Medicine.* 2004;66(1):79–84.
12. Kraemer HC, Kazdin AE, Offord DR, Kessler RC, Jensen PS, Kupfer DJ. Coming to terms with the terms of risk. *Archives of General Psychiatry.* 1997;54(4):337–343.
13. Kraemer HC, Stice E, Kazdin A, Offord D, Kupfer D. How do risk factors work together? Mediators, moderators, and independent, overlapping, and proxy risk factors. *American Journal of Psychiatry.* 2001;158(6):848–856.
14. Kraemer HC, Lowe KK, Kupfer DJ. *To Your Health: How to Understand What Research Tells Us About Risk.* Oxford University Press; 2005.
15. Stice E. Risk and maintenance factors for eating pathology: A meta-analytic review. *Psychological Bulletin.* 2002;128(5):825.
16. Baron RM, Kenny DA. The moderator–mediator variable distinction in social psychological research: Conceptual, strategic, and statistical considerations. *Journal of Personality and Social Psychology.* 1986;51(6):1173.
17. Dozois DJ, Seeds PM, Collins KA. Transdiagnostic approaches to the prevention of depression and anxiety. *Journal of Cognitive Psychotherapy.* 2009;23(1):44–59.
18. Barlow DH, Allen LB, Choate ML. Toward a unified treatment for emotional disorders—republished article. *Behavior Therapy.* 2016;47(6):838–853.
19. Taylor S. *Anxiety Sensitivity: Theory, Research, and Treatment of the Fear of Anxiety.* Mahwah, NJ, US: Lawrence Erlbaum Associates Publishers; 1999.
20. McNally RJ. Anxiety sensitivity and panic disorder. *Biological Psychiatry.* 2002;52(10):938–946.
21. Reiss S, Peterson RA, Gursky DM, McNally RJ. Anxiety sensitivity, anxiety frequency and the prediction of fearfulness. *Behaviour Research and Therapy.* 1986;24(1):1–8.
22. Zinbarg RE, Barlow DH, Brown TA. Hierarchical structure and general factor saturation of the anxiety sensitivity index: Evidence and implications. *Psychological Assessment.* 1997;9(3):277.
23. Reiss S. Expectancy model of fear, anxiety, and panic. *Clinical Psychology Review.* 1991;11(2):141–153.
24. Fedroff IC, Taylor S, Asmundson GJ, Koch WJ. Cognitive factors in traumatic stress reactions: Predicting PTSD symptoms from anxiety sensitivity and beliefs about harmful events. *Behavioural and Cognitive Psychotherapy.* 2000;28(1):5–15.

25. Taylor S, Koch WJ, Woody S, McLean P. Anxiety sensitivity and depression: How are they related? *Journal of Abnormal Psychology*. 1996;105(3):474.
26. Scott EL, Heimberg RG, Jack MS. Anxiety sensitivity in social phobia: Comparison between social phobics with and without panic attacks. *Depression and Anxiety*. 2000;12(4):189–192.
27. Spira AP, Zvolensky MJ, Eifert GH, Feldner MT. Avoidance-oriented coping as A predictor of panic-related distress: A test using biological challenge. *Journal of Anxiety Disorders*. 2004;18(3):309–323.
28. Vujanovic AA, Farris SG, Bartlett BA, et al. Anxiety sensitivity in the association between posttraumatic stress and substance use disorders: A systematic review. *Clinical Psychology Review*. 2018;62:37–55.
29. Timpano KR, Raines AM, Shaw AM, Keough ME, Schmidt NB. Effects of a brief anxiety sensitivity reduction intervention on obsessive compulsive spectrum symptoms in a young adult sample. *Journal of Psychiatric Research*. 2016;83:8–15.
30. Schmidt NB, Norr AM, Allan NP, Raines AM, Capron DW. A randomized clinical trial targeting anxiety sensitivity for patients with suicidal ideation. *Journal of Consulting and Clinical Psychology*. 2017;85(6):596–610.
31. Otto MW, Reilly-Harrington NA, Taylor S. The impact of treatment on anxiety sensitivity. *Anxiety Sensitivity: Theory, Research, and Treatment of the Fear of Anxiety*. 1999:321–336.
32. Avallone KM, McLeish AC, Luberto CM, Bernstein JA. Anxiety sensitivity, asthma control, and quality of life in adults with asthma. *Journal of Asthma*. 2012;49(1): 57–62.
33. Asmundson GJG, Wright KD, Hadjistavropoulos HD. Anxiety sensitivity and disabling chronic health conditions: State of the art and future directions. *Scandinavian Journal of Behaviour Therapy*. 2000;29(3–4):100–117.
34. Otto MW, Smits JAJ. Anxiety sensitivity, health behaviors, and the prevention and treatment of medical illness. *Clinical Psychology (New York)*. 2018;25(3):e12253.
35. Horenstein A, Potter CM, Heimberg RG. How does anxiety sensitivity increase risk of chronic medical conditions? *Clinical Psychology: Science and Practice*. 2018; 25(3):110.
36. Leyro TM, Zvolensky MJ, Bernstein A. Distress tolerance and psychopathological symptoms and disorders: A review of the empirical literature among adults. *Psychological Bulletin*. 2010;136(4):576–600.
37. Macatee RJ, Cougle JR. Development and evaluation of a computerized intervention for low distress tolerance and its effect on performance on a neutralization task. *Journal of Behavior Therapy and Experimental Psychiatry*. 2015;48:33–39.
38. Leventhal AM, Zvolensky MJ. Anxiety, depression, and cigarette smoking: A transdiagnostic vulnerability framework to understanding emotion-smoking comorbidity. *Psychological Bulletin*. 2015;141(1):176–212.
39. Laposa JM, Collimore KC, Hawley LL, Rector NA. Distress tolerance in OCD and anxiety disorders, and its relationship with anxiety sensitivity and intolerance of uncertainty. *Journal of Anxiety Disorders*. 2015;33:8–14.
40. Vujanovic AA, Rathnayaka N, Amador CD, Schmitz JM. Distress tolerance: Associations with posttraumatic stress disorder symptoms among trauma-exposed, cocaine-dependent adults. *Behavior Modification*. 2016;40(1–2):120–143.
41. Zvolensky MJ, Vujanovic AA, Bernstein A, Leyro T. Distress tolerance: Theory, measurement, and relations to psychopathology. *Current Directions in Psychological Science*. 2010;19(6):406–410.
42. Boffa JW, Short NA, Gibby BA, Stentz LA, Schmidt NB. Distress tolerance as a mechanism of PTSD symptom change: Evidence for mediation in a treatment-seeking sample. *Psychiatry Research*. 2018;267:400–408.

43. Zeifman RJ, Boritz T, Barnhart R, Labrish C, McMain SF. The independent roles of mindfulness and distress tolerance in treatment outcomes in dialectical behavior therapy skills training. *Personality Disorders: Theory, Research, and Treatment*. 2020; 11(3):181–190.

44. Kauffman BY, Garey L, Bakhshaie J, et al. Distress tolerance dimensions and smoking behavior among Mexican daily smokers: A preliminary investigation. *Addictive Behaviors*. 2017;69:59–64.

45. Kauffman BY, Bakhshaie J, Zvolensky MJ. The association between distress tolerance and eating expectancies among trauma-exposed college students with obesity. *Journal of American College Health*. 2020:1–6.

46. Veilleux JC. The relationship between distress tolerance and cigarette smoking: A systematic review and synthesis. *Clinical Psychology Review*. 2019;71:78–89.

47. Mattingley S, Youssef GJ, Manning V, Graeme L, Hall K. Distress tolerance across substance use, eating, and borderline personality disorders: A meta-analysis. *Journal of Affective Disorders*. 2022;300:492–504.

48. Brooks Holliday S, Pedersen ER, Leventhal AM. Depression, posttraumatic stress, and alcohol misuse in young adult veterans: The transdiagnostic role of distress tolerance. *Drug and Alcohol Dependence*. 2016;161:348–355.

49. Gratz KL, Roemer L. Multidimensional assessment of emotion regulation and dysregulation: Development, factor structure, and initial validation of the difficulties in emotion regulation scale. *Journal of Psychopathology and Behavioral Assessment*. 2004;26(1):41–54.

50. Gross JJ. The extended process model of emotion regulation: Elaborations, applications, and future directions. *Psychological Inquiry*. 2015;26(1):130–137.

51. Gratz KL, Roemer L. Multidimensional assessment of emotion regulation and dysregulation: Development, factor structure, and initial validation of the difficulties in emotion regulation scale. *Journal of Psychopathology & Behavioral Assessment*. 2004;26(1):41–54.

52. Aldao A, Nolen-Hoeksema S, Schweizer S. Emotion-regulation strategies across psychopathology: A meta-analytic review. *Clinical Psychology Review*. 2010;30(2): 217–237.

53. Berking M, Wupperman P. Emotion regulation and mental health: Recent findings, current challenges, and future directions. *Current Opinion in Psychiatry*. 2012;25(2): 128–134.

54. Cisler JM, Olatunji BO, Feldner MT, Forsyth JP. Emotion regulation and the anxiety disorders: An integrative review. *Journal of Psychopathology and Behavioral Assessment*. 2010;32(1):68–82.

55. Joormann J, Stanton CH. Examining emotion regulation in depression: A review and future directions. *Behaviour Research and Therapy*. 2016;86:35–49.

56. Sakiris N, Berle D. A systematic review and meta-analysis of the unified protocol as a transdiagnostic emotion regulation based intervention. *Clinical Psychology Review*. 2019;72:101751.

57. Weiss NH, Kiefer R, Goncharenko S, et al. Emotion regulation and substance use: A meta-analysis. *Drug and Alcohol Dependence*. 2022;230:109131.

58. Jones J, Kauffman BY, Rosenfield D, Smits JAJ, Zvolensky MJ. Emotion dysregulation and body mass index: The explanatory role of emotional eating among adult smokers. *Eating Behaviors*. 2019;33:97–101.

59. Roy B, Riley C, Sinha R. Emotion regulation moderates the association between chronic stress and cardiovascular disease risk in humans: A cross-sectional study. *Stress*. 2018;21(6):548–555.

3 Socioeconomic Determinants of Health

Jenny M. Cundiff, PhD and Robert D. Faulk, MA

KEY POINTS
- SEP-health disparities are ubiquitous and large enough to matter for population health.
- SEP is a complex social construct, and many factors contribute to disparities.
- Stress and negative affect are at the heart of psychological theories explaining differences in health by SEP.
- Interdisciplinary and longitudinal research will be important contributors to the next decade of knowledge on this pernicious social problem.

Significant disparities in health exist in the United States. Arguably the largest and most ubiquitous of these disparities are those attributable to differences in socioeconomic position (SEP). It is clear that our place in the social hierarchy shapes our mental and physical health, and differences in health by SEP are similar in magnitude to well-established risk factors for poor health that have been top public health priorities. For example, differences in health by SEP rival the effects of obesity, physical inactivity, hypertension, and alcohol intake.[1] Disparities by SEP are also not disease-specific. Both mental and physical diseases and acute and chronic conditions show significant disparities by SEP. For example, incidence of diseases such as hypertension, stroke, and Alzheimer's disease show associations with SEP,[2-5] as do most cancers, asthma, rheumatoid arthritis, the common cold, and depression.[6-11]

The disproportionate rates of poor mental health experienced by those with lower SEP are driven by a complex interplay of systemic, psychosocial, and biological factors.[12,13] For example, individuals of lower SEP evidence a higher risk of developing mental health disorders, and also have lower access to mental healthcare services, and both of these factors contribute to poorer mental health outcomes.[12,13] In addition to higher rates of frank mental illness, individuals of lower SEP also report lower rates of subjective well-being (e.g., happiness, life satisfaction) when compared to those of higher SEP.[14] Some research further delineates hedonic well-being – a measure of happiness or contentment – and eudaimonic well-being – a measure of self-actualization and fulfillment or life-purpose, both of which also show differences by SEP.[15]

We will often distinguish mental health from physical health in this chapter. Although mental and physical health differ in important ways (e.g., etiology, treatment) and can be useful as separate categories, they are, of course, not separate, divided systems within an individual. Both acute and chronic physical illness as well as changes in associated biological systems (e.g., inflammation) can affect basic

DOI: 10.1201/b22810-4

psychological processes such as affect (e.g., anhedonia), cognition, and behavior (e.g., social avoidance).[16,17] Similarly, mental illness as well as changes in associated psychological systems (e.g., affect, social behavior) can affect basic biological processes such as immune, cardiovascular, and neuroendocrine functioning.[18] Thus, psychological and biological processes are interconnected, and influence and are influenced by features of the social environment such as SEP. However, this is a complex and dynamic process that is not simply "one-to-one" (e.g., a specific psychological process having a specific biological signature or vice versa) and is still not precisely understood.

3.1   ONE CONCEPT, MANY MEASURES

There are many different terms that refer to the hierarchical ordering of individuals and groups within society. The term we favor in this chapter, *socioeconomic position* (SEP), is often used to capture broad social stratification based on economic resources and social rank, and it highlights the fact that both rank and resources may influence health.[19,20] The closely related and more traditional term *socioeconomic status* (SES) more typically refers to absolute levels of socioeconomic resources, some of which may also be rank- or prestige-based (e.g., occupation). SEP can be measured at multiple levels of analysis (e.g., individual, neighborhood, country), but this chapter focuses on the individual level.

Individual measures of SEP are only modestly correlated with one another and are not interchangeable.[21] The three most commonly used indicators of SEP are income, education, and occupation. *Income* is a measure of financial resources and is often assessed as self-reported annual income or household income (income considering the number of people it supports), but can also be assessed in a myriad of other ways (tax records, pay stubs, income relative to the poverty line, etc.). *Education* is a measure of one's potential to generate and access resources and to build human capital. Education is often assessed as the number of years of education or highest educational level achieved selected from predetermined categories (e.g., less than high school degree, high school completion or GED, some college, bachelor's degree, master's or doctoral degree). *Occupation*, often referred to as occupational prestige, is a measure of social rank and potential to generate income. Occupation is often assessed using coding schemes to hierarchically rank occupations.[22,23] Much of the literature examining occupational prestige and health (which is distinct from research on occupational stress and health) is based on research from European countries, where occupational classifications are more clearly hierarchical compared to US classification systems.[24,25] Employment status (whether one is employed full-time, part-time, or not employed) is also examined in SEP- health research and is often treated dichotomously (employed vs unemployed). Although somewhat less common, *wealth* is another measure of financial resources that indexes accumulated financial resources, rather than simply cash flow, thus indexing one's ability to weather potential financial hardships and disruption. Wealth is often assessed by self-reports or objective indicators of savings, property, and investments, sometimes minus debts.[26]

Subjective assessments of SEP are also useful and are being administered with increasing frequency. Perhaps the most commonly used measure of subjective SEP in psychological research is the MacArthur Scale of Subjective Social Status, which uses a visual analogue scale of a 10-rung ladder and asks individuals to rank themselves relative to a reference group. Epidemiological studies tend to use country of residence as the reference group (e.g., rank relative to others in the United States) and anchor ratings to traditional SES indicators; at the top are those who make the most money and who have the best jobs and the most education, and at the bottom are those who make the least money and who have the worst jobs and least education.[27] There is also a "community" version of this ladder which is used to assess social rank in individuals' more proximal social environment. In this version of the ladder, community is defined by participants, and rankings are not anchored to traditional socioeconomic indicators. The ladder scale has also been adapted in order to examine social rank at earlier stages of development (e.g., rank within your school), before individuals complete their education and enter the workforce.[28] Different measures of subjective SEP can also differ in their degree of subjectivity and degree to which they capture social rank and/or economic resources. For example, ladder measures that ask people to label their relative place in society without providing economic anchors (e.g., school- and community-based ladders of subjective social status) are more subjective and less anchored to economic resources compared to ladder measures (e.g., US ladder) which specifically assesses subjective SEP anchored to traditional socioeconomic indicators.

These distinctions in measurement have conceptual and practical implications. For example, SEP indicators that most closely assess objective economic resources may be most closely associated with exposure to stressors such as crowding and financial strain. On the other hand, SEP indicators that assess relative SEP, subjective perceptions, or social rank may be more closely associated with negative psychological states associated with downward social comparisons (shame, anxiety, depression) compared to SEP measures assessing absolute and objective SEP and measures of economic resources.

3.2 LEADING PSYCHOLOGICAL THEORIES REGARDING HOW SOCIAL HIERARCHY SHAPES HEALTH

3.2.1 STRESS AND NEGATIVE AFFECT

The psychological constructs of stress and negative affect have been, and continue to be, central to psychosocial explanations of SEP-health disparities.[29-31] Stress has been broadly defined as "a set of constructs representing stages in a process by which environmental demands that tax or exceed the adaptive capacity of an organism occasion psychological, behavioral, and biological responses that may place persons at risk for disease."[32] There has been growing criticism that the construct is operationalized so imprecisely as to make the term useless,[33] and the NIH stress network has recently summarized and organized the measurement of stress into typologies.[34]

Two guiding frameworks in the literature on SEP and mental health are the social causation and diathesis-stress frameworks, both of which focus on stress pathways.

Social causation holds that lower SEP is associated with disproportionate exposure to a variety of stressors that cause individuals to develop mental illness both acutely and over time.[35] This is how most researchers conceptualize disparate outcomes by SEP. The *diathesis-stress* framework also focuses on socioenvironmental stress pathways to developing mental disorders.[36,37] For example, lower SEP is associated with higher rates of exposure to a variety of stressors which are also associated with increased mental health risk: food insecurity, housing insecurity, traumatic life experiences, social exclusion or isolation, unemployment, high-demand/low-control work, childhood abuse or neglect, poor neighborhood conditions (e.g., living in a food desert or lacking access to community amenities), discrimination, poor access to and lower quality of healthcare and education, and low social support.[12,13,36,38–41]

There is still some debate in the literature concerning the idea of social selection, which argues that poorer health may precede lower SEP, rather than result from low SEP as suggested by theories of social causation. Social selection holds that developing mental illness reduces individuals' ability to obtain and maintain access to resources, causing them to "drift" into lower SEP.[35] A growing body of research has shown that causation and selection processes act in tandem, with SEP and mental health having reciprocal impacts on each other over time.[12] Indeed, physical illness and disability can lead to job loss and expensive medical treatments can result in poverty and loss of housing. Some social selection arguments suggest that health is better at higher levels of SEP due to "survival of the fittest" or "Social Darwinism" in which physical ability and vitality increase the probability of upward social mobility.[42,43] Health does not appear to be a major determinant of social mobility and increasing opportunities for social mobility appears to reduce health disparities, rather than exacerbate them as would be expected by a social Darwinist perspective.[43] Reviews suggest that there is more evidence for social causation than social selection in the literature on both mental[44] and physical health.[45] However, it is clear that both mental and physical health can influence and be influenced by indicators of SEP, leading some authors to suggest that accumulation models (accumulating risk factors for poor health over the life course) may most closely reflect the reality of bidirectional processes between SEP and health.[45]

In conceptual models focusing on physical health, stress exposure and associated affective and biological responses are ubiquitously referenced as important pathways linking lower SEP to poorer physical health.[46 47] Highly influential models of SEP-health associations incorporate higher stress and/or negative affect as mechanisms explaining how low SEP contributes to poor health outcomes. For example, Gallo's Reserve Capacity Model, posits that low SEP environments increase the probability of exposure to stressful and threatening situations and reduce the probability of exposure to rewarding and beneficial situations which together increase the likelihood of emotional disruption and negative affect.[30,48] This disruption in affect, and its precursors, disrupts biobehavioral pathways leading to poorer health and earlier death. Although stress is not named in Gallo's model, experiences of high demand and low control mirror seminal definitions of stress. See Figure 3.1.[49]

Other psychosocial models of SEP-health disparities also highlight stress and/ or negative affect. Psychological models such as Chen's shift-and-persist model focus on cognitive-behavioral and affective responses to stress that may promote

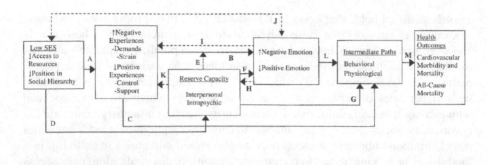

FIGURE 3.1   The Reserve Capacity Model. (Original figure from Gallo, Bogart, Vranceneau, and Matthews (2005).)

biobehavioral resilience in low SEP contexts.[50] Even epidemiological models examining the construct of "social capital" highlight that social environments can be characterized by support and social cohesion, which promote health, or stress and social distrust, which promote disease.[51] Epidemiological models of deprivation specifically state that stress and anxiety resulting from perceptions of having less than others are key mechanisms linking social hierarchy to health.[52,53]

Evidence supports this central role of stress. Lower SEP is associated with higher exposure to different types of stressors.[54] Measures of ambient stress exposure such as crowding, noise pollution, and crime are higher at lower levels of SEP, as are exposures such as traumatic life events, perceived stress, and daily hassles.[55–57] Less comprehensive assessments of stress appear to underestimate the role of stress exposure in shaping SEP disparities. For example, there are larger differences in stress exposure by SEP when stress exposure is assessed as a composite of multiple forms of stress (recent life events, major and potentially traumatic events, chronic stress, and discrimination) than when stress exposure is assessed simply with the life events checklist.[58] Further, such comprehensive measures of stress accounted for almost half of the variance in SEP disparities in depression.[58]

3.2.2 DOWNSTREAM PSYCHOSOCIAL FACTORS (RISK AND PROTECTIVE)

Many common psychosocial risk and resilience factors track with SEP and are thus potential mediators of the association between SEP and health. Not surprisingly, stressful aspects of work-life are more common at lower levels of SEP, and may contribute to SEP-health disparities.[31] Stressful aspects of home-life and other important forms of social connection such as social isolation, low social support, and conflict in intimate relationships also appear to be more common at lower levels of SEP,[59,60] and can contribute to SEP-health disparities.[1] Low SEP is also associated with higher levels of negative affective traits, symptoms, and disorders, and negative affect appears to contribute to SEP-health disparities.[30]

Social support is also commonly featured as a psychosocial resource (mediator) or buffer (moderator) in psychosocial models explaining SEP-health disparities. For example, interpersonal resources such as social support are part of individuals' "reserve capacity" in Gallo's model, social connection and support specific to a role model is a central feature of Chen's shift-and-persist model, and social support and cohesion are indicators of social environments that promote health in models of social capital. Hence, hypotheses suggest that social support may be harder to cultivate at lower SEP and that the effectiveness of social support to buffer the deleterious effects of stress may also vary across SEP hierarchies. These theorized mediating and moderating influences of social support in explaining SEP-health disparities mirror classic theories in health psychology about how the social world may come to influence our biology and ultimately our physical health; stress and its biobehavioral correlates wear us down and social support builds us up, with social support perhaps especially important in the face of high exposure to stress.[61]

Current evidence suggests that social support may be most accurately conceptualized as having a stronger beneficial effect on health at lower levels of SEP. Laboratory manipulations of stress and social support have shown that social support is a particularly effective buffer against cortisol and inflammatory reactivity to stress amongst lower SEP participants.[62,63] In a study of almost 30,000 US adults age 25 and older, social support and integration did not mediate associations between SEP and self-rated health, but social integration moderated associations between SEP and self-rated health.[64] Hence, although social support appears to decrease with decreasing SEP, higher levels of social support may indeed protect health at lower levels of SEP.

Perceived control, the belief that one's actions can directly influence life outcomes, also appears to play a role in associations between low SEP and poor health, including outcomes of mortality, incident disease, and biological risk factors.[65–67] While most studies suggest that perceived control mediates associations between SEP and poor health, others suggest that perceived control is a moderator, buffering the effects of low SEP on health.[68] For example, one large prospective study found that self-efficacy and mastery at baseline partially mediated the association between SEP and incident heart disease.[65] Another large prospective study found that low SEP individuals with high perceived control had lower mortality rates (14-year follow-up). In contrast, perceived control was not associated with mortality among high SEP individuals.[68]

Emotion regulation strategies (suppression, reappraisal), purpose in life, and personality traits (i.e., conscientiousness and neuroticism) have also been examined in the context of SEP-health disparities. Reappraisal (changing thoughts about a stimulus to decrease the emotional impact) is thought to promote better health particularly in low SEP contexts;[50] suppression (inhibiting the expression of felt emotions), the other primary response-focused emotion regulation strategy, is associated with, and reinforced by, lower rank in the social hierarchy. Suppression also relates to biological and psychosocial risk factors for poor health (e.g., parasympathetic functioning and receipt of social support), but few studies directly examine the potential mediating influence of suppression in the context of SEP-health associations.[69]

3.2.3 HEALTH BEHAVIORS (MOVING, EATING, SLEEPING, SUBSTANCES)

SEP-health disparities are not simply due to cognitive or emotional factors frequently associated with stress and social support. Health behaviors such as smoking, lower physical activity, poorer diet, and excess food consumption also play a role. For example, 25% of the SEP gradient in coronary heart disease could be attributed to traditional medical risk factors in the Whitehall study.[70] A more recent review of the literature similarly estimated that health behaviors account for approximately 25% of the variance in health due to SEP.[71] Thus, health behaviors in aggregate appear to be an important contributor to SEP-health associations.

3.3 SELECT LIMITATIONS OF CURRENT KNOWLEDGE

Our understanding of psychological and behavioral contributions to SEP-health disparities is still incomplete. Below we outline two important limitations and how they may be addressed.

3.3.1 MEASURING CONSTRUCTS WELL IN LARGE SAMPLES

We often begin scientific inquiry in search of a solution to a problem. We often identify problems based on large datasets from population sciences such as demography, epidemiology, and sociology. Research from these disciplines has important strengths, such as very large samples and detailed attention to obtaining a representative sample. However, careful attention to the measurement of psychological and social constructs is often missing (and not feasible) within population sciences. In contrast, psychology has a long tradition and commitment to rigorous conceptualization and measurement of psychological and social constructs, including relevant psychometric assessments. However, many of these studies with thorough and valid measurements fail to attend to sample representativeness, and, instead, are often carried out in small, homogeneous samples with limited external validity. Scientific advances on SEP-health disparities will require attending both to sampling features (ensuring population coverage and representation) and to valid assessment of constructs (e.g., stress, negative affect, social support) thought to play a key role in understanding mechanisms that are hypothesized to explain the association between SEP and health. Recruiting large samples for the examination of psychosocial factors on health disparities rather than relying on secondary data analysis of large samples where data were not collected for the purpose of examining health disparities may help move the field forward. Additionally, samples that specifically target a wide range of SEP and thoroughly assess psychosocial variables would complement studies that target low SEP individuals exclusively, which appears to be a more common sampling strategy in psychological research on health disparities. Multi-disciplinary teams of researchers will likely be necessary to harness these opposing strengths and weaknesses in future research on SEP-health disparities.

3.3.2 CAPTURING CHANGES

Up to this point we have mostly focused on static, one-time measures of SEP and its association with psychosocial factors and health. The bulk of the literature also takes this approach. However, SEP can change throughout the life course and examining such changes provides opportunities to test key assumptions of how SEP may influence health and whether changing SEP may be a viable avenue for reducing

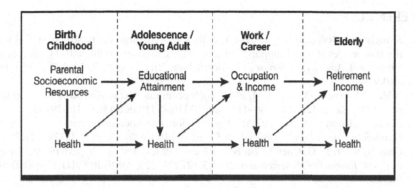

FIGURE 3.2 The dynamic relationship between SES and health across the lifespan. (Original figure from Adler and Stewart (2010).)

SEP-health disparities. SEP can influence health at all stages of the life course. Socioeconomic conditions in early life shape opportunities to develop high SEP in adulthood and also affect health via additional mechanisms. While disparities in health are present at all ages, the size of SEP disparities is not consistent across the life course. For example, physical health disparities tend to be largest in middle adulthood, and smaller in childhood, adolescence, and at old ages.[72] However, the strength and patterning of these associations can also vary depending on which measure of SEP is being examined. See Figure 3.2.

Our focus on one-time measures mirrors the literature. Most data on SEP-health associations are cross-sectional, most commonly measuring SEP at one point in time in adulthood. However, SEP can change over the life course, and changes in SEP may have unique implications for health.[73] Empirical studies generally support positive health effects of upward social mobility. One recent analysis of over 6,000 older adults from the nationally representative Health and Retirement Study found that upward mobility and stable high SEP between childhood and adulthood were similarly associated with markers of healthy aging in adulthood (walking speed, peak expiratory flow, and grip strength), suggesting protective effects of upward mobility.[74] A smaller study (N=311) of Black and White men that prospectively examined SEP mobility between ages 7 and 16 found that the degree of upward mobility (e.g., within-person slope) during three developmental periods (i.e., middle childhood, late childhood, middle adolescence) each independently predicted diagnosed physical health problems at age 32.[75] Further, there is a significant body of work suggesting that upward social mobility may be detrimental to health.[76] Some frameworks suggest that upward mobility may increase risk for poor physical health specifically for Black Americans who grew up in low SEP contexts.[77] However, adverse physical health outcomes associated with upward mobility have also been found in White Americans.[78] It will be important for future research to bring more longitudinal data to study social mobility, attending to the economic conditions that enable or inhibit mobility and likewise measuring relevant psychosocial mechanisms.

REFERENCES

1. Stringhini S, Berkman L, Dugravot A, et al. Socioeconomic status, structural and functional measures of social support, and mortality: The British Whitehall II Cohort Study, 1985–2009. *American Journal of Epidemiology.* 2012;175(12):1275–1283. doi:10.1093/aje/kwr461
2. Addo J, Ayerbe L, Mohan KM, et al. Socioeconomic status And stroke: An updated review. *Stroke.* 2012;43(4):1186–1191. doi:10.1161/STROKEAHA.111.639732
3. Grotto I, Huerta M, Sharabi Y. Hypertension and socioeconomic status. *Current Opinion in Cardiology.* 2008;23(4):335–339. doi:10.1097/HCO.0b013e3283021c70
4. Leng B, Jin Y, Li G, Chen L, Jin N. Socioeconomic status and hypertension: A meta-analysis. *Journal of Hypertension.* 2015;33(2):221–229. doi:10.1097/HJH.0000000000000428
5. Stern Y, Gurland B, Tatemichi TK, Tang MX, Wilder D, Mayeux R. Influence of education and occupation on the incidence of Alzheimer's disease. *JAMA.* 1994; 271(13):1004–1010.
6. Hoebel J, Kroll LE, Fiebig J, et al. Socioeconomic inequalities in total and site-specific cancer incidence in Germany: A population-based registry study. *Frontiers in Oncology.* 2018;8. Accessed February 23, 2023. https://www.frontiersin.org/articles/10.3389/fonc.2018.00402
7. Basagaña X, Sunyer J, Kogevinas M, et al. Socioeconomic status and asthma prevalence in young adults: The European community respiratory health survey. *American Journal of Epidemiology.* 2004;160(2):178–188. doi:10.1093/aje/kwh186
8. Bengtsson C, Nordmark B, Klareskog L, Lundberg I, Alfredsson LEIRA Study Group. Socioeconomic status and the risk of developing rheumatoid arthritis: Results from the Swedish EIRA study. *Annals of the Rheumatic Diseases.* 2005;64(11):1588–1594. doi:10.1136/ard.2004.031666
9. Cohen S, Janicki-Deverts D, Miller GE. Psychological stress and disease. *JAMA.* 2007;298(14):1685–1687. doi:10.1001/jama.298.14.1685
10. Domènech-Abella J, Mundó J, Leonardi M, et al. The association between socioeconomic status and depression among older adults in Finland, Poland and Spain: A comparative cross-sectional study of distinct measures and pathways. *Journal of Affective Disorders.* 2018;241:311–318. doi:10.1016/j.jad.2018.08.077
11. Schwartz DM, Kanno Y, Villarino A, Ward M, Gadina M, O'Shea JJ. JAK inhibition as a therapeutic strategy for immune and inflammatory diseases. *Nature Reviews Drug Discovery.* 2017;16(12):843–862. doi:10.1038/nrd.2017.201
12. Alegría M, NeMoyer A, Falgas I, Wang Y, Alvarez K. Social determinants of mental health: where we are and where we need to go. *Current Psychiatry Reports.* 2018;20(11):95. doi:10.1007/s11920-018-0969-9
13. Bell R, Marmot M, Bhugra D, Moussaoui D, Craig TJ. *Oxford Textbook of Social Psychiatry.* Oxford University Press; 2022.
14. Tan JJX, Kraus MW, Carpenter NC, Adler NE. The association between objective and subjective socioeconomic status and subjective well-being: A meta-analytic review. *Psychological Bulletin.* 2020;146(11):970–1020. doi:10.1037/bul0000258
15. Yan W, Zhang L, Li W, You X, Kong F. Associations of family subjective socioeconomic status with hedonic and eudaimonic well-being in emerging adulthood: A daily diary study. *Social Science & Medicine 1982.* 2022;298:114867. doi:10.1016/j.socscimed.2022.114867
16. Eisenberger NI, Moieni M. Inflammation affects social experience: Implications for mental health. *World Psychiatry.* 2020;19(1):109–110. doi:10.1002/wps.20724
17. Gassen J, Hill SE. Why inflammation and the activities of the immune system matter for social and personality psychology (and not only for those who study health). *Social and Personality Psychology Compass.* 2019;13(6):e12471. doi:10.1111/spc3.12471

18. Steptoe A, Kivimäki M. Stress And cardiovascular disease: An update on current knowledge. *Annual Review of Public Health.* 2013;34:337–354. doi:10.1146/annurev-publhealth-031912-114452

19. Galobardes B, Shaw M, Lawlor DA, Lynch JW, Davey Smith G. Indicators of socioeconomic position (part 1). *Journal of Epidemiology and Community Health.* 2006;60(1): 7–12. doi:10.1136/jech.2004.023531

20. Krieger N. A glossary for social epidemiology. *Journal of Epidemiology and Community Health.* 2001;55(10):693–700. doi:10.1136/jech.55.10.693

21. Geyer S, Hemström O, Peter R, Vågerö D. Education, income, and occupational class cannot be used interchangeably in social epidemiology. Empirical evidence against a common practice. *Journal of Epidemiology and Community Health.* 2006;60(9): 804–810. doi:10.1136/jech.2005.041319

22. Duncan O. A socioeconomic index for all occupations. *Occup Soc Status.* Published online 1961. Accessed February 21, 2023. https://cir.nii.ac.jp/crid/1570291225254986112

23. Joseph NT, Muldoon MF, Manuck SB, et al. The role of occupational status in the association between job strain and ambulatory blood pressure during working and nonworking days. *Psychosomatic Medicine.* 2016;78:940–949. doi:10.1097/PSY.0000000000000349

24. Marmot MG, Shipley MJ, Rose G. Inequalities in death–specific explanations of a general pattern. *The Lancet Lond England.* 1984;1(8384):1003–1006. doi:10.1016/s0140-6736(84)92337-7

25. Schieman S, Koltai J. Discovering pockets of complexity: Socioeconomic status, stress exposure, and the nuances of the health gradient. *Social Science Research.* 2017;63: 1–18. doi:10.1016/j.ssresearch.2016.09.023

26. Duncan GJ, Daly MC, McDonough P, Williams DR. Optimal indicators of socioeconomic status for health research. *American Journal of Public Health.* 2002;92(7):1151–1157.

27. Adler NE. Health disparities through a psychological lens. *American Psychologist.* 2009;64(8):663–673. doi:10.1037/0003-066X.64.8.663

28. Goodman E, Adler NE, Kawachi I, Frazier AL, Huang B, Colditz GA. Adolescents' perceptions of social status: Development and evaluation of a new indicator. *Pediatrics.* 2001;108(2):E31. doi:10.1542/peds.108.2.e31

29. Cundiff JM, Boylan JM, Muscatell KA. The pathway from social status to physical health: Taking a closer look at stress as a mediator. *Current Directions in Psychological Science.* 2020;29(2):147–153. doi:10.1177/0963721420901596

30. Gallo LC, Matthews KA. Understanding the association between socioeconomic status and physical health: Do negative emotions play a role? *Psychological Bulletin.* 2003;129(1):10–51. doi:10.1037/0033-2909.129.1.10

31. Matthews KA, Gallo LC. Psychological perspectives on pathways linking socioeconomic status and physical health. *Annual Review of Psychology.* 2011;62:501–530. doi:10.1146/annurev.psych.031809.130711

32. Cohen S, Gianaros PJ, Manuck SB. A stage model of stress and disease. *Perspectives on Psychological Science Journals – Association for Psychological Science.* 2016; 11(4):456–463. doi:10.1177/1745691616646305

33. Kagan J. Why stress remains an ambiguous concept: Reply to McEwen & McEwen (2016) and Cohen et al. (2016). *Perspectives on Psychological Science.* 2016;11(4): 464–465. doi:10.1177/1745691616649952

34. Epel ES, Crosswell AD, Mayer SE, et al. More than a feeling: A unified view of stress measurement for population science. *Frontiers in Neuroendocrinology.* 2018;49:146–169. doi:10.1016/j.yfrne.2018.03.001

35. Hudson CG. Socioeconomic status and mental illness: Tests of the social causation and selection hypotheses. *American Journal of Orthopsychiatry.* 2005;75(1):3–18. doi:10.1037/0002-9432.75.1.3

36. Fisher M, Baum F. The social determinants of mental health: Implications for research and health promotion. *Australian and New Zealand Journal of Psychiatry.* 2010;44(12):1057–1063. doi:10.3109/00048674.2010.509311

37. Zuckerman M. Diathesis-stress models. In: *Vulnerability to Psychopathology: A Biosocial Model.* American Psychological Association; 1999:3–23. doi:10.1037/10316-001

38. Kyle T, Dunn JR. Effects of housing circumstances on health, quality of life and healthcare use for people with severe mental illness: A review. *Health & Social Care in the Community.* 2008;16(1):1–15. doi:10.1111/j.1365-2524.2007.00723.x

39. Martin MS, Maddocks E, Chen Y, Gilman SE, Colman I. Food insecurity and mental illness: Disproportionate impacts in the context of perceived stress and social isolation. *Public Health.* 2016;132:86–91. doi:10.1016/j.puhe.2015.11.014

40. Shim R, Koplan C, Langheim FJP, Manseau MW, Powers RA, Compton MT. The social determinants of mental health: An overview and call to action. *Psychiatric Annals.* 2014;44(1):22–26. doi:10.3928/00485713-20140108-04

41. Silver E, Mulvey EP, Swanson JW. Neighborhood structural characteristics and mental disorder: Faris and Dunham revisited. *Social Science & Medicine 1982.* 2002;55(8):1457–1470. doi:10.1016/s0277-9536(01)00266-0

42. Black D. Inequalities in health: Report of a research working group. *DHSS.* Published online 1980:417.

43. Chandola T, Marmot MG. *The Handbook of Stress Science: Biology, Psychology, and Health.* 1st edition. (PhD RC, PhD AB, eds.). Springer Publishing Company; 2010.

44. Mossakowski KN. social causation and social selection. In: Cockerham WC, Dingwall R, Quah S, eds. John Wiley & Sons, Ltd; 2014:2154–2160. doi:10.1002/9781118410868. wbehibs262

45. Blane D, Smith GD, Bartley M. Social selection: What does it contribute to social class differences in health? *Sociology of Health and Illness.* 1993;15(1):1–15. doi:10.1111/j.1467-9566.1993.tb00328.x

46. Adler NE, Snibbe AC. The role of psychosocial processes in explaining the gradient between socioeconomic status and health. *Current Directions in Psychological Science.* 2003;12:119–123. doi:10.1111/1467-8721.01245

47. Seeman M, Stein Merkin S, Karlamangla A, Koretz B, Seeman T. Social status and biological dysregulation: The "status syndrome" and allostatic load. *Social Science & Medicine 1982.* 2014;118:143–151. doi:10.1016/j.socscimed.2014.08.002

48. Gallo LC, Bogart LM, Vranceanu AM, Matthews KA. Socioeconomic status, resources, psychological experiences, and emotional responses: A test of the reserve capacity model. *Journal of Personality and Social Psychology.* 2005;88(2):386–399. doi:10.1037/0022-3514.88.2.386

49. Lazarus RS, DeLongis A, Folkman S, Gruen R. Stress and adaptational outcomes: The problem of confounded measures. *American Psychologist.* 1985;40:770–779. doi:10.1037/0003-066X.40.7.770

50. Chen E, Miller GE. "Shift-and-persist" strategies: Why being low in socioeconomic status isn't always bad for health. *Perspectives on Psychological Science Journal of the Association for Psychological Science.* 2012;7(2):135–158. doi:10.1177/1745691612436694

51. Kawachi I, Kennedy BP, Lochner K, Prothrow-Stith D. Social capital, income inequality, and mortality. *American Journal of Public Health.* 1997;87(9):1491–1498. doi:10.2105/ajph.87.9.1491

52. Wilkinson RG, Pickett KE. Income inequality and population health: A review and explanation of the evidence. *Social Science & Medicine 1982.* 2006;62(7):1768–1784. doi:10.1016/j.socscimed.2005.08.036

53. Smith HJ, Pettigrew TF, Pippin GM, Bialosiewicz S. Relative deprivation: A theoretical and meta-analytic review. *Personality and Social Psychology Review.* 2012;16(3):203–232. doi:10.1177/1088868311430825

54. Lantz PM, House JS, Mero RP, Williams DR. Stress, life events, and socioeconomic disparities in health: Results from the Americans' changing lives study. *Journal of Health and Social Behavior.* 2005;46(3):274–288. doi:10.1177/002214650504600305

55. Cundiff JM, Bennett A, Carson AP, Judd SE, Howard VJ. Socioeconomic status and psychological stress: Examining intersection with race, sex and US geographic region in the reasons for geographic and racial differences in stroke study. *Stress and Health : Journal of the International Society for the Investigation of Stress.* 2022;38(2): 340–349. doi:10.1002/smi.3095

56. Hatch SL, Dohrenwend BP. Distribution of traumatic and other stressful life events by race/ethnicity, gender, SES and age: A review of the research. *American Journal of Community Psychology.* 2007;40(3–4):313–332. doi:10.1007/s10464-007-9134-z

57. Jahnel T, Ferguson SG, Shiffman S, Schüz B. Daily stress as link between disadvantage and smoking: An ecological momentary assessment study. *BMC Public Health.* 2019;19(1):1284. doi:10.1186/s12889-019-7631-2

58. Turner RJ, Avison WR. Status variations in stress exposure: Implications for the interpretation of research on race, socioeconomic status, and gender. *Journal of Health and Social Behavior.* 2003;44(4):488–505.

59. Conger RD, Conger KJ, Martin MJ. Socioeconomic status, family processes, and individual development. *Journal of Marriage and Family.* 2010;72(3):685–704. doi:10.1111/j.1741-3737.2010.00725.x

60. Roberts BW, Kuncel NR, Shiner R, Caspi A, Goldberg LR. The power of personality: The comparative validity of personality traits, socioeconomic status, and cognitive ability for predicting important life outcomes. *Perspectives on Psychological Science.* 2007;2(4):313–345. doi:10.1111/j.1745-6916.2007.00047.x

61. Cohen S, Wills TA. Stress, social support, and the buffering hypothesis. *Psychological Bulletin.* 1985;98:310–357. doi:10.1037/0033-2909.98.2.310

62. Hooker ED, Campos B, Zoccola PM, Dickerson SS. Subjective socioeconomic status matters less when perceived social support is high: A study of cortisol responses to stress. *Social Psychological and Personality Science.* 2018;9:981–989. doi:10.1177/1948550617732387

63. John-Henderson NA, Stellar JE, Mendoza-Denton R, Francis DD. socioeconomic status and social support: social support reduces inflammatory reactivity for individuals whose early-life socioeconomic status was low. *Psychological Science.* 2015;26(10): 1620–1629. doi:10.1177/0956797615595962

64. Gorman BK, Sivaganesan A. The role of social support and integration for understanding socioeconomic disparities in self-rated health and hypertension. *Social Science & Medicine 1982.* 2007;65(5):958–975. doi:10.1016/j.socscimed.2007.04.017

65. Bosma H, Van Jaarsveld CHM, Tuinstra J, et al. Low control beliefs, classical coronary risk factors, and socio-economic differences in heart disease in older persons. *Social Science & Medicine 1982.* 2005;60(4):737–745. doi:10.1016/j.socscimed.2004.06.018

66. Zilioli S, Imami L, Slatcher RB. Socioeconomic status, perceived control, diurnal cortisol, and physical symptoms: A moderated mediation model. *Psychoneuroendocrinology.* 2017;75:36–43. doi:10.1016/j.psyneuen.2016.09.025

67. Orton LC, Pennington A, Nayak S, et al. What is the evidence that differences in 'control over destiny' lead to socioeconomic inequalities in health? A theory-led systematic review of high-quality longitudinal studies on pathways in the living environment. *Journal of Epidemiology and Community Health.* 2019;73(10):929–934. doi: 10.1136/jech-2019-212565

68. Turiano NA, Chapman BP, Agrigoroaei S, Infurna FJ, Lachman M. Perceived control reduces mortality risk at low, not high, education levels. *Health Psychology.* 2014;33:883–890. doi:10.1037/hea0000022

69. Cundiff JM, Jennings JR, Matthews KA. Social stratification and risk for cardiovascular disease: Examination of emotional suppression as a pathway to risk. *Personality and Social Psychology Bulletin*. 2019;45:1202–1215. doi:10.1177/0146167218808504

70. Marmot MG, Smith GD, Stansfeld S, et al. Health inequalities among British civil servants: The Whitehall II study. The *Lancet Lond England*. 1991;337(8754):1387–1393. doi:10.1016/0140-6736(91)93068-k

71. Pampel FC, Krueger PM, Denney JT. Socioeconomic disparities in health behaviors. *Annual Review of Sociology*. 2010;36:349–370. doi:10.1146/annurev.soc.012809.102529

72. Adler NE, Stewart J. Health disparities across the lifespan: Meaning, methods, and mechanisms. *Annals of the New York Academy of Sciences*. 2010;1186:5–23. doi:10.1111/j.1749-6632.2009.05337.x

73. Johnson-Lawrence V, Galea S, Kaplan G. Cumulative socioeconomic disadvantage and cardiovascular disease mortality in the alameda county study 1965–2000. *Annals of Epidemiology*. 2015;25(2):65–70. doi:10.1016/j.annepidem.2014.11.018

74. Vable AM, Gilsanz P, Kawachi I. Is it possible to overcome the "long arm" of childhood socioeconomic disadvantage through upward socioeconomic mobility? *Journal of Public Health | Oxford Academic*. 2019;41(3):566–574. doi:10.1093/pubmed/fdz018

75. Cundiff JM, Boylan JM, Pardini DA, Matthews KA. Moving up matters: Socioeconomic mobility prospectively predicts better physical health. *Health Psychology: Official journal of the Division of Health Psychology, American Psychological Association*. 2017;36(6):609–617. doi:10.1037/hea0000473

76. Destin M. Socioeconomic mobility, identity, and health: Experiences that influence immunology and implications for intervention. *American Psychologist*. 2019;74(2):207–217. doi:10.1037/amp0000297

77. Miller GE, Cohen S, Janicki-Deverts D, Brody GH, Chen E. Viral challenge reveals further evidence of skin-deep resilience in African Americans from disadvantaged backgrounds. *Health Psychology: Official journal of the Division of Health Psychology, American Psychological Association*. 2016;35(11):1225–1234. doi:10.1037/hea0000398

78. Miller GE, Yu T, Chen E, Brody GH. Self-control forecasts better psychosocial outcomes but faster epigenetic aging in low-SES youth. *Proceedings of the National Academy of Sciences*. 2015;112(33):10325–10330. doi:10.1073/pnas.1505063112

4 Personality and Emotional Adjustment in Health Risk and Resilience

Paula G. Williams, PhD and Steven E. Carlson, MS

KEY POINTS

- Evidence-based dimensional frameworks of personality and mental health, as well as their hypothesized interconnections, can be utilized to better understand how the emotional adjustment correlates of personality are relevant to health outcomes.
- Personality factors and related emotional adjustment have high predictive utility with respect to mortality risk, disease onset and progression, health behavior, and stress regulation.
- Cumulative evidence of the relevance of personality to health-relevant behavior and disease outcomes suggest that these associations should now be considered in assessment and tailored intervention within lifestyle medicine.

4.1 INDIVIDUAL DIFFERENCES RELEVANT TO LIFESTYLE MEDICINE: PERSONALITY AND EMOTIONAL ADJUSTMENT IN HEALTH RISK AND RESILIENCE

Characteristic ways of thinking, feeling, and behaving—i.e., *personality*—and related variability in emotional adjustment are strongly related to the maintenance of health and the development of and adaptation to illness. Indeed, personality-health associations are often of the same or larger magnitude as other risk factors such as socioeconomic status,[1] solidifying the role of personality factors in health risk prediction models.[2] The focus of the current chapter is to provide an overview of the associations between personality, emotional adjustment, and health outcomes, as well as the relevance of personality to the six pillars of lifestyle medicine (i.e., healthful eating, physical activity, stress management, relationships, sleep, and substance use).

4.2 OVERVIEW OF PERSONALITY ASSESSMENT

Although historically, there was a lack of consensus on the definitive collection of traits in comprehensive personality assessment, the widely-accepted adoption of the "Big Five"[3] or Five-Factor Model (FFM)[4] has led to a "renaissance" of personality psychology generally.[5] Table 4.1 outlines the FFM traits, the two overarching

DOI: 10.1201/b22810-5

TABLE 4.1
Schematic of Five Factor Model Traits and Facets, Maladaptive Variant Examples, and Hypothesized Related Constructs from the Hierarchical Taxonomy of Psychopathology (HiTOP) and Research Domain Criteria (RDoC)

Meta-Trait[a]	Stability			Plasticity	
FFM Trait[b]	Neuroticism	Conscientiousness	Agreeableness	Extraversion	Openness
	(-) Emotional Stability	(-) Unreliability	(-) Antagonism	(-) Introversion	(-) Closed-minded
Aspects[c]	Volatility	Industriousness	Compassion	Assertiveness	Openness
	Withdrawal	Orderliness	Politeness	Enthusiasm	Intellect
Facets[b]	Anxiety	Competence	Trust	Warmth	Fantasy
	Angry Hostility	Order	Straightforwardness	Gregariousness	Aesthetics
	Depression	Dutifulness	Altruism	Assertiveness	Feelings
	Self-Consciousness	Achievement Striving	Compliance	Activity	Actions
	Impulsiveness	Self-Discipline	Modesty	Excitement-seeking	Ideas
	Vulnerability	Deliberation	Tender-Mindedness	Positive Emotion	Values
Exemplar Maladaptive Variants[d]	Shameful	Perfectionistic	Subservient	Attention Seeking	Eccentric
	Fearful	Workaholic	Gullible	Pushy	Magical thinking
	(-) Shameless	(-) Lax	(-) Arrogant	(-) Anhedonic	(-) Mechanical
	(-) Unrealistic	(-) Careless	(-) Callous	(-) Lethargic	(-) Concrete
HiTOP Domain[e]	Internalizing	(-) Disinhibited Externalizing	(-) Antagonistic Externalizing	(-) Detachment	Thought Disorder
Exemplar Psychopathology Correlates	Anxiety disorders	(-) Inattention/ADHD	(-) Narcissism	Bipolar disorder	Schizotypal
Hypothesized RDoC[f]	Negative Valence	Arousal/Regulatory	Social	Positive Valence Social	Cognitive

[a]DeYoung[6]; [b]McCrae and Costa[8]; [c]DeYoung[7]; [d]Rojas[97]; [e]Widiger et al.[32]; [f]Trull and Widiger[15]

Note: HiTOP = Hierarchical Taxonomy of Psychopathology; RDoC = Research Domain Criteria. Reprinted with permission from: Williams, P.G., & Carlson, S.E. (in press). Personality and emotional adjustment in health risk and resilience. T.W. Smith and N.B. Anderson (Eds.), *APA Handbook of Health Psychology (Vol. 1)*. Washington, D.C.: American Psychological Association meta-traits (stability and plasticity),[6] the hypothesized "aspects" within each FFM domain,[7] and the narrower "facets" of each of the five factor traits as labeled in validated personality measures, such as the NEO (neuroticism, extraversion, and openness) instruments.[8]

Importantly, personality is associated with mental health factors that also have central relevance to health and disease. Despite this known overlap, personality and psychopathology are often treated as separate research endeavors, and the associations between them are overlooked. Recent advancements that can help address this disparity have included the development of the National Institute of Mental Health (NIMH) Research Domain Criteria (RDoC),[9] the Hierarchical Taxonomy of Psychopathology (HiToP),[10,11] and FFM of personality disorders.[12,13] These evidence-based dimensional frameworks, as well as their hypothesized interconnections[14,15] can be utilized to better understand how the emotional adjustment correlates of FFM personality factors[16] are relevant to the maintenance of health, illness trajectories, and adjustment to chronic conditions (see Table 4.1 for hypothesized associations between FFM personality traits and psychopathology dimensions).

4.3   PERSONALITY ASSOCIATIONS WITH HEALTH OUTCOMES

When possible, we review exemplar studies of FFM personality factors, facets, and related emotional adjustment and objective health, emphasizing meta-analyses and large-scale studies using nationally representative databases. Unless otherwise noted, personality assessment is self-reported.

4.3.1   NEUROTICISM

Neuroticism, sometimes termed trait negative affectivity or emotional stability, involves proneness to anxiety and related emotions. It is reflected in the "negative valence" system in RDoC and the "internalizing" domain of HiToP;[16,17] as such, neuroticism is a vulnerability factor for the development of anxiety disorders and depression (see Table 4.1).

Despite a somewhat controversial history, there is now substantial evidence that neuroticism, along with related psychopathology, is a key factor in health risk and resilience, as well as successful aging.[18] Neuroticism is associated with objective health outcomes in multiple studies utilizing large nationally-representative databases, including all-cause mortality.[19,20] Related, transdiagnostic internalizing psychopathology is associated with mortality risk.[21] Importantly, however, some studies have found no association between neuroticism and mortality[22] and others have found *lower* mortality risk in relation to neuroticism,[23] the proneness to worry component in particular,[24] perhaps reflecting greater concern for maintaining health and/or propensity to seek medical care. In an examination of multi-informant reports of personality, the higher-order stability meta-trait (comprising shared variance among neuroticism, agreeableness, and conscientiousness)[6] was independently associated with aggregated cardiometabolic risk; neuroticism was (marginally) associated.[25]

4.3.2 EXTRAVERSION

The central feature of extraversion is proneness to positive affect and high reward drive, which manifests in sociability, excitement seeking, and high activity levels. On the opposite pole, introverts are reserved and independent, but not necessarily unhappy or shy.[8] Extraversion is best represented by the "positive valence" component of RDoC,[26] particularly reward sensitivity,[27] given associations with the dopamine reward system.[26] Introversion is represented in the "detachment" component of HiToP[28] (see Table 4.1). Specific mental health issues include proneness to mania/bipolar disorder, as well as to depression due to low behavioral activation/anhedonia (i.e., low positive emotions facet).[29] Two core aspects characterize extraversion: "communal" and "agentic" (also termed "enthusiasm" and "assertiveness"),[30] with separable mental health implications: the communal aspect is largely adaptive, whereas the agentic aspect is often maladaptive.[31,32] Further, positive affect may be largely adaptive for health,[33] whereas proneness to dominance, or excessive agency may be maladaptive.

The two-component issue described above may underlie the mixed findings related to mortality risk, with some studies finding increased risk.[34] However, positive affect is specifically associated with *lower* mortality risk in a meta-analysis[35] and a large longitudinal study.[36] In a large study that included both self- and informant-reports of personality, the activity facet was one of only two facets (with order from conscientiousness) that demonstrated method independent association with (lower probability of) diabetes diagnosis.[37]

4.3.3 OPENNESS TO EXPERIENCE

Openness has been described as "...the breadth, depth, and permeability of consciousness, and ... the recurrent need to enlarge and examine experience" (p826).[38] This personality factor is also described as reflecting comfort with novelty and motivation for cognitive exploration.[7] Openness is a broad factor with facets focused on openness to fantasy, aesthetics (i.e., art, nature, beauty), actions, ideas, and values. Although Openness is associated with the HiToP "thought disorder" domain,[16] this appears to be largely related to the fantasy facet (i.e., the potential for loss of reality testing, though see Widiger & Crego[39] for discussion of equivocal findings).

Although less studied in personality-health research, there is now evidence that higher openness is a protective factor in all-cause mortality,[40] incident coronary heart disease (CHD),[41] obesity risk,[42] and adverse lipid profiles.[43,44] Further, multi-informant assessed openness is independently associated with lower aggregated cardiometabolic risk.[25]

4.3.4 AGREEABLENESS

Agreeableness is an interpersonally-focused personality factor reflected in communal striving (i.e., motivation for interpersonal harmony, altruism, and cooperation) vs. antagonism (i.e., competitiveness, low trust, and skepticism of others' intentions). As shown in Table 4.1, Agreeableness is related to the "social processes" domain of RDoC and the "antagonistic externalizing" domain of HiToP. Low agreeableness is related to externalizing psychopathology (e.g., narcissism, antisocial behavior, substance abuse).[45] Notably, low agreeableness is related to the historically-significant "Type A behavior pattern" along with the angry hostility facet of neuroticism, making it a risk factor for coronary heart disease (see Smith et al[46] for discussion).

The broad agreeableness factor has not typically been implicated in mortality risk. However, the submissiveness and hostile submissiveness scales of the interpersonal circumplex, reflecting a combination of agreeableness and extraversion, are associated with elevated mortality risk.[47] As previously described, the stability meta-trait ([low] agreeableness, along with neuroticism and conscientiousness) appears to confer risk for cardiometabolic disease.[25]

4.3.5 CONSCIENTIOUSNESS

Fundamentally, conscientiousness reflects self-control (i.e., organizational skill, planning, deliberation, and self-assessed competence). Emotional adjustment correlates of (low) conscientiousness are subsumed within the "disinhibited externalizing" domain of HiToP,[16] including impulsivity and distractibility (i.e., attention deficit hyperactivity disorder) (see Table 4.1).

Conscientiousness has been consistently associated with (lower) mortality risk.[20,22,34] Conscientiousness has an (inverse) association with body mass index (BMI),[48,49] obesity risk,[42,50,51] and lipid profiles,[43,44,52] as well as cardiometabolic risk as part of the stability meta-trait.[25] Conscientiousness is also associated with lower C-reactive protein (CRP)—a marker of inflammation.[53] Further, the inflammation marker IL-6 may partially mediate the lower mortality risk among high conscientious individuals.[54]

4.4 PERSONALITY AND THE SIX PILLARS OF LIFESTYLE MEDICINE

As described above, personality factors have established associations with physical health outcomes, including chronic disease incidence and mortality risk. In the following sections, we provide a brief overview of the implications of personality for the six pillars of lifestyle medicine.

4.4.1 HEALTHFUL EATING

As reviewed previously, personality factors have demonstrated relations to lipids, adiposity, and BMI, as well as to metabolic disease. These findings suggest that personality may be associated with dietary behavior. Indeed, reports of eating unhealthy foods are related to lower agreeableness, conscientiousness, neuroticism, and openness.[55] Notably, lower conscientiousness is associated with increased leptin, a hormone implicated in appetite, even when controlling for BMI, waist circumference, and inflammatory markers.[56]

4.4.2 PHYSICAL ACTIVITY

With respect to physical activity, two meta-analyses have found positive associations for extraversion, openness, and conscientiousness, and a negative association for neuroticism.[57,58] Low neuroticism and high conscientiousness are also associated with less sedentary behavior.[57] Facet-level analyses of the NEO personality inventory revised (NEO PI-R) have shown that activity (extraversion) and self-discipline (conscientiousness) are particularly relevant to exercise behavior, whereas anxiety (neuroticism) moderates the intention-exercise behavior relationship.[59] Indeed, the activity facet—assessing propensity to a high energy, fast-paced lifestyle—is associated with lower mortality risk,[47] perhaps via higher physical activity. In addition, objectively-assessed physical activity has linked conscientiousness to cardiometabolic risk.[60] Further, conscientiousness and openness predict increases in physical activity over time, whereas agreeableness predicts decreases in physical activity; examination of longitudinal reciprocal associations indicates that increases in physical activity may lead to increased openness.[61]

4.4.3 STRESS MANAGEMENT

Given that stress, broadly considered, is a known mechanism for the development of illness,[62] stress management is a key component of lifestyle medicine. In recent years, a "stress process" framework has been suggested as a means to understand pathways to adverse health outcomes better.[63,64] Within such a framework, "stress" comprises *stress exposure, stress reactivity, stress recovery,* and *stress restoration.* Such explication can also inform tailored stress management strategies. As discussed in prior reviews,[46,65] personality factors figure prominently in variation across these stress processes. Because sleep is a key stress restoration process, personality associations are discussed below in a separate section.

With respect to *stress exposure,* personality factors constrain the probability of stressful events in a variety of ways including characteristic maladaptive behaviors such as difficulty with cognitive control or proneness to interpersonal conflict, as well as self-selection into stressful circumstances (e.g., excessive workload). For example, neuroticism is associated with daily hassles,[66] as well as interpersonal conflict.[67] There is also evidence that higher conscientiousness is associated with fewer "self-dependent episodic stressors,"[68] illustrating the extent to which difficulties with self-control and organization may lead to greater stress exposure. Stressful events can also be internal, including worry (i.e., anticipation of stressful circumstances) and rumination (i.e., re-living of past stressful events), collectively known as "perseverative cognition" or "repetitive thought." Not surprisingly, neuroticism has robust associations with perseverative cognition and repetitive thought[69,70] and aspects of internalizing psychopathology characterized by worry (e.g., generalized anxiety disorder) and rumination (e.g., depression).[16]

Personality is associated with variation in physiological, emotional, and cognitive responses to potentially stressful events (i.e., *stress reactivity*). For example, the inter-related personality traits including anger, hostility, aggressiveness, and variations of " Type A behavior" are significantly associated with cardiovascular reactivity.[71] With respect to cognitive reactivity to stressors, perseverative cognition—a key correlate, if not a defining feature, of neuroticism—is significantly associated with cardiovascular, endocrine, and autonomic activation.[72] Not surprisingly, neuroticism is also related to emotional stress reactivity.[73]

Although physiological reactivity has been a central focus of stress-health research, the *duration* of stress-related cardiovascular responses—or degree of *recovery* to baseline in laboratory stress studies—may be as important as the magnitude of initial reactivity.[74,75] Indeed, poor cardiovascular recovery has been prospectively associated with increases in blood pressure over a period of several years.[76,77] With respect to personality predictors of stress recovery, anxiety-related traits (i.e., neuroticism) have the strongest associations with prolonged cardiovascular recovery,[71] as well as poorer cardiovascular recovery following hostile laboratory social stressors.[78]

4.4.4 RELATIONSHIPS

Social relationship quality is a key predictor of health and illness[79] and virtually all personality factors that confer risk or resilience in studies of health outcomes also have robust associations with the quality and stability of personal relationships.[80] With respect to objective health outcomes, antagonism (low agreeableness) has hypothesized pathways to adverse health outcomes given the competitive striving and general mistrust of others which can lead to chronic interpersonal conflict and, potentially, degradation of health-protective social support. There are also reciprocal associations—for example, perceived social support predicts increases in conscientiousness in older adults.[81]

4.4.5 SLEEP

Sleep is a key—if not *the* key—factor in stress restoration. Sleep serves critical biological functions, most notably clearance of metabolic waste products in the brain[82] and is associated with virtually all adverse stress-related health outcomes. As with the term "stress," the broad term "sleep" can usefully be considered as comprising components, each of which may have unique associations with health as well as personality. These components are often framed as *duration, continuity, quality,* and *architecture*.[83] Sleep timing variability and sleep duration variability, beyond mean levels, have also been linked to disease risk.[84,85] In addition, chronotype—an individual's tendency towards early or late sleep timing[86]—is also relevant to personality-health research.

With respect to personality-sleep associations, agreeableness is related to longer sleep duration; higher neuroticism and lower extraversion is related to greater sleep "deficiency" (the discrepancy between duration and self-reported sleep need); and reported sleep problems are positively related to neuroticism and negatively associated with extraversion, agreeableness, and conscientiousness.[87] Chronotype appears to have distinct personality correlates, which may be relevant to the development of health risk. Indeed, "morningness-eveningness" has been considered a dimension of personality historically.[88] Early chronotype is associated with higher conscientiousness and, more modestly, with lower openness.[89–92] Not surprisingly, given associations with internalizing psychopathology, neuroticism is a key predictor of subjective sleep quality and insomnia, along with low openness and conscientiousness.[93]

4.4.6 SUBSTANCE USE

Because cigarette smoking remains a critical risk factor for the development of most types of chronic illness and, hence, all-cause mortality, it represents a putative mechanism for personality-health relations. In a nine-cohort study meta-analysis, higher neuroticism, higher extraversion, and lower conscientiousness were associated with current smoking status; longitudinally, higher neuroticism predicted greater relapse among non-smokers, as well as less smoking cessation, whereas higher extraversion and lower conscientiousness predicted smoking initiation.[94]

Alcohol use represents another potential pathway from personality to objective illness and mortality. In a prospective meta-analysis of alcohol use, higher extraversion and lower conscientiousness were associated with transition from moderate to heavy alcohol use, whereas lower extraversion, higher agreeableness, and lower openness predicted transition from moderate alcohol use to abstinence, as well as abstinence status.[95] Another meta-analysis indicated that high neuroticism, low agreeableness, and low conscientiousness were associated with alcohol involvement.[96] Turiano et al.[22] found that heavy drinking, smoking, and central adiposity mediated the conscientiousness-mortality risk association.

4.5 CONCLUSIONS

The last decade has seen an impressive increase in personality-health research, including many meta-analyses confirming the predictive utility of personality characteristics in mortality risk, disease risk, health behavior, and stress regulation. As outlined in this chapter, the major personality factors have implications for all aspects of lifestyle medicine. The known associations between personality and health outcomes, as well as the pillars of lifestyle medicine mean that practitioners might usefully consider these associations in tailored interventions. Indeed, the study of personality and health is now poised to be at the forefront of public health research and, therefore, a central consideration in lifestyle medicine.

REFERENCES

1. Roberts BW, Kuncel NR, Shiner R, Caspi A, Goldberg LR. The power of personality: The comparative validity of personality traits, socioeconomic status, and cognitive ability for predicting important life outcomes. *Perspectives on Psychological Science.* 2007;2(4):313–345. doi:10.1111/j.1745-6916.2007.00047.x
2. Chapman BP, Lin F, Roy S, Benedict RHB, Lyness JM. Health risk prediction models incorporating personality data: Motivation, challenges, and illustration. *Personality Disorders.* 2019;10(1):46–58. doi:10.1037/per0000300
3. Goldberg LR. An alternative "description of personality": The big-five factor structure. *Journal of Personality and Social Psychology.* 1990;59(6):1216–1229. doi:10.1037/0022-3514.59.6.1216
4. McCrae RR, John OP. An introduction to the five-factor model and its applications. *Journal of Personalized.* 1992;60(2):175–215. doi:10.1111/j.1467-6494.1992.tb00970.x
5. Roberts BW, Yoon HJ. Personality psychology. *Annual Review of Psychology.* 2022;73(1):489–516. doi:10.1146/annurev-psych-020821-114927

6. DeYoung CG. Higher-order factors of the big five in a multi-informant sample. *Journal of Personality and Social Psychology*. 2006;91(6):1138–1151. doi:10.1037/0022-3514. 91.6.1138

7. DeYoung CG. Openness/intellect: A dimension of personality reflecting cognitive exploration. In: *APA Handbook of Personality and Social Psychology, Volume 4: Personality Processes and Individual Differences*. American Psychological Association; 2015:369–399. *APA handbooks in psychology®*.

8. McCrae RR, Costa PT. *NEO Inventories: NEO Personality Inventory-3 (NEO-PI-3)*. Psychological Assessment Resources; 2010.

9. Cuthbert BN, Insel TR. Toward the future of psychiatric diagnosis: The seven pillars of RDoC. *BMC Medicine*. 2013;11(1):126. doi:10.1186/1741-7015-11-126

10. Kotov R, Krueger RF, Watson D, et al. The hierarchical taxonomy of psychopathology (HiTOP): A dimensional alternative to traditional nosologies. *Journal of Abnormal Psychology*. 2017;126(4):454–477. doi:10.1037/abn0000258

11. Mackin DM, Kotov R, Perlman G, et al. Reward processing and future life stress: Stress generation pathway to depression. *Journal of Abnormal Psychology*. 2019;128(4): 305–314. doi:10.1037/abn0000427

12. Krueger RF, Markon KE. The role of the dsm-5 personality trait model in moving toward a quantitative and empirically based approach to classifying personality and psychopathology. *Annual Review of Clinical Psychology*. 2014;10(1):477–501. doi:10.1146/annurev-clinpsy-032813-153732

13. Widiger TA, Lowe JR. Five-factor model assessment of personality disorder. *Journal of Personality Assessment*. 2007;89(1):16–29. doi:10.1080/00223890701356953

14. Michelini G, Palumbo IM, DeYoung CG, Latzman RD, Kotov R. Linking RDoC and HiTOP: A new interface for advancing psychiatric nosology and neuroscience. *Clinical Psychology Review*. 06/01/2021;86:102025. doi:10.1016/j.cpr.2021.102025

15. Trull TJ, Widiger TA. Dimensional models of personality: The five-factor model and the DSM-5. *Dialogues in Clinical Neuroscience*. 2013;15(2):135–146. doi:10.31887/DCNS.2013.15.2/ttrull

16. Widiger TA, Sellbom M, Chmielewski M, et al. Personality in a hierarchical model of psychopathology. *Clinical Psychological Science*. 2018;7(1):77–92. doi:10.1177/2167702618797105

17. Brandes CM, Tackett JL. Contextualizing neuroticism in the hierarchical taxonomy of psychopathology. *Journal of Research in Personality*. 2019;81:238–245. doi:10.1016/j.jrp.2019.06.007

18. Friedman HS. Neuroticism and health as individuals age. *Personality Disorders*. 2019; 10(1):25–32. doi:10.1037/per0000274

19. Graham EK, Rutsohn JP, Turiano NA, et al. Personality predicts mortality risk: An integrative data analysis of 15 international longitudinal studies. *Journal of Research in Personality*. 2017;70:174–186. doi:10.1016/j.jrp.2017.07.005

20. Jokela MA-O, Airaksinen J, Virtanen M, Batty GD, Kivimäki M, Hakulinen C. Personality, disability-free life years, and life expectancy: Individual participant meta-analysis of 131,195 individuals from 10 cohort studies. *Journal of Personalized*. 2020;88(3):596–605. doi:10.1111/jopy.12513

21. Kim H, Turiano NA, Forbes MK, et al. Internalizing psychopathology and all-cause mortality: A comparison of transdiagnostic vs. diagnosis-based risk prediction. *World Psychiatry*. 2021;20(2):276–282. doi:10.1002/wps.20859

22. Turiano NA, Chapman BP, Gruenewald TL, Mroczek DK. Personality and the leading behavioral contributors of mortality. *Health Psychology*. 2015;34(1):51–60. doi:10.1037/hea0000038

23. Weiss A, Gale CR, Batty GD, Deary IJ. A questionnaire-wide association study of personality and mortality: The Vietnam experience study. *Journal of Psychosomatic Research*. 2013;74(6):523–529. doi:10.1016/j.jpsychores.2013.02.010

24. Gale CR, Čukić I, Batty GD, McIntosh AM, Weiss A, Deary IJ. When is higher neuroticism protective against death? Findings from UK biobank. *Psychological Science.*
2017;28(9):1345–1357. doi:10.1177/0956797617709813
25. Dermody SS, Wright AGC, Cheong J, et al. Personality correlates of midlife cardiometabolic risk: The explanatory role of higher-order factors of the five-factor model.
Journal of Personalized. 2016;84(6):765–776. doi:10.1111/jopy.12216
26. Smillie LD, Jach HK, Hughes DM, Wacker J, Cooper AJ, Pickering AD. Extraversion
and reward-processing: Consolidating evidence from an electroencephalographic index
of reward-prediction-error. *Biological Psychology.* 2019;146:107735. doi:10.1016/j.
biopsycho.2019.107735
27. Blain SD, Sassenberg TA, Xi M, Zhao D, DeYoung CG. Extraversion but not depression predicts reward sensitivity: Revisiting the measurement of anhedonic phenotypes. *Journal of Personality and Social Psychology.* 2021;121(2):e1–e18. doi:10.1037/
pspp0000371
28. Suzuki T, Samuel DB, Pahlen S, Krueger RF. DSM-5 alternative personality disorder
model traits as maladaptive extreme variants of the five-factor model: An item-response
theory analysis. *Journal of Abnormal Psychology.* 2015;124(2):343–354. doi:10.1037/
abn0000035
29. Watson D, Stasik SM, Ellickson-Larew S, Stanton K. Extraversion and psychopathology: A facet-level analysis. *Journal of Abnormal Psychology.* 2015;124(2):432–446.
doi:10.1037/abn0000051
30. DeYoung CG, Carey BE, Krueger RF, Ross SR. Ten aspects of the big five in the personality inventory for DSM-5. *Personality Disorders.* 2016;7(2):113–123. doi:10.1037/
per0000170
31. Watson D, Clark LA, Khoo S. The temperamental basis of extraversion and its implications for psychopathology. *Personality and Individual Differences.* 2022;185:111302.
doi:10.1016/j.paid.2021.111302
32. Widiger TA, Bach B, Chmielewski M, et al. Criterion a of the AMPD in HiTOP.
Journal of Personality Assessment. 2019;101(4):345–355. doi:10.1080/00223891.2018.
1465431
33. Pressman SD, Jenkins BN, Moskowitz JT. Positive affect and health: What do we
know and where next should we go? *Annual Review of Psychology.* 2019;70:627–650.
doi:10.1146/annurev-psych-010418-102955
34. Jokela M, Pulkki-Råback L, Elovainio M, Kivimäki M. Personality traits as risk factors for stroke and coronary heart disease mortality: Pooled analysis of three cohort
studies. *Journal of Behavioral Medicine.* 2014;37(5):881–889. doi:10.1007/s10865-013-
9548-z
35. Zhang Y, Han B. Positive affect and mortality risk in older adults: A meta-analysis.
Psychology journal. 2016;5(2):125–138. doi:10.1002/pchj.129
36. Petrie KJ, Pressman SD, Pennebaker JW, Øverland S, Tell GS, Sivertsen B. Which
aspects of positive affect are related to mortality? Results from a general population
longitudinal study. *Annals of Behavioral Medicine.* 2018;52(7):571–581. doi:10.1093/
abm/kax018
37. Čukić I, Mõttus R, Realo A, Allik J. Elucidating the links between personality traits
and diabetes mellitus: Examining the role of facets, assessment methods, and selected
mediators. *Personality and Individual Differences.* 2016;94:377–382. doi:10.1016/j.
paid.2016.01.052
38. McCrae RR, Costa PT, Jr. Conceptions and correlates of openness to experience. In
R. Hogan, J. A. Johnson, & S. R. Briggs (Eds.), *Handbook of personality psychology*
1997; 825–847. Academic Press. https://doi.org/10.1016/B978-012134645-4/50032-9
39. Widiger TA, Crego C. The five factor model of personality structure: An update. *World
Psychiatry.* 2019;18(3):271–272. doi:10.1002/wps.20658

40. Ferguson E, Bibby PA. Openness to experience and all-cause mortality: A meta-analysis and requivalent from risk ratios and odds ratios. *British Journal of Health Psychology*. 2012;17(1):85–102. doi:10.1111/j.2044-8287.2011.02055.x
41. Lee HB, Offidani E, Ziegelstein RC, et al. Five-factor model personality traits as predictors of incident coronary heart disease in the community: A 10.5-year cohort study based on the Baltimore epidemiologic catchment area follow-up study. *Psychosomatics*. 2014;55(4):352–361. doi:10.1016/j.psym.2013.11.004
42. Sutin AR, Terracciano A. Five-factor model personality traits and the objective and subjective experience of body weight. *Journal of Personalized*. 2016;84(1):102–112. doi:10.1111/jopy.12143
43. Armon G. Personality and serum lipids: Does lifestyle account for their concurrent and long–term relationships. *European Journal of Personality*. 2014;28(6):550–559. doi:10.1002/per.1943
44. Roh SJ, Kim HN, Shim U, et al. Association between blood lipid levels and personality traits in young Korean women. *PLoS One*. 2014;9(9). doi:10.1371/journal.pone.0108406
45. Lynam DR, Miller JD. The basic trait of antagonism: An unfortunately underappreciated construct. *Journal of Research in Personality*. 2019;81:118–126. doi:10.1016/j.jrp.2019.05.012
46. Smith TW, Williams PG, Segerstrom SC. Personality and physical health. *APA Handbook of Personality and Social Psychology, Volume 4: Personality Processes and Individual Differences*. American Psychological Association; 2015:639–661. *APA handbooks in psychology®*.
47. Chapman BP, Elliot A, Sutin A, et al. Mortality risk associated with personality facets of the big five and interpersonal circumplex across three aging cohorts. *Psychosomatic Medicine*. 2020;82(1):64–73. doi:10.1097/psy.0000000000000756
48. Jokela M, Hintsanen M, Hakulinen C, et al. Association of personality with the development and persistence of obesity: A meta-analysis based on individual–participant data. *Obesity Reviews*. 2013;14(4):315–323. doi:10.1111/obr.12007
49. Vainik U, Dagher A, Realo A, et al. Personality-obesity associations are driven by narrow traits: A meta-analysis. *Obesity Reviews*. 2019;20(8):1121–1131. doi:10.1111/obr.12856
50. Sutin AR, Ferrucci L, Zonderman AB, Terracciano A. Personality and obesity across the adult life span. *Journal of Personality and Social Psychology*. 2011;101(3):579–592. doi:10.1037/a0024286
51. Terracciano A, A.R. S, McCrae RR, et al. Facets of personality linked to underweight and overweight. *Psychosomatic Medicine*. 2009;71(6):682–689. doi:10.1097/PSY.0b013e3181a2925b
52. Sutin AR, Terracciano A, Deiana B, et al. Cholesterol, triglycerides, and the five-factor model of personality. *Biological Psychology*. 2010;84(2):186–191. doi:10.1016/j.biopsycho.2010.01.012
53. Luchetti M, Barkley JM, Stephan Y, Terracciano A, Sutin AR. Five-factor model personality traits and inflammatory markers: New data and a meta-analysis. *Psychoneuroendocrinology*. 2014;50:181–193. doi:10.1016/j.psyneuen.2014.08.014
54. O'Súilleabháin PS, Turiano NA, Gerstorf D, et al. Personality pathways to mortality: Interleukin-6 links conscientiousness to mortality risk. *Brain, Behavior, and Immunity*. 2021;93:238–244. doi:10.1016/j.bbi.2021.01.032
55. Weston SJ, Edmonds GW, Hill PL. Personality traits predict dietary habits in middle-to-older adults. *Psychology, Health & Medicine*. 2020;25(3):379–387. doi:10.1080/13548506.2019.1687918
56. Sutin AR, Zonderman AB, Uda M, et al. Personality traits and leptin. *Psychosomatic Medicine*. 2013;75(5):505–509. doi:10.1097/PSY.0b013e3182919ff4

57. Sutin AR, Stephan Y, Luchetti M, Artese A, Oshio A, Terracciano A. The five-factor model of personality and physical inactivity: A meta-analysis of 16 samples. *Journal of Research in Personality.* 2016;63:22–28. doi:10.1016/j.jrp.2016.05.001

58. Wilson KE, Dishman RK. Personality and physical activity: A systematic review and meta-analysis. *Personality and Individual Differences.* 2015;72:230–242. doi:10.1016/j.paid.2014.08.023

59. Hoyt AL, Rhodes RE, Hausenblas HA, Giacobbi PR. Integrating five-factor model facet-level traits with the theory of planned behavior and exercise. *Psychology of Sport and Exercise.* 2009;10(5):565–572. doi:10.1016/j.psychsport.2009.02.008

60. Thomas MC, Duggan KA, Kamarck TW, Wright AGC, Muldoon MF, Manuck SB. Conscientiousness and cardiometabolic risk: A test of the health behavior model of personality using structural equation modeling. *Annals of Behavioral Medicine.* 2022; 56(1):100–111. doi:10.1093/abm/kaab027

61. Allen MS, Magee CA, Vella SA, Laborde S. Bidirectional associations between personality and physical activity in adulthood. *Health Psychology.* 2017;36(4)doi:10.1037/hea0000371

62. O'Connor DB, Thayer JF, Vedhara K. Stress and health: A review of psychobiological processes. *Annual Review of Psychology.* 2021;72(1):663–688. doi:10.1146/annurev-psych-062520-122331

63. Hawkley LC, Cacioppo JT. Loneliness and pathways to disease. *Brain, Behavior, and Immunity.* 2003;17(Supplement 1):98–105. doi:10.1016/S0889-1591(02)00073-9

64. Uchino BN, Smith TW, Holt-Lunstad J, Campo R, Reblin M. Stress and illness. In: *Handbook of Psychophysiology, 3rd ed.* Cambridge University Press; 2007:608–632.

65. Williams PG, Smith TW, Gunn HE, Uchino BN. Personality and stress: Individual differences in exposure, reactivity, recovery, and restoration. In: *The Handbook of Stress Science: Biology, Psychology, and Health.* Springer Publishing Company; 2011:231–245.

66. Vollrath M. Personality and hassles among university students: A three-year longitudinal study. *European Journal of Personality.* 2000;14(3):199–215. doi:10.1002/1099-0984(200005/06)14:3<199::AID-PER372>3.0.CO;2-B

67. Bolger N, Zuckerman A. A framework for studying personality in the stress process. *Journal of Personality and Social Psychology.* 1995;69(5):890–902. doi:10.1037//0022-3514.69.5.890

68. Murphy ML, Miller GE, Wrosch C. Conscientiousness and stress exposure and reactivity: A prospective study of adolescent females. *Journal of Behavioral Medicine.* 2013;36(2):153–164. doi:10.1007/s10865-012-9408-2

69. Segerstrom SC, Gloger EM, Hardy JK, Crofford LR. Exposure and reactivity to repetitive thought in the neuroticism-distress relationship. *Cognitive Therapy and Research.* 2020;44(3):659–667. doi:10.1007/s10608-020-10078-4

70. Van den Bergh O, Brosschot J, Critchley H, Thayer JF, Ottaviani C. Better safe than sorry: A common signature of general vulnerability for psychopathology. *Perspectives on Psychological Science.* 2020;16(2):225–246. doi:10.1177/1745691620950690

71. Chida Y, Hamer M. Chronic psychosocial factors and acute physiological responses to laboratory-induced stress in healthy populations: A quantitative review of 30 years of investigations. *Psychological Bulletin.* 2008;134(6):829–885. doi:10.1037/a0013342

72. Ottaviani C, Thayer JF, Verkuil B, et al. Physiological concomitants of perseverative cognition: A systematic review and meta-analysis. *Psychological Bulletin.* 2016; 142(3):231–259. doi:10.1037/bul0000036

73. Leger KA, Turiano NA, Bowling W, Burris JL, Almeida DM. Personality traits predict long-term physical health via affect reactivity to daily stressors. *Psychological Science.* 2021;32(5):755–765. doi:10.1177/0956797620980738

74. Brosschot JF, Gerin W, Thayer JF. The perseverative cognition hypothesis: A review of worry, prolonged stress-related physiological activation, and health. *Journal of Psychosomatic Research.* 2006;60(2):113–124. doi:10.1016/j.jpsychores.2005.06.074

75. Schwartz AR, Gerin W, Davidson KW, et al. Toward a causal model of cardiovascular responses to stress and the development of cardiovascular disease. *Psychosomatic Medicine.* 2003;65(1):22–35. doi:10.1097/01.psy.0000046075.79922.61

76. Moseley JV, Linden W. Predicting blood pressure and heart rate change with cardiovascular reactivity and recovery: Results from 3-year and 10-year follow up. *Psychosomatic Medicine.* 2006;68(6):833–843. doi:10.1097/01.psy.0000238453.11324.d5

77. Stewart JC, Janicki DL, Kamarck TW. Cardiovascular reactivity to and recovery from psychological challenge as predictors of 3-year change in blood pressure. *Health Psychology.* 2006;25(1):111–118. doi:10.1037/0278-6133.25.1.111

78. Hutchinson JG, Ruiz JM. Neuroticism and cardiovascular response in women: Evidence of effects on blood pressure recovery. *Journal of Personalized.* 2011;79(2):277–302. doi:10.1111/j.1467-6494.2010.00679.x

79. Holt-Lunstad J. Why social relationships are important for physical health: A systems approach to understanding and modifying risk and protection. *Annual Review of Psychology.* 2018;69(1):437–458. doi:10.1146/annurev-psych-122216-011902

80. Smith TW, Baucom BRW. Intimate relationships, individual adjustment, and coronary heart disease: Implications of overlapping associations in psychosocial risk. *American Psychologist.* 2017;72(6):578–589. doi:10.1037/amp0000123

81. Hill PL, Payne BR, Jackson JJ, Stine-Morrow EAL, Roberts BW. Perceived social support predicts increased conscientiousness during older adulthood. *The Journals of Gerontology.* 2014;69(4):543–547. doi:10.1093/geronb/gbt024

82. Fultz NE, Bonmassar G, Setsompop K, et al. Coupled electrophysiological, hemodynamic, and cerebrospinal fluid oscillations in human sleep. *Science.* 2019;366(6465): 628–631. doi:10.1126/science.aax5440

83. Hall MH. Behavioral medicine and sleep: Concepts, measures, and methods. In: Steptoe A, ed. *Handbook of Behavioral Medicine: Methods and Applications.* Springer: New York; 2010:749–765.

84. Baron KG, Reid KJ, Malkani RG, Kang J, Zee PC. Sleep variability among older adults with insomnia: Associations with sleep quality and cardiometabolic disease risk. *Behavioral Sleep Medicine.* 2017;15(2):144–157. doi:10.1080/15402002.2015.1120200

85. Bei B, Wiley JF, Trinder J, Manber R. Beyond the mean: A systematic review on the correlates of daily intraindividual variability of sleep/wake patterns. *Sleep Medicine Reviews.* 2016;28:108–124. doi:10.1016/j.smrv.2015.06.003

86. Adan A, Archer SN, Hidalgo MP, Di Milia L, Natale V, Randler C. Circadian typology: A comprehensive review. *Chronobiology International.* 2012;29(9):1153–1175. doi:10.3 109/07420528.2012.719971

87. Hintsanen M, Puttonen S, Smith K, et al. Five-factor personality traits and sleep: Evidence from two population-based cohort studies. *Health Psychology.* 2014;33(10):1214–1223. doi:10.1037/hea0000105

88. Matthews G. Morningness–eveningness as a dimension of personality: Trait, state, and psychophysiological correlates. *European Journal of Personality.* 1988;2(4):277–293. doi:10.1002/per.2410020405

89. Lenneis A, Vainik U, Teder-Laving M, et al. Personality traits relate to chronotype at both the phenotypic and genetic level. *Journal of Personalized.* 2021;89(6):1206–1222. doi:10.1111/jopy.12645

90. Lipnevich AA, Credè M, Hahn E, Spinath FM, Roberts RD, Preckel F. How distinctive are morningness and eveningness from the big five factors of personality? A meta-analytic investigation. *Journal of Personality and Social Psychology.* 2017;112(3):491–509. doi:10.1037/pspp0000099

91. Randler C, Schredl M, Göritz AS. Chronotype, sleep behavior, and the big five personality factors. *SAGE Open.* 2017;7(3). doi:10.1177/2158244017728321

92. Tsaousis I. Circadian preferences and personality traits: A meta-analysis. *European Journal of Personality.* 2010;24(4):356–373. doi:10.1002/per.754

93. Ellis JG, Perlis ML, Espie CA, et al. The natural history of insomnia: Predisposing, precipitating, coping, and perpetuating factors over the early developmental course of insomnia. *Sleep.* 2021;44(9):zsab095. doi:10.1093/sleep/zsab095

94. Hakulinen C, Hintsanen M, Munafò MR, et al. Personality and smoking: Individual-participant meta-analysis of nine cohort studies. *Addiction.* 2015;110(11):1844–1852. doi:10.1111/add.13079

95. Hakulinen C, Elovainio M, Batty GD, Virtanen M, Kivimäki M, Jokela M. Personality and alcohol consumption: Pooled analysis of 72,949 adults from eight cohort studies. *Drug and Alcohol Dependence.* 2015;151:110–114. doi:10.1016/j.drugalcdep.2015.03.008

96. Malouff JM, Thorsteinsson EB, Rooke SE, Schutte NS. Alcohol involvement and the five-factor model of personality: A meta-analysis. *Journal of Drug Education.* 2007;37(3):277–294. doi:10.2190/DE.37.3.d

97. Rojas SL, Crego C, Widiger TA. A conceptual dismantling of the five factor form: Lexical support for the bipolarity of maladaptive personality structure. *Journal of Research in Personality.* 2019;80:62–71. doi:10.13023/ETD.2017.216

5 Trauma Considerations

Gia Merlo, MD, MBA, MEd and
Steven G Sugden, MD, MPH, MSS

KEY POINTS

- Given the high prevalence of trauma exposures, trauma's impact affects the individual, his/her community, and the health care system.
- Many individuals who have experienced trauma do not have noticeable physical symptoms that suggest a trauma exposure. As such, providers are encouraged to adopt a trauma-informed care approach for all patients.
- In situations of significant trauma, complex trauma, and recurring triggering trauma, the hypothalamic-pituitary-adrenal (HPA) is unable to down-regulate, and the individual adopts a chronic trauma response.

5.1 INTRODUCTION

Trauma is a complex phenomenon that has varying degrees of intensity and impairment for individuals who experience it. While many factors affect human beings over their lifespan, trauma affects human functioning dramatically and sometimes permanently changes psychological functioning. Trauma can be physical, emotional, or sexual; it can be experienced directly, witnessed occurring to others, or experienced through learning that the event has happened to others.[1] While a single defining traumatic event is frequently linked to post-traumatic stress disorder (PTSD), complex trauma and other potentially sub-threshold traumatic events may still have long-lasting effects on individuals, which should be addressed appropriately by healthcare providers. The model of trauma-informed care provides a framework within which providers may leverage clients' trauma to guide treatment and enhance outcomes.

The impact of trauma and the development of PTSD-like symptoms have been described in literature as far back as Homer's *Iliad*. Austrian physician Josef Leopold in 1761 was one of the first to describe "nostalgia" among traumatized soldiers wanting to return home. Later U.S. physician Jacob Mendez Da Costa studied and followed Civil War soldiers, complaining of chest pain, shortness of breath, and worry, who were commonly diagnosed with "Soldier's heart" or "irritable heart." Throughout subsequent global conflicts, the diagnosis among soldiers changed (i.e., shell shock, battle fatigue, combat stress reaction), yet the symptoms were consistent with each era. It was not until the Diagnostic and Statistical Manual of Mental Disorders, Third Edition (DSM-III), that PTSD was introduced. Unlike previous diagnoses, the DSM-III highlighted how non-military veterans could develop these symptoms.[1] The Diagnostic and Statistical Manual of Mental Disorders, Fifth Edition (DSM 5) was the first to categorize PTSD as a trauma disorder, thereby removing it from the anxiety category.[2]

DOI: 10.1201/b22810-6

Historically, PTSD has centered on big traumatic events, which have commonly been called "Big T" trauma as they refer to combat veterans, survivors of rape, physical violence, or vehicle accidents, etc. Clinicians, however, noted that many individuals developed similar symptoms due to a series of repeated, prolonged, or multiple traumas. Individually, the events may not have produced the events, yet collectively, they did. Hence these series of events have been coined "little t" trauma. Herman was among the first to describe the complex nature of recurrent trauma on behavioral and physical health and coined the term complex post-traumatic stress disorder (CPTSD).[3] After years of following patients experiencing the long-term sequela of trauma, Van der Kolk et al. proposed a similar diagnosis, developmental trauma disorder, that takes into consideration the chronic long-term behavioral and physical health-related effects.[4]

Although these additions have not been reflected within the Diagnostic and Statistical Manual of Mental Disorders, Fifth Edition-Text Revision (DSM 5-TR), the eleventh revision of the International Classification of Diseases (ICD-11), adopted the diagnosis of CPTSD. The symptoms include those of PTSD with the addition of disturbances in self-organization symptoms, including affect dysregulation, impairments in self-concept and disturbances in relationships.[5] Population-based studies have shown that patients who meet the criteria of CPTSD experience more severe behavioral and physical symptom with lower levels of psychological well-being than PTSD. As such, individuals with CPTSD required a longer course of treatment, higher amounts of therapeutic interventions, and a greater likelihood that these symptoms return.[6]

Just as we are now coming to understand how socioeconomic determinants can affect healthcare, we can frame trauma in a similar way. Later in this volume, Chapter 27 will discuss PTSD. For this chapter, we are going to discuss general principles and specific effects and ways to approach trauma-informed care. This understanding and sensitivity to people suffering with a history of trauma is paramount for mental health providers, but also for primary care providers (PCP) who often treat such patients as difficult patients because they do not follow the prescribed paradigms and tax our healthcare systems.[7] Using trauma-informed care principles is not only sensitive and inclusive for this patient population, but also economically sound practice.

It is estimated that over 66% of children have experienced at least one complex trauma in their life.[8] Complex trauma has been shown to impact the functioning parts of the brain that regulate the neuroendocrine and limbic systems, which results in symptoms such as hyperarousal, attention and executive deficits, emotional and behavioral dysregulation, and dissociation from the activation of the survival-focused brain. While taken alone, these experiences may not be considered an adverse childhood experience nor meet the DSM 5-TR diagnostic criteria of PTSD or other psychiatric disorder(s), they can significantly impact the individual's ability to function throughout the lifespan.[9] The impact of trauma extends beyond the mental realm and frequently overlaps with elements of physical health and overall well-being.[10]

5.2   NEUROPLASTIC CHANGE DUE TO TRAUMA

Apart from the physical injury that may result from a kinetic physical injury, neuroplastic change centers on the chronic effects of the stress response within the brain and gut. In a non-stress environment, cortisol is released by the adrenal glands following the circadian rhythm in a steady, predictable manner.[11] The low-dose cortisol aids in recovery and daily repair within the cerebrum.[12] Cortisol is self-regulated via a negative feedback loop within the central nervous system, particularly the hypothalamic-pituitary-adrenal axis (HPA). Within the limbic system, the amygdala (AG), hippocampus (HC), and medial prefrontal cortex (PFC) constantly monitor the individual's environment. When a threat or a perceived threat is noticed, the limbic system activates the HPA axis, which regulates the production and secretion of cortisol. The higher than baseline levels of cortisol release epinephrine and norepinephrine, which further enhance the stress or autonomic response (also described as "fight or flight") and prevents the release of an inflammatory-immune response. Once the threat has passed, the HPA down-regulates the stress response, and the individual returns to his/her baseline.

In situations of significant trauma, complex trauma, and recurring triggering trauma, the HPA is unable to down-regulate, and the individual adopts a chronic trauma response. Instead of improving concentration and focus by increasing the release of dopamine from the nucleus accumbens (NA) to the PFC, chronic stress inhibits the release of dopamine.[13] This chronic release of epinephrine and norepinephrine within the PFC reduces cognitive abilities,[14] and may be linked with PFC atrophy in veteran populations with pervasive symptomatology.[15] Additionally, HC volume is inversely related to chronic cortisol exposure, which may explain further memory difficulties. Longitudinal studies within veteran populations showed a decline in facial recognition[16] and verbal decline.[15] Heightened cortisol also leads to heightened AG activations, which may explain some of the hyper-vigilant response.[11]

As mentioned, another aspect of cortisol impacts the inflammatory-immune response by the activation of inflammatory markers, particularly interferon gamma, interleukin 6, interleukin 1 beta, and tumor necrosis factor-alpha.[17] This activation process may affect epigenetic factors, correlate to higher than normal autoimmune disorders in individuals with chronic trauma, or relate to the development of gut dysbiosis.[18] Patients with chronic trauma and gut dysbiosis, whether due to inflammatory markers or higher levels of cortisol[19] that corresponded with high bacterial concentrations of Actinobacteria, Lentisphaerae, and Verrucomicrobia, also developed worsening trauma response symptomatology.[20] Another related factor of dysbiosis is the increased production of dopamine and norepinephrine and decreased the production of serotonin.[21]

5.3 TRAUMA-INFORMED CARE

Due to the pervasiveness of trauma exposure globally, its impact can be significant for communities as well as the individual.[9,22] As all health care providers will have direct contact with those who have experienced trauma, experts have urged the adoption of trauma-informed care[22] similar to the concept of universal precautions for bloodborne diseases. This approach recognizes that any individual seeking any type of treatment may be a survivor of trauma. Modern-day health care is perceived as a predominantly pragmatic and factual practice and focuses on "what is wrong with the individual." Whereas trauma-informed care encourages the provider to be patient, transparent, noncoercive, and corroborative and place greater emphasis on "what happened to the individual."[9] Although some have argued about the implementation of trauma-informed care and its practicality with every patient,[23] experts still advocate that all providers should avoid shaming tactics that belittle or devalue an individual's self-perception, social worth, identity, position or relationship within a social group.[9]

In addition to creating a more compassionate and empathetic atmosphere for the patient and decreasing the potential for retraumatization,[24] trauma-informed care leads to improved health outcomes[24] and significant economic benefits.[25] School-wide mental health interventions can be seen as trauma-informed care since they recognize the prevalence of traumatic experiences within the general population, particularly among adolescents and young adults, and thus condense the sample size to an academic setting. Studies done on the implementation of school-wide mental health interventions take into account all cost savings attributable to lower health care costs and increased productivity gains.[26] Additionally trauma-informed care has been shown to improve workplace satisfaction, organizational climate, and patient satisfaction and retention.[27]

5.4   IMPACT OF SHAME

Shame and guilt are emotions that frequently occur in trauma discourse and treatment.[9] While guilt represents a more objective evaluation of individuals' actions and behaviors (e.g., "I did a bad thing"), shame encompasses global assessments about the self (e.g., "I am a bad person"). Shame is often characterized as the "master or blanket emotion" or a negative self-conscious emotion because of its significance in personal relationships and within social situations.[9] Additionally, shame can often camouflage as various behaviors, so it is often difficult to determine the core issue.[28] Most traumatic experiences are mediated by shame, especially those with interpersonal components, which include inaccurate blame or responsibility, feeling unlovable, being broken, fear of judgment or overidentification with a label (e.g. survivor, victim, homeless, addict, etc.). As such, shame poses a significant barrier to patients in seeking treatment. Due to stigma and self-antagonization associated with shame, patients seeing healthcare providers for physiological issues may still avoid requesting mental health services as they fear potential judgment, labeling, or perceived rejection.[9] Dolezal and Gibson investigated the role of shame-sensitive practice towards trauma-informed care and noted that the trauma-informed approach inadequately addressed shame unless coupled with shame sensitivity.[9] Their analysis of shame sensitivity showed that understanding shame as a profound emotion associated with trauma may weaken its association with unhealthy lifestyle behaviors, such as a lack of social connectedness and defensive behaviors.[9] Therefore, they highlighted the importance of using a "shame lens" along with a "trauma lens" for providing ideal treatment that avoids retraumatization. The primary care clinic can guide a patient from the realm of physical problems into consideration for potential psychiatric evaluation by considering the impact of shame on the patient. Additionally, PCPs can link increased self-efficacy in self-care for health conditions to potential for change and improvement in mental health conditions and symptoms.

Addressing trauma through shame sensitivity is extremely important for regulating the "fight, flight, freeze, and fawn"[28] response. The fight response is when individuals face a threat aggressively; flight response is running away from danger; freeze response is being unable to move or act against a threat; and fawn response is immediately acting to please in order to avoid any conflict. There are two types of freeze response:[28] the orienting freeze that lasts only for a moment and the tonic immobility-emotional shutdown freeze when the individual cannot flee, and fighting is ineffective. When a provider notices his/her patient experiencing the freeze response, it is imperative that shame is reduced by highlighting how the mind, brain, and body protected rather than failed them at the time of the trauma.

5.5 THERAPEUTIC INTERVENTIONS

Treatment of complex trauma can be complex and challenging even for the most experienced clinician; yet all providers can assist in the process. As mentioned, a significant component of trauma-informed care is creating an environment of safety. Cognitive therapies (i.e., trauma-focused cognitive behavioral therapy, prolonged exposure, cognitive processing therapy, etc.), have been the mainstay of treatment for trauma-related symptoms;[29] however, many patients struggle to implement change due to the freeze/fawn nature of their symptoms. For many, motivational interviewing (MI) improves self-care in patients by helping them overcome ambivalence and enhance their readiness for change.[30] While most individuals are able to change, the challenge often rests on whether or not they are able to overcome obstacles that impede their ability to change.[31] During this process, MI respects patients' autonomy and allows them to make decisions according to their own maladaptive behaviors or cognitions.[32] A recent system review revealed that structure and respect for autonomous change were more effective in helping adolescents with trauma-achieved health behavior change compared to goal-setting behaviors.[32]By implementing a therapeutic approach that strives to improve self-efficacy, MI can be woven seamlessly into trauma-informed care. For example, patients may learn how to do breathing exercises or engage in yoga to help self-regulate and feel more comfortable in their own bodies, which will then allow them to experience other emotional discomfort as they engage in other life changes.[30] Tibbitts et al. analyzed the impact of trauma-informed yoga on emotional and physical well-being by establishing a trauma-informed yoga program where attendees completed optional questionnaires before and after class.[33] The results showed that attendees of multiple yoga classes reported noticing their feelings, making healthier choices to cope with their feelings, and being able to handle negative or stressful situations.[33] Therefore, Tibbitts et al. concluded that practicing trauma-informed yoga significantly improved physical and mental health, and this coping mechanism has substantial implications for treating trauma.

A large component of MI is helping the patient transition from sustain talk to change talk, reflecting their reasons, desire, and ability to change.[30] During the progression of MI treatment, healthcare providers echo this change talk back to patients to serve as a motivational tool that reflects the patient's own beliefs. This approach can have immense utility in a wide range of medical situations, including non-psychiatric ones. For example, Hettema, Steele, and Miller conducted a meta-analysis of the efficacy of MI in medical settings for smoking cessation. Results included the outperformance of MI on the treatment of tobacco dependence among nonpregnant patients and favorable short-term outcomes of MI with skills-based treatments for individuals with low tobacco dependence. Implementing MI in substance abuse treatment highlighted its efficacy for treating those with low motivation or low substance dependence. By considering the patient to be a crucial part of their own treatment and recovery, MI not only empowers self-care behavior, but creates the basis for a trusting, supportive relationship between client and provider.[30]

5.6 PREVENTION

Given the significant impact of trauma on mental and physical health,[1] factors which will be further explored in Chapter 27, efforts have been made to see if the severe symptoms may be ameliorated particularly with first responders, healthcare providers, and military personnel. These responders are particularly at risk given their exposure to the unpredictable traumatic events that may be a part of their employment[6] and developing sequelae following exposures.[6] Psychological Simple Triage and Rapid Treatment (PsySTART) is a self-triage tool designed to help identify risk factors in responders working within a disaster response. First responders participate in a pre-engagement assessment where they are guided into anticipating challenges within the future assignment (e.g., talking about the potential details, sights, and smells). Next, they plan how to respond to particularly self-identified challenging responses (e.g., the individual will step away to meditate for five minutes, or exercise in place, or stretch as a means of regulating their emotional response). Finally, responders are asked to monitor their daily exposure to 19 events. A sum of six or more exposures correlates with the potential development of future trauma-related symptoms. By making people more aware of their higher exposure rate, individuals have been effective in ameliorating and preventing the development of trauma-related symptoms.[34]

5.7 CONCLUSION

Trauma affects the emotional, physical, and social spheres of an individual. Individuals that experience variations of trauma adopt a chronic trauma response that may reduce cognitive ability and result in dysbiosis of gut microbiota. As these symptoms may be long-lasting and impact physiological functioning, understanding the optimal treatment for trauma is dire for engaging patients and reducing the risk of retraumatization. Trauma-informed care as a reinforcing and patient approach focuses on understanding what has happened to the individual rather than placing blame. By incorporating shame-sensitive and shame-informed practices to trauma-informed care, the clinician (including mental and behavioral health providers, specialists, and primary care clinicians) is better suited for addressing the needs of the individual without shame or emotional harm. Additional examples of trauma-informed treatments include Motivational Interviewing (MI), trauma-informed yoga, and mindfulness practices. Implementing these treatments may establish positive coping mechanisms and increased self-efficacy. Trauma coupled with shame is a complex mechanism with severe implications, so the need for implementing patient-centered treatments aimed at shame sensitivity and promoting self-efficacy is imminent.

REFERENCES

1. History of PTSD in Veterans: Civil War to DSM-5 | BrainLine. Published May 31, 2017. Accessed April 20, 2023. https://www.brainline.org/article/history-ptsd-veterans-civil-war-dsm-5

2. Shalev A, Liberzon I, Marmar C. Post-traumatic stress disorder. *The New England Journal of Medicine.* 2017;376(25):2459–2469. doi:10.1056/NEJMra1612499

3. Herman JL. Complex PTSD: A syndrome in survivors of prolonged and repeated trauma. *Journal of Traumatic Stress.* 1992;5:377–391. doi:10.1002/jts.2490050305

4. van Der Kolk B, Ford JD, Spinazzola J. Comorbidity of developmental trauma disorder (DTD) and post-traumatic stress disorder: Findings from the DTD field trial. *European Journal of Psychotraumatology.* 10(1):1562841. doi:10.1080/20008198.2018.1562841

5. Condon M, Bloomfield MAP, Nicholls H, Billings J. Expert international trauma clinicians' views on the definition, composition and delivery of reintegration interventions for complex PTSD. *European Journal of Psychotraumatology.* 2023;14(1):2165024. doi:10.1080/20008066.2023.2165024

6. Cloitre M, Hyland P, Bisson JI, et al. ICD-11 posttraumatic stress disorder and complex posttraumatic stress disorder in the United States: A population-based study. *Journal of Traumatic Stress.* 2019;32(6):833–842. doi:10.1002/jts.22454

7. Merlo G. *Principles of Medical Professionalism.* Oxford University Press; 2021.

8. Benjet C, Bromet E, Karam EG, et al. The epidemiology of traumatic event exposure worldwide: Results from the world mental health survey consortium. *Psychological Medicine.* 2016;46(2):327–343. doi:10.1017/S0033291715001981

9. Dolezal L, Gibson M. Beyond a trauma-informed approach and towards shame-sensitive practice. *Humanities and Social Sciences Communications.* 2022;9:214. doi:10.1057/s41599-022-01227-z

10. Oh DL, Jerman P, Silvério Marques S, et al. Systematic review of pediatric health outcomes associated with childhood adversity. *BMC Pediatrics.* 2018;18(1):83. doi:10.1186/s12887-018-1037-7

11. Dedovic K, Duchesne A, Andrews J, Engert V, Pruessner JC. The brain and The stress axis: The neural correlates of cortisol regulation in response to stress. *NeuroImage.* 2009;47(3):864–871. doi:10.1016/j.neuroimage.2009.05.074

12. Loonen AJM, Ivanova SA. Circuits regulating pleasure and happiness—Mechanisms of depression. *Frontiers in Human Neuroscience.* 2016;10:571. doi:10.3389/fnhum.2016.00571

13. Baik JH. Stress and the dopaminergic reward system. *Experimental & Molecular Medicine.* 2020;52(12):1879–1890. doi:10.1038/s12276-020-00532-4

14. Arnsten AFT. Stress weakens prefrontal networks: Molecular insults to higher cognition. *Nature Neuroscience.* 2015;18(10):1376–1385. doi:10.1038/nn.4087

15. Cardenas VA, Samuelson K, Lenoci M, et al. Changes in brain anatomy during the course of PTSD. *Psychiatry Research.* 2011;193(2):93–100. doi:10.1016/j.pscychresns.2011.01.013

16. Samuelson KW, Neylan TC, Lenoci M, et al. Longitudinal effects of PTSD on memory functioning. *Journal of the International Neuropsychological Society.* 2009;15(6):853–861. doi:10.1017/S1355617709990282

17. Passos IC, Vasconcelos-Moreno MP, Costa LG, et al. Inflammatory markers in post-traumatic stress disorder: A systematic review, meta-analysis, and meta-regression. *Lancet Psychiatry.* 2015;2(11):1002–1012. doi:10.1016/S2215-0366(15)00309-0

18. Bersani FS, Mellon SH, Lindqvist D, et al. Novel pharmacological targets for combat PTSD—Metabolism, inflammation, the gut microbiome, and mitochondrial dysfunction. *Military Medicine.* 2020;185(Suppl 1):311–318. doi:10.1093/milmed/usz260

19. Tetel MJ, de Vries GJ, Melcangi RC, Panzica G, O'Mahony SM. Steroids, stress and the gut microbiome-brain axis. *Journal of Neuroendocrinology.* 2018;30(2). doi:10.1111/jne.12548

20. Hemmings SMJ, Malan-Müller S, van den Heuvel LL, et al. The microbiome in post-traumatic stress disorder and trauma-exposed controls: An exploratory study. *Psychosomatic Medicine.* 2017;79:936–946. doi:10.1097/PSY.0000000000000512

21. Horn J, Mayer DE, Chen S, Mayer EA. Role of diet and its effects on the gut microbiome in the pathophysiology of mental disorders. *Translational Psychiatry.* 2022;12(1):164. doi:10.1038/s41398-022-01922-0

22. Magruder KM, McLaughlin KA, Elmore Borbon DL. Trauma is a public health issue. *The European Journal of Psychotraumatology.* 2017;8(1):1375338. doi:10.1080/20008198.2017.1375338

23. Donisch K, Bray C, Gewirtz A. Child welfare, juvenile justice, mental health, and education Providers' conceptualizations of trauma-informed practice. *Child Maltreat.* 2016;21(2):125–134. doi:10.1177/1077559516633304

24. Piotrowski CC. Chapter 15 - ACEs and trauma-informed care. In: Asmundson GJG, Afifi TO, eds. *Adverse Childhood Experiences.* Academic Press; 2020:307–328. doi:10.1016/B978-0-12-816065-7.00015-X

25. Dugan J, Booshehri LG, Phojanakong P, et al. Effects of a trauma-informed curriculum on depression, self-efficacy, economic security, and substance use among TANF participants: Evidence from the building health and wealth network phase II. *Social Science & Medicine.* 2020;258:113136. doi:10.1016/j.socscimed.2020.113136

26. Lee YY, Barendregt JJ, Stockings EA, et al. The population cost-effectiveness of delivering universal and indicated school-based interventions to prevent the onset of major depression among youth in Australia. *Epidemiology and Psychiatric Sciences.* 2017;26(5):545–564. doi:10.1017/S2045796016000469

27. Hales TW, Green SA, Bissonette S, et al. Trauma-informed care outcome study. *Research on Social Work Practice.* 2019;29(5):529–539. doi:10.1177/1049731518766618

28. Reddon AR, Ruberto T, Reader SM. Submission signals in animal groups. *Behaviour.* 2021;159(1):1–20. doi:10.1163/1568539X-bja10125

29. Roberts NP, Kitchiner NJ, Kenardy J, Bisson JI. Early psychological interventions to treat acute traumatic stress symptoms. *Cochrane Database of Systematic Reviews.* 2010;(3):CD007944. Published 2010 Mar 17. doi:10.1002/14651858.CD007944.pub2

30. Hettema J, Steele J, Miller WR. Motivational interviewing. *Annual Review of Clinical Psychology.* 2005;1:91–111. doi:10.1146/annurev.clinpsy.1.102803.143833

31. Porges SW. Polyvagal theory: A science of safety. *Frontiers in Integrative Neuroscience.* 2022;16:871227. doi:10.3389/fnint.2022.871227

32. Mutschler C, Naccarato E, Rouse J, Davey C, McShane K. Realist-informed review of motivational interviewing for adolescent health behaviors. *Systematic Reviews.* 2018;7(1):109. doi:10.1186/s13643-018-0767-9

33. Tibbitts DC, Aicher SA, Sugg J, et al. Program evaluation of trauma-informed yoga for vulnerable populations. *Evaluation and Program Planning.* 2021;88:101946. doi:10.1016/j.evalprogplan.2021.101946

34. Schreiber M, Cates DS, Formanski S, King M. Maximizing the resilience of healthcare workers in multi-hazard events: Lessons from the 2014-2015 Ebola response in Africa. *Military Medicine.* 2019;184(Suppl 1):114–120. doi:10.1093/milmed/usy400

6 Emotion Regulation Approaches

Pauline N. Goodson*, BA, Eva E. Dicker*, MA,
and Bryan T. Denny, PhD

KEY POINTS

- Emotion regulation is a key deficit in many forms of psychopathology.
- Emotion regulation is a key ingredient in many psychotherapies.
- Using a personalized medicine approach to target training in specific emotion regulation strategies holds promise in developing effective novel, scalable, and accessible emotion regulation interventions.

6.1 INTRODUCTION

Emotion regulation is the ability to modulate the experience and expression of an emotional response, and it is essential to daily life and well-being.[1,2] Research has elucidated important ties between emotion regulation and emotional, mental, and physical health,[3-5] where adaptive emotion regulation practices predict greater life satisfaction,[6] less negative affect,[7,8] and greater physical well-being.[7,9] Further, several psychopathologies can be characterized by emotion dysregulation, particularly concerning how individuals interpret a situation or stimulus. This cognitive interpretation or evaluation process of events and stimuli in one's environment reflects appraisal, which is a crucial component of theoretical frameworks for emotion.[1,10,11] For example, borderline personality disorder (BPD) is a mental illness characterized by instability in managing emotions; signs and symptoms of the disorder include, but are not limited to, mood swings, uncertainty in self-image, extreme perspectives (e.g., things are either all good or all bad), and unstable relationships with others.[12-15] Mood and anxiety disorders, such as major depressive disorder, have also been characterized by emotion dysregulation.[16-18] Across many psychopathologies, many efficacious treatments, including cognitive behavioral therapies, leverage cognitive change via change in appraisal as a key training target.[19]

This chapter aims to elucidate ways in which emotion regulation, particularly from the perspective of appraisal theory, is central to diagnostic and treatment frameworks for psychopathology and serves as an experimentally-tractable, transdiagnostic set of processes through which the mechanisms underlying psychopathology may be further examined. To do so, we will first define core constructs, including emotion and

---

* Denotes equal authorship.

DOI: 10.1201/b22810-7

emotion regulation, from the perspective of appraisal theory.[1,10,11] Appraisal theory posits that emotions are elicited by our evaluations (i.e., appraisals) of the situations we encounter.[11] We will then discuss how emotion dysregulation is central in many forms of psychopathology. Finally, we'll discuss how emotion regulation plays an important role in many current psychotherapies and the utility of emotion regulation interventions in transdiagnostic approaches toward improved mental and physical health.

6.2 DEFINING CORE CONSTRUCTS

For this chapter, emotions and emotion regulation are subcategories of the superordinate category *affect*, which involves valenced states, emotion behaviors, moods, dispositional states, and valenced traits.[1] In essence, affect is an umbrella term that encompasses feelings and emotions. Constructs such as emotion and mood are distinct subcategories of affect, where emotions (e.g., anger) are transient, acute, and specific to a stimulus. Moods, by contrast, are differentiated by typically longer duration and difficulty in attribution to specific eliciting stimuli.[1]

Emotions may be modified by altering one or more emotion-generative processes. A useful theoretical framework for understanding emotion regulation is James Gross's process model of emotion regulation, which posits there are different points in the emotion generative process at which emotion regulation can occur.[1,2] This iterative process begins at the point of the emotion-eliciting stimulus (either internal or external to the observer), followed by selective attention to aspects of that stimulus, which is then crucially followed by an appraisal valuation of the meaning of that stimulus to oneself, which leads to a multifaceted emotional response encompassing behavioral, experiential, and physiological response tendencies. These emotional responses may then influence subsequent situations and emotion-eliciting stimuli, and the appraisal valuations derived from them, in an iterative cascade.[1,2] Each process along this model provides opportunities to regulate emotion (i.e., via selecting or modifying the situation itself, changing the focus of one's attention within a situation, engaging cognitive change about the meaning of that situation, or modulating one's emotion response). Emotion regulation can be brought to bear in the service of either downregulating or upregulating either negative or positive emotion, according to one's emotion goals.[1,20]

A large volume of emotion regulation research has examined cognitive change and response modulation strategies in particular. Specifically, cognitive reappraisal is a cognitive change emotion regulation strategy that involves changing how one thinks about an emotional stimulus or how we interpret its meaning. When downregulating negative emotion (e.g., feeling sadness at a child moving away to college), reappraisal can be operationalized to, for example, involve reframing a situation so that one imagines that the outcome will be good or not as bad as it first seemed (i.e., reinterpret the situation, for example by appreciating how much happiness adulthood and independence may bring the child). Alternatively, one could reappraise a negative situation by engaging in psychological distancing, whereby one appraises the situation as an objective, impartial observer (e.g., by understanding that these feelings are natural in this situation).[21,22]

Expressive suppression, on the other hand, is a response modulation strategy that occurs after the emotion has already been generated and involves attempts to modulate the outward expression of that emotion,[23] such as fighting to hold back tears in response to one's child leaving for college, as in the above example. Generally, research has yielded evidence of the adaptiveness of using cognitive reappraisal compared to expressive suppression; cognitive reappraisal has been associated with more positive mental and physical health outcomes.[3,23] For example, cognitive reappraisal may act as a buffer between high stress experiences and symptoms of depression.[24] Further, as suggested earlier, our appraisal of a stimulus or situation can significantly impact whether we perceive and react to that stimulus in healthy or maladaptive ways. Emotion dysregulation has been shown to be a critical component in multiple psychopathologies, particularly in the interpretation of a stimulus.[15-18,25] Thus, emotion regulation shows promise as a transdiagnostic framework through which to consider interventions to improve mental and physical health.

6.3 ROLE OF EMOTION REGULATION IN HEALTH AND HEALTH BEHAVIORS

Emotion regulation has ties to health and health behaviors, and emotion dysregulation has been connected to poor health behaviors. Adaptive emotion regulation strategy choice may be a key component to healthy behavior management. For example, emotion dysregulation plays an important role in eating disorders and in smoking habits.[26-28] In an ecological momentary assessment study in adult women, negative affect was strongly predictive of unhealthy eating episodes.[44] However, in another study, young adult smokers instructed to engage in cognitive reappraisal reported higher distress tolerance, reduced cravings, and reduced attentional bias towards smoking than those told to suppress or accept thoughts about smoking.[28]

Emotion regulation is also linked to perceived stress, where adaptive emotion regulation can buffer against negative psychological effects of stress[29] and physiological stress indicators, such as the hypothalamic-pituitary-adrenal (HPA) axis functioning in stressful situations.[30] Specifically, engaging in cognitive reappraisal has been shown to have longitudinal benefits for perceived stress, whereas engaging in expressive suppression has been shown as a longitudinal risk factor for the negative impacts of stress, such as internalizing symptoms.[29] Emotion regulation may impact physiological mechanisms of stress and health, such as diurnal cortisol levels (i.e., cortisol awakening response and cortisol slopes).[30] These factors are non-exhaustive points of interest which may be buffered against or bolstered through emotion regulation interventions, thus contributing to improved mental health and health behaviors.

6.4 EMOTION REGULATION AS A KEY DEFICIT IN MANY FORMS OF PSYCHOPATHOLOGY

Emotion regulation has been implicated as a shared underlying psychological mechanism across a variety of different psychopathologies.[19,31] Maladaptive emotion regulation is present in, but not limited to (i) mood and anxiety disorders such as depression, general anxiety disorder (GAD), and post-traumatic stress disorder (PTSD), as well as (ii) personality disorders such as borderline personality disorder (BPD) and bipolar disorder (BD).[31] Effects of maladaptive appraisals in these disorders have been observed within and across diagnostic category boundaries. Evidence has shown that in mood and anxiety disorders, individuals appraise stimuli as more negative than controls.[18] In the specific case of PTSD, these extreme appraisals can result from specific memories, thus explaining individual differences observed in individuals diagnosed with PTSD. Trauma experiences create salient autobiographical memories, which can be highly disruptive to future threat appraisals and coping strategies.[32] In all three disorders, however, the common thread is the highly negative appraisal given to a situation or stimulus that may drive or underlie the disordered thinking and behaviors associated with each disorder, such as over-interpreting threat or consequence of a particular situation and reacting following that interpretation.

Similarly, maladaptive appraisals provide a shared mechanism of understanding for BPD and BD. BPD is characterized by emotional instability, where individuals show increases in emotional reactivity to their appraisals of a situation (i.e., experience more intense emotional states due to their interpretation of what's occurring in a given situation). BD is different from BPD in that its characterization lies in the extreme shifts in mood, energy, and activity, categorized by variations of depressive and manic states.[33] Elevated emotional reactivity associated with extreme negative and positive appraisals tends to occur in individuals with BD.[34] Hence, intervening to modulate appraisal processes represents a key target of many current psychotherapies.[19]

6.5 EMOTION REGULATION AS A KEY INGREDIENT IN MANY PSYCHOTHERAPIES

Since emotion regulation can be conceptualized as a set of skills targeting different emotion processes that can be learned, psychotherapeutic treatment often includes teaching emotion regulation skills in either therapeutic or psychoeducational settings.[35] Cognitive behavioral therapy (CBT), for example, is based on the premise that maladaptive thoughts contribute emotional distress and behavioral difficulties, and altering these thoughts may in turn ameliorate the emotional and behavioral problems.[36] In this way, in part, CBT involves training individuals in cognitive reappraisal tactics. Additionally, individuals work collaboratively with a therapist to better understand maladaptive behavior patterns and learn new behaviors that will be most helpful to them in developing the ability to regulate their emotions. This aspect of CBT most closely resembles emotion regulation strategies such as situation selection and situation modification in the process model of emotion regulation.[1,2,35]

6.5.1. ACCEPTANCE AND COMMITMENT THERAPY

Acceptance and commitment therapy (ACT) is an action-oriented approach to psychotherapy that stems from CBT.[37] In contrast to traditional cognitive behavioral therapeutic approaches, ACT does not emphasize challenging and changing unhelpful thoughts but rather accepting and adapting to the reality of the current cognitive and affective experience of the patient.[37] ACT incorporates many aspects of psychological distancing by encouraging patients to view a negative stimulus or situation with an impartial, objective mindset that engages with the negative content as opposed to avoiding it.[1,2,38]

6.5.2 MINDFULNESS-BASED THERAPIES

Mindfulness-based cognitive therapy (MBCT) is a modified form of cognitive therapy that incorporates mindfulness practices such as meditation and breathing exercises.[39] MBCT differs from CBT as it does not emphasize changing belief in the content of thought. The focus in MBCT is on a systematic training to be more aware, moment by moment, of physical sensations and of thoughts and feelings as mental events.[40] This therapeutic approach is similar, yet distinct from, Mindfulness-based stress reduction (MBSR). MBCT focuses on specific vulnerabilities or conditions under a cognitive framework, while MBSR is a more generalized training in skills necessary to respond to a variety of stress and does not emphasize psychological or cognitive aspects of experience.[41] "Decentering," a central process to MBCT and MBSR involving objective and impartial appraisal of thoughts, feelings, and physical sensations, is also importantly akin to psychological distancing. This suggests that emotion regulation strategies and tactics, like psychological distancing, are key processes to further examine in the context of MBCT and MBSR and other psychotherapies to determine the extent to which they may influence or drive psychotherapeutic benefits.[35,39,42–44]

6.6 EMOTION REGULATION INTERVENTIONS USING A PERSONALIZED MEDICINE APPROACH

Importantly, current evidence-based, validated psychotherapies such as those above typically incorporate heterogeneous approaches that leverage training in multiple emotion regulation strategies and education, acceptance, and adaptive behavior change to address a multitude of clinical symptoms. We argue that focusing on training in particular emotion regulation strategies holds promise for developing novel, accessible, and scalable interventions to improve mental and physical health within a personalized medicine framework.[35,45,46] Successful emotion regulation from a personalized medicine approach relies on adaptive interactions of person, situation, and strategy factors.[45] Existing evidence supports the promise of targeted emotion regulation interventions in adaptively changing emotional responses with both short and long-term durability.[22, 35, 46–48] Hypothesis-driven, empirically-validated emotion regulation interventions that take this personalized medicine approach can provide scalable, relatively low cost/burden intervention options that may increase access to adaptive emotion regulation skills training across clinical and non-clinical populations.

6.7 FUTURE DIRECTIONS

As described above, emotion regulation is a promising target for developing novel, scalable interventions to improve mental and physical health. Longitudinal, experimental research is needed to help determine causality of training in particular emotion regulation strategies/tactics, or potentially adaptive combinations of strategies, in bringing about adaptive changes in mental or physical health.[21,35,45,49] Additionally, it will be essential to understand if these particular strategies or combination of strategies are differentially adaptive within or across different categories of disorders (e.g., internalizing versus externalizing disorders), and more broadly, according to transdiagnostic individual differences and other person factors (e.g., age, gender, race, ethnicity, personality, culture, etc.). In addition, it will be crucial to continue to explore these relationships between emotion regulation and mental and physical health from a translational social cognitive neuroscience and psychoneuroimmunology perspective to elucidate the underlying neural and other biobehavioral mechanisms of change.

6.8 CONCLUSION

Managing one's emotions adaptively is an essential skill in maintaining psychological and physical health. Emotion dysregulation is a transdiagnostic factor underlying various psychopathologies. Current validated, evidence-based psychotherapies primarily take a multi-componential approach; cognitive behavioral-based therapies, mindfulness-based therapies, and emotion regulation skill-building interventions promote adaptive strategy choice and success and reduce maladaptive strategy choice. However, interventions that target specific emotion regulation strategies and tactics have also shown positive short- and long-term promise. Investigating hypothesis-driven, targeted, shorter-duration interventions focused on training in particular emotion regulation strategies may yield adaptive outcomes that are more scalable and accessible within and across ranges of individuals, in keeping with a personalized medicine approach.

REFERENCES

1. Gross JJ. The emerging field of emotion regulation: An integrative review. *Review of General Psychology*. 1998;2(3):271–299. doi:10.1037/1089-2680.2.3.271
2. Gross JJ. The extended process model of emotion regulation: Elaborations, applications, and future directions. *Psychological Inquiry*. 2015;26(1):130–137. doi:10.1080/1047840X.2015.989751
3. Hu T, Zhang D, Wang J, Mistry R, Ran G, Wang X. Relation between emotion regulation and mental health: A meta-analysis review. *Psychological Reports*. 2014;114(2):341–362. doi:10.2466/03.20.PR0.114k22w4
4. Nelis SM, Clare L, Whitaker CJ. Attachment in people with dementia and their caregivers: A systematic review. *Dementia*. 2014;13(6):747–767. doi:10.1177/1471301213485232
5. Ostir GV, Markides KS, Black SA, Goodwin JS. Emotional well-being predicts subsequent functional independence and survival. *Journal of the American Geriatrics Society*. 2000;48(5):473–478. doi:10.1111/j.1532-5415.2000.tb04991.x

6. Quoidbach J, Berry EV, Hansenne M, Mikolajczak M. Positive emotion regulation and well-being: Comparing the impact of eight savoring and dampening strategies. *Personality and Individual Differences.* 2010;49(5):368–373. doi:10.1016/j.paid.2010.03.048

7. Lopez RB, Denny BT. Negative affect mediates the relationship between use of emotion regulation strategies and general health in college-aged students. *Personality and Individual Differences.* 2019;151:109529. doi:10.1016/j.paid.2019.109529

8. Egloff B, Schmukle SC, Burns LR, Schwerdtfeger A. Spontaneous emotion regulation during evaluated speaking tasks: Associations with negative affect, anxiety expression, memory, and physiological responding. *Emotion.* 2006;6(3):356–366. doi:10.1037/1528-3542.6.3.356

9. DeSteno D, Gross JJ, Kubzansky L. Affective science and health: The importance of emotion and emotion regulation. *Health Psychology.* 2013;32(5):474–486. doi:10.1037/a0030259

10. Roseman IJ, Smith CA. Appraisal theory: Overview, assumptions, variety, controversies. In: Scherer K, Schorr A, Johnstone T, eds. *Appraisal Processes in Emotion: Theory, Methods, Research.* OUP USA; 2001:3–19.

11. Lazarus RS. Cognition and emotion. In: Lazarus RS, ed. *Emotion and Adaptation.* Oxford University Press; 1991:127–170.

12. Skodol AE, Gunderson JG, Pfohl B, Widiger TA, Livesley WJ, Siever LJ. The borderline diagnosis I: Psychopathology, comorbidity, and personality structure. *Biological Psychiatry.* 2002;51(12):936–950. doi:10.1016/s0006-3223(02)01324-0

13. Tomko RL, Trull TJ, Wood PK, Sher KJ. Characteristics of borderline personality disorder in a community sample: Comorbidity, treatment utilization, and general functioning. *Journal of Personality Disorders.* 2014;28(5):734–750. doi:10.1521/pedi_2012_26_093

14. Carpenter RW, Trull TJ. Components of emotion dysregulation in borderline personality disorder: A review. *Current Psychiatry Reports.* 2013;15(1):335. doi:10.1007/s11920-012-0335-2

15. Houben M, Claes L, Sleuwaegen E, Berens A, Vansteelandt K. Emotional reactivity to appraisals in patients with A borderline personality disorder: A daily life study. *Borderline Personality Disorder and Emotion Dysregulation.* 2018;5(1):18. doi:10.1186/s40479-018-0095-7

16. Bradley B, DeFife JA, Guarnaccia C, et al. Emotion dysregulation and negative affect: Association with psychiatric symptoms. *The Journal of Clinical Psychiatry.* 2011;72(5):685–691. doi:10.4088/JCP.10m06409blu

17. Hofmann SG, Sawyer AT, Fang A, Asnaani A. Emotion dysregulation model of mood and anxiety disorders. *Depress Anxiety.* 2012;29(5):409–416. doi:10.1002/da.21888

18. Espejo EP, Hammen C, Brennan PA. Elevated appraisals of the negative impact of naturally occurring life events: A risk factor for depressive and anxiety disorders. *Journal of Abnormal Child Psychology.* 2012;40(2):303–315. doi:10.1007/s10802-011-9552-0

19. Berking M, Wupperman P, Reichardt A, Pejic T, Dippel A, Znoj H. Emotion-regulation skills as a treatment target in psychotherapy. *Behaviour Research and Therapy.* 2008;46(11):1230–1237. doi:10.1016/j.brat.2008.08.005

20. Tamir M, Vishkin A, Gutentag T. Emotion regulation is motivated. *Emotion.* 2020;20(1):115–119. doi:10.1037/emo0000635

21. McRae K, Ciesielski B, Gross JJ. Unpacking cognitive reappraisal: Goals, tactics, and outcomes. *Emotion.* 2012;12(2):250–255. doi:10.1037/a0026351

22. Denny BT, Ochsner KN. Behavioral effects of longitudinal training in cognitive reappraisal. *Emotion.* 2014;14(2):425–433. doi:10.1037/a0035276

23. Gross JJ, John OP. Individual differences in two emotion regulation processes: Implications for affect, relationships, and well-being. *Journal of Personality and Social Psychology.* 2003;85(2):348–362. doi:10.1037/0022-3514.85.2.348

24. Troy AS, Wilhelm FH, Shallcross AJ, Mauss IB. Seeing the silver lining: Cognitive reappraisal ability moderates the relationship between stress and depressive symptoms. *Emotion.* 2010;10(6):783–795. doi:10.1037/a0020262

25. Borderline Personality Disorder. National Institute of Mental Health (NIMH). Accessed April 22, 2022. https://www.nimh.nih.gov/health/topics/borderline-personality-disorder

26. Munsch S, Meyer AH, Quartier V, Wilhelm FH. Binge eating in binge eating disorder: A breakdown of emotion regulatory process? *Psychiatry Research.* 2012;195(3): 118–124. doi:10.1016/j.psychres.2011.07.016

27. Harrison A, Genders R, Davies H, Treasure J, Tchanturia K. Experimental measurement of the regulation of anger and aggression in women with anorexia nervosa. *Clinical Psychology & Psychotherapy.* 2011;18(6):445–452. doi:10.1002/cpp.726

28. Szasz PL, Szentagotai A, Hofmann SG. Effects of emotion regulation strategies on smoking craving, attentional bias, and task persistence. *Behaviour Research and Therapy.* 2012;50(5):333–340. doi:10.1016/j.brat.2012.02.010

29. Zahniser E, Conley CS. Interactions of emotion regulation and perceived stress in predicting emerging adults' subsequent internalizing symptoms. *Motivation and Emotion.* 2018;42(5):763–773. doi:10.1007/s11031-018-9696-0

30. Gilbert K, Mineka S, Zinbarg RE, Craske MG, Adam EK. Emotion regulation regulates more than emotion: Associations of momentary emotion regulation with diurnal cortisol in current and past depression and anxiety. *Clinical Psychological Science.* 2017;5(1):37–51. doi:10.1177%2F2167702616654437

31. Sloan E, Hall K, Moulding R, Bryce S, Mildred H, Staiger PK. Emotion regulation as a transdiagnostic treatment construct across anxiety, depression, substance, eating and borderline personality disorders: A systematic review. *Clinical Psychology Review.* 2017;57:141–163. doi:10.1016/j.cpr.2017.09.002

32. Gómez de La Cuesta G, Schweizer S, Diehle J, Young J, Meiser-Stedman R. The relationship between maladaptive appraisals and posttraumatic stress disorder: A meta-analysis. *European Journal of Psychotraumatology.* 10(1):1620084. doi:10.1080/20008198. 2019.1620084

33. Grande I, Berk M, Birmaher B, Vieta E. Bipolar disorder. *Lancet.* 2016;387(10027): 1561–1572. doi:10.1016/S0140-6736(15)00241-X

34. Kelly RE, Dodd AL, Mansell W. When my moods drive upward there is nothing I can do about it": A review of extreme appraisals of internal States and the bipolar spectrum. *Frontiers in Psychology.* 2017;8:1235. doi:10.3389/fpsyg.2017.01235

35. Denny BT. Getting better over time: A framework for examining the impact of emotion regulation training. *Emotion.* Published online 2020. doi:psycnet.apa.org/record/2020-03346-019

36. Hofmann SG, Asnaani A, Vonk IJJ, Sawyer AT, Fang A. Efficacy of cognitive behavioral therapy: A review of meta-analyses. *Cognitive Therapy and Research.* 2012;36(5):427–440. doi:10.1007/s10608-012-9476-1

37. Hayes SC. Acceptance and commitment therapy, relational frame theory, and the third wave of behavioral and cognitive therapies. *Behavior Therapy.* Published online 2004. doi:www.sciencedirect.com/science/article/pii/S0005789404800133

38. Kross E, Ayduk O. Self-distancing: Theory, research, and current directions. *Advances in Experimental Social Psychology.* Published online 2017. doi:www.sciencedirect.com/science/article/pii/S0065260116300338

39. Farb N, Anderson A, Irving J, Segal ZV. Mindfulness interventions and emotion regulation. *Handbook of Emotion Regulation.* Published online January 1, 2014: 548–567.

40. Segal ZV, Williams JMG, Teasdale JD. *Mindfulness-Based Cognitive Therapy for Depression: A New Approach to Preventing Relapse.* Guilford Press; 2002:xiv, 351.

41. Garland E, Gaylord S, Fredrickson B. Positive reappraisal mediates the stress-reduc-
    tive effects of mindfulness: An upward spiral process. *Mindfulness.* 2011;2:59–67.
    doi:10.1007/s12671-011-0043-8
42. Garand L, Rinaldo DE, Alberth MM, et al. Effects of problem solving therapy on
    mental health outcomes in family caregivers of persons with A new diagnosis of mild
    cognitive impairment or early dementia: A randomized controlled trial. *The American
    Journal of Geriatric Psychiatry.* 2014;22(8):771–781.
43. Teper R, Segal ZV, Inzlicht M. Inside the mindful mind: How mindfulness enhances
    emotion regulation through improvements in executive control. *Current Directions in
    Psychological Science.* 2013;22(6):449–454. doi:10.1177/0963721413495869
44. Hanley AW, de Vibe M, Solhaug I, et al. Modeling the mindfulness-to-meaning theo-
    ry's mindful reappraisal hypothesis: Replication with longitudinal data from a random-
    ized controlled study. *Stress Health.* 2021;37(4):778–789. doi:10.1002/smi.3035
45. Doré BP, Silvers JA, Ochsner KN. Toward a personalized science of emotion regu-
    lation. *Social and Personality Psychology Compass.* 2016;10(4):171–187. doi:10.1111/
    spc3.12240
46. Cohen N, Ochsner KN. From surviving to thriving in the face of threats: The emerg-
    ing science of emotion regulation training. *Current Opinion in Behavioral Sciences.*
    2018;24:143–155. doi:10.1016/j.cobeha.2018.08.007
47. Denny BT, Inhoff MC, Zerubavel N, Davachi L, Ochsner KN. Getting over it: Long-
    lasting effects of emotion regulation on amygdala response. *Psychological Science.*
    2015;26(9):1377–1388. doi:10.1177/0956797615578863
48. Gross JJ, Halperin E, Porat R. Emotion regulation in intractable conflicts. *Current
    Directions in Psychological Science.* 2013;22(6):423–429. doi:10.1177/0963721413495871
49. Ford BQ, Gross JJ, Gruber J. Broadening our field of view: The role of emotion poly-
    regulation. *Emotion Review.* 2019;11(3):197–208. doi:10.1177/1754073919850314

7 Cognitive and Behavioral Approaches

Alyssa M. Vela, PhD and Allison J. Carroll, PhD

KEY POINTS

- Cognitive behavioral therapy is one of the most well-studied and empirically validated psychotherapeutic approaches for a wide range of populations and conditions.
- Specific cognitive and behavioral strategies can be utilized to support mental health and promote health behavior change.
- Cognitive behavioral therapy is an evidence-based treatment for common conditions, such as depression, anxiety, insomnia, and chronic pain.

7.1 INTRODUCTION

While there are many theories applied to the conceptualization of mental health and the prevention and treatment of mental disorders, cognitive behavioral approaches are among the most common and well-studied. Mental disorders, clinical conditions characterized by emotional, cognitive, or behavioral disturbances that result in impairments in daily functioning, are influenced by a variety of intersectional factors, including genetics, chemical and structural changes in the brain, psychological characteristics, and social functioning.[1] Moreover, lifestyle factors ranging from substance use to eating behaviors to sleep habits can have an immense impact on mental health and quality of life. These multifactorial influences on health and well-being also allow for multiple approaches to prevention and treatment. Cognitive behavioral approaches leverage these pathways to effectively change the thoughts and behaviors that interfere with lifestyle goals or exacerbate mental health symptoms. The current chapter will provide an overview of cognitive behavioral theory and cognitive behavioral therapy (CBT), select cognitive and behavioral strategies to address mental health, and specific applications of CBT, such as for insomnia.

7.2 THEORETICAL UNDERPINNINGS

Cognitive behavioral theory, which first emerged in the 1960s, draws on both cognitive and behavioral theories in an effort to more fully explain and address emotional and behavioral concerns. Although behavioral and cognitive theories both seek to explain human learning processes, behavioral theory focuses on external, observable actions while cognitive theory focuses on internal mental processes. Behavioral theory, also known as behaviorism, emerged in the late 19th and early 20th centuries

DOI: 10.1201/b22810-8

in response to early introspective methods of understanding behavior. Cognitive theory boomed in the 1970s and early 1980s in response to some of the limitations of behavioral theory.[2] Both serve as important underpinnings to cognitive behavioral theory, which combines elements of each to further understanding the human experience. The equal emphasis of behavioral and cognitive contributions to emotional disturbance (i.e., mental health conditions), is the foundation of cognitive behavioral theory, and highlights how thoughts, emotions, and behaviors are all connected.

7.2.1 BEHAVIORAL THEORY

Behavioral theory explains human behavior by attending to the antecedents and consequences of one's environment, as well as the learned associations developed through historical experiences. Psychologist John B. Watson contributed to this work by critiquing the subjective nature of psychodynamic theory and arguing for a focus on objective actions (i.e., what humans and animals *do*), rather than internal states.[3] This perspective led to applied behavioral theory and the development of foundational behavioral models, including classical and operant conditioning. Importantly, behavioral theory does not dismiss the importance of thoughts and feelings, but sees them as a byproduct of behavior—some behaviorists have gone so far as to conceptualize thoughts and feelings as mental or internal behaviors.[3]

Much of the initial work to apply behavioral theory focused on depression.[3] Early behavioral models of depression were developed by Lewisohn and colleagues in the 1970s and were based on assumptions that response-contingent positive reinforcement is environmentally influenced, can elicit depressive behavior, and can be a sufficient explanation for depression.[2,4] This behavioral model led to the development of clinical approaches such as behavioral activation, which was designed to increase engagement in pleasurable activities to reduce depressive symptoms.[2]

7.2.2 COGNITIVE THEORY

Cognitive theory developed as a response to behaviorism and the belief that behavior alone was insufficient to understand internal psychological processes, highlighting the importance of one's interpretation of events or stimuli and how they influence emotional functioning. Cognitive theory views people as more than blank slates, emphasizing that one's unique lived experiences, knowledge, and viewpoint influence their thoughts and feelings. Thus, cognitive theory posits that thinking, attitude, logic, and reasoning all influence behavior. Foundational to cognitive theory is the concept of schemas (i.e., persistent semantic representation of ideas or constructs) that guide cognitive processes related to information gathering, storage, and retrieval. Schemas influence one's beliefs and attitudes, which results in the development of core beliefs—those rigid and overgeneralized beliefs that develop early in life and persist in influencing one's perception of him- or herself and the world.[5-7]

Similar to behaviorism, much of the foundational research on cognitive theory focused on understanding and addressing depression.[5,6] Aaron T. Beck, one of the most influential cognitive scientists, theorized that psychological disturbance results from the long-standing mental representations of oneself and the world that manifest in maladaptive behaviors, thoughts, physiological responses, and affect, and ulti-mately into symptoms of mental disorders. The theory then outlines that remediation of this biased processing of information is essential to addressing and treating men-tal disorders.[5,7] Thus, the clinical application of cognitive theory involves identifying and then changing one's thoughts, core beliefs, and schemas to a more positive and accurate perspective of oneself and the world.

7.2.3 COGNITIVE BEHAVIORAL THEORY

Eventually, clinicians and scholars sought to integrate behavior modification and cognitive processing approaches to support therapeutic change, leading to the devel-opment of cognitive behavioral theory.[8] Cognitive behavioral theory emphasizes the interconnected nature of behaviors, thoughts, and emotions. From behavioral theory, it utilizes activity pacing, pleasure-seeking, and reinforcement.[9] From cog-nitive theory, it draws on the concepts of automatic thoughts, cognitive distortions, and schemas. Distinct from both, cognitive behavioral theory prioritizes the role and influence of cognitions, particularly patterns of thinking, in the maintenance of behavioral and emotional reactions. Cognitive behavioral theory posits that how we react to stimuli is related to how we think about and make sense of our reality.[9] Central tenants of cognitive behavioral theory include that our thoughts mediate our response to external stimuli, and that it is possible to access and understand our cognitive processes, as well as to then target and change such thoughts (or patterns of thinking). As researchers found that behavioral theory alone could not account for behavior change, cognitive behavioral theory includes key aspects of behavior-ism with cognitive approaches by emphasizing positive reinforcement for behavior modification and self-efficacy, one's sense of his or her own ability to manage a problem or situation, as foundational for change.[8] Overall, the theory emphasizes environmental influences on thoughts and feelings and their relation to behaviors.

The cognitive behavioral triangle represents the theoretical connections between behaviors, thoughts, and emotions.[7] As depicted in Figure 7.1, feelings are the changes

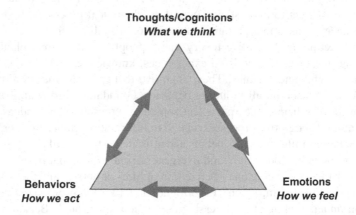

FIGURE 7.1 Theoretical underpinnings of cognitive behavioral theory and cognitive behavioral therapy.

one experiences in response to an emotion, often the physical manifestations of emotions. The behavior corner of the triangle represents both actions and inactions, in both internal and external states. The cognitive corner of the triangle indicates the in-the-moment thoughts as well as deep-seated beliefs about oneself and the world. All relationships between behaviors, thoughts, and emotions are bidirectional—in one direction, thoughts trigger feelings, feelings result in behaviors, and behaviors (action, or inaction) reinforce our thoughts and patterns of thinking.[7]

7.3 COGNITIVE BEHAVIORAL THERAPY (CBT)

The therapeutic application of cognitive behavioral theory is structured, time-limited, educational, and goal-oriented, with some customization to the individual needs of the patient.[10] CBT typically involves regularly scheduled 30 to 60 minute sessions with a licensed and trained professional, with better outcomes associated with 16 to 20 sessions.[11,12] CBT attends to unhelpful patterns of cognitions and behaviors that trigger distress. Specifically, CBT focuses on changing patterns of thinking, such as re-evaluating and restructuring cognitive distortions, improving coping skills, and reducing behavioral avoidance.[13] CBT guides patients to identify the connections between their thoughts, behaviors, and given situations or environments, and how those connections ultimately influence emotions. Key therapeutic change occurs in recognizing patterns of thinking and behaviors that reinforce negative or problematic emotional states, and addressing such patterns to minimize negative emotions and improve overall well-being.[9,13] Unlike other treatment modalities, CBT tends to focus on current issues and factors that contribute to thoughts and behaviors, rather than prioritizing past or early-life experiences. Additionally, patients or clients are typically given "homework" or exercises to practice outside of treatment to encourage utilization of skills and strategies in day-to-day activities and contexts, which increases the likelihood that patients maintain the gains made in treatment.[14] Given the breadth of research on CBT, the modality has emerged as the gold-standard psychological treatment for myriad medical and mental health conditions across the lifespan, including and extending far beyond depression.[13,15,16]

7.3.1 COGNITIVE AND BEHAVIORAL STRATEGIES FOR MENTAL HEALTH

Foundational cognitive and behavioral strategies that are widely employed within CBT and may also be used as brief interventions in other clinical contexts (see Table 7.1). Strategies to address coping skills, problem-solving, and cognitive restructuring, are frequently paired with broader approaches, such as psychoeducation (i.e., providing knowledge to the patient about their condition and treatment, often using the CBT triangle [Figure 7.1] as a guide), Socratic questioning (i.e., probing the patient in a manner that gently challenges beliefs, assumptions, and behaviors), and guided discovery (i.e., engaging the patient in treatment by encouraging them to develop their own conclusions).[17,18] The specific strategies to be used may

TABLE 7.1

Key Cognitive and Behavioral Strategies for Mental and Behavioral Health

Strategy	Description
Coping Skills Training	Development of specific behavioral and cognitive techniques to self-soothe, reduce stress, and shift thinking.
Problem-Solving	A systematic approach to slow down and address problems. Steps include: identifying the problem, generating solutions and their strengths and weaknesses, choosing a solution, and implementing the solution.
Cognitive Restructuring	Positively changing one's mindset by identifying cognitive distortions, or faulty patterns in thinking (e.g., all-or-nothing thinking), monitoring when they occur, and proposing alternative (positive) thoughts based on contextual evidence.
Self-Monitoring	Daily monitoring of a behavior, including when, where, how, the context, and relevant thoughts or emotions.
Exposure and Systematic Desensitization	Graded exposure, typically slowly over time and in a controlled manner, to a stressor, trigger, or whatever may elicit a compulsive, avoidance, or stress response.
Behavioral Activation	Intentional scheduling of pleasant activities (e.g., taking a walk), with a focus on consistency. Also known as activity scheduling.
Relaxation Training	Skills training to learn and apply specific relaxation strategies, such as diaphragmatic breathing, progressive muscle relaxation, guided imagery, and mindfulness exercises.

be indicated in a particular protocol or may be selected by a clinician based on the patient's needs.

Coping Skills Training focuses on learning or improving behavioral processes that are more adaptive. This often occurs through cognitive approaches, such as self-guided training.[13]

Problem-Solving teaches a patient to approach problems through an adaptative lens to assess how best to solve the problem. The process involves applying four primary skills: defining the problem, developing alternative solutions, making a decision, and implementing a solution.[13]

Cognitive Restructuring is the process of strengthening one's mindset. This restructuring starts by identifying thoughts and beliefs that impede functioning and quality of life and are considered as hypotheses rather than truth. Such thoughts are then examined in the context of all information to allow for intentional, positive change.[19,20] Cognitive restructuring is a particular instance of the broader concept of *cognitive reframing*, which can be a positive or negative change in one's mindset that may occur subconsciously.

Self-Monitoring is a strategy in which an individual keeps a record of their behavior over time, typically documenting the time spent engaging in a behavior, location/setting, context, and sometimes co-occurring emotions or thoughts.[1] Self-monitoring is often an initial approach to improve awareness and identify patterns related to a behavior and may be utilized as part of treatment to improve self-regulation.[13]

Exposure and Systematic Desensitization are behavioral approaches that use gradual exposure over time to reduce cognitive, emotional, and behavioral responses to a stimulus, or trigger, with the goal to support improvement of distress tolerance.[13-15] Specific applications of exposure treatment include exposure and response prevention for obsessive-compulsive disorder and prolonged exposure for post-traumatic stress disorder.[21,22]

Behavioral Activation is a strategy that prioritizes scheduling pleasant activities to reduce distress. Of note, Behavioral Activation is also a specific treatment that can involve multiple components (e.g., self-monitoring, skills training, contingency management) that ultimately support the goal of reducing avoidance behaviors.[23]

Relaxation Training involves education and practice of specific relaxation techniques. Examples of relaxation techniques include deep or diaphragmatic breathing, progressive muscle relaxation, guided imagery, and mindful exercises (e.g., journaling, gentle movement). The goal of these techniques is to manage and cope with stress and other symptoms that interfere with mental and behavioral health. These strategies also help individuals identify signs of stress, such as muscle tension or shallow breathing, so they can intervene and prevent major state changes.[24]

7.4 APPLICATIONS OF CBT FOR VARIOUS CONDITIONS AND POPULATIONS

While it is beyond the scope of this chapter to review all applications of CBT, there are some conditions for which CBT protocols and strategies have been especially well-studied. For example, relaxation training has been highly studied in the treatment of anxiety disorders.[25] A 2013 study found cognitive restructuring plus relaxation to be more effective than relaxation alone in addressing symptoms of depression and anxiety related to academic performance.[26] Self-monitoring has been highly utilized for health behavior changes related to diet and physical activity, and has been shown to be useful to address behavior change independently, or within the context of therapist-guided CBT.[27] Additionally, CBT has been adapted and tested for specific health conditions or populations. Some of the most established applications include, but are not limited to, depression, anxiety, chronic pain, and insomnia.

7.4.1 CBT FOR DEPRESSION

The literature overwhelmingly supports the efficacy of CBT for major depressive disorder, with research supporting treatment in a variety of clinical settings. A 2019 study found CBT to be effective for both clinically significant depression and subclinical depressive symptoms when offered by trained professionals within a primary care setting. The study also indicated CBT was effective for depression across individual, group, or self-guided modalities.[28] CBT is effective in relapse prevention for those with a history of major depressive disorder, which is important as historical episodes of depression are one of the greatest predictors of future episodes.[29] Further, a 2019 meta-analysis not only found that CBT was effective for depression, but that it was effective regardless of delivery method, including face-to-face, telehealth, or hybrid treatment.[30]

7.4.2 CBT FOR ANXIETY

CBT as a treatment for anxiety is supported by several meta-analyses, with efficacy and effectiveness in both real-life settings and randomized controlled trials. The approach has been studied and supported across various anxiety disorders, such as panic disorder and social anxiety disorder, with strongest outcomes for generalized anxiety disorder and post-traumatic stress disorder. Exposure therapy and relaxation training alone or in combination have also demonstrated efficacy across anxiety disorders.[31] Moreover, CBT for anxiety has been shown to be significantly more effective than no treatment or waitlist control, other forms of therapy (e.g., psychodynamic approaches), and, for some forms of anxiety, medications.[32] Recent research has also indicated that CBT for anxiety delivered remotely via telephone or video conferencing had similar outcomes to in-person treatment.[33]

7.4.3 CBT FOR CHRONIC PAIN

Symptoms of depression and anxiety occur at higher rates for those living with chronic pain, and these mental health conditions increase the risk of worse pain outcomes. CBT has emerged as the first-line treatment for chronic pain, with CBT interventions demonstrating efficacy in symptom reduction and improved quality of life when delivered both in-person and virtually.[34,35] Research has established the efficacy of CBT for various pain conditions, such as back or neck pain, knee or other joint pain, and fibromyalgia. Similar to other research on CBT, greater number of sessions was associated with greater improvement of symptoms, including effective reduction of pain intensity.[34,35]

7.4.4 CBT OF INSOMNIA (CBT-I)

CBT-I uses a semi-structured treatment protocol, typically lasting between six and eight sessions, to improve sleep quality and decrease sleep-related distress. Treatment focuses narrowly on the connection between sleep-related thoughts, feelings, and behaviors and uses cognitive behavioral strategies, including sleep restriction, stimulus control, cognitive restructuring, and relaxation training. CBT-I is the most effective treatment for insomnia, with outcomes similar to, or better than, sleep medications, without the detriment of treatment side effects.[36] Research indicates that 70% to 80% of patients have an immediate benefit from CBT-I, and that treatment effects can have positive long-term effects.[37] Studies have also indicated CBT-I is effective for diverse populations such as the following: those with chronic insomnia; comorbid psychiatric conditions such as anxiety, depression, and PTSD; and cancer survivors.[38–40] Despite the efficacy of CBT-I and low risk compared to pharmacotherapy, it remains underutilized.[36]

7.5   CBT FOR HEALTH BEHAVIORS AND LIFESTYLE CHANGE

CBT is an ideal intervention to address health behaviors, given that behavioral change is a core tenet. Stress is also a primary risk factor for poor health behaviors (e.g., sedentary behavior, poor diet, cigarette smoking) and impedes making health behavior changes.[41] CBT for behavior changes focuses on problem-solving and developing new coping skills to replace or adapt unhealthy behaviors, as well as cognitive restructuring of automatic thoughts. For example, CBT for smoking cessation may start with self-monitoring and identifying high-risk situations for smoking, develop strategies to change those situations in an attempt to break the associations they have with cigarettes, and increase coping skills for managing distress related to physical and psychological withdrawal.[42] CBT for smoking cessation has demonstrated effectiveness broadly and for specific populations (e.g., pregnant people, people with fewer socioeconomic resources), may be used as an adjuvant therapy to other treatment protocols, and remains efficacious when provided via telehealth.[43]

CBT is frequently used to support patients with serious and chronic health conditions who may need to make lifestyle changes, adjust to diagnosis, and cope with illness. These CBT interventions support secondary and tertiary disease prevention through health behavior change. For example, among patients with type 2 diabetes mellitus, CBT is associated with improved glycemic control, as well as improvements in anxiety and depression, which are common among those with diabetes.[44] As another example, a 2018 meta-analysis of CBT interventions among patients with cardiovascular disease and comorbid depression or anxiety found that CBT interventions were associated with decreased symptoms of depression, decreased anxiety, and greater quality of life, as well as reduced risk for cardiovascular disease-related morbidity and mortality.[45] In many cases of chronic disease, CBT is coupled with typical lifestyle interventions, such as dietary change, to allow for more sustainable health behavior changes and improved outcomes.

The influence of health behaviors on lifestyle is multifactorial, including health beliefs, cultural influences, health literacy, and access to resources. Health behaviors are also influenced by social determinants of health, which include the institutions, ideologies, and situational factors that impact health biologically, psychologically, and socially.[46] Thus, while health behavior change and lifestyle maintenance may seem simple in theory, they are often challenging to put into practice. Common barriers to lifestyle changes include the following: poor food environment (e.g., low accessibility to grocery stores, high availability of fast food restaurants), financial limitations, time pressures, and unsafe environments. These factors can be exacerbated by family or household factors, such as maintaining consistency and balancing autonomy versus social support.[47] Given these complex and intersecting risk factors, CBT practitioners help patients to identify and change thoughts and behaviors within the context of their unique biopsychosocial influences to support lifestyle change.

7.6   SUMMARY AND CONCLUSION

CBT approaches have shown consistent efficacy to support the treatment of mental health conditions, symptoms of mental distress (e.g., stress), and health behaviors.

CBT approaches have been applied to a wide range of populations and conditions, from depression and serious mental illness, to health behaviors and lifestyle factors, and including adults managing chronic medical conditions. Unfortunately, a persistent barrier to patients accessing CBT is that evidence-based practice requires a highly trained provider with clinical expertise.[25,26] For those without such training, there is an opportunity to utilize cognitive behavioral skills and support specific skill building, which has also been shown to support patient outcomes.[27] With the appropriate adaptations, CBT is a powerful treatment to support the mental health and lifestyle change goals of many patients.

REFERENCES

1. American Psychiatric Association, American Psychiatric Association DSM-5 Task Force. *Diagnostic and Statistical Manual of Mental Disorders: DSM-5.* 5th ed. American Psychiatric Association; 2013.
2. Dimidjian S, Barrera M, Martell C, Muñoz RF, Lewinsohn PM. The origins and current status of behavioral activation treatments for depression. *Annual Review of Clinical Psychology.* 2011;7(1):1–38. doi:10.1146/annurev-clinpsy-032210-104535
3. Angell B. Behavioral theory. In: *Encyclopedia of Social Work.* Oxford University Press; 2008. Accessed December 22, 2022. http://www.oxfordreference.com/display/10.1093/acref/9780195306613.001.0001/acref-9780195306613-e-30
4. Lewinsohn PM. A behavioral approach to depression. *Essent Pap Depress.* Published online 1974:150–172.
5. Meyering TC. *Historical Roots of Cognitive Science: The Rise of a Cognitive Theory of Perception from Antiquity to the Nineteenth Century,* vol. 208. Springer Science & Business Media; 2012.
6. Grider C. Foundations of Cognitive Theory: A Concise Review. Published online 1993.
7. Clark DA, Beck AT, Alford BA, Bieling PJ, Segal ZV. *Scientific Foundations of Cognitive Theory and Therapy of Depression.* Springer; 2000.
8. Schultz DP, Schultz SE. *A History of Modern Psychology.* Cengage Learning; 2015.
9. González-Prendes AA, Resko SM. Cognitive- behavioral theory. In: *Trauma: Contemporary Directions in Theory, Practice, and Research*; 2019. https://dx.doi.org/10.4135/9781452230597
10. Chand SP, Kuckel DP, Huecker MR. Cognitive behavior therapy. In: *StatPearls.* StatPearls Publishing; 2022. Accessed December 22, 2022. http://www.ncbi.nlm.nih.gov/books/NBK470241/
11. Pybis J, Saxon D, Hill A, Barkham M. The comparative effectiveness and efficiency of cognitive behaviour therapy and generic counselling in the treatment of depression: Evidence from the 2nd UK national audit of psychological therapies. *BMC Psychiatry.* 2017;17(1):215. doi:10.1186/s12888-017-1370-7
12. Lincoln TM, Jung E, Wiesjahn M, Schlier B. What is the minimal dose of cognitive behavior therapy for psychosis? An approximation using repeated assessments over 45 sessions. *European Psychiatry: Official journal of the European Psychiatric.* 2016;38:31–39. doi:10.1016/j.eurpsy.2016.05.004
13. Dobson KS, Backs-Dermott BJ, Dozois DJA. Cognitive and cognitive behavioral therapies. In: *Handbook of Psychological Change: Psychotherapy Processes and Practices for the 21st Century.* John Wiley & Sons; 2000:409–428.
14. Craske MG. *Cognitive–Behavioral therapy.* American Psychological Association; 2010.
15. Dozois DJ, Dobson KS, Rnic K. Historical and philosophical bases of the cognitive-behavioral therapies. Published online 2019.

16. Hofmann SG, Asnaani A, Vonk IJ, Sawyer AT, Fang A. The efficacy of cognitive behavioral therapy: A review of meta-analyses. *Cognitive Therapy and Research.* 2012;36(5):427–440.
17. Kazantzis N, Luong HK, Usatoff AS, Impala T, Yew RY, Hofmann SG. The processes of cognitive behavioral therapy: A review of meta-analyses. *Cognitive Therapy and Research.* 2018;42(4):349–357.
18. Mansell W, Harvey A, Watkins E, Shafran R. Conceptual foundations of the transdiagnostic approach to CBT. *Journal of Cognitive Psychotherapy.* 2009;23(1):6–19. doi:10.1891/0889-8391.23.1.6
19. Young JE, Rygh JL, Weinberger AD, Beck AT. Cognitive therapy for depression. Published online 2014.
20. Beck AT, Weishaar M. Cognitive therapy. In: *Comprehensive Handbook of Cognitive Therapy.* Springer; 1989:21–36.
21. Koran LM. Treatment of patients with obsessive-compulsive disorder. Published online 2010.
22. American Psychological Association. Clinical practice guideline for the treatment of posttraumatic stress disorder (PTSD) in adults. Published online 2017.
23. Kanter JW, Manos RC, Bowe WM, Baruch DE, Busch AM, Rusch LC. What is behavioral activation? A review of the empirical literature. *Clinical Psychology Review.* 2010;30(6):608–620. doi:10.1016/j.cpr.2010.04.001
24. Benhamou K, Piedra A. CBT-informed interventions for essential workers during the COVID-19 pandemic. *Journal of Contemporary Psychotherapy.* 2020;50(4):275–283. doi:10.1007/s10879-020-09467-3
25. Manzoni GM, Pagnini F, Castelnuovo G, Molinari E. Relaxation training for anxiety: A ten-years systematic review with meta-analysis. *BMC Psychiatry.* 2008;8(1):41. doi:10.1186/1471-244X-8-41
26. Akinsola EF, Nwajei AD. Test anxiety, depression and academic performance: Assessment and management using relaxation and cognitive restructuring techniques. *Psychology.* 2013;04(06):18. doi:10.4236/psych.2013.46A1003
27. Cohen JS, Edmunds JM, Brodman DM, Benjamin CL, Kendall PC. Using self-monitoring: Implementation of collaborative empiricism in cognitive-behavioral therapy. *Cognitive and Behavioral Practice.* 2013;20(4):419–428. doi:10.1016/j.cbpra.2012.06.002
28. Santoft F, Axelsson E, Öst LG, Hedman-Lagerlöf M, Fust J, Hedman-Lagerlöf E. Cognitive behaviour therapy for depression in primary care: Systematic review and meta-analysis. *Psychological Medicine.* 2019;49(8):1266–1274.
29. Zhang Z, Zhang L, Zhang G, Jin J, Zheng Z. The effect of CBT and its modifications for relapse prevention in major depressive disorder: A systematic review and meta-analysis. *BMC Psychiatry.* 2018;18(1):50. doi:10.1186/s12888-018-1610-5
30. López-López JA, Davies SR, Caldwell DM, et al. The process and delivery of CBT for depression in adults: A systematic review and network meta-analysis. *Psychological Medicine.* 2019;49(12):1937–1947. doi:10.1017/S003329171900120X
31. Norton PJ, Price EC. A meta-analytic review of adult cognitive-behavioral treatment outcome across the anxiety disorders. *The Journal of Nervous and Mental Disease.* 2007;195(6):521. doi:10.1097/01.nmd.0000253843.70149.9a
32. Loerinc AG, Meuret AE, Twohig MP, Rosenfield D, Bluett EJ, Craske MG. Response rates for CBT for anxiety disorders: Need for standardized criteria. *Clinical Psychology Review.* 2015;42:72–82. doi:10.1016/j.cpr.2015.08.004
33. Krzyzaniak N, Greenwood H, Scott AM, et al. The effectiveness of telehealth versus face-to face interventions for anxiety disorders: A systematic review and meta-analysis. *Journal of Telemedicine and Telecare.* Published online December 3, 2021: 1357633X211053738. doi:10.1177/1357633X211053738

34. Knoerl R, Lavoie Smith EM, Weisberg J. Chronic pain and cognitive behavioral therapy: An integrative review. *Western Journal of Nursing Research.* 2016;38(5):596–628.
doi:10.1177/0193945915615869
35. Ehde DM, Dillworth TM, Turner JA. Cognitive-behavioral therapy for individuals with
chronic pain: Efficacy, innovations, and directions for research. *American Psychologist.*
2014;69(2):153.
36. Rossman J. Cognitive-behavioral therapy for insomnia: An effective and underutilized
treatment for insomnia. *American Journal of Lifestyle Medicine.* 2019;13(6):544–547.
doi:10.1177/1559827619867677
37. Morin CM, Benca R. Chronic insomnia. *Lancet London England.* 2012;379(9821):
1129–1141. doi:10.1016/S0140-6736(11)60750-2
38. Johnson JA, Rash JA, Campbell TS, et al. A systematic review and meta-analysis of
randomized controlled trials of cognitive behavior therapy for insomnia (CBT-I) in
cancer survivors. *Sleep Medicine Reviews.* 2016;27:20–28.
39. Taylor DJ, Pruiksma KE. Cognitive and behavioural therapy for insomnia (CBT-I)
in psychiatric populations: A systematic review. *International Review of Psychiatry.*
2014;26(2):205–213. doi:10.3109/09540261.2014.902808
40. Trauer JM, Qian MY, Doyle JS, Rajaratnam SMW, Cunnington D. Cognitive behavioral therapy for chronic insomnia. *Annals of Internal Medicine.* 2015;163(3):191–204.
doi:10.7326/M14-2841
41. Smyth JM, Sliwinski MJ, Zawadzki MJ, et al. Everyday stress response targets in
the science of behavior change. *Behaviour Research and Therapy.* 2018;101:20–29.
doi:10.1016/j.brat.2017.09.009
42. Caroll AJ, Veluz-Wilkins AK, Hintsman B. Smoking cessation in clinical practice. In:
Mechanick JI, Kushner RF, eds. *Lifestyle Medicine: A Manual for Clinical Practice.*
Springer; 2016:135–150.
43. Vinci C. Cognitive behavioral and mindfulness-based interventions for smoking cessation: A review of the recent literature. *Current Oncology Reports.* 2020;22(6):58.
doi:10.1007/s11912-020-00915-w
44. Uchendu C, Blake H. Effectiveness of cognitive–behavioural therapy on glycaemic
control and psychological outcomes in adults with diabetes mellitus: A systematic
review and meta-analysis of randomized controlled trials. *Diabetic Medicine.* 2017;
34(3):328–339.
45. Reavell J, Hopkinson M, Clarkesmith D, Lane DA. Effectiveness of cognitive
behavioral therapy for depression and anxiety in patients with cardiovascular disease: A systematic review and meta-analysis. *Psychosomatic Medicine.* 2018;80(8):
742–753.
46. Short SE, Mollborn S. Social determinants and health behaviors: Conceptual frames
and empirical advances. *Current Opinion in Psychology.* 2015;5:78–84. doi:10.1016/j.
copsyc.2015.05.002
47. Wild CE, Rawiri NT, Willing EJ, Hofman PL, Anderson YC. Challenges of making healthy lifestyle changes for families in Aotearoa/New Zealand. *Public Health
Nutrition.* 2021;24(7):1906–1915. doi:10.1017/S1368980020003699

8 Positive Psychology Approaches

Liana Lianov, MD, MPH and
Jolanta Burke, CPsychol, PhD

KEY POINTS

- Studies of positive psychology interventions show an association with improved subjective and psychological well-being.
- Positive psychology approaches contribute to the effectiveness of health behavior coaching.
- Positive affect, when associated with health behavior changes, increases motivation for and has a reinforcing, reciprocal link with these behaviors.
- Flourishing, achieved by healthy behaviors and positive activities and mindsets, can be experienced by individuals despite having mental and physical illness.
- Prescriptions of positive psychology-based activities, in conjunction with a healthy lifestyle, can be incorporated into psychiatric and other medical practices to bolster mental health and manage mental illness.

8.1 POSITIVE PSYCHOLOGY FOR MENTAL HEALTH

The field of positive psychology has significantly evolved since its inception a few decades ago by Martin Seligman and other leaders who made the case that promoting mental and emotional health involves more than addressing illness, stress, and negative emotions. They strongly argued that clinical practitioners need to also apply techniques that enhance positive emotions to help individuals become their best selves and reach a state of well-being beyond that achieved by treating and preventing poor mental and physical health.[1]

A review article by Waters and other positive psychology leaders laid out three roles for positive psychology in mental health. These behavioral strategies, mindsets, and interventions can buffer mental health against negative events, bolster mental health in the face of adversity, and build mental health resources for thriving despite stressful daily life challenges and traumatic events. In fact, positive psychology approaches can play a key role in promoting post-traumatic growth.[2]

In recognition of the accumulating evidence that positive psychology interventions can boost subjective and psychological well-being,[3–8] as well as serve as a primary driver of health behavior change,[9,10] positive psychology approaches should be considered as part of psychiatric treatment and management and of health care more broadly, including lifestyle medicine and self-care. When healthy lifestyles and

DOI: 10.1201/b22810-9

positive psychology are combined as the underpinnings of care, we can help patients move toward positive health with a set of behaviors that can support them regardless of underlying mental and physical conditions.

8.2 THE ROLE OF POSITIVE PSYCHOLOGY IN HEALTH BEHAVIOR CHANGE

One of the most robust areas of positive psychology research demonstrates a link between positive emotions, especially ones experienced during healthy behaviors, and repeating those behaviors. According to the upward spiral of lifestyle change, positive emotions can trigger unconscious motivation for healthy behaviors, and, in turn, healthy behaviors boost positive emotions. Moreover, additional resources are built to reinforce this reciprocal cycle, leading to an upward and outward spiral of lifestyle change.[9] Positive emotions can also help individuals with problem solving to overcome barriers to making change.[10]

Happier people tend to engage in healthier behaviors, such as exercise, not smoking, using seat belts, eating healthy food, and avoiding risky alcohol use.[11] One key positive psychology construct is developing and maintaining life purpose. For example, people with purpose in life tend to adhere to preventive services recommendations.[12] In addition, positive affect enhances engagement in self-care.[13,14]

As the literature has mounted on the key role of positive psychology constructs in behavior change, health professionals who offer health coaching and counseling can apply positive psychology best practices for helping their patients both achieve and maintain health behaviors and other recommended treatments.

8.2.1 COACHING HEALTH BEHAVIORS WITH POSITIVE PSYCHOLOGY APPROACHES

One of the early groups adopting positive psychology in health care has been health coaches. Traditional behavior change techniques, such as motivational interviewing, were bolstered by a reframing of the approach to leveraging positive psychology principles.[15–17] Psychology leaders argue that positive psychology is a natural construct for counseling psychology. Applying the positive psychology techniques not only has the potential to help address psychological issues of psychology and psychiatry patients, as evidenced by the effect on subjective and psychological well-being, but also can indirectly nudge health behaviors and treatment adherence.[18]

The PERMA framework for flourishing--positive emotions, engagement, relationships, meaning, and achievement-- can be incorporated into health coaching and behavior change strategies. This process involves engaging in activities that elicit positive emotions (P), immersing oneself in activities that produce a sense of engagement or flow (E), involving others in the desired behaviors to increase support and accountability (R), paying attention to how desired behaviors align with one's sense of meaning and life purpose (M), and tracking progress towards goals and celebrating achievements (A).[19]

In addition to PERMA elements, future visioning, appreciative inquiry, and leveraging character strengths are positive psychology constructs that can be integrated into health coaching. Positive images of the future fuel individuals with hope and nudge them to identify solutions to barriers so they can reach their desired goals.[20,21] Developing a clear image of one's best self produces positive emotions that can motivate behavior change.[22] Moreover, use of signature character strengths can empower the individual. For example, strengths, such as self-regulation and perseverance, provide support during challenges.

Studies have shown that positive psychology interventions are well accepted in patient populations and associated with substantial improvements in behavioral and psychological outcomes.[23] Moreover, positive psychology constructs can be interwoven with traditional coaching approaches, such as integrating the PERMA model, to enhance the overall approach for addressing a range of behaviors in treating both mental and physical illness.

8.3 THE IMPACT OF POSITIVE PSYCHOLOGY INTERVENTIONS (PPIs) ON MENTAL HEALTH

Even though PPIs have been created for the non-clinical population, they are valuable tools for clinicians to introduce to their patients. The interventions are free from mental illness stigma and can be self-administered. Thus, patients are more willing to use them and more importantly, they can involve their families on their journey of a meaningful pursuit of well-being.[24] Furthermore, existing evidence indicates that PPIs reduce the symptoms of mental illness and enhance the resources that either protect individuals from experiencing mental health issues or provide them with tools that help them recover faster.

Concerning reduction of illness symptoms, most research evaluates the effect of PPIs on mood disorders. For example, a recent systematic review of PPIs practiced with over 72,000 participants across 41 countries from clinical and non-clinical populations showed that PPIs indicated small to medium effects on enhancing well-being and reducing depression, anxiety and stress.[4] The outcomes were maintained at a 3-month follow-up. Another review explicitly focused on a clinical population and found that apart from improving subjective and psychological well-being, PPIs had a small effect on reducing symptoms of depression.[3] Both reviews emphasized the importance of longer-term programs for ensuring robust results rather than ad hoc interventions.

Similar results were shown for patients with severe mental illness. A systematic review of nine studies that used PPIs with patients experiencing schizophrenia indicated that the interventions significantly improved their well-being (e.g., life satisfaction, self-esteem, self-acceptance, subjective well-being, and quality of life); some studies also noted a decrease in symptoms sustained at 3- or 6-month follow-ups.[25] Another systematic review extended beyond schizophrenia into 16 studies with patients experiencing other severe mental illnesses (e.g., major depressive disorder, bipolar disorder, borderline personality disorder, schizoaffective disorder), and the results showed a moderate effect of PPIs on enhancing patients' well-being and a large effect on reducing the symptoms of psychopathology.[26] Thus, despite the evidence still emerging on the effectiveness of PPIs in psychiatric conditions, these studies offer hopeful results.

Furthermore, given that mental illness is not exclusive to psychological flourishing,[27,28] it is essential to acknowledge the role that well-being (as an outcome of PPI practice) plays in protecting individuals against mental health issues and helping them cope effectively with adversities. Flourishing is a state of optimal human functioning and high emotional and social well-being levels.[29] It is a fluid condition that extends from mental illness through languishing (feeling unwell but not having enough symptoms to be diagnosed with mental illness as per DSM [Diagnostic and Statistical Manual of Mental Disorders]), moderate health, and flourishing. Over a decade, approximately half of the flourishers' well-being declined, and half of the languishers' well-being improved.[30] A longitudinal study showed that a decline from flourishing to moderate health (where most of the population resides) makes individuals seven times more likely to experience depression within two years.[31] At the same time, despite experiencing depression or anxiety, 14-19% of individuals flourish psychologically, and their positive mental state assists them in recovering faster from a psychiatric illness, as measured three years later.[28] Thus, using PPIs with psychiatric patients can potentially speed up their recovery.

Most importantly, however, helping individuals use PPIs can protect them against developing symptoms of poor mental health. As such, PPIs are early interventions that can be applied in non-clinical populations to enhance their hope and optimism, improve their experiences of positive emotions, relationships, engagement, accomplishment, and many other components of well-being that lead to an upward spiral of mental health,[32-35] all of which act as protective mechanisms during adversity. Using PPIs can improve the population's health by increasing flourishing symptoms and reducing mental illness symptoms.[36] Thus, encouraging patients' families to use PPIs may protect them from developing mental health conditions in the future.

Although emerging research applied to the clinical population is promising, many studies cannot be generalized to the psychiatric population. Thus, more research is required to identify the role of PPIs in psychiatric practice. In the meantime, sufficient evidence exists to consider PPIs as complementary methods for preventing mental health illness and helping the clinical population reduce their symptoms of mental health issues. That said, care needs to be taken to ensure that interventions offer choices and variety (mix and match) to prevent adverse outcomes of PPIs.[37]

8.4   THE LIFESTYLE MEDICINE (LM) PILLARS AND MENTAL HEALTH

While PPIs are one way to improve well-being and help individuals reach psychological well-being, i.e., flourishing, recently, LM demonstrated an alternative route towards reaching flourishing. In a study with 1,112 participants, flourishers were three times more likely to use 3+ LM pillars than individuals with moderate health; equally, they were nine times more likely to use 3+ LM pillars than languishers.[38] Moreover, a new 10-week program for a non-clinical population that mixed PPIs with LM tools was designed and showed a significant improvement in participants' flourishing.[39] In addition, Burke and colleagues[27] reviewed the literature and identified over 100 research-based PPIs and LM interventions that showed evidence of flourishing among clinical and non-clinical populations.

In addition to blending PPIs and LM interventions, the pillars of LM interventions can expand positive outcomes by from integrating positive psychology constructs. For example, emerging research indicates that positive affect created by such interventions as gratitude expression can support individuals in improving their sleep quality.[40] Thus, gratitude can be a tool for helping people flourish and eliciting sleep. Another example comes from the LM stress management tools that could be supplemented with stress mindset changes. A stress mindset relates to appraising stressful events as opportunities to grow, which results in participants using more effective approaches to coping.[41] As such, stress mindset interventions can help participants manage their stress more effectively and result in positive outcomes of stress.[42] These examples highlight alternatives to PPIs to help individuals flourish and improve physiological outcomes.

8.5 INCORPORATING POSITIVE PSYCHOLOGY INTO HEALTH CARE

Health care, including psychiatry, can harness positive psychology in a range of clinical processes, such as assessing positive emotions and life satisfaction, monitoring positive activity habits, coaching with positive psychology constructs, and prescribing PPIs as part of the health management plan. Referrals to community programs and digital apps that promote positive activities provide ongoing support outside the medical/psychiatric practice.[43]

As the current state of the evidence does not provide specificity on how to implement positive psychology interventions in psychiatric or general medical care, practitioners can engage in open discussions with patients about their cultural preferences, interests, and life situations to identify whether positive activities are appropriate and hone down the desired activities.

Early research investigating the influence of culture on well-being gains from PPIs suggests that individualistic versus collectivist cultures may garner different benefits. For example, in a rotating intervention (gratitude letter or acts of kindness) study of US and South Korean participants, greater benefits were observed for the US participants who wrote a gratitude letter before performing acts of kindness, while the reverse was found for the South Korean participants.[44,45]

Moreover, self-selection can influence success with PPIs. An 8-month intervention study of the immediate and longer-term effects of regularly practicing two assigned positive activities - expressing optimism and gratitude - on well-being indicated that initial self-selection of the activity conditions impacted the intervention, but not the control group. Those who self-selected the activity condition made a greater effort to engage in the activities.[46]

Lyubomirsky and Layous posited a model in which several factors moderate the effect of positive activities on well-being, including the features of the activities, such as dosing, frequency and variety; characteristics of the individuals, such as their level of motivation and effort; and person-activity fit, how much the activity feels natural, enjoyable or valuable versus triggers shame and feelings of being forced to do it.[37,44,47] When prescribing these activities, the potential for habituation to the activity needs to be considered; hence prescribers should make a concerted effort to recommend a variety of activities to help avoid this effect.[48,49] Future studies need to examine the influence of such prescriptions and behavioral supports in a variety of settings and for diverse populations.

8.6 CONCLUSION

In this chapter, we make the case for incorporating positive psychology approaches into psychiatric and medical care to increase successful health behavior change and boost mental health. Meta-analyses pointing to the link between positive psychology interventions and subjective and psychological well-being are discussed. The scientific literature offers support for the role of positive emotions in facilitating and sustaining healthy behaviors.

The reciprocal, reinforcing link between positive emotions and healthy behaviors in the upward spiral theory of lifestyle change explains the foundation of the power of positive emotions. Moreover, positive emotions can lead to additional, independent physiologic benefits and can enhance outcomes of the lifestyle medicine intervention pillars.

A variety of PPIs have been studied with varying mental health and well-being effects. Prescribing these activities is worthy of consideration for interested patients as part of their health and well-being management plans. However, further research is needed to show which activities create the greatest benefits for diverse mental health conditions and subpopulations.

REFERENCES

1. Seligman MEP. Positive health. *Applied Psychology.* 2008;57(s1):3–18. doi:10.1111/j.1464-0597.2008.00351.x
2. Waters L, Algoe SB, Dutton J, et al. Positive psychology in a pandemic: Buffering, bolstering, and building mental health. *The Journal of Positive Psychology.* 2022; 17(3):303–323. doi:10.1080/17439760.2021.1871945
3. Bolier L, Haverman M, Westerhof GJ, Riper H, Smit F, Bohlmeijer E. Positive psychology interventions: A meta-analysis of randomized controlled studies. *BMC Public Health.* 2013;13:119. doi:10.1186/1471-2458-13-119
4. Carr A, Cullen K, Keeney C, et al. Effectiveness of positive psychology interventions: A systematic review and meta-analysis. *The Journal of Positive Psychology.* 2021;16:749–769. doi:10.1080/17439760.2020.1818807
5. Chakhssi F, Kraiss JT, Sommers-Spijkerman M, Bohlmeijer ET. The effect of positive psychology interventions on well-being and distress in clinical samples with psychiatric or somatic disorders: A systematic review and meta-analysis. *BMC Psychiatry.* 2018;18(1):211. doi:10.1186/s12888-018-1739-2
6. Hendriks T, Schotanus-Dijkstra M, Hassankhan A, Jong J, de Bohlmeijer E. The efficacy of multi-component positive psychology interventions: A systematic review and meta-analysis of randomized controlled trials. *Journal of Happiness Studies.* 2020;21(1):357–390. doi:10.1007/s10902-019-00082-1
7. van Agteren J, Iasiello M, Lo L, et al. A systematic review and meta-analysis of psychological interventions to improve mental wellbeing. *Nature Human Behaviour.* 2021;5(5):631–652. doi:10.1038/s41562-021-01093-w

8. White CA, Uttl B, Holder MD. Meta-analyses of positive psychology interventions: The effects are much smaller than previously reported. *PLoS One.* 2019;14(5):e0216588. doi:10.1371/journal.pone.0216588

9. Van Cappellen P, Rice EL, Catalino LI, Fredrickson BL. Positive affective processes underlie positive health behavior change. *Psychology Health.* 2018;33(1):77–97. doi:10.1080/08870446.2017.1320798

10. Fredrickson BL. Positive emotions broaden and build. In: *Advances in Experimental Social Psychology*, vol. 47. Elsevier; 2013:1–53. doi:10.1016/B978-0-12-407236-7.00001-2

11. Kansky J, Diener E. Benefits of well-being: Health, social relationships, work, and resilience. *Journal of Positive Psychology and Wellbeing.* 2017;1(2):129–169.

12. Kim ES, Strecher VJ, Ryff CD. Purpose in life and use of preventive health care services. *Proceedings of the National Academy of Sciences.* 2014;111(46):16331–16336. doi:10.1073/pnas.1414826111

13. Carrico AW, Moskowitz JT. Positive affect promotes engagement in care after HIV diagnosis. *Health Psychology: Official Journal of the Society for Health Psychology Association* . 2014;33(7):686–689. doi:10.1037/hea0000011

14. Gonzalez JS, Penedo FJ, Antoni MH, et al. Social support, positive states of mind, and HIV treatment adherence in men and women living with HIV/AIDS. *Health Psychology: Official Journal of the Division of Health Psychology, American Psychological Association.* 2004;23(4):413–418. doi:10.1037/0278-6133.23.4.413

15. Huffman JC, Golden J, Massey CN, et al. A positive psychology-motivational interviewing program to promote physical activity in type 2 diabetes: The BEHOLD-16 pilot randomized trial. *General Hospital Psychiatry.* 2021;68:65–73. doi:10.1016/j.genhosppsych.2020.12.001

16. Biswas-Diener R. *Practicing Positive Psychology Coaching: Assessment, Activities and Strategies for Success.* 1st edition. Wiley; 2010.

17. Kauffman C. Positive psychology: The science at the heart of coaching. In: *Evidence Based Coaching Handbook: Putting Best Practices to Work for Your Clients.* John Wiley & Sons, Inc; 2006:219–253.

18. Magyar-Moe JL, Owens RL, Conoley CW. Positive psychological interventions in counseling: What every counseling psychologist should know. *Counseling Psychology.* 2015;43(4):508–557. doi:10.1177/0011000015573776

19. Falecki D, Leach C, Green S. PERMA-powered coaching: Building foundations for a flourishing life. In: *Positive Psychology Coaching in Practice.* Routledge; 2018.

20. McQuaid M, Niemiec R, Doman F. A character strengths-based approach to positive psychology coaching. In: *Positive Psychology Coaching in Practice.* Routledge; 2018.

21. Reynolds R, Palmer S, Green S. *Positive Psychology Coaching in Practice*; 2018. doi:10.4324/9781315716169

22. Boyatzis RE, Rochford K, Taylor SN. The role of the positive emotional attractor in vision and shared vision: Toward effective leadership, relationships, and engagement. *Frontiers in Psychology.* 2015;6:670. doi:10.3389/fpsyg.2015.00670

23. Celano CM, Albanese AM, Millstein RA, et al. Optimizing a positive psychology intervention to promote health behaviors after an acute coronary syndrome: The positive emotions after acute coronary events III (PEACE-III) randomized factorial trial. *Psychosomatic Medicine.* 2018;80(6):526–534. doi:10.1097/PSY.0000000000000584

24. Waters L. Using positive psychology interventions to strengthen family happiness: A family systems approach. *The Journal of Positive Psychology.* 2020;15:645–652. doi: 10.1080/17439760.2020.1789704

25. Pina I, Braga C de M, de Oliveira TFR, de Santana CN, Marques RC, Machado L. Positive psychology interventions to improve well-being and symptoms in people on the schizophrenia spectrum: A systematic review and meta-analysis. *Rev Bras Psiquiatr Sao Paulo Braz 1999.* 2021;43(4):430–437. doi:10.1590/1516-4446-2020-1164

26. Geerling B, Kraiss JT, Kelders SM, Stevens AWMM, Kupka RW, Bohlmeijer ET. The effect of positive psychology interventions on well-being and psychopathology in patients with severe mental illness: A systematic review and meta-analysis. *The Journal of Positive Psychology*. 2020;15:572–587. doi:10.1080/17439760.2020.1789695

27. Burke J, Dunne PJ, Meehan T, O'Boyle CA, van Nieuwerburgh C. *Positive Health: 100+ Research-Based Positive Psychology and Lifestyle Medicine Tools to Enhance Your Wellbeing*. Routledge; 2022. doi:10.4324/9781003279594

28. Schotanus-Dijkstra M, Keyes CLM, de Graaf R, Ten Have M. Recovery from mood and anxiety disorders: The influence of positive mental health. *Journal of Affective Disorders*. 2019;252:107–113. doi:10.1016/j.jad.2019.04.051

29. Keyes CLM. The mental health continuum: From languishing to flourishing in life. *Journal of Health and Social Behavior*. 2002;43(2):207–222.

30. Keyes CLM, Dhingra SS, Simoes EJ. Change in level of positive mental health as a predictor of future risk of mental illness. *American Journal of Public Health*. 2010;100(12):2366–2371. doi:10.2105/AJPH.2010.192245

31. Keyes CLM, Yao J, Hybels CF, Milstein G, Proeschold-Bell RJ. Are changes in positive mental health associated with increased likelihood of depression over a two year period? A test of the mental health promotion and protection hypotheses. *Journal of Affective Disorders*. 2020;270:136–142. doi:10.1016/j.jad.2020.03.056

32. Diener E. New findings and future directions for subjective well-being research. *American Psychologist*. 2012;67(8):590–597. doi:10.1037/a0029541

33. Huppert FA, So TTC. Flourishing across Europe: Application of a new conceptual framework for defining well-being. *Social Indicators Research*. 2013;110(3):837–861. doi:10.1007/s11205-011-9966-7

34. Ryff CD. Psychological well-being revisited: Advances in the science and practice of eudaimonia. *Psychotherapy and Psychosomatics*. 2014;83(1):10–28. doi:10.1159/000353263

35. Seligman MEP. *Flourish: A Visionary New Understanding of Happiness and Well-Being*. Reprint edition. Atria; 2012.

36. Felicia AH, Nick B, Barry K, eds. *The Science of Well-Being*. Oxford University Press; 2006.

37. Lyubomirsky S, Sheldon KM, Schkade D. Pursuing happiness: The architecture of sustainable change. *Review of General Psychology*. 2005;9(2):111–131. doi:10.1037/1089-2680.9.2.111

38. Burke J, Dunne PJ. Lifestyle medicine pillars as predictors of psychological flourishing. *Frontiers in Psychology*. 2022;13:963806. doi:10.3389/fpsyg.2022.963806

39. Przybylko G, Morton DP, Morton JK, Renfrew ME, Hinze J. An interdisciplinary mental wellbeing intervention for increasing flourishing: Two experimental studies. *The Journal of Positive Psychology*. 2022;17(4):573–588. doi:10.1080/17439760.2021.1897868

40. Jackowska M, Brown J, Ronaldson A, Steptoe A. The impact of a brief gratitude intervention on subjective well-being, biology and sleep. *Journal of Health Psychology*. 2016;21(10):2207–2217. doi:10.1177/1359105315572455

41. Crum AJ, Akinola M, Martin A, Fath S. The role of stress mindset in shaping cognitive, emotional, and physiological responses to challenging and threatening stress. *Anxiety, Stress, & Coping*. 2017;30(4):379–395. doi:10.1080/10615806.2016.1275585

42. Jamieson JP, Crum AJ, Goyer JP, Marotta ME, Akinola M. Optimizing stress responses with reappraisal and mindset interventions: An integrated model. *Anxiety, Stress, & Coping*. 2018;31(3):245–261. doi:10.1080/10615806.2018.1442615

43. Lianov L. *Roots of Positive Change: Optimizing Health Care With Positive Psychology*. HealthType; 2019.

44. Layous K, Lee H, Choi I, Lyubomirsky S. Culture matters when designing a successful happiness-increasing activity: A comparison of the United States and South Korea. *Journal of Cross-Cultural Psychology*. 2013;44:1294–1303. doi:10.1177/0022022113487591

45. Boehm JK, Lyubomirsky S, Sheldon KM. A longitudinal experimental study comparing the effectiveness of happiness-enhancing strategies in Anglo Americans and Asian Americans. *Cognition and Emotion*. 2011;25(7):1263–1272. doi:10.1080/02699931.2010.541227

46. Lyubomirsky S, Dickerhoof R, Boehm JK, Sheldon KM. Becoming happier takes both a will and a proper way: An experimental longitudinal intervention to boost well-being. *Emotion*. 2011;11(2):391–402. doi:10.1037/a0022575

47. Lyubomirsky S, Layous K. How do simple positive activities increase well-being? *Current Directions in Psychological Science*. 2013;22(1):57–62. doi:10.1177/0963721412469809

48. Sheldon KM, Lyubomirsky S. The challenge of staying happier: Testing the hedonic adaptation prevention model. *Personality and Social Psychology Bulletin*. 2012;38(5):670–680. doi:10.1177/0146167212436400

49. Sheldon KM, Lyubomirsky S. Achieving sustainable gains in happiness: Change your actions, not your circumstances. *Journal of Happiness Studies*. 2006;7(1):55–86. doi:10.1007/s10902-005-0868-8

9 Burnout
Risk Factors and Associations

*Kristin M. Davis, PhD, Lauren E. Chu, BA,
and Kyle W. Murdock, PhD*

KEY POINTS

- Burnout is a work-related syndrome characterized by emotional exhaustion, depersonalization, and reduced personal and professional accomplishment.
- Individuals who report higher burnout are also more likely to experience depression, anxiety, and physical health problems.
- Intervention research on burnout has produced promising but inconsistent results; additional studies are needed.

9.1 WHAT IS BURNOUT?

Burnout was formally defined in the 1970s[1] and has subsequently been recognized as a significant problem in various workplaces worldwide.[2] Burnout involves work-related symptoms of physical, emotional, and social exhaustion that negatively impact work performance and self-perception.[3] These symptoms occur within three dimensions of burnout: 1) emotional exhaustion, or the degree to which an individual has exceeded their ability to cope with stress; 2) depersonalization, or the tendency to detach from and objectify other humans; and 3) reduced personal accomplishment, or feeling less competent and successful.[4] No specific diagnostic criteria for burnout have been delineated,[5] and the nosological value of burnout remains controversial due to substantial overlap with other psychological phenomena, including depression.[6,7,39] Despite these concerns, burnout was classified as a syndrome by the World Health Organization (WHO) in 2019.[8] The WHO defines burnout (QD85) as "a syndrome conceptualized as resulting from chronic workplace stress that has not been successfully managed," stating that burnout is specific to occupational exhaustion and does not apply to other life areas.[8]

9.2 RISK AND PROTECTIVE FACTORS

Many factors either promote or protect from burnout. Chronic, unmanaged workplace stress is an important risk factor,[9,10] but not all forms of workplace stress lead to burnout.[6] Widespread burnout has been observed in healthcare workers, such as physicians,[11] mental health professionals,[12] nurses,[13] and emergency medical service providers.[14] However, burnout has been observed in a variety of professionals, including social workers,[15] athletes,[16] teachers,[17] students,[18] military personnel,[19]

DOI: 10.1201/b22810-10

hospitality workers,[20] and farmers.[21] Burnout has even been seen outside the professional workplace, in parents,[22,23] informal caregivers,[24,25] and social and political activists.[26-28] According to the existential perspective, burnout involves a combination of chronic workplace stress and the loss of a sense of personal meaning.[6] Maintaining a sense of personal meaning under high-stress conditions can reduce burnout risk, while losing this sense may yield burnout even in lower-stress circumstances.[6,29]

Maslach and Leiter (1977) described six antecedents of burnout in the work environment: excessive workload, lack of control over work activities, effort-reward imbalance, lack of community at work, lack of fairness or trust, and conflicting values.[30] While excessive workload can lead to burnout, boredom can contribute to feelings of meaninglessness and lack of value at work, also potentially leading to burnout.[1,10,31] Certain personality traits also confer an increased risk of burnout, including high neuroticism, low conscientiousness, and low agreeableness.[23] Overcommitment to work,[32] poor emotion regulation,[33] a history of depression,[34] and a lack of social support[35] are also risk factors. The relationship between gender and burnout is complex, with women experiencing more emotional exhaustion and men experiencing more depersonalization.[36]

9.3   BURNOUT AND MENTAL HEALTH

Whether burnout is a unique disorder or not remains hotly contested, with evidence supporting both possibilities.[11] Burnout could be a phase in the development of depression, with prospective studies finding that higher burnout predicts an increase in depressive symptoms.[37] However, greater depressive symptoms also prospectively predict the development of burnout.[40] It has additionally been argued that burnout is a form of depression due to overlapping symptoms, including anhedonia, fatigue, feelings of worthlessness, changes in appetite or sleep, loss of interest, and difficulty concentrating.[7] Symptoms of burnout and depression are moderately[41] to strongly[7,38] correlated. Further, individuals with burnout and depression have similar symptom severity in 8 out of 9 major depressive episode diagnostic criteria; self-blame appears to be higher among those who are depressed.[38]

Despite their shared characteristics, a growing body of evidence suggests that burnout and depression may be unique.[41] The primary distinction centers around burnout being specific to job or career contexts, while depression is a more pervasive condition that impacts all domains of life, both in and out of work.[10] Supporting this, lack of reciprocity in intimate partner relationships predicts the development of depression but not burnout, while a lack of reciprocity in work relationships directly predicts burnout but only indirectly predicts depression.[42] Similarly, lack of control at work[43] and job strain[34] are directly associated with burnout, but indirectly associated with depression. Further research is needed to disentangle the constructs of burnout and depression.

The relationship between burnout and anxiety is also unclear. Individuals with high trait anxiety are more prone to developing burnout,[41] possibly because reacting to job stress with anxiety is emotionally exhausting. Similarly, individuals with social anxiety are more likely to experience burnout,[44] underscoring the interpersonal aspects of burnout development. Anxiety and burnout also share some predictors, such as high job demands and over-commitment.[41] Despite these similarities, the correlation between burnout and anxiety symptoms is moderate, explaining approximately 21% of the variance.[41] Consequently, there may be differences between the two; additional studies are needed.

Efforts to identify biomarkers that differentiate burnout from other mental health concerns have yielded mixed results.[9] Evidence suggests that hypothalamic-pituitary-adrenal axis dysregulation is a key feature of burnout physiology,[45] but this is also true of depression[46] and anxiety disorders.[47] DNA methylation patterns have been identified as a promising biomarker for differentiating burnout.[5] Decreased methylation of the glucocorticoid receptor gene (NR3C1) and the serotonin transporter gene (SLC6A4) has been observed in burnout,[48] and the methylation pattern differs significantly from that seen in depression or stress.[5] Differences in methylation patterns in the brain-derived neurotrophic factor (BDNF) gene have also been observed between burnout, stress, and depression,[5] with burnout being associated with increased methylation of promoter regions I and IV.[49] Potential differences in DNA methylation patterns between burnout and anxiety disorders are unknown.

9.4   BURNOUT AND PHYSICAL HEALTH

Prospective studies suggest that burnout may increase risk of many health problems, including type 2 diabetes[50] and coronary heart disease.[51] Health behaviors may underlie, in part, associations between burnout and physical health. Cross-sectional studies suggest that those reporting greater burnout are more likely to consume more fast food[52] have a sleep disorder,[53] and consume excessive alcohol.[52] For example, each one-point increase in burnout is associated with an 80% increase in alcohol dependence among women, and a 51% increase among men.[54] Those with high burnout may also exercise less often than those with lower burnout,[52,55] such that a one standard deviation increase in burnout is associated with a 21% increase in odds of low physical activity.[55] In contrast, a longitudinal investigation did not identify an association between burnout and exercise over time.[56] A cross-sectional study of more than 3,300 participants reported that those with burnout were 10% more likely to have a physical illness, and results remained significant when accounting for health behaviors.[57] Whether associations between burnout and physical health differ from those identified for depression and anxiety is unknown. Initial evidence suggests that burnout may be associated with obesity and coronary heart disease above and beyond depressive symptoms;[51] however, prospective research is needed to determine whether burnout independently predicts long-term disease risk.

Several biological mechanisms that may link burnout and health have been evaluated, with inconsistent results. For example, increased burnout was associated with higher production of pro-inflammatory cytokines among school teachers,[58] but this association was only observed among women in a separate study.[59] Diurnal cortisol patterns may differ between those who report high vs. lower levels of burnout,[60] but some studies have reported no significant associations between burnout and cortisol.[45] Similarly, evidence both for and against an association between burnout and allostatic load has been observed.[61,62] Given the inconsistent findings, and overlap with biomarkers of depression and anxiety,[63] prospective longitudinal studies that recruit individuals prior to burnout development are needed to differentiate the physiological mechanisms and consequences of burnout.[9]

9.5 INTERVENTIONS FOR BURNOUT

Research suggests that burnout may be receptive to intervention: across 25 intervention studies, 80% effectively reduced burnout.[56] Preventing burnout before it develops is also an emerging area of research. Primordial prevention attempts to alleviate risk factors before they impact an individual; emerging evidence suggests that primordial interventions targeting social support, health behaviors, and coping strategies may effectively prevent burnout development.[64] Primary, secondary, and tertiary interventions have also been tested to reduce burnout after it has developed. Primary interventions, which seek to identify and reduce sources of burnout, are possible at both the system- and individual-level.[64] At the system-level, six key goals have been identified for the primary prevention of burnout: encouraging a positive work environment, creating positive learning environments, reducing administrative burden, enabling the use of technology solutions, providing support to employees, and investing in research.[65] Because burnout is a work-related phenomenon, person-level primary prevention also typically involves the workplace. For example, a biweekly peer support group for clinicians in a Veterans Affairs hospital qualitatively reduced symptoms of burnout, suggesting that providing individuals with adequate institutional support in the workplace may be beneficial.[66]

Secondary and tertiary interventions focus on reducing symptoms and negative consequences of burnout after it has developed. A variety of person-level secondary and tertiary interventions for burnout have been tested, including exercise programs and mindfulness practices, as well as cognitive behavioral therapy, gratitude practices, and art therapy.[67] Exercise-based interventions appear promising, but results are mixed. One meta-analysis reported that no clear differences were seen between experimental and control groups across exercise-based burnout interventions.[68] A more recent meta-analysis of interventions to reduce burnout in students reported that group counseling was the most widely used design, but exercise-based interventions were the most effective.[69] Mindfulness-based interventions may also be beneficial. One systematic review reported that 6 out of 8 studies found significant improvement in burnout after mindfulness training.[70] A separate systematic review and meta-analysis of 17 articles on the efficacy of mindfulness interventions on burnout in nurses also reported beneficial results.[71] Even brief mindfulness interventions may be useful, with 9 out of 14 brief interventions (≤4 hours of training) achieving significant improvement in burnout symptoms.[72] However, two recent systematic reviews on mindfulness interventions for burnout reported inconclusive results, stating that the evidence is low-quality due to methodological issues and a high risk of bias.[73,74] Further research using higher-quality study designs is warranted.

While some evidence suggests that reductions in burnout may remain significant for six months or more,[67] the effects diminish over time and refresher interventions may be necessary.[67] Further, strategies that have been effective in some professions[75] have been ineffective in others.[76] Thus, even if an intervention is successful in one job domain, additional research is required to test efficacy in other fields. Researchers have made progress in developing interventions to reduce burnout, but research to date is limited by small sample sizes, inconsistent methodologies, poor generalizability, and short follow-up periods.[67,73] Measurement concerns and heterogeneous study designs make it difficult to compare the efficacy of interventions.[73] Higher-quality studies that implement randomized controlled designs would help move the field forward.

9.6 CONCLUSIONS

Burnout, a psychological reaction to chronic workplace stress with inadequate coping resources, is characterized by emotional exhaustion, depersonalization, and reduced personal accomplishment.[4,8,77,78] Diagnostic criteria for burnout have not been specified,[5] and it is difficult to differentiate burnout from other mental health concerns.[41] Still, burnout is classified as a unique syndrome by the WHO,[8] and evidence suggests that burnout is common across a wide range of professions, from physicians to police officers.[10]

The literature on burnout and burnout interventions is vast and rapidly growing, yet inconsistent results make interpretation of this body of work challenging. Further complicating the situation, reviews and meta-analyses suggest that much of the evidence regarding the efficacy of burnout interventions is low-quality, with small samples, poorly defined constructs, and substantial heterogeneity in implementation.[73,74] Additional prospective longitudinal studies are sorely needed to advance the field and reduce the burden of burnout on society.

REFERENCES

1. Freudenberger HJ. Staff burn-out. *Journal of Social Issues*. 1974;30(1):159–165.
2. Maslach C, Leiter MP. Understanding burnout: New models. In: Cooper CL, Quick JC, eds. *The Handbook of Stress and Health: A Guide to Research and Practice*. Wiley Blackwell Hoboken, NJ; 2017:36–56.
3. Nabizadeh-Gharghozar Z, Adib-Hajbaghery M, Bolandianbafghi S. Nurses' job burnout: A hybrid concept analysis. *J Caring Sci*. 2020;9(3):154–161.
4. Maslach C, Jackson SE. The measurement of experienced burnout. *J Organ Behav*. 1981;2(2):99–113.
5. Bakusic J, Schaufeli W, Claes S, Godderis L. Stress, burnout and depression: A systematic review on DNA methylation mechanisms. *J Psychosom Res*. 2017;92:34–44.
6. Pines AM, Keinan G. Stress and burnout: The significant difference. *Pers Individ Dif*. 2005;39(3):625–635.
7. Schonfeld IS, Bianchi R. Burnout and depression: Two entities or one? *J Clin Psychol*. 2016;72(1):22–37.
8. World Health Organization. ICD-10: International statistical classification of diseases and related health problems. In: 10th ed. 2019. Available from: https://icd.who.int/browse11/l-m/en#/http://id.who.int/icd/entity/129180281
9. Bayes A, Tavella G, Parker G. The biology of burnout: Causes and consequences. *World J Biol Psychiatry*. 2021;22(9):686–698.

10. Maslach C, Schaufeli WB, Leiter MP. Job burnout. *Annu Rev Psychol.* 2001;52: 397–422. doi:10.1146/annurev.psych.52.1.397.
11. Yates SW. Physician stress and burnout. *Am J Med.* 2020;133(2):160–164.
12. Connor KO, Muller D, Pitman S, O', Connor K, Muller Neff D, Pitman S. Burnout in mental health professionals : A systematic review and meta-analysis of prevalence and determinants. *Eur Psychiatry.* 2018;53:74–99.
13. Gama G, Barbosa F, Vieira M. Personal determinants of nurses' burnout in end of life care. *Eur J Oncol Nurs.* 2014;18(5):527–533.
14. Crowe RP, Fernandez AR, Pepe PE, Cash RE, Rivard MK, Wronski R, et al. The association of job demands and resources with burnout among emergency medical services professionals. *J Am Coll Emerg Physicians Open.* 2020;1(1):6–16.
15. Schwartz RH, Tiamiyu MF, Dwyer DJ. Social worker hope and perceived burnout: The effects of age, years in practice, and setting. *Adm Soc Work.* 2007;31(4):103–119.
16. Eklund RC, DeFreese JD. Athlete burnout. In: Tenenbaum G, Eklund RC, Boiangin N, eds. *Handbook of Sport Psychology.* 2020;II:1220–1240.
17. Hultell D, Melin B, Gustavsson JP. Getting personal with teacher burnout: A longitudinal study on the development of burnout using a person-based approach. *Teach Teach Educ.* 2013;32:75–86.
18. Madigan DJ, Curran T. Does burnout affect academic achievement? A meta-analysis of over 100,000 students. *Educ Psychol Rev.* 2021;33(2):387–405.
19. Wilcox VL. Burnout in military personnel. In: Jones FD, ed. *Military Psychiatry: Preparing in Peace for War.* Washington (DC): Government Printing Office; 2000:31–49.
20. Ayachit M, Chitta S. A systematic review of burnout studies from the hospitality literature. *J Hosp Mark Manag.* 2022;31(2):125–144.
21. Truchot D, Andela M. Burnout and hopelessness among farmers: The farmers stressors inventory. *Soc Psychiatry Psychiatr Epidemiol.* 2018;53(8):859–867.
22. Roskam I, Raes ME, Mikolajczak M. Exhausted parents: Development and preliminary validation of the parental burnout inventory. *Front Psychol.* 2017;8(FEB):1–12.
23. Le Vigouroux S, Scola C, Raes ME, Mikolajczak M, Roskam I. The big five personality traits and parental burnout: Protective and risk factors. *Pers Individ Dif.* 2017;119:216–219.
24. Truzzi A, Valente L, Ulstein I, Engelhardt E, Laks J, Engedal K. Burnout in familial caregivers of patients with dementia. *Rev Bras Psiquiatr.* 2012;34(4):405–412.
25. Gérain P, Zech E. Do informal caregivers experience more burnout? A meta-analytic study. *Psychol Heal Med.* 2021;26(2):145–161.
26. Chen CW, Gorski PC. Burnout in social justice and human rights activists: Symptoms, causes and implications. *J Hum Rights Pract.* 2015;7(3):366–390.
27. Gorski PC. Racial battle fatigue and activist burnout in racial justice activists of color at predominately White colleges and universities. *Race Ethn Educ.* 2019;22(1):1–20.
28. Pines AM. Burnout in political activism: An existential perspective. *J Health Hum Resour Adm.* 1994;16(4):381–394.
29. Hooker SA, Post RE, Sherman MD. Awareness of meaning in life is protective against burnout among family physicians. *Fam Med.* 2020;52(1):11–16.
30. Maslach C, Leiter MP. *The Truth About Burnout: How Organizations Cause Personal Stress and What to Do About It.* John Wiley & Sons; 1997.
31. Sousa T, Neves P. Two tales of rumination and burnout: Examining the effects of boredom and overload. *Appl Psychol.* 2021;70(3):1018–1044.
32. Violanti JM, Mnatsakanova A, Andrew ME, Allison P, Gu JK, Fekedulegn D. Effort–reward imbalance and overcommitment at work: Associations with police burnout. *Police Q.* 2018;21(4):440–460.
33. Jackson-Koku G, Grime P. Emotion regulation and burnout in doctors: A systematic review. *Occup Med (Chic Ill).* 2019;69(1):9–21.

34. Ahola K, Hakanen J. Job strain, burnout, and depressive symptoms: A prospective study among dentists. *J Affect Disord.* 2007;104(1–3):103–110.
35. Newton TL, Ohrt JH, Guest JD, Wymer B. Influence of mindfulness, emotion regulation, and perceived social support on burnout. *Couns Educ Superv.* 2020;59(4): 252–266.
36. Purvanova RK, Muros JP. Gender differences in burnout: A meta-analysis. *J Vocat Behav.* 2010;77(2):168–185.
37. Bianchi R, Schonfeld IS, Laurent E. Burnout-depression overlap: A review. *Clin Psychol Rev.* 2015;36:28–41.
38. Bianchi R, Boffy C, Hingray C, Truchot D, Laurent E. Comparative symptomatology of burnout and depression. *J Health Psychol.* 2013;18(6):782–787.
39. Brenninkmeyer V, Van Yperen NW, Buunk BP. Burnout and depression are not identical twins: Is decline of superiority a distinguishing feature? *Pers Individ Dif.* 2001;30(5):873–880.
40. Toker S, Biron M. Job burnout and depression: Unraveling their temporal relationship and considering the role of physical activity. *J Appl Psychol.* 2012;97(3):699–710.
41. Koutsimani P, Montgomery A, Georganta K. The relationship between burnout, depression, and anxiety: A systematic review and meta-analysis. *Front Psychol.* 2019;10(284):1–19.
42. Bakker AB, Schaufeli WB, Demerouti E, Janssen PP, Van Der Hulst R, Brouwer J. Using equity theory to examine the difference between burnout and depression. *Anxiety, Stress Coping.* 2000;247–268.
43. Glass DC, McKnight JD. Perceived control, depressive symptomatology, and professional burnout: A review of the evidence. *Psychol Health.* 1996;11(1):23–48.
44. Vassilopoulos SP. Job burnout and its relation to social anxiety in teachers of primary education. *Hell J Psychol.* 2012;9(1):18–44.
45. Sertoz OO, Binbay IT, Koylu E, Noyan A, Yıldırım E, Mete HE. The role of BDNF and HPA axis in the neurobiology of burnout syndrome. *Prog Neuro-Psychopharmacol Biol Psychiatry.* 2008;32(6):1459–1465.
46. Belvederi Murri M, Pariante C, Mondelli V, Masotti M, Atti AR, Mellacqua Z, et al. HPA axis and aging in depression: Systematic review and meta-analysis. *Psychoneuroendocrinology.* 2014;41:46–62.
47. Faravelli C, Lo Sauro C, Lelli L, Pietrini F, Lazzeretti L, Godini L, et al. The role of life events and HPA axis in anxiety disorders: A review. *Curr Pharm Des.* 2012; 18(35):5663–5674.
48. Bakusic J, Ghosh M, Polli A, Bekaert B, Schaufeli W, Claes S, et al. Role of NR3C1 and SLC6A4 methylation in the HPA axis regulation in burnout. *J Affect Disord.* 2021; 295(January):505–512.
49. Bakusic J, Ghosh M, Polli A, Bekaert B, Schaufeli W, Claes S, et al. Epigenetic perspective on the role of brain-derived neurotrophic factor in burnout. *Transl Psychiatry.* 2020;10(1):1–9.
50. Melamed S, Shirom A, Toker S, Shapira I. Burnout and risk of type 2 diabetes: A prospective study of apparently healthy employed persons. *Psychosom Med.* 2006;68(6): 863–869.
51. Toker S, Melamed S, Berliner S, Zeltser D, Shapira I. Burnout and risk of coronary heart disease: A prospective study of 8838 employees. *Psychosom Med.* 2012; 74(8):840–847.
52. Alexandrova-Karamanova A, Todorova I, Montgomery A, Panagopoulou E, Costa P, Baban A, et al. Burnout and health behaviors in health professionals from seven European countries. *Int Arch Occup Environ Health.* 2016;89(7):1059–1075.
53. Armon G. Do burnout and insomnia predict each other's levels of change over time independently of the job demand control-support (JDC-S) model? *Stress Heal.* 2009; 25(4):333–342.

54. Ahola K, Honkonen T, Pirkola S, Isometsä E, Kalimo R, Nykyri E, et al. Alcohol dependence in relation to burnout among the Finnish working population. *Addiction.* 2006;101(10):1438–1443.

55. Ahola K, Pulkki-râback L, Kouvonen A, Rossi H, Aromaa A. Burnout and behavior-related health risk factors: Results from the population-based Finnish health 2000 study. *J Occup Environ Med.* 2012;54(1):17–22.

56. de Vries JD, Bakker AB. The physical activity paradox: A longitudinal study of the implications for burnout. *Int Arch Occup Environ Health.* 2021;95(1):1–15.

57. Honkonen T, Ahola K, Pertovaara M, Isometsä E, Kalimo R, Nykyri E, et al. The association between burnout and physical illness in the general population-results from the Finnish health 2000 study. *J Psychosom Res.* 2006;61(1):59–66.

58. von Känel R, Bellingrath S, Kudielka BM. Association between burnout and circulating levels of pro- and anti-inflammatory cytokines in schoolteachers. *J Psychosom Res.* 2008;65(1):51–59.

59. Toker S, Shirom A, Shapira I, Berliner S, Melamed S. The association between burnout, depression, anxiety, and inflammation biomarkers: C-reactive protein and fibrinogen in men and women. *J Occup Health Psychol.* 2005;10(4):344–362.

60. Marchand A, Durand P, Juster RP, Lupien SJ. Workers' psychological distress, depression, and burnout symptoms: Associations with diurnal cortisol profiles. *Scand J Work Environ Heal.* 2014;40(3):305–314.

61. Juster RP, Sindi S, Marin MF, Perna A, Hashemi A, Pruessner JC, et al. A clinical allostatic load index is associated with burnout symptoms and hypocortisolemic profiles in healthy workers. *Psychoneuroendocrinology.* 2011;36(6):797–805.

62. Langelaan S, Bakker AB, Schaufeli WB, Van Rhenen W, Van Doornen LJP. Is burnout related to allostatic load? *Int J Behav Med.* 2007;14(4):213–221.

63. O'Connor DB, Thayer JF, Vedhara K. Stress and health: A review of psychobiological processes. *Annu Rev Psychol.* 2021;72:663–688.

64. Merlo G, Rippe J. Physician burnout: A lifestyle medicine perspective. *Am J Lifestyle Med.* 2021;15(2):148–157.

65. National Academies of Sciences Engineering and Medicine, Committee on Systems Approaches to Improve Patient Care by Supporting Clinician Well-Being. Taking Action Against Clinician Burnout: A Systems Approach to Professional Well-being. National Academies Press; 2019. Accessed November 27, 2020. 2019. Available from: https://www.ncbi.nlm.nih.gov/books/NBK552618/

66. Schwartz R, Shanafelt TD, Gimmler C, Osterberg L. Developing institutional infrastructure for physician wellness: Qualitative insights from VA physicians. *BMC Health Serv Res.* 2020;20(1):1–9.

67. Awa WL, Plaumann M, Walter U. Burnout prevention: A review of intervention programs. *Patient Educ Couns.* 2010;78(2):184–190.

68. Ochentel O, Humphrey C, Pfeifer K. Efficacy of exercise therapy in persons with burnout. A systematic review and meta-analysis. *J Sport Sci Med.* 2018;17(3):475–484.

69. Tang L, Zhang F, Yin R, Fan Z. Effect of interventions on learning burnout: A systematic review and meta-analysis. *Front Psychol.* 2021;12(February):1–13.

70. Luken M, Sammons A. Systematic review of mindfulness practice for reducing job burnout. *Am J Occup Ther.* 2016;70(2):p1-7002250020.

71. Suleiman-Martos N, Gomez-Urquiza JL, Aguayo-Estremera R, Cañadas-De La Fuente GA, De La Fuente-Solana EI, Albendín-García L. The effect of mindfulness training on burnout syndrome in nursing: A systematic review and meta-analysis. *J Adv Nurs.* 2020;76(5):1124–1140.

72. Gilmartin H, Goyal A, Hamati MC, Mann J, Saint S, Chopra V. Brief mindfulness practices for healthcare providers: A systematic literature review. *Am J Med.* 2017;130(10):1219.e1–1219.e17.

73. Klein A, Taieb O, Xavier S, Baubet T, Reyre A. The benefits of mindfulness-based interventions on burnout among health professionals: A systematic review. *Explore*. 2020;16:35–43.

74. Salvado M, Marques DL, Pires IM, Silva NM. Mindfulness-based interventions to reduce burnout in primary healthcare professionals: A systematic review and meta-analysis. *Healthcare*. 2021;9(10), 1–15.

75. Darban F, Balouchi A, Narouipou A, Safarzaei E, Shahdadi H. Effect of communication skills training on the burnout of nurses: A cross-sectional study. *J Clin Diagnostic Res*. 2016;10(4):IC01–IC04.

76. Bragard I, Etienne AM, Merckaert I, Libert Y, Razavi D. Efficacy of a communication and stress management training on medical residents' self-efficacy, stress to communicate and burnout: A randomized controlled study. *J Health Psychol*. 2010;15(7): 1075–1081.

77. Golembiewski RT, Munzenrider RF. Phases of burnout, modes and social support: Contributions to explaining differences in physical symptoms. *J Manag Issues*. 1990; 2(2):176–183.

78. Gryskiewicz N, Buttner EH. Testing the robustness of the progressive phase burnout model for a sample of entrepreneurs. *Educ Psychol Meas*. 1992;52(3):747–751.

Section II

Biopsychosocial Processes
Basic Concepts and Disease Implications

10 Neurobiology

Lorena A. Ferguson, MA and
Stephanie L. Leal, PhD

KEY POINTS

- Neurobiology is essential for understanding the biopsychosocial processes underlying mental and neurological health.
- Advances in human neuroimaging methods have substantially increased our understanding of the neural mechanisms underlying disease states such as depression, anxiety, and dementia.
- Neuroimaging biomarkers have become a key component of measuring the impact of disease on brain health as well as informing the development of more targeted interventions.
- Lifestyle factors may augment mental and neurological health in clinical populations, and offer affordable, non-invasive means of both preventing and managing symptoms.

10.1 INTRODUCTION

Neurobiology is the study of cells of the nervous system and their organization into the functional circuits that process information and mediate behavior. It is an essential component of biopsychosocial processes, which considers biological, psychological, and social factors and their complex interactions in understanding health and disease. Understanding how the brain works, from the cellular to the cognitive level, is essential for unraveling the complexities of human experience. In this chapter, we will review basic concepts of neurobiology and describe their implications for understanding mental health and neurological disorders. We will then discuss advances in neuroimaging techniques, which have allowed unprecedented access to the neural mechanisms underlying health and disease.

10.2 BASIC CONCEPTS IN NEUROBIOLOGY

10.2.1 THE CENTRAL NERVOUS SYSTEM

The *central nervous system* (CNS) comprises the brain and spinal cord. The *brainstem* comprises the *medulla, pons,* and *midbrain* and is involved in essential physiological processes such as breathing, blood pressure, heart rate, and sleep.[1] The *peripheral nervous system* (PNS), which includes all the nerve fibers in the body outside of the brain and spinal cord, relays information to and from the CNS. The brain is made up of *grey and white matter. Grey matter* refers to the unmyelinated

DOI: 10.1201/b22810-12

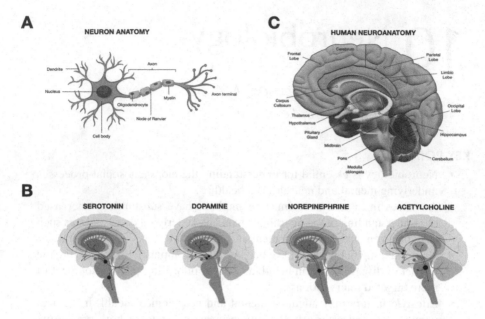

FIGURE 10.1 Neurobiology of the human brain. A) Neuron structure, B) Neurotransmitter systems, C) Human neuroanatomy.

cell bodies that make up the brain's outer cortex and innermost regions. *White matter* refers to the *fiber tracts* that connect cell bodies. They are wrapped in a fatty layer, called myelin, which allows electrical impulses to travel quickly.[2]

10.2.2 Cell Types in the Human Brain

The human brain contains approximately 86 billion neurons and 85 billion glial cells.[3]. *Neurons* are the nerve cells of the brain and are responsible for everything from receiving external sensory input to communicating with the rest of the body.[4] *Glial cells* are the support cells of the brain and are involved in a variety of different functions, such as maintaining homeostasis and helping keep unwanted substances out of the brain.[5] Oligodendrocytes are responsible for creating the myelin sheaths that surround white matter tracts[6] (Figure 10.1A).

10.2.3 Neuron Structure & Function

All *neurons* contain three basic features: the *cell body* (which houses the DNA of the cell), *dendrites* (which receive information), and an *axon* (which sends information) (Figure 10.1A). Dendrites branch from the cell body, and at the end of each dendrite are receptors that become activated by neurotransmitters. The axon is a long structure that extends from the cell body.

Information travels down the axon through an *action potential*, an electrical signal that triggers the release of neurotransmitters into the *synapse*, the gap between neurons. On the other side of the synapse are the dendrites of another neuron, which allows neurons to communicate with one another.[7]

10.2.4 NEUROTRANSMITTERS

Neurotransmitters are the chemical messengers generated within neurons that transmit information from neuron to neuron (Figure 10.1B). Different kinds of neurotransmitters serve different functions. *Glutamate* is an excitatory neurotransmitter that is associated with neural plasticity, or the ability of neurons to change activity in response to stimuli.[8] Plasticity is essential for functions such as learning, memory, and recovery from brain injury.[9] Gamma-aminobutyric acid (*GABA*) is the primary inhibitory neurotransmitter in the brain and controls the excessive firing of neurons, which can in turn do such things as inhibiting motor movement.[7,10] *Serotonin* (5-HT) is secreted from the Raphe nuclei of the brainstem and plays a role in regulating emotion, memory, and mood.[4,11] *Dopamine* (DA) is secreted from the substantia nigra and ventral tegmental area of the brainstem and plays an important role in reward, executive function, and motor function.[4] DA can have both excitatory and inhibitory effects.[12] *Norepinephrine* (NE) is produced in the locus coeruleus (LC) of the brainstem and is involved in learning, memory, emotion, and fight-or-flight functions.[13,14] *Acetylcholine* (ACh) is synthesized in the basal forebrain and plays a role in learning, memory, and arousal.[15]

10.2.5 FUNCTIONAL NEUROANATOMY

The brain can be broadly divided into four lobes: frontal, parietal, temporal, and occipital (Figure 10.1C). The *frontal lobe* is the largest lobe in the brain, accounting for roughly 40% of the total brain volume.[16] The *prefrontal cortex* (PFC) is responsible for executive functions such as inhibition, goal-directed behavior, and working memory.[17] The PFC can be subdivided into smaller anatomical areas, with two common divisions being the *dorsolateral* (DLPFC) and *ventromedial* (VMPFC) cortices.[18,19] The DLPFC is broadly involved in cognitive control processes,[20] while the VMPFC is responsible for reward and emotion processing.[21-23] Another important region is the *anterior cingulate cortex* (ACC), which is involved in both cognitive and emotional processes, such as error detection.[24] The *parietal lobe* is located posterior to the frontal lobe and is involved in the integration of sensory information processing. A parietal region of note is the *posterior cingulate cortex* (PCC), which is involved in internally focused cognition.[25,26]

The *temporal lobes* support a wide variety of functions, including memory, emotion, and language. The *medial temporal lobe* (MTL) includes the hippocampus, extrahippocampal cortices, and amygdala, and is crucial for memory and emotion processing.[27,28] The *hippocampus* is essential for creating new episodic memories, or memories for events.[29] However, memories are not stored within the hippocampus. Instead, it acts as an index to memories distributed throughout the cortex.[30,31] The hippocampus is composed of several subfields, including hippocampal cornu ammonis (CA1-4), the subiculum, and the dentate gyrus (DG). Two hippocampal computations play an important role in memory: pattern completion and pattern separation.[32].

Pattern completion is the process of remembering an event when partial cues are present (e.g., recognizing your friend even though they got a haircut) and relies on hippocampal CA3. *Pattern separation* is the process of reducing interference across similar experiences (e.g., remembering where you parked your car today versus yesterday) and relies on hippocampal DG. Balancing between these two computations is essential for memory. Adjacent to the hippocampus is the *amygdala*, which is responsive to emotionally salient events[33] and can modulate memory.[13]. Finally, the *occipital lobe* is responsible for visual processing. The primary visual cortex, or V1, is involved in early processing of visual stimuli. Different visual elements are extracted and sent to other, more specialized areas for further processing of specific features (e.g., V2 for color, V5 for motion).[34,35]

10.2.6 Neuroimaging Methodology

Historically, psychology has relied on patients with lesions to determine which brain areas were involved in which functions. Take, for instance, the famous case of Phineas Gage, a railroad worker who had an iron spike driven through his frontal lobe. He subsequently suffered from executive dysfunction and erratic behavior, thus suggesting that the frontal lobe was essential for regulation of executive function.[36] Thankfully, the advent of neuroimaging technologies allows for less invasive measures than an iron spike through regions of interest.

Magnetic Resonance Imaging (MRI) is a neuroimaging technique that generates detailed structural brain images (Figure 10.2A). It does so through the use of a powerful magnet, which briefly aligns hydrogen protons to the MRI scanner's magnetic field.[37] Weak electromagnetic pulses then misalign the hydrogen protons from the magnetic field. When the pulse ends, the protons realign to the magnetic field and produce radiofrequency signals. These signals are then captured by the MRI scanner and translated into images of the brain, which are grouped into 3D squares called *voxels*.[37] High-resolution MRI scans allow unprecedented visualization of small cortical structures, such as the hippocampal subfields, that are not possible to visualize using traditional MRI.[38] Another way to assess brain structure is through *Diffusion Tensor Imaging* (DTI), which measures white matter tracts in the brain. It assesses the directionality and motion of water molecules within axons and provides images of white matter tract integrity (Figure 10.2B).[39]

A   B   C

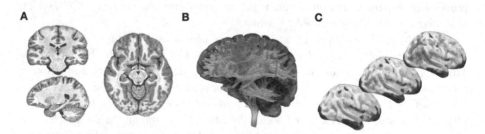

FIGURE 10.2 Neuroimaging methods of the human brain. A) Structural magnetic resonance imaging (MRI) scan, B) diffusion tensor imaging (DTI) scan, C) longitudinal PET imaging using the [18F]AV-1451 tau tracer.

Functional MRI (fMRI) scans assess the functional properties of the brain. fMRI does not directly measure neural activity but instead relies on an indirect measure of blood flow.[40] Brain regions that are active and involved in a cognitive process should consume higher levels of oxygen. The differences in the magnetic properties of oxygenated and deoxygenated blood are what generate the Blood Oxygen-Level Dependent (BOLD) response,[41] which can then be used to determine brain function during a particular task relative to a control condition.

Resting-state fMRI scans are used to measure the functional properties of the brain at rest. This provides insight into networks of brain regions, such as the *default mode network* (DMN), that are active when no explicit task is being performed. The DMN is composed of the PCC, precuneus, medial PFC, and MTL.[25] The DMN plays an important role in self-referential processing, such as autobiographical memory and theory of mind.[25,42]

Positron Emission Tomography (PET) can be used to measure metabolism, glucose uptake, proteins, and neurotransmitters.[43] Participants are injected with a radioactive tracer, which binds to the ligand or tissue of interest. As the radioactive tracer decays, positrons are emitted and collide with nearby electrons, producing gamma rays. The PET scanner analyzes these gamma rays to determine the rate and location of the decay.[43] One commonly used tracer is [^{18}F]FDG, which is used to measure glucose metabolism.[44] Some PET tracers are specialized for binding to beta-amyloid (Aβ) and tau proteins, which are implicated in Alzheimer's disease (AD)[45,46] (Figure 10.2C). However, PET has relatively poor temporal resolution compared to MRI, and the tracers are susceptible to off-target binding.[47]

Electroencephalography (EEG) measures the electrical signals of the brain. EEG directly measures neural activity rather than relying on indirect methods. As neurons fire, electrodes placed on the scalp sum the charges of the surrounding neurons to generate a neural signal.[48] This gives rise to patterns of oscillations, which are dependent on neural firing rates. There is evidence that these oscillations are tied to specific cognitive functions.[48,49] However, it can be difficult to measure the neural signals from deep cortical structures, limiting the brain regions that can be measured with this technique.

Transcranial magnetic stimulation (TMS) is the process of magnetically stimulating areas of the cortex to selectively inhibit, and occasionally excite, neurons in a given area. This is done by holding a small magnetic coil over an individual's head and inducing a focal magnetic field. This creates a sort of virtual lesion, where the affected region is briefly incapable of performing its functions.[50] TMS is a relatively affordable, non-invasive way of determining whether a cortical region is necessary for a given cognitive process. However, a limitation of this method is that TMS can only stimulate brain regions close to the skull.

10.3 DISEASE IMPLICATIONS

10.3.1 DEPRESSION

10.3.1.1 Neurobiological Impairments

Depression is characterized by emotional dysregulation (such as depressed mood and anhedonia), sleep and concentration problems, and memory impairment[51,52] Neurobiological changes include reduced neuroplasticity, particularly in the MTL and frontal lobe,[53] as well as neuroinflammation[54] and dysregulation of neurotransmitters.[55,56] The frontal lobe is vulnerable in depressed individuals,[57,58] who show VMPFC hyperactivity and dorsolateral cortex (DLPFC) hypoactivity while viewing emotional stimuli.[59] This PFC dysfunction is associated with changes in self-referential processing, such as guilt, self-dislike, and rumination,[23,60,61] impaired emotion regulation, and symptoms such as lack of motivation and flat affect.[23,62] The ACC is also impacted in depression and is associated with apathy and impaired response inhibition[63] as well as reductions in amygdala-ACC connectivity when viewing emotional stimuli.[64] These frontal disruptions provide a neural basis for some of the emotional dysfunction present in depression.

Within the MTL, the amygdala shows heightened activity in response to negative stimuli in depressed individuals.[65,66] Depression is also associated with reduced hippocampal volume[67,68] and declines in hippocampal neurogenesis, the process of generating new neurons.[69] These hippocampal changes are associated with worse memory and greater symptom severity[70,71] However, memory for negative stimuli is enhanced in depression.[72,73] This negativity bias may be due to increased connectivity between the amygdala and hippocampus.[65] Mnemonic discrimination tasks that tax hippocampal pattern separation have found that depressed individuals show decreased hippocampal DG/CA3 activity and increased amygdala activity when remembering negative stimuli.[74] It has been proposed that hippocampal pattern separation deficits may be indicative of depression[75] and offer a more sensitive framework for detecting neural changes in clinical populations.[76]

10.3.1.2 Treatments and Interventions

Depression is commonly treated through psychotherapy and pharmacological approaches.[77] Some of the most common pharmacological treatments are *antidepressants*, such as selective serotonin reuptake inhibitors (SSRIs). However, not all patients respond to pharmacological treatment,[78] with beneficial effects potentially being limited only to those with the most severe depressive symptoms.[79] Recent evidence has suggested it may be more accurate to classify depression as a neuroplasticity disorder, where stress causes reduced neuroplasticity in the hippocampus and PFC.[53] SSRIs can induce synaptic plasticity and hippocampal neurogenesis and improve memory, especially when combined with other behaviors that induce neuroplasticity, such as exercise.[80–82]

Another treatment for depression is *electroconvulsive therapy* (ECT), which is reserved for those with severe or treatment-resistant depression.[83] ECT works by sending brief electrical pulses to the brain through electrodes applied to the scalp, causing mild seizures. This stimulates greater neurotransmitter transmission and promotes neuroplasticity, which can lead to increased hippocampal and amygdala volume and reductions in depressive symptoms.[83,84] A more recently developed treatment is *repetitive TMS* (rTMS), in which a series of electromagnetic currents are delivered to cortical regions, such as the PFC, over time to regulate brain activity.[85] However, rTMS may be more efficacious for certain types of depressive symptoms. A recent study found that resting-state functional connectivity patterns in depressed participants could be clustered into four distinct biotypes, each of which was associated with certain behavioral features of depression such as anxiety, fatigue, and anhedonia.[86] These depression biotypes can then be used to predict rTMS treatment responsiveness.[86]

Lifestyle interventions such as exercise, social engagement, sleep, and diet have shown promise as a means of preventing depression and alleviating depressive symptoms.[87–91] Exercise stimulates hippocampal neurogenesis and has been associated with improvements in memory and mood.[92,93] Furthermore, engaging in more social activity and having more social ties may also reduce symptoms of depression.[94,95] However, only high-quality relationships appear to be associated with improvements in mental health.[96] In contrast, sleep disturbances have been associated with increases in neuroinflammation and disruptions in cortical function, both of which can increase the risk of depression and exacerbate depressive symptoms.[97] Thus, a good night's sleep is an important factor in promoting well-being. Finally, there is also emerging evidence that diets high in foods such as whole grains, vegetables, and fish, such as the Mediterranean diet, are associated with reductions in depressive symptoms.[98,99] Healthier diets can reduce inflammation, regulate cortisol levels, and promote hippocampal neurogenesis.[98] Thus, lifestyle interventions offer a promising method for alleviating depressive symptoms and improving quality of life.

Training emotion regulation skills has also shown promise in treating depressive symptoms[100,101] and may provide a method to normalize memory[102,103] and aberrant brain activity in depression. Previous work has shown that brief training in cognitive reappraisal via distancing – which involves appraising an emotional situation as an objective, rational observer (third person) – can reduce self-reported negative affect,[104,105] perceived stress,[104] and amygdala activity when viewing negative stimuli[105] in both healthy[104–106] and depressed populations.[106,107] Reappraisal via immersion – which involves appraising an emotional situation from a first-person perspective – may be especially beneficial for improving older adults' well-being when processing positive stimuli.[108] These strategies offer an innovative and practical way to modify affect, memory, and brain dysfunction. Another promising intervention strategy is increasing heart rate variability through breathing exercises. This has been associated with improvements in inhibitory control, a critical feature of emotion regulation, in both younger and older adults.[109] These treatment methods could potentially be enhanced by *real-time fMRI neurofeedback training* (fMRI-NF), where participants are shown their neural activity in real-time and are trained to regulate their brain activity, typically through depictions of their neural activity as a kind of thermometer that needs to be kept in an ideal range.[110] Using fMRI-NF, depressed patients can upregulate PFC activity,[111] a region important for emotion regulation,[112] and amygdala responses to positive autobiographical memories,[113] thereby improving mood and emotion regulation abilities and reducing depressive symptom severity. This is promising evidence for development of more personalized and nuanced approaches to treating mood disorders.

10.3.2 ANXIETY

10.3.2.1 Neurobiological Impairments

Anxiety is characterized by excessive worry, which can include symptoms of irritability, sleep disturbances, and concentration difficulty.[114] There is significant overlap in the neurobiological mechanisms underlying depression and anxiety, and these disorders are often comorbid.[115] There is reduced PFC and ACC activation in response to negative stimuli in anxious patients, suggesting difficulties recruiting top-down emotion regulation processes.[116,117] Anxiety is also associated with alterations in amygdala volume as well as amygdala hyperactivity in response to negative stimuli.[118] There is reduced connectivity between the amygdala and the VMPFC and ACC[119, 120] and increased connectivity between the hippocampus and PFC, which is associated with greater symptom severity.[121] Additionally, anxiety is associated with higher levels of glutamate[122,123] and declines in GABA, which may result in reduced top-down regulation.[124] This dysregulation of excitatory and inhibitory systems may lead to the overgeneralized fear response to nonthreatening stimuli characteristic of anxiety.[125] A recent study utilizing a mnemonic discrimination task (which taxes hippocampal pattern separation) in those with anxiety found that anxiety symptoms were associated with impaired recognition of negative stimuli.[126] This is in contrast to the enhanced memory for negative stimuli observed in depression,[72,73] suggesting that while there is a lot of overlap between these conditions, there are points of differentiation that could be useful when developing more targeted treatments.

Neuroimaging methods have been a valuable means of studying the structural and functional changes associated with anxiety. A recent study utilized MRI to determine how state (transient) and trait (stable personability characteristics) anxiety differentially affected brain structure and function. They found evidence of a neuroanatomical and functional distinction between state and trait anxiety, suggesting these neural features (namely grey matter measures and resting-state functional connectivity) may be important markers when evaluating treatment effects in anxiety disorders.[127]

10.3.2.2 Treatment and Interventions

Many of the pharmacological treatments for anxiety overlap with those for depression. Each of these treatments has its limitations, although there is promising evidence that targeting glutamate and GABA may be particularly beneficial as they are the core source of neurophysiological dysfunction in anxiety.[125,128] As with depression, exercise, social connection, good relationship quality, undisturbed sleep, healthy diets, and emotion regulation training may augment these effects.[96,97,129–132] Imaging techniques could also provide predictive value as to which treatments work best. For example, PTSD patients who responded well to either psychotherapeutic or pharmacological treatments had reduced functional connectivity across DMN and saliency network regions compared to non-responders, suggesting that resting-state functional connectivity may be predictive of treatment response.[133] This offers exciting promise for the utility of neuroimaging measures in informing treatment plans.

10.3.3 Alzheimer's Disease and Related Dementias (ADRD)

10.3.3.1 Neurobiological Impairments

Alzheimer's disease (AD) is the most common form of dementia, accounting for about 60-80% of dementia cases.[134] It is a progressive neurodegenerative disease that is characterized by severe memory impairment, Aβ plaques and tau tangles throughout the brain, and neurodegeneration.[135] Aβ are neurotoxic extracellular plaque deposits,[136] and tau is a protein that becomes phosphorylated and aggregates to form neurofibrillary tangles in AD.[137] However, tau pathology is not unique to AD, as it is also found in frontotemporal dementia (FTD) and dementia with Lewy bodies (DLB)[138,139] According to the *amyloid cascade hypothesis*, Aβ is the initiating event of AD that causes tau accumulation, which then leads to neurodegeneration.[140] However, this hypothesis has been hotly debated, as evidence has shown that Aβ is not strongly associated with cognitive decline[141] and begins to develop decades before clinical symptom onset.[142] Tau appears to be more predictive of clinical severity than Aβ.[143] More recent evidence has suggested that the interaction between these pathologies offers a better explanation for cognitive decline than Aβ alone.[144,145]

An official diagnosis of AD has traditionally relied on postmortem analyses of brain tissue to determine the presence of characteristic AD pathology. However, advances in neuroimaging technology allow us to now examine these pathologies *in vivo*. Structural MRI has been useful for imaging cortical atrophy (neurodegeneration) and determining which regions are affected early in the disease, often before clinical symptoms manifest.[146] PET imaging allows for the visualization of tau and Aβ pathology in the living brain. There is recent evidence that tau PET tracer uptake predicts the rate of later cortical atrophy in patients with early AD.[147] Neuroimaging methods have also been critical for differentiating types of dementias, such as FTD from AD. FTD encompasses a broad group of dementias that affect the frontal and temporal lobes[148] and is often misdiagnosed as AD, which has implications for treatment.[149]

Memory declines are a characteristic feature of aging and AD.[150] There are a host of age-related changes in the MTL, such as reduced hippocampal volume[151,152] and hippocampal hyperactivity,[153] which has been associated with greater Aβ accumulation and increased cognitive decline.[154] There are also alterations in hippocampal subfield dynamics, which leads to a shift away from pattern separation to pattern completion in aging.[32,155] Therefore, older adults have a harder time distinguishing the details of an experience and instead overgeneralize memories.[32] This pattern separation deficit appears early in aging, making it a useful measure of early age-related memory decline.[156,157] One of the first regions to show tau pathology is the LC.[158,159] The LC has extensive projections to the MTL, which may be how tau travels into the MTL, another early site of tau pathology in AD.[160,161] Novel imaging techniques using neuromelanin-sensitive MRI have only recently been developed to visualize LC integrity in humans.[162] Assessing LC integrity in conjunction with sensitive cognitive tasks will be necessary for the early detection of pathological changes.

10.3.3.2 Treatment and Interventions

Current treatments for AD are largely ineffective, mainly because we still do not know the underlying cause of AD. *Cholinesterase inhibitors* are the primary form of treatment for the symptoms of AD.[163] The cholinergic hypothesis of aging states that dysfunction in the cholinergic system, which is integral for learning and memory, contributes to the cognitive declines present in AD.[164] While not curative, cholinesterase inhibitors may offer a viable solution for prolonging memory and cognitive function in AD.[165] A recent target for treatment is *hippocampal hyperactivity*. *Levetiracetam*, an antiepileptic drug, can reduce hippocampal hyperactivity and improve pattern separation ability in patients with mild cognitive impairment, MCI.[166] Another approach is to target Aβ, such as through the drug *aducanumab*.[167] However, while effective in removing Aβ, it is unclear whether aducanumab improves cognitive function.[168] This may be because the drug is given too late, once irreversible damage has already been done, or perhaps because there is a better target for rescuing cognition, such as tau.[143] Neuroimaging techniques are crucial for understanding how pathology progresses over the development of AD, but also for detecting early neural changes before clinical symptoms appear. The earlier we can detect age-related changes, the earlier we can intervene to prevent or slow the progression of dementia.[169]

Modifiable risk factors have been identified, such as low levels of education, social isolation, and infrequent exercise, that offer promising means of protecting against dementia and slowing disease progression.[170] Psychological stress also increases the risk of developing dementia,[171,172] but exercise[173] and social support[174] show promise in buffering these detrimental effects. Greater educational attainment early in life is a protective factor in the development of AD, and remaining cognitively active throughout life can reduce dementia risk.[172,175] Additionally, exercise promotes hippocampal neurogenesis, reduces neuroinflammation, and can slow accumulation of AD pathology.[176] Light to moderate levels of aerobic exercise, such as walking several times a week, show promise as a means of slowing cognitive decline and protecting against dementia.[177,178] Loneliness is common in late life and has been associated with dementia risk.[179] Thus, remaining socially active and maintaining high-quality relationships[180] are important for preserving cognition.[172] Interventions promoting community engagement may help protect cognition and promote neuroplasticity in older adults.[181,182] Sleep is another important intervention target in aging and dementia. Sleep is important for clearing toxins, including pathological AD proteins, from the brain, but older adults frequently experience sleep disruptions which can reduce the efficacy of this clearing process.[183,184] Thus, enhancing sleep quality, such as through cognitive behavioral therapy or exercise,[185] may help reduce the risk of AD.[172] Diets high in fish, caffeine, and green vegetables, such as the Mediterranean diet, have been associated with increased cortical thickness, preserved cognition, reduced neuroinflammation, and a lower burden of AD pathology.[186] Implementing these lifestyle practices across the lifespan may prove to be an important way of reducing the incidence of dementia later in life.[187] Finally, environment is a factor that is not as easily modifiable but is nonetheless important when considering dementia risk. Environmental issues such as pollution[188] and low neighborhood socioeconomic status[189,190] can increase the risk of developing dementia, while exposure to more green space may be associated with reduced risk of AD.[191]

10.3.3.3 Comorbidities across Neurological and Mental Health

Finally, it is important to note that dementia and mood disorders, particularly depression, are highly comorbid.[192] These disorders share many neural and behavioral pathologies, such as hippocampal volume decline, apathy, and memory impairment.[193–195] Research has shown that depression and anxiety may both be risk factors for dementia,[196,197] as well as signs of early cognitive impairment,[193,198] suggesting a bidirectional relationship. Early treatment of mood disorders may be important for reducing the risk of developing dementia.[196]

10.4 CONCLUSION

The brain is an immensely complex organ. There remains much to be discovered about how it functions in both healthy and disease populations. Thankfully, neuro-imaging techniques have enabled a wave of new research that is making scientific advances at an unprecedented pace. We are now able to utilize whole-brain functional and structural connectivity techniques *in vivo* to assess complex brain networks in healthy and clinical populations, as well as apply high-resolution imaging techniques that allow for a deeper understanding of the subtle neurobiological changes that may accompany the disease. Novel imaging measures have been developed to explore previously inaccessible areas of the human brain. For example, the advent of neuromelanin-sensitive MRI has allowed us to measure small brainstem regions such as the LC. With PET imaging, we can now measure AD pathology in the human living brain. These new methods give researchers and clinicians hope for developing effective, personalized treatments to promote mental and neurological health. It is important to consider how biological, psychological, and social factors interact to influence mental and neurological health (Figure 10.3). Factors such as emotion regulation, exercise, and sleep may offer affordable, accessible means of fostering health and well-being. These social factors are inherently linked to psychological factors such as cognition and memory, which in turn depend on underlying neurobiological factors. Importantly, these neurobiological factors are flexible and plastic, allowing various

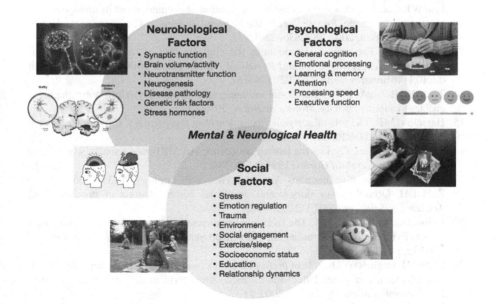

FIGURE 10.3 Biopsychosocial factors impacting mental and neurological health.

treatment and intervention strategies to impact both brain function and behavior. Thus, a biopsychosocial framework may help to elucidate the complex interactions across these factors, allowing for a richer understanding of mental and neurological disorders as a whole, which is greater than the sum of its parts.

REFERENCES

1. Basinger H, Hogg JP. Neuroanatomy, Brainstem. *StatPearls*; 2021.
2. Bunge RP. *Glial cells and the central myelin sheath.* 1968;48:197–251. doi:10.1152/physrev.1968.48.1.197
3. Azevedo FAC, et al. Equal numbers of neuronal and nonneuronal cells make the human brain an isometrically scaled-up primate brain. *Journal of Comparative Neurology.* 2009;513:532–541.
4. Squire LR, et al. Fundamental neuroscience: Fourth edition. *Fundamental Neuroscience: Fourth Edition.* 2012:1–1127. doi:10.1016/C2010-0-65035-8
5. Jessen KR. Glial cells. *The International Journal of Biochemistry & Cell Biology.* 2004;36:1861–1867.
6. Baumann N, Pham-Dinh D. Biology of oligodendrocyte and myelin in the mammalian central nervous system. *Physiological Reviews.* 2001;81:871–927.
7. Nicholls JG, et al. *From Neuron to Brain.* Sinauer Associates; 2012.
8. Nakanishi S. Metabotropic glutamate receptors: Synaptic transmission, modulation, and plasticity. *Neuron.* 1994;13:1031–1037.
9. Mateos-Aparicio P, Rodríguez-Moreno A. The impact of studying brain plasticity. *Frontiers in Cellular Neuroscience.* 2019;13:66.
10. Coxon JP, Stinear CM, Byblow WD. Intracortical inhibition during volitional inhibition of prepared action. *Journal of Neurophysiology.* 2006;95:3371–3383.
11. Lucki I. The spectrum of behaviors influenced by serotonin. *Biological Psychiatry.* 1998;44:151–162.
12. Gao WJ, Goldman-Rakic PS. Selective modulation of excitatory and inhibitory microcircuits by dopamine. *Proceedings of the National Academy of Sciences of the United States of America.* 2003;100:2836–2841.
13. McGaugh JL The amygdala modulates the consolidation of memories of emotionally arousing experiences. *Annual Review of Neuroscience.* 2004;27:1–28 Preprint at doi:10.1146/annurev.neuro.27.070203.144157.
14. Tully K, Bolshakov VY. Emotional enhancement of memory: How norepinephrine enables synaptic plasticity. *Molecular Brain.* 2010;3:1–9.
15. Hasselmo ME. The role of acetylcholine in learning and memory. *Current Opinion in Neurobiology.* 2006;16:710–715.
16. Kennedy DN et al. Gyri of the human neocortex: An MRI-based analysis of volume And variance. *Cerebral Cortex.* 1998;8:372–384.
17. Diamond A. Executive functions. *Annual Review of Psychology.* 2013;64:135.
18. Zald DH. Orbital versus dorsolateral prefrontal cortex. *Annals of the New York Academy of Sciences.* 2007;1121:395–406.
19. Kringelbach ML, Rolls ET. The functional neuroanatomy of the human orbitofrontal cortex: Evidence from neuroimaging and neuropsychology. *Progress in Neurobiology.* 2004;72:341–372.
20. Kane MJ, Engle RW. The role of prefrontal cortex in working-memory capacity, executive attention, and general fluid intelligence: An individual-differences perspective. *Psychonomic Bulletin & Review.* 2002;9:637–671.
21. Lin A, Adolphs R, Rangel A. Social and monetary reward learning engage overlapping neural substrates. *Social Cognitive and Affective Neuroscience.* 2012;7:274–281.

22. Nejati V, Majdi R, Salehinejad MA, Nitsche MA. The role of dorsolateral and ventro-medial prefrontal cortex in the processing of emotional dimensions. *Scientific Reports.* 2021;11:1–12.

23. Koenigs M, Grafman J. The functional neuroanatomy of depression: Distinct roles for ventromedial and dorsolateral prefrontal cortex. *Behavioural Brain Research.* 2009; 201:239–243.

24. Bush G, Luu P, Posner MI. Cognitive and emotional influences in anterior cingulate cortex. *Trends in Cognitive Sciences.* 2000;4:215–222.

25. Buckner RL, Andrews-Hanna JR, Schacter DL. The brain's default network. *Annals of the New York Academy of Sciences.* 2008;1124:1–38.

26. Leech R, Kamourieh S, Beckmann CF, Sharp DJ. Fractionating the default mode network: Distinct contributions of the ventral and dorsal posterior cingulate cortex to cognitive control. *Journal of Neuroscience.* 2011;31:3217–3224.

27. Squire LR, Zola-Morgan S. The medial temporal lobe memory system. *Science (1979).* 1991;253:1380–1386.

28. Dolcos F, Labar KS, Cabeza R. Remembering one year later: Role of the amygdala and the medial temporal lobe memory system in retrieving emotional memories. *Proceedings of the National Academy of Sciences of the United States of America.* 2005;102:2626–2631.

29. Tulving E, Markowitsch HJ. Episodic and declarative memory: Role of the hippocampus. *Hippocampus.* 1998;8:198–204.

30. McClelland JL, McNaughton BL, O'Reilly RC. Why there are complementary learning systems in the hippocampus and neocortex: Insights from the successes and failures of connectionist models of learning and memory. *Psychological Review.* 1995;102:419–457.

31. Squire LR, Stark CEL, Clark RE. The medical temporal lobe*. 2004;27:279–306. doi:10.1146/annurev.neuro.27.070203.144130

32. Yassa MA, Stark CEL. Pattern separation in the hippocampus. *Trends in Neurosciences.* 2011;34:515–525. doi:10.1016/j.tins.2011.06.006.

33. Anderson AK, Phelps EA. Lesions of the human amygdala impair enhanced perception of emotionally salient events. *Nature.* 2001;411:305–309.

34. Felleman DJ, Van Essen DC. Distributed hierarchical processing in the primate cerebral cortex. *Cerebral Cortex.* 1991;1:1–47.

35. Tootell RBH et al. Functional analysis of primary visual cortex (V1) in humans. *Proceedings of the National Academy of Sciences of the United States of America.* 1998;95:811–817.

36. Damasio H, Grabowski T, Frank R, Galaburda AM, Damasio AR. The return of Phineas gage: Clues about the brain from the skull of a famous patient. *Science (1979).* 1994;264:1102–1105.

37. Lerch JP et al. Studying neuroanatomy using MRI. *Nature Neuroscience.* 2017;20: 314–326.

38. Iglesias JE et al. A computational atlas of the hippocampal formation using ex vivo, ultra-high resolution MRI: Application to adaptive segmentation of in vivo MRI. *Neuroimage.* 2015;115:117–137.

39. Alexander AL, Lee JE, Lazar M, Field AS. Diffusion tensor imaging of the brain. *Neurotherapeutics.* 2007;4:316.

40. Arthurs OJ, Boniface S. How well do we understand the neural origins of the fMRI BOLD signal? *Trends Neuroscience.* 2002;25:27–31.

41. Logothetis NK, Pfeuffer J. On the nature of the BOLD fMRI contrast mechanism. *Magnetic resonance imaging.* 2004;22:1517–1531.

42. Gusnard DA, Raichle ME. Searching for a baseline: Functional imaging and the resting human brain. *Nature Reviews Neuroscience.* 2001;2:685–694.

43. Berger A. How does it work?: Positron emission tomography. *BMJ : British Medical Journal.* 2003;326:1449.
44. Zimmer L, Luxen A. PET radiotracers for molecular imaging in the brain: Past, present and future. *Neuroimage.* 2012;61:363–370.
45. Okamura N et al. The development and validation of tau PET tracers: Current status and future directions. *Clinical and Translational Imaging.* 2018;6:305–316.
46. Morris E et al. Diagnostic accuracy of 18F amyloid PET tracers for the diagnosis of Alzheimer's disease: A systematic review and meta-analysis. *European Journal of Nuclear Medicine and Molecular Imaging.* 2016;43:374–385.
47. Lemoine L, Leuzy A, Chiotis K, Rodriguez-Vieitez E, Nordberg A. Tau positron emission tomography imaging in tauopathies: The added hurdle of off-target binding. *Alzheimer's & Dementia: Diagnosis, Assessment & Disease Monitoring.* 2018;10:232–236.
48. Jackson AF, Bolger DJ. The neurophysiological bases of EEG and EEG measurement: A review for the rest of us. *Psychophysiology.* 2014;51:1061–1071.
49. Herrmann CS, Strüber D, Helfrich RF, Engel AK. EEG oscillations: From correlation to causality. *International Journal of Psychophysiology.* 2016;103:12–21.
50. Siebner HR, Hartwigsen G, Kassuba T, Rothwell JC. How does transcranial magnetic stimulation modify neuronal activity in the brain? - Implications for studies of cognition. *Cortex.* 2009;45:1035.
51. Gotlib IH, Joormann J. *Cognition and Depression: Current Status and Future Directions.* 2010;6:285–312. doi:10.1146/annurev.clinpsy.121208.131305.
52. Fried EI, Nesse RM. Depression sum-scores don't add up: Why analyzing specific depression symptoms is essential. *BMC Medicine.* 2015;13:1–11.
53. Serafini G. Neuroplasticity and major depression, the role of modern antidepressant drugs. *World Journal of Psychiatry.* 2012;2:49.
54. Majd M, Saunders EFH, Engeland CG. Inflammation and the dimensions of depression: A review. *Frontiers in Neuroendocrinology.* 2020;56:100800.
55. Philip NS, Carpenter LL, Tyrka AR, Price LH. Nicotinic acetylcholine receptors and depression: A review of the preclinical and clinical literature. *Psychopharmacology (Berl).* 2010;212:1–12.
56. Nutt DJ. Relationship of neurotransmitters to the symptoms of major depressive disorder. *The Journal of Clinical Psychiatry.* 2008;69:18494537.
57. George MS, Ketter TA, Post RM. Prefrontal cortex dysfunction in clinical depression. *Depression.* 1994;2:59–72.
58. Bremner JD et al. Reduced volume of orbitofrontal cortex in major depression. *Biological Psychiatry.* 2002;51:273–279.
59. Jaworska N, Yang XR, Knott V, Macqueen G. *A review of fMRI studies during visual emotive processing in major depressive disorder.* 2014;16:448–471. doi:10.3109/15622975.2014.885659.
60. Drevets WC, et al. A functional anatomical study of unipolar depression. *Journal of Neuroscience.* 1992;12:3628–3641.
61. Kühn S, Gallinat J. Resting-state brain activity in schizophrenia and major depression: A quantitative meta-analysis. *Schizophrenia Bulletin.* 2013;39:358–365.
62. Galynker II, et al. Hypofrontality and negative symptoms in major depressive disorder. *J Nucl Med.* 1998;39(4):608–612.
63. Rogers MA, et al. Executive and prefrontal dysfunction in unipolar depression: A review of neuropsychological and imaging evidence. *Journal of Neuroscience Research.* 2004;50:1–11.
64. Carballedo A, et al. Functional connectivity of emotional processing in depression. *Journal of Affective Disorders.* 2011;134:272–279.
65. Hamilton JP, Gotlib IH. Neural substrates of increased memory sensitivity for negative stimuli in major depression. *Biological Psychiatry.* 2008;63:1155–1162.

66. Laeger I, et al. Amygdala responsiveness to emotional words is modulated by subclinical anxiety and depression. *Behavioural Brain Research.* 2012;233:508–516.
67. Campbell S, MacQueen G. The role of the hippocampus in the pathophysiology of major depression. *Journal of Psychiatry and Neuroscience.* 2004;29:417.
68. Sheline YI. Depression and the hippocampus: Cause or effect? *Biological Psychiatry.* 2011;70:308.
69. McEwen BS, Magarinos AM. Stress and hippocampal plasticity: Implications for the pathophysiology of affective disorders. *Human Psychopharmacology: Clinical and Experimental.* 2001;16:S7–S19.
70. Hickie I, et al. Reduced hippocampal volumes and memory loss in patients with early- and late-onset depression. *British Journal of Psychiatry.* 2005;186:197–202.
71. Brown ES, et al. Association of depressive symptoms with hippocampal volume in 1936 adults. *Neuropsychopharmacology.* 2013;39:770–779.
72. Ridout N, Astell AJ, Reid IC, Glen T, O'Carroll RE. *Memory bias for emotional facial expressions in major depression.* 2010;17:101–122. doi:10.1080/02699930302272.
73. Bradley BP, Mogg K, Williams R. Implicit and explicit memory for emotion-congruent information in clinical depression and anxiety. *Behaviour Research and Therapy.* 1995;33:755–770.
74. Leal SL, Tighe SK, Jones CK, Yassa MA. Pattern separation of emotional information in hippocampal dentate and CA3. *Hippocampus.* 2014;24:1146–1155.
75. Gandy K, et al. Pattern separation: A potential marker of impaired hippocampal adult neurogenesis in major depressive disorder. *Frontiers in Neuroscienc.* 2017;11:571.
76. Leal SL, Yassa MA. Integrating new findings and examining clinical applications of pattern separation. *Nature Neuroscience.* 2018;21:163–173. Preprint at doi:10.1038/s41593-017-0065-1.
77. Broquet KE. Status of treatment of depression. *Southern Medical Journal.* 1999;92:846–856.
78. Voineskos D, Daskalakis ZJ, Blumberger DM. Management of treatment-resistant depression: Challenges and strategies. *Neuropsychiatric Disease and Treatment.* 2020;16:221.
79. Kirsch I, et al. Initial severity and antidepressant benefits: A meta-analysis of data submitted to the food and drug administration. *PLOS Medicine.* 2008;5:e45.
80. Duman RS. Pathophysiology of depression: The concept of synaptic plasticity. *European Psychiatry.* 2002;17:306–310.
81. Malberg JE, Duman RS. Cell proliferation in adult hippocampus is decreased by inescapable stress: Reversal by fluoxetine treatment. *Neuropsychopharmacology.* 2003;28:1562–1571.
82. Kraus C, Castrén E, Kasper S, Lanzenberger R. Serotonin and neuroplasticity – Links between molecular, functional and structural pathophysiology in depression. *Neuroscience & Biobehavioral Reviews.* 2017;77:317–326.
83. Kellner CH, et al. *ECT in treatment-resistant depression.* 2012;169:1238–1244. doi:10.1176/appi.ajp.2012.12050648
84. Joshi SH, et al. Structural plasticity of the hippocampus and amygdala induced by electroconvulsive therapy in major depression. *Biological Psychiatry.* 2016;79:282–292.
85. George MS, Taylor JJ, Short EB. The expanding evidence base for rTMS treatment of depression. *Current Opinion in Psychiatry.* 2013;26:13.
86. Drysdale AT, et al. Resting-state connectivity biomarkers define neurophysiological subtypes of depression. *Nature Medicine.* 2016;23:28–38.
87. Jacka FN, Berk M. Depression, diet and exercise. *Medical Journal of Australia.* 2013;199:S21–S23.
88. Stubbs B, Schuch F. Physical activity and exercise as a treatment of depression: Evidence and neurobiological mechanism. *Neurobiology of Depression: Road to Novel Therapeutics.* 2019;293–299. doi:10.1016/B978-0-12-813333-0.00026-3

89. Harvey SB, et al. Exercise and the prevention of depression: Results of the HUNT cohort study. *American Journal of Psychiatry.* 2018;175:28–36.
90. Josefsson T, Lindwall M, Archer T. Physical exercise intervention in depressive disorders: Meta-analysis and systematic review. *Scandinavian Journal of Medicine & Science in Sports.* 2014;24:259–272.
91. Sarris J, O'Neil A, Coulson CE, Schweitzer I, Berk M. Lifestyle medicine for depression. *BMC Psychiatry.* 2014;14:1–13.
92. Déry N, et al. Adult hippocampal neurogenesis reduces memory interference in humans: Opposing effects of aerobic exercise and depression. *Frontiers in Neuroscience.* 2013;0:66.
93. Ernst C, et al. Antidepressant effects of exercise: Evidence for an adult-neurogenesis hypothesis? *Review Psychiatry and Neuroscience.* 200631:84–92.
94. Cruwys T, et al. Social group memberships protect against future depression, alleviate depression symptoms and prevent depression relapse. *Social Science & Medicine.* 2013;98:179–186.
95. Nagy E, Moore S. Social interventions: An effective approach to reduce adult depression? *Journal of Affective Disorders.* 2017;218:131–152.
96. Leach LS, Butterworth P, Olesen SC, Mackinnon A. Relationship quality and levels of depression and anxiety in a large population-based survey. *Social Psychiatry and Psychiatric Epidemiology.* 2012;48:417–425.
97. Freeman D, Sheaves B, Waite F, Harvey AG, Harrison PJ. Sleep disturbance and psychiatric disorders. *Lancet Psychiatry.* 2020;7:628–637.
98. Marx W, et al. Diet and depression: Exploring the biological mechanisms of action. *Molecular Psychiatry.* 2020;26:134–150.
99. Sanchez-Villegas A, Martínez-González MA. Diet, a new target to prevent depression? *BMC Medicine.* 2013;11:1–4.
100. Berking M, Ebert D, Cuijpers P, Hofmann SG. Emotion regulation skills training enhances the efficacy of inpatient cognitive behavioral therapy for major depressive disorder: A randomized controlled trial. *Psychother Psychosom.* 2013;82:234–245.
101. Gross JJ, Muñoz RF. Emotion regulation and mental health. *Clinical Psychology: Science and Practice.* 1995;2:151–164.
102. Holland AC, Kensinger EA. An fMRI investigation of the cognitive reappraisal of negative memories. *Neuropsychologia.* 2013;51:2389–2400.
103. Richards JM, Gross JJ. Emotion regulation and memory: The cognitive costs of keeping one's cool. *Journal of Personality and Social Psychology.* 2000;79:410–424.
104. Denny BT, Ochsner KN. Behavioral effects of longitudinal training in cognitive reappraisal. *Emotion.* 2014;14:425–433.
105. Denny BT, Inhoff MC, Zerubavel N, Davachi L, Ochsner KN. Getting over it: Long-lasting effects of emotion regulation on amygdala response. *Psychological Science.* 2015;26:1377–1388.
106. Kross E, Ayduk O. Self-distancing: Theory, research, and current directions. In: *Advances in Experimental Social Psychology;* 2017:81–136. doi:10.1016/bs.aesp.2016.10.002.
107. Kross E, Gard D, Deldin P, Clifton J, Ayduk O. Asking Why' from a distance: Its cognitive and emotional consequences for people with major depressive disorder. *Journal of Abnormal Psychology.* 2012;121:559–569.
108. Nowlan JS, Wuthrich VM, Rapee RM. Positive reappraisal in older adults: A systematic literature review. *Aging and Mental Health.* 2014;19:475–484.
109. Nashiro K, et al. Effects of a randomised trial of 5-week heart rate variability biofeedback intervention on cognitive function: Possible benefits for inhibitory control. *Applied Psychophysiology and Biofeedback.* 2022;1:1–14.
110. Sulzer J, et al. Real-time fMRI neurofeedback: Progress and challenges. *Neuroimage.* 2013;76:386–399.

111. Linden DEJ, et al. Real-time self-regulation of emotion networks in patients with depression. *PLoS One.* 2012;7:e38115.
112. Ochsner KN, Gross JJ. *Cognitive emotion regulation.* 2008;17:153–158. doi:10.1111/j.1467-8721.2008.00566.x
113. Young KD, et al. Real-time fMRI neurofeedback training of amygdala activity in patients with major depressive disorder. *PLoS One.* 2014;9:e88785.
114. Stein MB, Sareen J. Generalized anxiety disorder. *The New England Journal of Medicine.* 2015;373:2059–68.
115. Kalin NH. *The critical relationship between anxiety and depression.* 2020;177: 365–367. doi: 10.1176/appi.ajp.2020.20030305
116. Bishop S, Duncan J, Brett M, Lawrence AD. Prefrontal cortical function and anxiety: Controlling attention to threat-related stimuli. *Nature Neuroscience.* 2004;7:184–188.
117. Manber Ball T, Ramsawh HJ, Campbell-Sills L, Paulus MP, Stein MB. Prefrontal dysfunction during emotion regulation in generalized anxiety and panic disorders. *Psychological Medicine.* 2013;43:1475–1486.
118. Martin EI, Ressler KJ, Binder E, Nemeroff CB. The neurobiology of anxiety disorders: Brain imaging, genetics, and psychoneuroendocrinology. *Psychiatric Clinics.* 2009;32:549–575.
119. Jalbrzikowski M, et al. Development of white matter microstructure and intrinsic functional connectivity between the amygdala and ventromedial prefrontal cortex: Associations with anxiety and depression. *Biological Psychiatry.* 2017;82:511–521.
120. Etkin A, Prater KE, Hoeft F, Menon V, Schatzberg AF. Failure of anterior cingulate activation and connectivity with the amygdala during implicit regulation of emotional processing in generalized anxiety disorder. *American Journal of Psychiatry.* 2010;167:545–554.
121. Wang W, et al. Aberrant regional neural fluctuations and functional connectivity in generalized anxiety disorder revealed by resting-state functional magnetic resonance imaging. *Neuroscience Letters.* 2016;624:78–84.
122. Bergink V, Van Megen HJGM, Westenberg HGM. Glutamate and anxiety. *European Neuropsychopharmacology.* 2004;14:175–183.
123. Riaza Bermudo-Soriano C, Perez-Rodriguez MM, Vaquero-Lorenzo C, Baca-Garcia E. New perspectives in glutamate and anxiety. *Pharmacology Biochemistry and Behavior.* 2012;100:752–774.
124. Nuss P. Anxiety disorders and GABA neurotransmission: A disturbance of modulation. *Neuropsychiatric Disease and Treatment.* 2015;11:165.
125. Nasir M, et al. glutamate systems in DSM-5 anxiety disorders: Their role and a review of glutamate and GABA psychopharmacology. *Frontiers in Psychiatry.* 2020;11:1186.
126. Granger SJ, et al. Latent anxiety in clinical depression is associated with worse recognition of emotional stimuli. *Journal of Affective Disorders.* 2022;301:368–377.
127. Saviola F, et al. Trait and state anxiety are mapped differently in the human brain. *Scientific Reports.* 2020;10:1–11.
128. Swanson CJ, et al. Metabotropic glutamate receptors as novel targets for anxiety and stress disorders. *Nature Reviews Drug Discovery.* 2005;4:131–144.
129. Stonerock GL, Hoffman BM, Smith PJ, Blumenthal JA. Exercise as treatment for anxiety: Systematic review and analysis. *Annals of Behavioral Medicine.* 2015;49: 542–556.
130. Cisler JM, Olatunji BO. Emotion regulation and anxiety disorders. *Current Psychiatry Reports.* 2012;14:182–187.
131. Taylor CT, Pearlstein SL, Kakaria S, Lyubomirsky S, Stein MB. Enhancing social connectedness in anxiety and depression through amplification of positivity: Preliminary treatment outcomes and process of change. *Cognitive Therapy and Research.* 2020; 44:788–800.

132. Sarris J, et al. Complementary medicine, exercise, meditation, diet, and lifestyle modification for anxiety disorders: A review of current evidence. *Evidence-Based Complementary and Alternative Medicine.* 2012;2012:1–20.
133. Sheynin J, et al. Associations between resting-state functional connectivity and treatment response in a randomized clinical trial for posttraumatic stress disorder. *Depress Anxiety.* 2020;37:1037–1046.
134. Alzheimer's Association. 2022 Alzheimer's disease facts and figures. *Alzheimer's & Dementia.* 2023;19:700–789.
135. Jack CR et al. NIA-AA research framework: Toward a biological definition of Alzheimer's disease. *Alzheimers Dement.* 2018;14:535–562.
136. Masters CL, Selkoe DJ. Biochemistry of amyloid β-protein and amyloid deposits in Alzheimer disease. *Cold Spring Harbor Perspectives in Medicine.* 2012;2:a006262.
137. Grundke-Iqbal I, et al. Abnormal phosphorylation of the microtubule-associated protein tau (tau) in Alzheimer cytoskeletal pathology. *Proceedings of the National Academy of Sciences of the United States of America.* 1986;83:4913–4917.
138. Arai H, et al. Cerebrospinal fluid tau levels in neurodegenerative diseases with distinct tau-related pathology. *Biochem Biophys Res Commun* 236, 262–264 (1997).
139. Gomperts SN, et al. Tau PET imaging in the Lewy body diseases. *JAMA Neurology.* 2016;73:1334.
140. Hardy J, Selkoe DJ. The amyloid hypothesis of Alzheimer's disease: Progress and problems on the road to therapeutics. *Science (1979).* 2002;297:353–356.
141. Davis DG, Schmitt FA, Wekstein DR, Markesbery WR. Alzheimer neuropathologic alterations in aged cognitively normal subjects. *Journal of Neuropathology & Experimental Neurology.* 1999;58:376–388.
142. Villemagne VL, et al. Amyloid β deposition, neurodegeneration, and cognitive decline in sporadic Alzheimer's disease: A prospective cohort study. *Lancet Neurology.* 2013;12:357–367.
143. Villemagne VL, Doré V, Burnham SC, Masters CL, Rowe CC. Imaging tau and amyloid-β proteinopathies in Alzheimer disease and other conditions. *Nature Reviews Neurology.* 2018;14:225–236.
144. Jack CR, et al. Associations of amyloid, tau, and neurodegeneration biomarker profiles with rates of memory decline among individuals without dementia. *JAMA.* 2019;321:2316–2325.
145. Sperling RA, et al. The impact of amyloid-beta and tau on prospective cognitive decline in older individuals. *Annals of Neurology.* 2019;85:181–193.
146. Jack CR, et al. Rates of hippocampal atrophy correlate with change in clinical status in aging and AD. *Neurology.* 2000;55:484–490.
147. Joie RL, et al. Prospective longitudinal atrophy in Alzheimer's disease correlates with the intensity and topography of baseline tau-PET. *Science Translational Medicine.* 2020;12:5732.
148. Neary D, Snowden J, Mann D. Frontotemporal dementia. *Lancet Neurology.* 2005;4:771–780.
149. Harris JM, et al. Sensitivity and specificity of FTDC criteria for behavioral variant frontotemporal dementia. *Neurology.* 2013;80:1881–1887.
150. Small GW. What we need to know about age related memory loss. *British Medical Journal.* 2002;324:1502–1505. Preprint at doi:10.1136/bmj.324.7352.1502.
151. Golomb J, et al. Hippocampal formation size in normal human aging: A correlate of delayed secondary memory performance. *Learning Memory.* 1994;1:45–54.
152. Persson J, et al. Structure-function correlates of cognitive decline in aging. *Cerebral Cortex.* 2006;**16**:907–915.
153. Furst AJ, Mormino EC A BOLD move: Clinical application of fMRI in aging. *Neurology.* 2010;74;1940–1941. Preprint at doi:10.1212/WNL.0b013e3181e533f8.

154. Leal SL, Landau SM, Bell RK, Jagust WJ. Hippocampal activation is associated with longitudinal amyloid accumulation and cognitive decline. *Elife*. 2017;6:1–15.

155. Wilson IA, Gallagher M, Eichenbaum H, Tanila H. Neurocognitive aging: Prior memories hinder new hippocampal encoding. *Trends in Neurosciences*. 2006; 29:662–670.

156. Stark SM, Yassa MA, Tark CEL. Individual differences in spatial pattern separation performance associated with healthy aging in humans. *Learning and Memory*. 2010;17:284–288.

157. Leal SL, Yassa MA. Effects of aging on mnemonic discrimination of emotional information. *Behavioral Neuroscience*. 2014;128:539–547.

158. Braak H, Thal DR, Ghebremedhin E, Del Tredici K. Stages of the pathologic process in Alzheimer disease: Age categories from 1 to 100 years. *Journal of Neuropathology & Experimental Neurology*. 2011;70:960–969.

159. Stratmann K, et al. Precortical phase of Alzheimer's disease (AD)-related tau cytoskeletal pathology. *Brain Pathology*. 2016;26:371–386.

160. Braak H, Braak E. Frequency of stages of Alzheimer-related lesions in different age categories. *Neurobiology of Aging*. 1997;18:351–357.

161. Lewis J, Dickson DW. Propagation of tau pathology: Hypotheses, discoveries, and yet unresolved questions from experimental and human brain studies. *Acta Neuropathologica*. 2015;131:27–48.

162. Sasaki M, et al. Neuromelanin magnetic resonance imaging of locus ceruleus and substantia nigra in Parkinson's disease. *Neuroreport*. 2006;17:1215–1218.

163. Waldemar G, et al. Recommendations for the diagnosis and management of Alzheimer's disease and other disorders associated with dementia: EFNS guideline. *European Journal of Neurology*. 2007;14:e1–e26.

164. Francis PT, Palmer AM, Snape M, Wilcock GK. The cholinergic hypothesis of Alzheimer's disease: A review of progress. *Journal of Neurology, Neurosurgery, and Psychiatry*. 1999;66:137–147.

165. Anand P, Singh B. A review on cholinesterase inhibitors for Alzheimer's disease. *Archives of Pharmacal Research*. 2013;36:375–399.

166. Bakker A, et al. Reduction of hippocampal hyperactivity improves cognition in amnestic mild cognitive impairment. *Neuron*. 2012;74:467–474.

167. Sevigny J, et al. The antibody aducanumab reduces Aβ plaques in Alzheimer's disease. *Nature*. 2016;537:50–56.

168. Walsh S, Merrick R, Milne R, Brayne C. Aducanumab for Alzheimer's disease? *BMJ*. 2021;374:1–2.

169. Amanatkar HR, Papagiannopoulos B, Grossberg GT. *Analysis of recent failures of disease modifying therapies in Alzheimer's disease suggesting a new methodology for future studies*. 2016;17:7–16. doi:10.1080/14737175.2016.1194203

170. Livingston G, et al. Dementia prevention, intervention, and care: 2020 report of the lancet commission. *The Lancet*. 2020;396:413–446.

171. Johansson L, et al. Midlife psychological stress and risk of dementia: A 35-year longitudinal population study. *Brain*. 2010;133:2217–2224.

172. Kivipelto M, Mangialasche F, Ngandu T. Lifestyle interventions to prevent cognitive impairment, dementia and Alzheimer disease. *Nature Reviews Neurology 2018 14:11*. 2018;14:653–666.

173. Salmon P. Effects of physical exercise on anxiety, depression, and sensitivity to stress: A unifying theory. *Clinical Psychology Review*. 2001;21:33–61.

174. Cohen S, McKay G. Social support, stress and the buffering hypothesis: A theoretical analysis. *Handbook of Psychology and Health, Volume IV: Social Psychological Aspects of Health*. 2020;253–267. doi:10.1037/0033-2909.98.2.310

175. Stern Y. Cognitive reserve in ageing and Alzheimer's disease. *The Lancet Neurology*. 2012;11:1006–1012. Preprint at doi:10.1016/S1474-4422(12)70191-6.

176. Valenzuela PL, et al. Exercise benefits on Alzheimer's disease: State-of-the-science. *Ageing Research Reviews*. 2020;62:101108. Preprint at doi:10.1016/j.arr.2020.101108.

177. Andel R, et al. Physical exercise at midlife and risk of dementia three decades later: A population-based study of Swedish twins. *The Journals of Gerontology: Series A*. 2008;63:62–66.

178. López-Ortiz S et al. Exercise interventions in Alzheimer's disease: A systematic review and meta-analysis of randomized controlled trials. *Ageing Research Reviews*. 2021;72:101479.

179. Kuiper JS, et al. Social relationships and risk of dementia: A systematic review and meta-analysis of longitudinal cohort studies. *Ageing Research Reviews*. 2015;22:39–57.

180. Amieva H, et al. What aspects of social network are protective for dementia? Not the quantity but the quality of social interactions is protective up to 15 years later. *Psychosomatic Medicine*. 2010;72:905–911.

181. Fried LP, et al. Experience corps: A dual trial to promote the health of older adults and children's academic success. *Contemporary Clinical Trials*. 2013;36:1–13.

182. Carlson MC, et al. Evidence for neurocognitive plasticity in at-risk older adults: The experience corps program. *The Journals of Gerontology Series A Biological Sciences and Medical Sciences*. 2009;64A:1275.

183. Xie L, et al. Sleep drives metabolite clearance from the adult brain. *Science (1979)*. 2013;342:373–377.

184. Mander BA, Winer JR, Jagust WJ, Walker MP. Sleep: A novel mechanistic pathway, biomarker, and treatment target in the pathology of Alzheimer's disease? *Trends in Neurosciences*. 2016;39:552–566. Preprint at doi:10.1016/j.tins.2016.05.002

185. Gencarelli A, Sorrell A, Everhart CM, Zurlinden T, Everhart DE. Behavioral and exercise interventions for sleep dysfunction in the elderly: A brief review and future directions. *Sleep Breath*. 2021;25:2111.

186. Solfrizzi V, et al. Relationships of dietary patterns, foods, and micro- and macronutrients with Alzheimer's disease and late-life cognitive disorders: A systematic review. *Journal of Alzheimer's Disease*. 2017;59:815–849.

187. Poscia A, et al. Effectiveness of nutritional interventions addressed to elderly persons: umbrella systematic review with meta-analysis. *European Journal of Public Health*. 2018;28:275–283.

188. Peters R, et al. Air pollution and dementia: A systematic review. *Journal of Alzheimer's Disease*. 2019;70:S145–S163.

189. Pase MP, et al. Association of neighborhood-level socioeconomic measures with cognition and dementia risk in Australian adults. *JAMA Network Open*. 2022;5: e224071–e224071.

190. Wu YT, Prina AM, Brayne C. The association between community environment and cognitive function: A systematic review. *Social Psychiatry and Psychiatric Epidemiology*. 2015;50:351–362.

191. Paul LA, et al. Urban green space and the risks of dementia and stroke. *Environmental Research*. 2020;186:109520.

192. Lyketsos CG, Olin J. Depression in Alzheimer's disease: Overview and treatment. *Biological Psychiatry*. 2002;52:243–252.

193. Panza F, et al. Late-life depression, mild cognitive impairment, and dementia: Possible continuum? *American Journal of Geriatric Psychiatry*. 2010;18:98–116.

194. Huey ED, Lee S, Cheran G, Grafman J, Devanand DP. Brain regions involved in arousal and reward processing are associated with apathy in Alzheimer's disease and frontotemporal dementia. *Journal of Alzheimer's Disease*. 2017;55:551–558.

195. Shimoda K, Kimura M, Yokota M, Okubo Y. Comparison of regional gray matter volume abnormalities in Alzheimer's disease and late life depression with hippocampal atrophy using VSRAD analysis: A voxel-based morphometry study. *Psychiatry Res Neuroimaging.* 2015;232:71–75.
196. Butters MA, et al. Pathways linking late-life depression to persistent cognitive impairment and dementia. *Dialogues in Clinical Neuroscience.* 2008;10:345–357.
197. Beaudreau SA, OHara R. Late-life anxiety and cognitive impairment: A review. *The American Journal of Geriatric Psychiatry.* 2008;16:790–803.
198. Seignourel PJ, Kunik ME, Snow L, Wilson N, Stanley M. Anxiety in dementia: A critical review. *Clinical Psychology Review.* 2008;28:1071–1082.

11 Neuroendocrine and Immune Pathways

Molly A. Wright, BS and
Christopher G. Engeland, PhD

KEY POINTS

- The stress response involves the integrated and carefully orchestrated actions of the SAM-axis, HPA-axis, ANS, and immune system.
- Prolonged stress can result in dysregulation of these pathways and is rarely isolated to a single pathway.
- Dysregulation of stress systems promotes non-optimal immune responses.
- Critical developmental periods exist (e.g., childhood) in which prolonged stress may exert permanent changes to these pathways.
- Evaluation and treatment of stress should be considered in clinical practice.

List of Abbreviations

ANS	Autonomic nervous system
CAP	Cholinergic anti-inflammatory pathway
CVD	Cardiovascular disease
ELA	Early life adversity
Epi	Epinephrine
GC	Glucocorticoid
GR	Glucocorticoid receptor
HRV	Heart rate variability
HPA	Hypothalamic-pituitary-adrenal
NE	Norepinephrine
NF-ƙB	Nuclear factor-kappa B
PNS	Parasympathetic nervous system
PVN	Paraventricular nucleus
PTSD	Post-traumatic stress disorder
SAM	Sympathetic-adrenal-medullary
SNS	Sympathetic nervous system
TNF-α	Tumor-necrosis factor-alpha
vmHRV	Vagally mediated heart rate variability (HRV)
VNS	Vagal nerve stimulation

DOI: 10.1201/b22810-13

11.1 INTRODUCTION

The human stress response is highly evolved and critical to our survival. It serves many adaptive and beneficial purposes, particularly when encountering an imminent threat or challenge. This stress response works best when it is activated and then deactivated quickly. It is when we experience *prolonged* stress (i.e., extended or continuous activation of stress pathways) that this response can become maladaptive, deleteriously affecting immunity and health.[1] This chapter will outline some of integral pathways by which stress has effects on human health: the sympathetic-adrenal-medullary (SAM) pathway, the hypothalamic-pituitary-adrenal (HPA) pathway, the cholinergic anti-inflammatory pathway (CAP), and the parasympathetic nervous system (PNS) branch of the autonomic nervous system (ANS). Many of the negative effects of stress on health occur via interactions of these pathways with the immune system. The implications of dysregulation of these pathways for mental health and chronic disease, particularly in developmental periods (e.g., childhood) where the consequences are most profound, will also be discussed.

11.2 SYMPATHETIC-ADRENAL-MEDULLARY (SAM) PATHWAY

Upon exposure to a stressor, the *flight-fight response* is quickly activated. This occurs in seconds and involves activation of the sympathetic nervous system (SNS) (specifically, the SAM-axis), which innervates practically every part of the body. This early stress response involves the perception of a stressor by the integrative cortex, followed by activation of the locus coeruleus, which in turn initiates norepinephrine (NE) release both centrally and from nerve endings into the periphery. The adrenal glands are directly innervated by sympathetic nerves; hence, signaling is very quick when it occurs and promotes the release (from the adrenal medulla) of both NE and epinephrine (Epi; i.e., adrenalin) into blood circulation. Activation of the SAM-axis is an evolved and adaptive response to perceived threat, culminating in increases in (1) heart and respiratory rates, (2) blood pressure (due to vasoconstriction), (3) blood flow to the periphery, and (4) circulating glucose levels (from glycogen in liver), along with pupil dilation and the inhibition of other bodily functions (e.g., digestion – e.g., dry mouth; sexual urges). Combined, these changes promote a high energy state, providing increased oxygen and nutrients to both skeletal muscle and brain, ultimately instilling greater readiness/ability to deal with the threat. As will be discussed, other stress-related systems subsequently become activated (HPA-axis, ANS) along with aspects of the immune system due to the higher chance of injury and infection in these moments.

Today, in developed countries, rather than physical danger we mainly face social and mental threats. Importantly, the stress elicited by such threats is often greatly prolonged by our tendencies to *ruminate* about past events and *worry* about future events. Unlike the zebra, which may escape from a predator and then resume peacefully grazing, the stress response in humans today is often much more protracted. This response is optimally designed to turn on and off quickly, and prolonged activation of stress pathways (hours to days to weeks) can have maladaptive effects on health. For instance, NE induces vasoconstriction. As a result, extended activation of the SAM-axis can (1) delay tissue repair due to reduced transport/delivery of oxygen, glucose, and white blood cells to the area of injury, and (2) increase blood pressure, causing wear and tear over time on the body's vasculature.[2,3] In addition, high blood pressure is a known risk factor for many chronic conditions and diseases.

Sympathetic nerves innervate immune storage areas (e.g., lymph nodes, organs) and immune cells express receptors for NE, Epi, and glucocorticoids (GCs).[4] Hence, the immune system is very responsive to perceived stress/threat. Prolonged psychological stress can suppress the function of T cells and natural killer cells, lymphocyte proliferation, and cytokine production.[1,4] It also lowers antibody responses to vaccines, thereby reducing the effectiveness of vaccination (e.g., pneumonia, influenza) regardless of age.[5] Stress also slows both dermal and mucosal wound closure, thereby increasing the risk of infection and post-operative complications.[2,3,6] Note that this is far from a complete listing of the deleterious effects of prolonged stress on immunity. All arms of the immune system are affected – innate, humoral, and cellular; even mucosal immunity is weakened in times of stress (e.g., reduced IgA1 in saliva with higher perceived stress).[1-3,7,8]

11.3 HYPOTHALAMIC-PITUITARY-ADRENAL (HPA) PATHWAY

Approximately 15-20 minutes after activation of the SAM-axis (described above), the HPA-axis becomes activated. This involves the release of corticotropin releasing factor from the paraventricular nucleus (PVN) of the hypothalamus into the hypophyseal portal, which is a local blood supply to the pituitary gland. This induces the release of adrenocorticotropic hormone into the general circulation which, in turn, stimulates the release of corticosteroids (mainly cortisol) from the adrenal glands. A negative feedback loop exists to the hypothalamus and the pituitary which then limits further activation of this axis. Cortisol is potently immunosuppressive and is the largest brake on inflammation that the human body produces; hence, the release of cortisol not only liberates energy but regulates the immune system so that immune responses (e.g., inflammation) remain modulated and do not get out of control.

Stress physiology and the immune system are tightly connected. Hence, dysregulation of one system typically results in dysregulation of the other. As an example, cortisol has a distinct circadian rhythm that is characterized by elevated levels when we wake which peak shortly afterwards and then drop throughout the day. This has a direct effect on pro-inflammatory cytokines, which generally exhibit an inverse rhythm and peak in the evening/night when cortisol is lowest.[9] As a result, cold/flu symptoms are often the worst at night when our immune system is relatively untethered from the inhibitory effects of cortisol; night, which is relatively quiescent, is also the time when we are most effective at fighting off illness/infection. In sum, cortisol is a potent down-regulator of immunity; as such, long-term alterations in cortisol can have direct effects on health via alterations in immunity.

All immune cells express GC receptors (GRs), enabling cortisol to have broad strong immunosuppressive effects and allowing it to play a critical role in regulating and limiting immune responses. Persistently elevated levels of cortisol (e.g., due to repeated or chronic stress) result in reduced responsiveness of immune cells to GCs via reduced GC receptor expression.[2,3,10] This in turn lowers immune inhibition, allowing for larger immune responses to occur relatively unchecked. This *GC resistance* is a key mechanism by which chronic stress can negatively affect health. For this reason, individuals with inflammatory conditions (e.g., rheumatoid arthritis, lupus, multiple sclerosis, inflammatory bowel syndrome, Crohn's disease) often exhibit inflammatory flare-ups and a worsening of symptoms during times of stress. In a separate example, latent viral loads (e.g., cytomegalovirus, Epstein-Barr virus) often increase (reactivate) under times of prolonged or severe stress, resulting in outbreaks of symptoms (e.g., cold sores due to herpes simplex virus type 1).[4,11] Here, this reactivation of latent viruses by stress is not due to GC resistance but instead a reduced ability of the immune system to suppress viral loads; as a result, antibody titers increase under times of ongoing or severe stress.[11]

The well-established relationship between prolonged or chronic stress and heightened inflammation is a prime example of how stress can dysregulate immunity and adversely affect health. Inflammation is an adaptive response to pathogen exposure, injury, perceived environmental threats, and psychological stress (i.e., threat of injury) that is counter-regulated by several endogenous mechanisms. These counter-regulatory pathways, including the hypothalamic-pituitary- adrenal (HPA) axis and parasympathetic nervous system (PNS), serve to terminate the inflammatory response once a threat has passed and to prevent the potentially damaging or lethal consequences of unrestrained inflammation. The harmful effects of prolonged high inflammation stem from cumulative damage (e.g., blood vessel walls) and, as discussed previously, non-optimal immune responses. This dysregulation by stress can result in inflammatory responses that are too high (and often prolonged) or too low. Heightened inflammation is a risk factor for many prevalent diseases and conditions (e.g., cardiovascular disease (CVD), type 2 diabetes, Alzheimer's disease).[12] Conversely, an underactive immune system can leave one more susceptible to a broad range of illnesses, from the common cold to cancer.[13]

11.4 CHOLINERGIC ANTI-INFLAMMATORY PATHWAY (CAP)

The cholinergic anti-inflammatory pathway (CAP) has garnered increasing attention in recent years for its role in modulating the neuroimmune and endocrine response to stress and in restoring homeostasis. The specific anti-inflammatory mechanisms of this pathway are delineated in this section, and health implications are discussed.

11.4.1 VAGUS-NEURAL COMMUNICATION

The vagus nerve, the primary constituent of the PNS, is the longest nerve in the body and innervates many visceral organs, including the gastrointestinal tract, heart, liver, and lungs. Composed of 80% afferent nerve fibers, it is a key immunosensory pathway for transmitting signals of bodily states to the brain. Peripheral cytokines bind to receptors present on vagal afferent nerve endings that project to the nucleus of the solitary tract and the area postrema of the dorsal vagal complex in the brainstem. These, in turn, project to higher order regions integral to stress responsivity, including the hypothalamic paraventricular nucleus, the amygdala, and the prefrontal cortex.[14,15] The immunosensory role of the vagus was first discovered in animals that failed to develop sickness behaviors (social withdrawal, anorexia, reduced exploration) that typically follow intraperitoneal lipopolysaccharide (LPS) injection after subdiaphragmatic vagotomy.[16] Thus, the vagus has been suggested to serve as an interface between peripheral inflammation and behavior.[15]

11.4.2 INFLAMMATORY REFLEX

The discovery that stimulation of vagus nerve efferent fibers attenuates tumor-necrosis factor-α (TNF-α) release in the periphery during endotoxemia lead to the proposition of an inflammatory reflex that counter-regulates excessive pro-inflammatory cytokine production.[17] This anti-inflammatory reflex is composed of an immunosensory component from vagal afferents coupled with the subsequent activation of a vagal motor efferent arc, which constitutes the cholinergic anti-inflammatory pathway (CAP).[18] Activation of the CAP inhibits further peripheral cytokine release; this occurs via binding of acetylcholine to α-7 nicotinic acetylcholine receptors located on macrophages and other immune cells and the resulting deactivation of nuclear factor-kappa B (NF-$\mathcal{k}$B) transcription factor.[18] Numerous studies in humans employing the use of vagus nerve stimulation (VNS) have confirmed the significance of the CAP in reducing the deleterious effects of inflammation in chronic inflammatory diseases and treatment-resistant depression.[19] The most frequently used measure of vagal tone in humans, heart rate variability (HRV), is consistently shown to be reduced in individuals with low grade systematic inflammation.[20,21] This suggests that insufficient vagal regulation of inflammation may contribute to the etiology of chronic inflammatory disease.

11.4.3 VAGAL MODULATION OF HPA-AXIS STRESS RESPONSE

The stress response requires coordinated activity between the HPA-axis, SAM-axis, and ANS via overlapping and interconnected neural networks.[14] For instance, activation of vagal afferents has a stimulatory effect on HPA activity via signaling through the PVN.[14] This connection between the vagus nerve and HPA-axis stress response is illustrated by findings from animal models that have found that lesions of neural pathways implicated in vagus to HPA-axis communication reduce activation of the HPA-axis following interleukin-1β administration.[22] This suggests that disruption of vagal signaling pathways may impair the ability of the HPA-axis to counter-regulate inflammation. In addition, human studies have found that VNS normalizes the altered HPA-axis response seen in depressed individuals and that low vagally mediated HRV (vmHRV) is associated with impaired recovery following stress of both cortisol and TNF-α.[23,24] Such findings indicate that reduced vagal efficiency can alter both HPA-axis functionality and inflammation.

11.4.4 VAGAL TONE: IMPLICATIONS FOR CHRONIC INFLAMMATION AND MENTAL HEALTH

Low vagal tone, as typically indexed by vmHRV, has been implicated as a salient marker of both physical and mental health. This has been consistently exemplified by studies finding vmHRV to be reduced in CVD,[25] rheumatoid arthritis,[26] post-traumatic stress disorder (PTSD),[27] and major depressive disorder. VmHRV has been posited to represent top-down inhibitory control of subcortical brain regions by higher-order cortical regions.[28,29] Given that these subcortical brain regions have been found to be overreactive in individuals with maladaptive stress responsivity, high vmHRV is suggested to be a marker of stress resilience.[29] There is also growing evidence that stress may dysregulate the CAP. For instance, traumatic life events and history of child maltreatment are associated with lower measures of vmHRV and a pro-inflammatory phenotype.[27,30] Reduced vagal activity and reduced efficiency of the CAP following chronic stress may, in turn, contribute to a less restrained inflammatory response which can further worsen chronic inflammatory conditions.

11.4.5 CONCLUSIONS

Dysregulation of the CAP may negatively affect chronic inflammatory disease development and mental health. This is supported by (1) the immunoregulatory role of the vagus, (2) its projections to cortical regions that subserve mood regulation and stress responsivity, and (3) vagal modulation of the HPA-axis stress response. Interventions designed to increase vagal tone, such as VNS and HRV biofeedback, may serve as promising treatment modalities in the future for individuals with diseases with an inflammatory component.

11.5 EARLY LIFE ADVERSITY: RE-PROGRAMMING OF NEUROENDOCRINE AND NEUROIMMUNE PATHWAYS

Exposure to stress or perceived environmental threat involves the concurrent actions of the HPA-axis, SAM-axis, ANS, and immune system. Given their interconnections, dysregulation of one pathway or system is rarely seen in isolation. Early life adversity (ELA) (e.g., childhood trauma, deprivation, neglect, maltreatment, abuse, pre/postnatal stress) has been posited to "re-program" and sensitize these pathways in such a way that confers greater risk for the emergence of psychological disorders and chronic stress-related disease.[31-33] The re-programming of these pathways, in response to ELA, and long-term implications are outlined below.

11.5.1 EARLY LIFE ADVERSITY (ELA) AND HPA-SAM AXIS DYSREGULATION

Rat pups exposed to prolonged maternal separation, or whose mothers show low maternal care, show elevated SAM and HPA-axis responsivity, reduced GC negative feedback, and a downregulation of hippocampal GRs.[34] In humans, similar alterations have been seen for ELA experienced at distinct developmental time periods. Early life disruption of caregiving has been linked with higher basal cortisol levels, impaired GC negative feedback, and slower HPA-axis recovery following stress.[32] In addition, adolescents and adults who had experienced ELA exhibited elevated cortisol and exaggerated SAM- and HPA-axis stress reactivity.[31,32,35] Conversely, experiences of severe childhood trauma or deprivation, or prenatal stress, have been associated with a blunted HPA-axis response to challenge,[35,36] which may be a consequence of ongoing chronic HPA-axis activation or reflect deficient HPA-axis regulation.[35] Importantly, very early childhood (before age 1) may be a particularly vulnerable time-window for later-life HPA dysregulation.[37] Importantly, these effects of ELA on the HPA-axis are often not evident until adolescence or adulthood.[31,35]

11.5.2 PRIMING AND SENSITIZATION OF INNATE IMMUNE CELLS

Early life adversity has been linked to notable changes in immune development and functioning. In adolescents and adults with a history of ELA, there have been consistent reports of a pro-inflammatory phenotype, increased NF-ƙB expression,[38] insensitivity to anti-inflammatory signaling, and deficits in adaptive immunity.[33] Such findings led to the notion that adversity experienced in early life primes macrophages to be especially sensitive to signals of distress initiated in response to infection or stress, thus leading to an exaggerated pro-inflammatory response.[33] The formation of GC resistance by immune cells, due to early-life immune activation and stress-induced HPA alterations, likely contributes to this heightened inflammatory response and to the state of chronic low-grade inflammation frequently observed in adults with history of ELA.[39,40] In concordance with this theory, ELA is associated with (1) a progressive increase in pro-inflammatory cytokine production and glucocorticoid insensitivity following microbial challenge, and (2) an elevated inflammatory response to an acute psychosocial stressor in adolescence and adulthood.[41,42] To sum, ELA appears to promote a pro-inflammatory phenotype that manifests more prominently later in life and is particularly apparent following exposure to physiological or psychosocial stress. A reprogramming of stress pathway sensitivities at the time of ELA likely underlies these changes in immunity.

11.5.3 AUTONOMIC NERVOUS SYSTEM DYSFUNCTION

Early life adversity is also associated with ANS dysfunction and reduced vagal tone. Specifically, lower resting HRV (i.e., vagal tone),[30] higher SNS activity coupled with lower HRV,[43] delayed vagal regulation of heart rate following stress,[43] and atypical vagal reactivity to an emotional stressor have been seen in individuals with a history of child maltreatment or early life deprivation.[43] Importantly, these reductions in vagal tone are more pronounced when measured in adulthood versus in adolescence or childhood, and for individuals with psychopathology in addition to ELA.[44] As described earlier, the vagus plays an important role in regulating both inflammation and the HPA-axis, and the feed-forward mechanism between the SAM-axis and HPA-axis in conditions of stress.[14,45] Hence, these ANS alterations seen in individuals with ELA may potentiate the alterations observed in other stress response pathways.

11.5.4 IMPLICATIONS FOR LATER LIFE DISEASE

ELA is consistently linked with detrimental health outcomes, poor overall well-being, and mortality risk.[46] Dysregulation of stress and immune pathways has been implicated as a potential mechanism by which ELA confers greater risk for psychopathology and chronic disease in later life.[40,46] While alterations in these pathways serves an adaptive purpose at the time of adversity (i.e., in the short term), the long-term consequences for both physical and mental health are often dire. For instance, dysregulation of these pathways by ELA increases risk for the development of chronic diseases of aging, as extensively reviewed elsewhere.[46] Note that chronic low-grade inflammation, seen in individuals with history of ELA, is a common feature of many prevalent diseases typically occurring in mid to late life. Dysregulated HPA-axis functionality and reduced vagal efficiency result in impaired counter-regulatory effects on inflammation, further contributing to the pro-inflammatory phenotype seen in adults with experiences of ELA. The manner by which ELA affects these endocrine and neuroimmune pathways illustrates the intricate connections between these systems; this overlap must be considered when trying to identify intermediary biological pathways influencing disease development. Importantly, early life adversity can put an individual on a different trajectory throughout life that promotes non-optimal responses to future stressors, accelerated aging, and poorer health.

11.6 OTHER RELEVANT FACTORS

11.6.1 AGING

Prolonged stress can negatively affect both the function and lifespan of various cells in our body. For example, telomere length can be shortened by stress;[3,47] in turn, this reduces the replicative ability and, ultimately, the lifespan of our cells. Stress can also promote immunosuppression in a manner normally seen with chronological age (e.g., antibody responses to vaccines, latent virus activation, susceptibility to infection, slower wound healing rates), and can promote "inflammaging."[48] Inflammaging is a phenomenon that describes the chronic low-grade systemic inflammation often seen as adults get older. The result is a chronic micro-inflammatory state in the body. As previously discussed, this higher inflammation produces wear and tear on structures such as blood vessels and can promote sub-optimal immune responses. It is considered a measure of immunosenescence and is strongly associated with many diseases related to aging (e.g., Alzheimer's disease, atherosclerosis, CVD, type 2 diabetes, cancer). Notably, the ANS also undergoes substantial changes with age, with large declines in vmHRV observed.[49] Given that chronic stress can increase inflammation (described above) and is associated with lower vmHRV, stress can potentially elicit or aggravate many disease conditions prevalent with increased age. To sum, prolonged stress promotes aging in the human body at both the cellular and systems level and does so through many of the same biological processes that aging affects. Through these mechanisms, psychological stress can literally age us.

11.6.2 Mental Health

The term "stress" in this chapter is not limited solely to psychological stress and per-
tains to many distinct psychosocial factors and conditions (e.g., loneliness, negative
mood, bereavement, caregiving for a loved one). In addition, all mental health conditions (e.g., depression, anxiety, PTSD) can be brought on and/or worsened by stress.
Mental health (e.g., depression) is also a unique stressor of its own. This positive
feedback loop can create a downward spiral, promoting further stress and reducing
the efficacy of therapy. Hence, efforts to reduce stress in patients with mental illness
is highly warranted.

11.6.3 Health Behaviors

Many of the detrimental consequences of chronic stress on health can occur from
an increased disposition of stressed individuals to display certain health behaviors.
Examples include poor sleep quality, unhealthy diet, reduced exercise, inactivity, and
increased substance use (e.g., alcohol, tobacco, illicit drugs). Many of these behaviors can promote each other (e.g., alcohol use and poor sleep quality), producing a
cycle that can be difficult to break. These behaviors are strong *indirect* pathways
through which stress can have a negative impact on health.

11.7 CONCLUSIONS AND CLINICAL IMPLICATIONS

Prolonged psychological stress can have many harmful effects on health. Some
of these effects occur via *direct* biological pathways, i.e., through modulation
of the immune system, and some through *indirect* pathways such as changes
in health behaviors. In addition, by promoting changes in the same biological
mechanisms that are altered as we get older, stress can literally age us. Severe
stress, especially early life adversity, can result in alterations (reprogramming) of
the various stress pathways described in this chapter, which can cause permanent
changes to the immune system. Ultimately, this increases health risks throughout
the lifespan.

The assessment of psychological stress should be a customary practice in
patients with inflammatory conditions or chronic disease. Given that prolonged
stress can increase a myriad of health risks, the clinical assessment and alle-
viation of stress is particularly important for patients who fall into other high-
risk categories. While assessing and alleviating stress in all individuals prior to a
major surgery would be ideal, this is arguably more important in an *older* woman
with *diabetes* (each being a risk factor for delayed healing) than in a younger
woman with no comorbidity. This is pertinent to many clinical scenarios. Risks
for poorer clinical outcomes and other medical complications are substantially
higher in chronically stressed individuals. The presence of high psychological
stress levels, especially in combination with other known risk factors and comorbidities, should serve as a red flag to the clinician, and attempts should be made
to address and minimize this stress prior to major surgery or other substantive
medical procedures.

REFERENCES

1. Hawkley L, Engeland C, Marucha PT. Loneliness, dysphoria, stress, and immunity: A role for cytokines. In: *Cytokines: Stress and Immunity*; 2006:67–85. doi:www.researchgate.net/publication/228361741

2. Engeland CG, Marucha PT. Wound healing and stress. In: *Neuroimmunology of the Skin*. Springer Berlin Heidelberg; 2009:233–247. doi:10.1007/978-3-540-35989-0_21

3. Engeland CG. Stress, aging, and wound healing. In: Bosch JA, Phillips AC, Lord JM, eds. *Immunosenescence: Psychosocial and Behavioral Determinants*. Springer New York; 2013:63–79. doi:10.1007/978-1-4614-4776-4_5

4. Glaser R, Kiecolt-Glaser JK. Stress-induced immune dysfunction: Implications for health. *Nature Reviews Immunology*. 2005;5(3):243–251. doi:10.1038/nri1571

5. Pedersen AF, Zachariae R, Bovbjerg DH. Psychological stress and antibody response to influenza vaccination: A meta-analysis. *Brain, Behavior, and Immunity*. 2009;23(4):427–433. doi:10.1016/j.bbi.2009.01.004

6. Engeland CG, Bosch JA, Cacioppo JT, Marucha PT. Mucosal wound healing: The roles of age and sex. *Archives of Surgery (Chicago 1960)*. 2006;141(12):1193–1197. doi:10.1001/archsurg.141.12.1193

7. Engeland CG, Hugo FN, Hilgert JB, et al. Psychological distress and salivary secretory immunity. *Brain, Behavior, and Immunity*. 2016;52:11–17. doi:10.1016/j.bbi.2015.08.017

8. Segerstrom SC, Miller GE. Psychological stress and the human immune system: A meta-analytic study of 30 years of inquiry. *Psychological Bulletin*. 2004;130(4):601–630. doi:10.1037/0033-2909.130.4.601

9. Petrovsky N, McNair P, Harrison LC. Diurnal rhythms of pro-inflammatory cytokines: Regulation by plasma cortisol and therapeutic implications. *Cytokine (Philadelphia, Pa)*. 1998;10(4):307–312. doi:10.1006/cyto.1997.0289

10. Jung SH, Wang Y, Kim T, et al. Molecular mechanisms of repeated social defeat-induced glucocorticoid resistance: Role of microRNA. *Brain, Behavior, and Immunity*. 2014;44:195–206. doi:10.1016/j.bbi.2014.09.015

11. Padgett DA, Sheridan JF, Dorne J, Berntson GG, Candelora J, Glaser R. Social stress and the reactivation of latent herpes simplex virus type 1. *Proceedings of the National Academy of Sciences - PNAS*. 1998;95(12):7231–7235. doi:10.1073/pnas.95.12.7231

12. Furman D, Campisi J, Verdin E, et al. Chronic inflammation in the etiology of disease across the life span. *Nature Medicine*. 2019;25(12):1822–1832. doi:10.1038/s41591-019-0675-0

13. Godbout JP, Glaser R. Stress-induced immune dysregulation: Implications for wound healing, infectious disease and cancer. *Journal of Neuroimmune Pharmacology*. 2006;1(4):421–427. doi:10.1007/s11481-006-9036-0

14. Mueller B, Figueroa A, Robinson-Papp J. Structural and functional connections between the autonomic nervous system, hypothalamic–pituitary–adrenal axis, and the immune system: A context and time dependent stress response network. *Neurological Sciences*. 2022;43(2):951–960. doi:10.1007/s10072-021-05810-1

15. Marvel FA, Chen CC, Badr N, Gaykema RPA, Goehler LE. Reversible inactivation of the dorsal vagal complex blocks lipopolysaccharide-induced social withdrawal and c-Fos expression in central autonomic nuclei. *Brain, Behavior, and Immunity*. 2004;18(2):123–134. doi:10.1016/j.bbi.2003.09.004

16. Bluthe RM, Walter V, Parnet P, et al. Lipopolysaccharide induces sickness behaviour in rats by a vagal mediated mechanism. *Comptes Rendus de l'Académie des Sciences III*. 1994;317(6):499–503.

17. Tracey KJ. The inflammatory reflex. *Nature(London)*. 2002;420:853–859.

18. Huston JM, Tracey KJ. The pulse of inflammation: Heart rate variability, the cholinergic anti-inflammatory pathway and implications for therapy. *Journal of Internal Medicine*. 2011;269:45–53. doi:10.1111/j.1365-2796.2010.02321.x

19. Johnson RL, Wilson CG. A review of vagus nerve stimulation as a therapeutic intervention. *Journal of Inflammation Research*. 2018;11:203–213. doi:10.2147/JIR.S163248

20. Sloan RP, Cole SW. Parasympathetic neural activity and the reciprocal regulation of innate antiviral and inflammatory genes in the human immune system. *Brain, Behavior, and Immunity*. 2021;98:251–256. doi:10.1016/j.bbi.2021.08.217

21. Williams DWP, Koenig J, Carnevali L, et al. Heart rate variability and inflammation: A meta-analysis of human studies. *Brain, Behavior, and Immunity*. 2019;80:219–226. doi:10.1016/j.bbi.2019.03.009

22. Buller K, Xu Y, Dayas C, Day T. Dorsal and ventral medullary catecholamine cell groups contribute differentially to systemic interleukin-1β-induced hypothalamic pituitary adrenal axis responses. *Neuroendocrinology*. 2001;73(2):129–138. doi:10.1159/000054629

23. O'Keane V, Dinan TG, Scott L, Corcoran C. Changes in hypothalamic-pituitary-adrenal axis measures after vagus nerve stimulation therapy in chronic depression. *Biological Psychiatry*. 2005;58(12):963–968. doi:10.1016/j.biopsych.2005.04.049

24. Weber CS, Thayer JF, Rudat M, et al. Low vagal tone is associated with impaired post stress recovery of cardiovascular, endocrine, and immune markers. *European Journal of Applied Physiology*. 2010;109(2):201–211. doi:10.1007/s00421-009-1341-x

25. Kemp AH, Quintana DS. The relationship between mental and physical health: Insights from the study of heart rate variability. *International Journal of Psychophysiology*. 2013;89(3):288–296. doi:10.1016/j.ijpsycho.2013.06.018

26. Adlan AM, Lip GYH, Paton JFR, Kitas GD, Fisher JP. Autonomic function and rheumatoid arthritis-a systematic review. *Seminars in Arthritis and Rheumatism*. 2014;44(3):283–304. doi:10.1016/j.semarthrit.2014.06.003

27. Ge F, Yuan M, Li Y, Zhang W. Posttraumatic stress disorder and alterations in resting heart rate variability: A systematic review and meta-analysis. *Psychiatry Investig*. 2020;17(1):9–20. doi:10.30773/pi.2019.0112

28. Thayer JF, Hansen AL, Saus-Rose E, Johnsen BH. Heart rate variability, prefrontal neural function, and cognitive performance: The neurovisceral integration perspective on self-regulation, adaptation, and health. *Annals of Behavioral Medicine*. 2009;37(2):141–153. doi:10.1007/s12160-009-9101-z

29. Carnevali L, Koenig J, Sgoifo A, Ottaviani C. Autonomic and brain morphological predictors of stress resilience. *Frontiers in Neuroscience*. 2018;12(APR). doi:10.3389/fnins.2018.00228

30. Kuzminskaite E, Vinkers CH, Elzinga BM, Wardenaar KJ, Giltay EJ, Penninx BWJH. Childhood trauma and dysregulation of multiple biological stress systems in adulthood: Results from the Netherlands study of depression and anxiety (NESDA). *Psychoneuroendocrinology*. 2020;121. doi:10.1016/j.psyneuen.2020.104835

31. Lupien SJ, McEwen BS, Gunnar MR, Heim C. Effects of stress throughout the lifespan on the brain, behaviour and cognition. *Nature Reviews Neuroscience*. 2009;10(6):434–445. doi:10.1038/nrn2639

32. Kuhlman KR, Chiang JJ, Horn S, Bower JE. Developmental psychoneuroendocrine and psychoneuroimmune pathways from childhood adversity to disease. *Neuroscience & Biobehavioral Reviews*. 2017;80:166–184. doi:10.1016/j.neubiorev.2017.05.020

33. Miller GE, Chen E, Parker KJ. Psychological stress in childhood and susceptibility to the chronic diseases of aging: Moving toward a model of behavioral and biological mechanisms. *Psychological Bulletin*. 2011;137(6):959–997. doi:10.1037/a0024768

34. Meaney MJ. Maternal care, gene expression, and the transmission of individual differences in stress reactivity across generations. *Annual Review of Neuroscience*. 2001;24(1):1161–1192. doi:10.1146/annurev.neuro.24.1.1161

35. Danese A, McEwen BS. Adverse childhood experiences, allostasis, allostatic load, and age-related disease. *Physiology & Behavior.* 2012;106(1):29–39. doi:10.1016/j.physbeh. 2011.08.019

36. Entringer S, Buss C, Wadhwa PD. Prenatal stress and developmental programming of human health and disease risk: Concepts and integration of empirical findings. *Current Opinion in Endocrinology, Diabetes and Obesity.* 2010;17(6):507–516. doi:10.1097/ MED.0b013c3283405921

37. Kuhlman KR, Vargas I, Geiss EG, Lopez-Duran NL. Age of trauma onset and HPA axis dysregulation among trauma-exposed youth. *Journal of Traumatic Stress.* 2015;28(6):572–579. doi:10.1002/jts.22054

38. Miller GE, Chen E, Fok AK, et al. Low early-life social class leaves a biological resi-due manifested by decreased glucocorticoid and increased pro-inflammatory signaling. *Proceedings of the National Academy of Sciences - PNAS.* 2009;106(34):14716–14721. doi:10.1073/pnas.0902971106

39. Danese A, Pariante CM, Caspi A, Taylor A, Poulton R. Childhood maltreatment pre-dicts adult inflammation in a life-course study. 2007. doi:10.1073/pnas.0610362104

40. Danese A, J Lewis S. Psychoneuroimmunology of early-life stress: The hidden wounds of childhood trauma. *Neuropsychopharmacology.* 2017;42(1):99–114. doi:10.1038/npp. 2016.198

41. Carpenter LL, Gawuga CE, Tyrka AR, Lee JK, Anderson GM, Price LH. Association between plasma IL-6 response to acute stress and early-life adversity in healthy adults. *Neuropsychopharmacology.* 2010;35(13):2617–2623. doi:10.1038/ npp.2010.159

42. Miller GE, Chen E. Harsh family climate in early life presages the emergence of a pro-inflammatory phenotype in adolescence. *Psychological Science: a Journal of the American Psychological Society/APS.* 2010;21(6):848–856. doi:10.1177/ 0956797610370161

43. Dale LP, Shaikh SK, Fasciano LC, Watorek VD, Heilman KJ, Porges SW. College females with maltreatment histories have atypical autonomic regulation and poor psychological wellbeing. *Psychological Trauma.* 2018;10(4):427–434. doi:10.1037/ tra0000342

44. Sigrist C, Mürner-Lavanchy I, Peschel SKV, Schmidt SJ, Kaess M, Koenig J. Early life maltreatment and resting-state heart rate variability: A systematic review and meta-analysis. *Neuroscience & Biobehavioral Reviews.* 2021;120:307–334. doi:10.1016/j. neubiorev.2020.10.026

45. Elenkov IJ, Wilder RL, Chrousos GP, Vizi ES. The sympathetic nerve–an inte-grative interface between two supersystems: The brain and the immune system. *Pharmacological Reviews.* 2000;52(4):595–638.

46. Ehrlich KB, Miller GE, Chen E. Childhood adversity and adult physical health. In: D. Cicchetti, ed. *Developmental Psychopathology: Risk, Resilience, and Intervention* John Wiley & Sons, Inc; 2016. doi: 10.1002/9781119125556.devpsy401.

47. Epel ES, Blackburn EH, Lin J, et al. Accelerated telomere shortening in response to life stress. *Proceedings of the National Academy of Sciences - PNAS.* 2004;101(49): 17312–17315. doi:10.1073/pnas.0407162101

48. Franceschi C, Bonafe M, Valensin S, et al. Inflamm-aging: An evolutionary perspec-tive on immunosenescence. *Annals of the New York Academy of Sciences.* 2000;908(1): 244–254. doi:10.1111/j.1749-6632.2000.tb06651.x

49. Kuo TB, Lin T, Yang CC, Li CL, Chen CF, Chou P. Effect of aging on gender differ-ences in neural control of heart rate. *American Journal of Physiology.* 1999;277(6): H2233–H2239. doi:10.1152/ajpheart.1999.277.6.h2233

12 Health Neuroscience

Emma Moughan, BA and Richard B. Lopez, PhD

KEY POINTS

- Health neuroscience, a burgeoning interdisciplinary field that examines links between brain function and mental and physical health, holds promise for lifestyle medicine practitioners.
- Practitioners and patients alike can benefit from learning about neural mechanisms that underlie regulation of eating behaviors, stress and negative emotions, and drug use.
- These behavioral domains can serve as targets of interventions that promote and enhance health and well-being.

12.1 INTRODUCTION

When the COVID-19 pandemic started to sweep the world in early 2020, life as we knew it changed dramatically. Significant scale shutdowns restricted people's social interactions and mobility, with many abruptly switching to remote learning and working. Rates of depression and anxiety jumped from 8.5% prior to the pandemic to 27.8% and have only gotten worse, rising to 32.8% in 2021.[1] These trends have put mental health—and overall health and well-being—in the spotlight, as individuals, businesses, and governments have realized that health has often been sacrificed in the service of overwork, burnout, and chronic stress. Throughout the pandemic, businesses have begun to take steps to promote and advocate for their employees' health actively. For example, in 2020, Google completely revamped its work schedule by transitioning to remote work, incorporating "work from anywhere" hours, and adding extended vacation hours and reset days.[2,3] Although these changes in the workplace are laudable, the healthcare system is one of the primary and more regular points of contact where people receive counsel on how to change their behaviors in the service of health. Finding holistic and innovative ways to support those individuals with poor mental health and other health concerns has been a persistent challenge for medical providers. Still, the pandemic added a sense of urgency to an already complex issue.

One way in which doctors have tackled this issue is by incorporating lifestyle medicine into their practice, emphasizing a multi-faceted approach to overall health and wellness. According to the American College of Lifestyle Medicine, lifestyle medicine is defined as "an evidence-based approach to treating and reversing disease by replacing unhealthy behaviors with positive ones,"[4] and it incorporates six fundamental pillars—nutrition, exercise, alcohol and tobacco use, stress management, sleep, and healthy relationships—into a general practice that relies on actionable behavior and lifestyle modifications, such as reducing stress, or making mindful and

DOI: 10.1201/b22810-14

healthy diet decisions. By actively pursuing these modifications, people can proactively maintain or enhance their health before disease ever takes hold. Although all six abovementioned factors are important, proper nutrition, stress management, and curbing substance use have direct and significant impacts on one's health.

In this chapter, we will focus on these three factors in light of recent findings from health neuroscience, a burgeoning interdisciplinary field that examines reciprocal links between brain function and mental and physical health. Health neuroscience holds significant promise for lifestyle medicine because it sheds light on the neural mechanisms that underlie behavior change. These mechanisms include brain systems associated with reward processing, regulation, and valuation, which we discuss at greater length below. By targeting these mechanisms, a person can minimize maladaptive behaviors (e.g., poor diet, chronic stress, and substance abuse), replace them with adaptive ones, and improve health and well-being.

12.2   NUTRITION AND EATING BEHAVIORS

One of lifestyle medicine's primary aims is to provide medical providers with practical, preventative measures to alter people's behaviors and habits to reduce the burden of chronic conditions such as diabetes and cardiovascular disease. One popular domain in which this occurs is the eating domain. Links between patterns of overeating and/or unhealthy eating and diseases such as cancer, cardiovascular disease, and type 2 diabetes are well established,[5,6] but effective interventions to promote healthier eating patterns less so.

We believe that medical practitioners would greatly benefit from learning more about the neural bases of the generation and regulation of eating behaviors, as this can inform the development of interventions to alter eating and nutritional intake in the service of health.

Many factors contribute to a person's overall nutritional wellness, but neural mechanisms that underlie impulsivity and self-control, respectively, play a significant role in how people approach their dietary decisions.[7] One of the key components of eating and appetitive behaviors is, put quite simply, control. Control can be broken down into different areas in the brain, with executive control being housed in our dorsolateral prefrontal cortex and inhibitory control in both our ventrolateral prefrontal cortex and inferior frontal gyrus.[8-11] Like most brain systems, these regions impact our functioning in many ways, but they play a seminal role in how humans engage in self-regulation and, ultimately, make decisions regarding their food intake. One of the primary goals of executive control (and, thus, the dorsolateral prefrontal cortex) is to lead a long and healthy life.[8] To lead that long and healthy life, a person would then need to engage in self-regulatory behaviors regarding food (and other areas like stress and substance abuse, which will be discussed later) not only to reach that goal but also to maintain it as well. Many factors contribute to why a person may make an "unhealthy" choice regarding their food intake, such as heavy cognitive load (using more cognitive resources and, thus, using more mental effort) and the subsequent ego depletion.[7] This concept forms the basis of the connection between one's idea of control and one's perception of the ensuing effects of nutritional decision-making on overall health.[6] These "unhealthy" decisions may be facilitated by our orbitofrontal cortex, which houses pleasantness and satiation centers, among others, as a way to derive pleasure from the food a person may eat.[12] The neural bases of eating and other food behaviors allow practitioners, researchers, and medical professionals to understand not only how decisions are made with food, but also why some people may make "unhealthy" decisions regarding their health and food intake.

While neural and brain bases are imperative to our understanding of how and why food-based decisions are made, there is growing evidence (and subsequent literature) that details the connection between the gut biome and brain and neural pathways and how their interaction influences these decisions. The connection between the gut and the brain, formally called the gut-brain axis (GBA), has been the interest of mental health and wellness research in the past and presents many interesting intersections between the brain and other biological systems.[13] Specifically, there is a link between a disrupted GBA and anxiety and depression, highlighting how changes in other areas of the body impact neural pathways.[13] This idea is also present in the stress response and hypothalamic-pituitary-adrenal (HPA) axis, where gut microbiota plays a large role in the programming of the HPA and how we react to stress in our lives.[14] Knowing this allows interventions curated by medical professionals to be more specific, as understanding that the GBA has implications in both food-related neural bases and stress-related neural bases opens the door for more exploration. The link between the central nervous system (CNS) function and the GBA is also relevant, as the CNS also triggers the stress response through stress circuits.[14] This link indicates that the bacteria within the gastrointestinal (GI) tract have the ability to elicit these stress circuits within the CNS, prompting a reaction that starts outside of the neural networks.[15,16] With the GBA and bacteria present in the GI tract able to elicit stress responses and contribute to the psychological and physiological symptoms of anxiety and depression (through these stress responses), mental health and GBA stability have more in common than was previously thought. The perspective health neuroscience and, more broadly, neuroscience, have on these important neural-body connections allows researchers and medical professionals to continue to dive deeper into the different brain-body interactions and continue to research how interventions within the GBA can be helpful in reducing stress and improving overall well-being.

12.3 STRESS AND EMOTION REGULATION

Appetitive cues represent a physical aspect to the domains of lifestyle medicine, but what about emotionally-laden cues, and affective responses they engender, that are so prevalent in our daily lives? By examining the importance of stress and emotion regulation in both mental and physical health fields, medical professionals and other personnel can expand knowledge of how and why stress is maintained. When discussing neural and brain pathways associated with stress and emotion regulation, there are a few imperative pathways that contribute to the response seen, including the sympathetic nervous system (SNS), the hypothalamus-adrenal-pituitary (HPA) axis, and the sympathetic-adreno-medullary (SAM) axis.[17–20] To break these down a little more specifically, the SNS supports bodily functions like blood pressure and heart rate;[19] the HPA axis helps to regulate cortisol levels throughout the body;[19] the SAM axis releases noradrenaline and norepinephrine to ensure the body is prepared for the stressor.[20] Much like the brain bases present in nutrition, these neural pathways have multiple functions outside of the stress response but are integral to how our body prepares to process the stressor. Another connection comes from a broader place, where it has been established that the dorsal anterior cingulate cortex (dACC) and the amygdala, both associated with our body's threat response, have been linked to similar physiological symptoms seen in the SNS and HPA axis, as well as our body's inflammatory system (which will be detailed below).[19] The intersection of neural pathways (and responses, such as symptomatic reactions) in both the stress and threat response highlights how brain systems can work together to create a response to protect our survival; an example of this type of response would be a person feeling threatened (life at risk or feeling rejected) and the SNS and HPA axis subsequently being stimulated (increased heart rate, increased cortisol levels, raised blood pressure, etc.).

Stress and emotion regulation are not new to the neural, or medical, world, as they both highlight the importance of understanding how negatively perceived situations in life can influence a person's brain and neural network. High stress and cortisol levels have been linked to greater risk in cardiovascular diseases, arthritis, and even cancer,[19,21–23] indicating a strong relation between one's mental health and one's physical health. Much of this speculation comes from the fact that inflammation and the sympathetic nervous system are influential in infection and illness response, as well as stress response.[19] Inflammation is a response our body elicits when under attack, and based on findings from,[19] stress is considered an attack worthy enough to see a response. Similarly, this is seen in the sympathetic nervous system, where a response is enacted when under stress.[19] In other words, the same mechanisms in place to help fight infection are also involved in the stress response.

Looking more broadly at the neural pathways present in the stress response, researchers have found that the neural pathways work together with other physiological responses to elicit a reaction. For example, strong cardiovascular reactions (quickening heart rate or increased blood pressure) to acute psychological stressors lead to activations in the amygdala[24] and the medial prefrontal cortex,[25] indicating that more than one process is at play when a stress response is prompted.[26] This idea is not only important in the field of health neuroscience, but gives researchers, doctors, and other medical and mental health professionals the ability to develop interventions as a way to incorporate healthy coping mechanisms into a person's everyday life. There is also evidence that, beyond physiological responses, social factors and interpersonal mechanisms are also interwoven into the stress response, indicating that emotional systems also impact health outcomes of those experiencing stress.[26] Knowing this, different types of intervention methods targeting specific types of stress would greatly benefit a person attempting to combat a stressor. As stated above, there are many different neural bases at play when a stress or threat response is prompted. Having the knowledge and understanding that different types of stress responses may be coming from the same neural pathway(s) allows medical professionals and researchers to target and intervene in specific responses.

12.4 SUBSTANCE ABUSE

Substance abuse, whether involving licit or illicit drugs, can have an immense impact on the medical field and all fields (like health neuroscience) related to it. The way drugs and substances influence and alter the brain and neural pathways within it has been a seminal research question for decades and remains an integral interaction between neuroscience and medical practice.

Reliance on various substances has been a large-scale societal problem, especially in the United States, where 12.5% of people ages 18 and above smoke cigarettes and 25.8% of people binge drink and/or engage in heavy alcohol use.[27,28] Alcohol, nicotine, and other drugs raise questions regarding why people enjoy drugs, especially when cognitive dissonance (i.e., knowing that smoking cigarettes is bad for your health and wellness but continuing to do it) and other self-violations (i.e., knowing that drinking alcohol in excess goes against personal goals but continuing to partake in the behavior) are present?[29] By examining the neural bases of substance abuse, we can begin to understand the underpinnings of these maladaptive behaviors while also recognizing why they may be maintained.

Reward and pleasure centers in the brain, specifically the mesolimbic dopamine pathway, play a large role in the maintenance of substance abuse and may provide some more context to the question "why do people enjoy drugs?"[29] The chronic use of certain drugs can change the brain's chemistry, creating a cycle of dependence and addiction that becomes extremely difficult to break.[29] This is because most drugs mimic the natural neurotransmitters in the brain, leading to a decrease in the natural production when a drug is abused.[29] When the reward and pleasure pathways have been altered by the drug of choice, you begin to see withdrawal symptoms. The withdrawal symptoms associated with motivation are dysphoria, anhedonia, and subsequent cravings, leading to a need for the drug to overtake all other needs a person may experience.[29] While these responses are typically seen in people abusing opiates or stimulants like cocaine, these same principles still apply to people abusing alcohol or nicotine. People going through alcohol withdrawal experience symptoms like tremors, hallucinations/delusions, and tachycardia,[29] illustrating the mind-body connection present in substance abuse.

Much like with stress and emotion regulation, similar brain regions are activated when people are dependent on substances. This is due to the connection between substance abuse and self-control, as well as a person's ability to self-soothe and regulate when under stress. Specifically, subcortical regions such as the ventral striatum and the amygdala play significant roles by supporting drug-seeking behaviors and emotional appraisals associated with those behaviors.[30] Higher-order cognition, such as self-related processing, also plays a role in the maintenance and regulation of substance abuse.[31] People who may abuse a substance, like alcohol or nicotine, may only be able to quit if long-term, negative health consequences are actively brought to mind to alter appraisals of the substance. This kind of reappraisal process is seen in Whelan and colleagues' 2017 study, which demonstrated short-term behavioral changes when participants were shown pictures of darkened lungs, as such images can be interpreted as self-relevant (i.e., "this can happen to me").[11] This bolsters the idea of how self-related processing impacts substance abuse, as Falk and colleagues[32] found that self-reflection and self-related processing have the potential for behavior change, which is imperative as we begin to research stronger and healthier interventions for smoking cessation and to lower the number of people that partake in binge drinking.

12.5 CONCLUSION

The importance of proper mental health practices is an integral aspect of both lifestyle medicine and health neuroscience. Lifestyle medicine, an evidence-based approach that aims to treat and reverse disease by replacing unhealthy behaviors with positive ones, can help mitigate maladaptive behaviors that undermine mental health and well-being. Health neuroscience presents the necessary theoretical grounding to pave the way for future interventions targeting physical and mental health problems. Indeed, lifestyle medicine practitioners will benefit greatly from an enhanced understanding of the neural bases underlying nutrition and eating behaviors, stress and emotion regulation, and substance abuse. By implementing such brain-based interventions, medical practitioners can develop more detailed and personalized treatment plans that help mitigate the physical and emotional symptoms of poor nutrition, stress, and substance abuse they observe in their patient population. Health neuroscience and lifestyle medicine allow this all to be possible and open new avenues to connections between the mental and physical health fields.

REFERENCES

1. Crawford G. Depression Rates in US Tripled When the Pandemic First Hit—Now, They're Even Worse. Boston University. Published October 13, 2021. Accessed February 21, 2023. https://www.bu.edu/sph/news/articles/2021/depression-rates-tripled-and-symptoms-intensified-during-first-year-of-covid/
2. Gurchiek K. Google Extends Work-from-Home Policy Through June 2021. SHRM. Published July 7, 2021. Accessed February 21, 2023. https://www.shrm.org/resourcesandtools/hr-topics/technology/pages/google-extends-work-from-home-policy-through-june-2021.aspx
3. Main K. How Google's Reimagined "Work from Anywhere" Policy Gets Staff Back in the Office. Inc.com. Published October 4, 2022. Accessed February 21, 2023. https://www.inc.com/kelly-main/how-googles-reimagined-work-from-anywhere-policy-gets-staff-back-in-office.html
4. Burke J, Dunne PJ. Lifestyle medicine pillars as predictors of psychological flourishing. *Frontiers in Psychology*. 2022;13:963806. doi:10.3389/fpsyg.2022.963806
5. World Health Organization. *Global Report on Diabetes*. World Health Organization; 2016. Accessed February 22, 2023. https://apps.who.int/iris/handle/10665/204871
6. Hall PA. Executive-control processes in high-calorie food consumption. *Current Directions in Psychological Science*. 2016;25(2):91–98. doi:10.1177/0963721415625049
7. Hofmann W, Friese M, Strack F. Impulse and self-control from a dual-systems perspective. *Perspectives on Psychological Science*. 2009;4(2):162–176. doi:10.1111/j.1745-6924.2009.01116.x

8. Lopez RB, Cruz-Vespa I. The brain bases of regulation of eating behaviors: The role of reward, executive control, and valuation processes, and new paths to propel the field forward. *Current Opinion in Behavioral Sciences.* 2022;48:101214. doi:10.1016/j.cobeha.2022.101214

9. Enax L, Hu Y, Trautner P, Weber B. Nutrition labels influence value computation of food products in the ventromedial prefrontal cortex. *Obesity Silver Spring Md.* 2015;23(4):786–792. doi:10.1002/oby.21027

10. Gearhardt AN, Yokum S, Stice E, Harris JL, Brownell KD. Relation of obesity to neural activation in response to food commercials. *Social Cognitive and Affective Neuroscience.* 2014;9(7):932–938. doi:10.1093/scan/nst059

11. Whelan ME, Morgan PS, Sherar LB, Orme MW, Esliger DW. Can functional magnetic resonance imaging studies help with the optimization of health messaging for lifestyle behavior change? A systematic review. *Preventive Medicine.* 2017;99:185–196. doi:10.1016/j.ypmed.2017.02.004

12. Kringelbach ML, O'Doherty J, Rolls ET, Andrews C. Activation of the human orbitofrontal cortex to a liquid food stimulus is correlated with its subjective pleasantness. *Cerebral Cortex New York, N.Y.* . 2003;13(10):1064–1071. doi:10.1093/cercor/13.10.1064

13. Clapp M, Aurora N, Herrera L, Bhatia M, Wilen E, Wakefield S. Gut microbiota's effect on mental health: The gut-brain axis. *Clinics and Practice.* 2017;7(4):987. doi:10.4081/cp.2017.987

14. Foster JA, McVey Neufeld KA. Gut-brain axis: How the microbiome influences anxiety and depression. *Trends in Neurosciences.* 2013;36(5):305–312. doi:10.1016/j.tins.2013.01.005

15. Goehler LE, Park SM, Opitz N, Lyte M, Gaykema RPA. Campylobacter jejuni infection increases anxiety-like behavior in the holeboard: Possible anatomical substrates for viscerosensory modulation of exploratory behavior. *Brain, Behavior, and Immunity.* 2008;22(3):354–366. doi:10.1016/j.bbi.2007.08.009

16. Lyte M, Li W, Opitz N, Gaykema RPA, Goehler LE. Induction of anxiety-like behavior in mice during the initial stages of infection with the agent of murine colonic hyperplasia *Citrobacter* rodentium. *Physiology & Behavior.* 2006;89(3):350–357. doi:10.1016/j.physbeh.2006.06.019

17. Gruenewald TL, Seeman TE, Ryff CD, Karlamangla AS, Singer BH. Combinations of biomarkers predictive of later life mortality. *Proceedings of the National Academy of Sciences.* 2006;103(38):14158–14163. doi:10.1073/pnas.0606215103

18. Miller GE, Chen E, Sze J, et al. A functional genomic fingerprint of chronic stress in humans: Blunted glucocorticoid and increased NF-kappaB signaling. *Biological Psychiatry.* 2008;64(4):266–272. doi:10.1016/j.biopsych.2008.03.017

19. Muscatell KA, Eisenberger NI. A social neuroscience perspective on stress and health. *Social and Personality Psychology Compass.* 2012;6(12):890–904. doi:10.1111/j.1751-9004.2012.00467.x

20. Godoy LD, Rossignoli MT, Delfino-Pereira P, Garcia-Cairasco N, de Lima Umeoka EH. A comprehensive overview on stress neurobiology: Basic concepts and clinical implications. *Frontiers in Behavioral Neuroscience.* 2018;12. Accessed February 21, 2023. https://www.frontiersin.org/articles/10.3389/fnbeh.2018.00127

21. Cohen S, Janicki-Deverts D, Miller GE. Psychological stress and disease. *JAMA.* 2007;298(14):1685–1687. doi:10.1001/jama.298.14.1685

22. Juster RP, McEwen BS, Lupien SJ. Allostatic load biomarkers of chronic stress and impact on health and cognition. *Neuroscience & Biobehavioral Reviews.* 2010;35(1):2–16. doi:10.1016/j.neubiorev.2009.10.002

23. Slavich GM, O'Donovan A, Epel ES, Kemeny ME. Black sheep get the blues: A psychobiological model of social rejection and depression. *Neuroscience & Biobehavioral Reviews.* 2010;35(1):39–45. doi:10.1016/j.neubiorev.2010.01.003

24. Gianaros PJ, Sheu LK, Matthews KA, Jennings JR, Manuck SB, Hariri AR. Individual differences in stressor-evoked blood pressure reactivity vary with activation, volume, and functional connectivity of the amygdala. *The Journal of Neuroscience : The Official Journal of the Society for Neuroscience*. 2008;28(4):990–999. doi:10.1523/JNEUROSCI.3606-07.2008

25. Wager TD, Waugh CE, Lindquist M, Noll DC, Fredrickson BL, Taylor SF. Brain mediators of cardiovascular responses to social threat: Part I: Reciprocal dorsal and ventral sub-regions of the medial prefrontal cortex and heart-rate reactivity. *NeuroImage*. 2009;47(3):82–835. doi:10.1016/j.neuroimage.2009.05.043

26. Erickson KI, Creswell JD, Verstynen TD, Gianaros PJ. Health neuroscience: Defining a new field. *Current Directions in Psychological Science*. 2014;23(6):446–453. doi:10.1177/0963721414549350

27. CDCTobaccoFree. Fast Facts. Centers for Disease Control and Prevention. Published December 1, 2022. Accessed February 21, 2023. https://www.cdc.gov/tobacco/data_statistics/fact_sheets/fast_facts/index.htm

28. National Institute on Alcohol Abuse and Alcoholism. Alcohol Facts and Statistics | National Institute on Alcohol Abuse and Alcoholism (NIAAA). Published March 2022. Accessed February 21, 2023. https://www.niaaa.nih.gov/publications/brochures-and-fact-sheets/alcohol-facts-and-statistics

29. Johnson HC. Neuroscience in social work practice and education. *Journal of Social Work Practice in the Addictions*. 2001;1:81–102. doi:10.1300/J160v01n03_06

30. Tang DW, Fellows LK, Small DM, Dagher A. Food and drug cues activate similar brain regions: A meta-analysis of functional MRI studies. *Physiology & Behavior*. 2012;106(3):317–324. doi:10.1016/j.physbeh.2012.03.009

31. Lieberman MD. Social cognitive neuroscience. In: *Handbook of Social Psychology, Vol. 1, 5th* Ed. John Wiley & Sons, Inc.; 2010:143–193. doi:10.1002/9780470561119.socpsy001005

32. Falk EB, O'Donnell MB, Tompson S, et al. Functional brain imaging predicts public health campaign success. *Social Cognitive and Affective Neuroscience*. 2016;11(2): 204–214. doi:10.1093/scan/nsv108

13 Mental Health and Cellular Aging through the Lifespan

Elissa J. Hamlat, PhD, Anthony Zannas, PhD, and Elissa Epel, PhD

KEY POINTS

- Psychological trauma, PTSD, and depression have been linked to indices of cell aging, including shorter telomeres and accelerated epigenetic clocks.
- A growing number of lifestyle and mind–body interventions have examined effects on cell aging indices (i.e., telomere length, telomerase activity, and epigenetic clocks) with promising initial results.
- Few psychosocial or behavioral interventions that target psychiatric disorders or psychopathology have been examined to see if they also beneficially influence cell aging indices.

13.1 INTRODUCTION

Psychiatric disorders are associated with significantly shorter healthspan and lifespan. For instance, depression is linked to greater premature mortality, largely from causes associated with diseases that more commonly occur with advanced age (e.g., CVD, T2DM, stroke, dementia).[1-3] The field of geroscience posits that if interventions slow the rate of cellular aging, we can prevent the onset or progression of disease and increase healthspan.[4] Given the comorbidity between psychopathology and chronic diseases of aging, it is important to understand how interventions might improve both mental and physical health at multiple levels. For example, integrative interventions may reduce stress-related dimensions of psychopathology, such as rumination, sleep dysregulation, and exaggerated threat reactivity, and at the same time influence stress mediators, such as oxidative stress, excessive exposure to hypothalamic-pituitary-adrenal (HPA) axis mediators (e.g., adrenocorticotropic hormone (ACTH), cortisol), and inflammation, which can influence cellular aging (see Figure 13.1).

This chapter reviews links between mental health and cellular aging as well as the current evidence and gaps in understanding of how psychosocial and behavioral interventions can impact these relationships. Examining indices of cellular aging before disease develops may eventually be used to design more beneficial mental health interventions. At the cellular level, both symptoms and disorders of psychopathology, particularly distress-related disorders (e.g., anxiety and depression), are

DOI: 10.1201/b22810-15

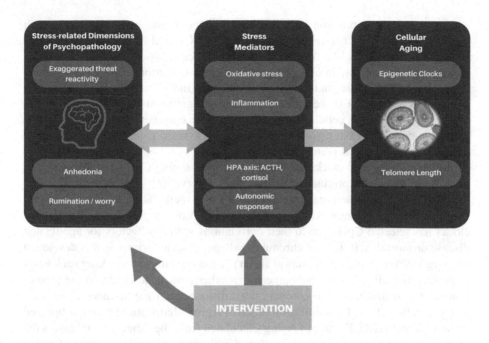

FIGURE 13.1 Theoretical model by which psychosocial interventions may reduce clinical manifestations of psychopathology and, at the same time, induce beneficial changes in stress mediators and cellular aging. Although the pathways in this model are speculative, evidence underlies the relationships between stress mediators and cellular aging. The associations between inflammation and both epigenetic aging and telomere length have been documented.[5-8] Another mediator with established links to cell aging is glucocorticoid signaling; Zannas and colleagues found that the CpGs utilized in the Horvath DNAm clock colocalize with glucocorticoid response elements and change in response to synthetic glucocorticoid exposure.[9]

linked to cellular aging. Two indices of cellular aging that have been studied concerning mental health are the epigenetic clock and immune cell telomere length. Although there are several indices of cellular aging, for illustrative purposes, we focus on two that have been widely studied and can be easily measured in humans. In this chapter, we review associations of mental health with epigenetic aging and telomere length, as well as the existing evidence on whether lifestyle, mind-body, and psychotherapeutic intervention can impact these indices of aging. We do not cover pharmacological interventions here as they are beyond the scope of this chapter.

13.2   THE EPIGENETIC CLOCK AS A BIOMARKER OF AGING AND DISEASE

Epigenetic clocks are composite markers of cellular aging that are derived by combining multiple DNA methylation sites. DNA methylation (DNAm) occurs when a methyl group (CH_3) attaches to cytosine-guanine dinucleotides (CpGs). DNAm can regulate gene expression by activating or silencing the genes associated with the sites.[10] Patterns of age-related alterations in DNA methylation can function as a cellular clock, much like "counting rings on a tree to assess its age" (Dr. Steve Horvath).[11] The magnitude of an epigenetic clock's deviation from an individual's chronological age is thought to reflect how much the individual is aging faster (if the deviation is positive) or slower (if the deviation is negative) than expected at the cellular level. Accelerated cellular aging measured with epigenetic clocks is associated with a greater risk for age-associated diseases such as cancer, cardiovascular disease, and dementia, as well as premature mortality.[12]

Different epigenetic clocks use largely non-overlapping CpG sites to assess cellular aging. Horvath's original epigenetic clock (Horvath)[13,14] was developed across different cell and tissue types by combining DNA methylation levels at 353 CpG sites that correlate strongly with chronological age. A newer generation of epigenetic clocks has selected CpGs due to their correlations with risk factors for age-related disease or mortality instead of chronological age. DNAm GrimAge was developed by using DNAm surrogate markers of seven plasma proteins and smoking pack years to predict mortality.[15] GrimAge outperforms other epigenetic clocks in the prediction of time-to-death, time-to-coronary heart disease, and time-to-cancer.[15] Another new generation clock, DunedinPoAm (Pace of Aging Methylation),[16] and its updated version, DunedinPACE (Pace of Aging Calculated from the Epigenome),[17] assess the rate of epigenetic aging and were developed with many clinical indicators of multiorgan system integrity across multiple time points.

13.2.1 ASSOCIATIONS BETWEEN EPIGENETIC AGING AND MENTAL HEALTH

Accelerated cellular aging as assessed with epigenetic clocks has been associated with a greater risk for psychopathology, particularly stress-related pathology. Consistent associations with accelerated epigenetic aging have been found for trauma exposure, post-traumatic stress disorder (PTSD), and major depression. Trauma exposure in childhood, particularly abuse or threat-related trauma, has been associated with accelerated epigenetic aging in children (Horvath[18-20]; Hannum clock[21]) and in adults (GrimAge[22]; Horvath[23]; Hannum[24]). Cumulative lifetime stress was associated with accelerated epigenetic aging in an urban, African American cohort (Horvath).[9] Further, accelerated epigenetic aging was identified in World Trade Center responders who had developed PTSD (GrimAge)[25] as well as war veterans diagnosed with PTSD (Hannum),[26] and for veterans, the severity of symptoms was correlated with epigenetic aging. Even exposure in utero may impact epigenetic aging; prenatal exposure to stress during the Great Depression predicted age acceleration (GrimAge, DunedinPoAm).[27]

For depression, having a current diagnosis of major depressive disorder (MDD) was associated with accelerated epigenetic aging, and individuals who had more severe symptoms of depression were the most accelerated (Horvath).[28] Other studies have replicated these associations between the current diagnosis of MDD and depression severity with accelerated epigenetic aging (Jansen clock,[29] GrimAge[30]). Moreover, a large nationally representative study of older adults found an association between depressive symptoms and accelerated epigenetic aging, assessed via multiple clocks (GrimAge, DunedinPoAm, PhenoAge, Horvath),[31] as did a twin study (Hannum, PhenoAge).[32] Studies of post-mortem brain tissue found that the epigenetic age of regions BA10 (anterior prefrontal cortex, involved in executive functioning)[33] and BA25 (subgenual cingulate area, found to be overactive in treatment-resistant depression)[34] of those with MDD was approximately a year older than that of healthy controls (Horvath).[28]

Most studies of epigenetic aging and mental health are cross-sectional. A few longitudinal studies support that experiencing trauma and depression, particularly at the clinical level, accelerates epigenetic aging. For war veterans, having PTSD symptoms or an alcohol-use disorder predicted an accelerated pace of epigenetic aging over two years (Horvath).[35] In the same sample, having a diagnosis of MDD or general anxiety disorder (GAD) did not impact the pace of epigenetic aging. In combat-exposed veterans diagnosed with PTSD, increases in PTSD symptoms were correlated with increases in epigenetic age acceleration over three years (GrimAge).[36]

One benefit of cell aging measures is that they can be examined in children. As with adults, psychopathology has been associated with accelerated epigenetic aging in children and adolescents (Horvath,[37] pediatric-buccal-epigenetic (PedBE) clock,[38] DNAm GA[39]). Internalizing symptoms at ages 2.5 and 4 predicted accelerated epigenetic aging at age 6, which in turn predicted internalizing symptoms at ages 6–10 (Horvath).[40] Maternal transmission effects of psychopathology on the epigenetic aging of offspring have been documented. Evidence suggests that maternal depressive symptoms during pregnancy may predict the epigenetic aging of offspring at birth (Knight clock).[41,42] Suarez and colleagues found that the effect of maternal depression on the internalizing problems of young boys (ages 3–4) was through gestational epigenetic age acceleration (DNAm GA).[39] In two cohorts, maternal anxiety during pregnancy predicted child epigenetic age acceleration: results appeared to be largely restricted to male children (PedBE clock).[38] One of these cohorts displayed a weak association between depression during pregnancy and child epigenetic age acceleration, and the other cohort showed no association.

Overall, research supports that accelerated epigenetic aging accompanies some forms of psychopathology. So far, epigenetic aging has not predicted the new incidence of mental illness with any specificity and so may be better thought of as a marker of future morbidity risk. Future research is clearly needed before any conclusive statements about the effects of epigenetic aging on psychopathology are made.

13.3 TELOMERE LENGTH AS A BIOMARKER OF AGING AND DISEASE

Telomeres are non-coding DNA sequences at the end of chromosomes that help maintain DNA and cell integrity.[43] Telomeres naturally shorten with cell division, so telomere length provides a useful metric of cellular aging.[44] The enzyme telomerase buffers the shortening of telomeres and replaces the lost base pairs to decrease telomere attrition.[45,46] As first established by Epel, Blackburn, and colleagues,[47] chronic stress is associated with shorter telomeres and reduced telomerase activity. We now understand how psychological stress can "get into the cell" – through cortisol, inflammation, and the tight relationship between telomere length and mitochondria.[46]

When a cell reaches a critically short telomere length, the cell is programmed to induce its senescence or cell death (apoptosis).[48] As with epigenetic clocks, accelerated telomere shortening has been associated with and can predict aging-related diseases such as cardiometabolic disease, stroke, cancer, and premature mortality.[49–51]

13.3.1 ASSOCIATIONS BETWEEN TELOMERE LENGTH AND MENTAL HEALTH

As with accelerated epigenetic aging, telomere shortening has been associated with psychopathology. A meta-analysis found accelerated telomere shortening across psychiatric disorders; effects were larger for PTSD, anxiety disorders, and depressive disorders than for bipolar and psychotic disorders.[52] Another meta-analysis found relationships between telomere shortening and PTSD, depression, and anxiety.[53] Multiple studies have found an association between trauma in early life and telomere length,[54] and there is a link between PTSD and telomere shortening in adults. A diagnosis of PTSD and PTSD symptoms have been associated with shorter telomeres, in both military and civilian samples.[55–57]

MDD has also been associated with telomere shortening,[58,59] and a dose-response relationship has been supported for individuals diagnosed with MDD. Those with the most severe and chronic episodes had the shortest telomeres.[60] Wolkowitz and colleagues[61] found that lifetime depression correlates with telomere length, as individuals above the median were approximately seven years older than those below the median. Severity of depressive episodes has also been negatively correlated with telomere length in older adults with late-life depression.[62] Individuals with current/remitted depression or anxiety disorders demonstrated shorter telomeres than healthy controls; however, changes in disorder status or symptoms did not correlate with telomere attrition over six years.[63] The latter finding suggests telomere shortening may be a consequence of psychopathology or a pre-existing vulnerability factor.

Discrepancies exist for some of the findings across studies. For example, Simon and colleagues[64] did not find a significant association between MDD and telomere length. To conclude that depression exposure predated accelerated shortening would require large longitudinal studies of individuals without MDD at baseline followed by regular measurements of telomere length and diagnostic assessments. As with epigenetic aging, most work is cross-sectional, but a few studies have found longitudinal associations between psychopathology and telomere shortening. In one study, men diagnosed with an internalizing disorder experienced telomere attrition over eight years;[65] however, effects were not found for women. In addition, there has been evidence that longer telomeres may protect against future depression; middle-aged women with longer telomeres had lower risk of worsening depressive symptoms later in life.[66]

Associations have been found between psychopathology and telomere length in children and adolescents. In a longitudinal study with multiple assessments of telomere length, internalizing symptoms at ages 8 to 10 predicted telomere shortening at ages 12 to 14, with no reciprocal effects.[67] As with epigenetic aging, prenatal stress exposure and parental psychopathology may also impact the telomere shortening of children. Maternal stress during pregnancy predicted shorter telomeres in newborns,[68] children aged 6 to 16,[69] and young adults.[70] Further, girls of depressed mothers had shorter telomeres, even if they had never experienced depression themselves;[71] this vulnerability appeared to have been inherited through prenatal experience or direct "telotype" transmission.[46,72]

13.4 CAN INTERVENTIONS SLOW CELLULAR AGING?

Most interventions that have been examined for their effect on cellular aging are lifestyle modifications, primarily diet and physical activity. The first such lifestyle study was by Dr. Dean Ornish, in which intensive lifestyle modification (nutrition, diet, activity, stress reduction) in thirty men with prostate cancer[73] was associated with increase in telomerase activity, which was correlated with decrease in psychological distress. A systematic review of lifestyle behaviors found associations of being less sedentary, good sleep habits, and not smoking with less telomere shortening.[74] A meta-analysis of 12 studies on physical activity found a positive effect on slowing telomere attrition, and that strength and endurance training may be the most beneficial.[75] Cross-sectional studies show that moderate-intensity aerobic exercise is reliably associated with longer telomeres.[76] A randomized controlled trial (RCT) of a nutrition and exercise intervention for obesity did not directly impact average telomere length across the sample; however, a small subsample who successfully maintained weight loss for one year demonstrated telomere lengthening.[77] Exercise may have a stronger impact on telomeres for individuals under chronic stress. Elderly caregivers of patients with dementia under high stress who were randomized to engage in aerobic exercise for six months showed telomere lengthening compared to controls.[78] Much available research demonstrates heterogeneity across interventions, and there is a need for more targeted interventions and standardized protocols.

Examinations of lifestyle intervention on epigenetic clocks are few, but we expect many such studies are in progress or will be published soon. Early evidence demonstrates some initial promise. The RCT of an eight-week intervention of diet, exercise, sleep, and relaxation guidance led to a reduction of approximately two years in the epigenetic age of men (Horvath).[79] Similarly, the RCT of a two-year dietary intervention slowed the epigenetic clock of women (GrimAge).[80]

Mindfulness-based, mind-body, or meditation interventions have been found to reduce the expression of inflammation-related genes,[81,82] and such interventions may also impact aspects of cellular aging, particularly telomerase levels. A review by Conklin and colleagues[83] found only two of nine studies of meditation interventions showed increases in telomere length; however, nine of eleven studies demonstrated increases in telomerase activity, the enzyme that stabilizes telomere length and protects them from stress-related shortening.[46] Another review concluded that it is unclear if meditation can reliably impact telomere length and that well-designed RCTs with larger sample sizes are needed to advance the field.[84]

There have been some indications that decreases in stress and symptoms of depression or anxiety may be correlated with changes in telomerase activity. A small RCT of an 8-week yoga meditation for caregivers resulted in reduced depressive symptoms as well as increased telomerase activity.[85] A pilot study on mindfulness for stress eating did not lead to intervention-related differences in telomerase activity; however, decreases in chronic stress and anxiety were correlated with increases in telomerase activity.[86] To our knowledge, the effects of meditation as an intervention on epigenetic aging have yet to be assessed. The epigenetic clock may be decelerated in long-term meditators (Horvath)[87] compared to controls, but RCTs are needed to address this possibility.

The effect of psychosocial group-based interventions on cellular aging of youth and their parents has a small evidence base. A ten-session family-based intervention for divorced families was associated with longer telomere length in parents six years later; there was no intervention effect on the telomere length of their children.[88] Brody and colleagues[89,90] designed Adults in the Making (AIM) as a family-based intervention for rural African American adolescents that would increase emotional support, instrumental assistance, vocational coaching and advocacy, and racial socialization. Adolescents who experienced non-supportive parenting at age 17 had shorter telomeres at age 22; however, adolescents that participated in AIM at age 17 did not show this association between parenting and telomere length.[91] Brody and colleagues[92] also implemented the Strong African American Families (SAAF) program to enhance supportive parenting and evaluated the effect on epigenetic aging (Horvath). In the control group, parental depressive symptoms when children were age 11 predicted the epigenetic aging of children at age 22; children in the SAAF treatment group did not show this association. There also appeared to be an indirect effect of treatment on epigenetic aging through reductions in harsh parenting.

Whether interventions that target psychopathology influence cellular aging remains an open question as very few studies of interventions have included cell aging outcomes. In one study of cognitive behavioral therapy for social anxiety disorder, neither telomere length nor telomerase changed significantly after treatment; however, an increase in telomerase activity across treatment was associated with reduced anxiety symptoms.[93] While the preliminary evidence that interventions can impact epigenetic age or telomere activity is promising, it is not clear how durable the effects on cellular aging will be or how effects will vary long, distinct mental health trajectories over longer time periods. To clarify these queries, the field needs more rigorous studies of interventions for psychiatric disorders that target cellular aging.

13.5   FUTURE DIRECTIONS IN MENTAL HEALTH AND CELLULAR AGING

Along with detrimental effects on functioning and well-being, psychopathology may prematurely age an individual at the cellular level, increasing the risk for chronic diseases of aging. Research supports a robust relationship for trauma and depression, particularly at the clinical level, with accelerated cellular aging as assessed by epigenetic clocks and telomere length.[6,9,18–32,52–60,62,63] With the cross-sectional nature of most studies, we cannot rule out that premorbid accelerated cellular aging increases the risk of later psychopathology, that effects are bi-directional over time, or that psychopathology and cellular aging have a common genetic antecedent.

The literature on lifestyle interventions supports that aerobic activity may stabilize telomere length and several studies of mindfulness-based interventions show an increase in telomerase. Only two studies have examined if lifestyle interventions impacted epigenetic clocks and, to our knowledge, no studies have assessed the effect of mindfulness, mind-body, or meditation interventions on epigenetic aging. Given that trauma and depression appear to result in accelerated cellular aging, preventing the onset of psychopathology could protect the body from the negative consequences of premature morbidity and mortality. There is a lack of research on the effects of evidence-based treatment for psychopathology on epigenetic aging and telomere length. To advance the field, research on interventions that target both psychiatric disorders and cellular aging is needed. Stored whole blood or DNA from already existing longitudinal studies could be newly used for assays of telomere length or epigenetic methylation. Although not without challenges, piggybacking cell aging assessments into existing trials should be considered when possible.

Most current research on mental health and cellular aging is cross-sectional or uses small samples. Along with rigorous study design and methodology, studies need to integrate multiple biomarkers of cellular aging in the same study, and measurements of cellular aging biomarkers need to be standardized. The National Institute on Aging (NIA) and the National Institute of Environmental Health Sciences have funded a Telomere Research Network in order to identify gold-standard measurement protocols (https://trn.tulane.edu/). Epigenetic clock research may have progressed quickly due to the use of shared technology and publicly available tools (such as from the Horvath lab, https://dnamage.genetics.ucla.edu/),[94] and research on telomeres may similarly benefit from shared resources. Research collaboration to determine standardization and share resources will facilitate well-powered intervention trials of the systemic and individual factors that impact cellular aging as well as mental health.

An association that needs further exploration is the one between childhood adversity and cellular aging.[72] Evidence suggests that it is adversity during childhood and not during adulthood that is most responsible for accelerated telomere shortening.[95] In both patient and post-mortem samples, those diagnosed with MDD who also experienced childhood trauma demonstrated the most advanced epigenetic aging.[28] In addition, telomere length was significantly shorter only in individuals diagnosed with PTSD who also had exposure to trauma in childhood.[96] Similarly, telomere attrition only predicted child behavior problems, if the mother had experienced a high number of childhood adverse experiences (ACEs).[97] The former surgeon general of California has initiated universal screening of ACEs in primary care, along with referrals and psychoeducation, which could reduce the impact and occurrence of these experiences on biological aging.

13.5.1 ARE TELOMERES AND EPIGENETIC CLOCKS EFFECTIVE FOR INDIVIDUAL CLINICAL USE?

For clinical use, it would be helpful to have accurate markers of cellular aging we could measure over the course of an intervention as changes in telomere activity or epigenetic aging could provide an early indication that a given treatment is working. However, telomere length changes over years, which is not a useful time frame for most interventions, and the time frame for changes in the epigenetic clock is not clear. Measures of malleable clinical biomarkers for short-term indices of health that can change in shorter periods include level of insulin resistance, inflammation, and aspects of autonomic nervous system balance such as heart rate variability. Testing kits to measure telomere length and epigenetic aging are now sold commercially. In our opinion, these kits are not warranted for clinical use at the present time – given the measurement error at an individual level, which may be equivalent to (or larger than) the average change seen after one year of aging. Currently, telomere activity and epigenetic aging are best interpreted at the population rather than at the individual level.

13.6 CONCLUSION

Psychological trauma, PTSD, and depression have been linked to shorter telomere length and accelerated epigenetic clocks. As shown in Figure 13.1, we hypothesize that stress-related dimensions of psychopathology drive stress mediators that lead to accelerated cell aging. Interventions could impact dimensions of psychopathology or their mediators and result in changes in cellular aging. Existing research suggests that lifestyle, mind–body interventions, and improving family functioning may impact cellular aging in the form of telomere length, telomerase activity, and epigenetic clocks. Few studies targeting stress and affective disorders have examined potential improvements in cell aging indices. Most studies are small-scale, and larger controlled clinical trials are needed. In addition to focusing on just symptom reduction, promoting emotional well-being (in line with the tenets of positive psychology and psychiatry) is a relatively new aim in public health.[98] Along with examinations of whether interventions on well-being facilitate changes in telomere activity and epigenetic aging, future research should determine if social and public health measures (e.g., decreases in air pollution, increases in education) could impact cellular aging on a larger scale.[99]

Indices of aging, such as telomeres and epigenetic clocks, provide evidence of the accelerated aging phenotype seen in MDD and other disorders. There is currently insufficient evidence to support a causal role for cellular aging in psychiatric disorders; our model in Figure 13.1 suggests that improvements in psychopathology may decelerate cellular aging by dampening the effects of stress mediators. Due to the overlap between the biological aging changes seen in MDD and those observed during the aging process, some researchers are suggesting the use of geroscience-guided interventions to improve treatment outcomes or lessen the negative consequences of MDD.[100] Interventions that successfully slow cell aging (e.g., physical exercise, senolytic drugs)[100] may lessen the impact of psychiatric disorders. This idea is largely unexplored, but such interventions might prevent the somatic consequences of cell aging and so interrupt a bidirectional cycle between psychopathology and aging-related outcomes (healthspan, dementia, physical disability). Longitudinal RCTs that assess biomarkers at multiple timepoints would be necessary to take the next step to modifying epigenetic aging and telomere length as an effective way to impact mental health.

REFERENCES

1. Byers AL, Yaffe K. Depression and risk of developing dementia. *Nat Rev Neurol.* 2011; 7(6):323–331.
2. Han X, Hou C, Yang H, Chen W, Ying Z, Hu Y, Sun Y, Qu Y, Yang L, Valdimarsdóttir UA, Zhang W. Disease trajectories and mortality among individuals diagnosed with depression: A community-based cohort study in UK biobank. *Mol Psychiatry.* 2021; 26(11):6736–6746.

3. Sariaslan A, Sharpe M, Larsson H, Wolf A, Lichtenstein P, Fazel S. Psychiatric comorbidity and risk of premature mortality and suicide among those with chronic respiratory diseases, cardiovascular diseases, and diabetes in Sweden: A nationwide matched cohort study of over 1 million patients and their unaffected siblings. *PLoS Med.* 2022 Jan 27;19(1):e1003864.

4. Sierra F, Caspi A, Fortinsky RH, Haynes L, Lithgow GJ, Moffitt TE, Olshansky SJ, Perry D, Verdin E, Kuchel GA. Moving geroscience from the bench to clinical care and health policy. *J Am Geriatr Soc.* 2021;69(9):2455–2463.

5. Epel ES, Prather AA. Stress, telomeres, and psychopathology: Toward a deeper understanding of a triad of early aging. *Annu Rev Clin Psychol.* 2018;14:371–397. doi:10.1146/annurev-clinpsy-032816-045054. Epub 2018 Mar 1. PMID: 29494257; PMCID: PMC7039047.

6. Stevenson AJ, McCartney DL, Harris SE, Taylor AM, Redmond P, Starr JM, Zhang Q, McRae AF, Wray NR, Spires-Jones TL, McColl BW. Trajectories of inflammatory biomarkers over the eighth decade and their associations with immune cell profiles and epigenetic ageing. *Clin Epigenetics.* 2018;10:159.

7. Irvin MR, Aslibekyan S, Do A, Zhi D, Hidalgo B, Claas SA, Srinivasasainagendra V, Horvath S, Tiwari HK, Absher DM, Arnett DK. Metabolic and inflammatory biomarkers are associated with epigenetic aging acceleration estimates in the GOLDN study. *Clin Epigenetics.* 2018;10:56.

8. Xiao C, Beitler JJ, Peng G, Levine ME, Conneely KN, Zhao H, Felger JC, Wommack EC, Chico CE, Jeon S, Higgins KA. Epigenetic age acceleration, fatigue, and inflammation in patients undergoing radiation therapy for head and neck cancer: A longitudinal study. *Cancer.* 2021 Sep 15;127(18):3361–3371.

9. Zannas AS, Arloth J, Carrillo-Roa T, Iurato S, Röh S, Ressler KJ, Nemeroff CB, Smith AK, Bradley B, Heim C, Menke A. Lifetime stress accelerates epigenetic aging in an urban, African American cohort: Relevance of glucocorticoid signaling. *Genome Biol.* 2015;16:266.

10. Moore LD, Le T, Fan G. DNA methylation and its basic function. *Neuropsychopharmacol.* 2013;38(1):23–38.

11. Park, 2016 https://time.com/4422860/menopause-accelerates-aging/

12. Fransquet PD, Wrigglesworth J, Woods RL, Ernst ME, Ryan J. The epigenetic clock as a predictor of disease and mortality risk: A systematic review and meta-analysis. *Clin Epigenetics.* 2019;11(1):62.

13. Horvath S. DNA methylation age of human tissues and cell types. *Genome Biol.* 2013; 14(10):3156.

14. Horvath S, Levine AJ. HIV-1 infection accelerates age according to the epigenetic clock. *J Infect Dis.* 2015 Nov 15;212(10):1563–1573.

15. Lu AT, Quach A, Wilson JG, Reiner AP, Aviv A, Raj K, Hou L, Baccarelli AA, Li Y, Stewart JD, Whitsel EA. DNA methylation GrimAge strongly predicts lifespan and healthspan. *Aging (Albany NY).* 2019 Jan 31;11(2):303.

16. Belsky DW, Caspi A, Arseneault L, Baccarelli A, Corcoran DL, Gao X, Hannon E, Harrington HL, Rasmussen LJ, Houts R, Huffman K. Quantification of the pace of biological aging in humans through a blood test, the DunedinPoAm DNA methylation algorithm. *Elife.* 2020;9:e54870.

17. Belsky DW, Caspi A, Corcoran DL, Sugden K, Poulton R, Arseneault L, Baccarelli A, Chamarti K, Gao X, Hannon E, Harrington HL. DunedinPACE, a DNA methylation biomarker of the pace of aging. *Elife.* 2022 Jan 14;11:e73420.

18. Jovanovic T, Vance LA, Cross D, Knight AK, Kilaru V, Michopoulos V, Klengel T, Smith AK. Exposure to violence accelerates epigenetic aging in children. *Sci Rep.* 2017 Aug 21;7(1):8962.

19. Sumner JA, Colich NL, Uddin M, Armstrong D, McLaughlin KA. Early experiences of threat, but not deprivation, are associated with accelerated biological aging in children and adolescents. *Biol Psychiatry.* 2019;85(3):268–278.

20. Tang R, Howe LD, Suderman M, Relton CL, Crawford AA, Houtepen LC. Adverse childhood experiences, DNA methylation age acceleration, and cortisol in UK children: A prospective population-based cohort study. *Clin Epigenetics.* 2020;12:55.

21. Marini S, Davis KA, Soare TW, Zhu Y, Suderman MJ, Simpkin AJ, Smith AD, Wolf EJ, Relton CL, Dunn EC. Adversity exposure during sensitive periods predicts accelerated epigenetic aging in children. *Psychoneuroendocrinology.* 2020;113:104484.

22. Hamlat EJ, Prather AA, Horvath S, Belsky J, Epel ES. Early life adversity, pubertal timing, and epigenetic age acceleration in adulthood. *Dev Psychobiol.* 2021;63(5): 890–902.

23. Lawn RB, Anderson EL, Suderman M, Simpkin AJ, Gaunt TR, Teschendorff AE, Widschwendter M, Hardy R, Kuh D, Relton CL, Howe LD. Psychosocial adversity and socioeconomic position during childhood and epigenetic age: Analysis of two prospective cohort studies. *Hum Mol Genet.* 2018;27(7):1301–1308.

24. Wolf EJ, Logue MW, Stoop TB, Schichman SA, Stone A, Sadeh N, Hayes JP, Miller MW. Accelerated DNA methylation age: Associations with PTSD and mortality. *Psychosom Med.* 2018;80(1):42–48.

25. Kuan PF, Ren X, Clouston S, Yang X, Jonas K, Kotov R, Bromet E, Luft BJ. PTSD is associated with accelerated transcriptional aging in world trade center responders. *Transl Psychiatry.* 2021 May 24;11:311.

26. Wolf EJ, Logue MW, Hayes JP, Sadeh N, Schichman SA, Stone A, Salat DH, Milberg W, McGlinchey R, Miller MW. Accelerated DNA methylation age: Associations with PTSD and neural integrity. *Psychoneuroendocrinology.* 2016;63:155–162.

27. Schmitz LL, Duque V. In utero exposure to the great depression is reflected in late-life epigenetic aging signatures. *V Proc Natl Acad Sci.* 2022;1:e2208530119.

28. Han LK, Aghajani M, Clark SL, Chan RF, Hattab MW, Shabalin AA, Zhao M, Kumar G, Xie LY, Jansen R, Milaneschi Y. Epigenetic aging in major depressive disorder. *Am J Psychiatry.* 2018;175(8):774–82.

29. Jansen R, Han LK, Verhoeven JE, Aberg KA, van den Oord EC, Milaneschi Y, Penninx BW. An integrative study of five biological clocks in somatic and mental health. *Elife.* 2021;10:e59479.

30. Protsenko E, Yang R, Nier B, Reus V, Hammamieh R, Rampersaud R, Wu GW, Hough CM, Epel E, Prather AA, Jett M. "GrimAge," an epigenetic predictor of mortality, is accelerated in major depressive disorder. *Transl Psychiatry.* 2021;11(1):193.

31. Beydoun MA, Beydoun HA, Hooten NN, Maldonado AI, Weiss J, Evans MK, Zonderman AB. Epigenetic clocks and their association with trajectories in perceived discrimination and depressive symptoms among US middle-aged and older adults. *Aging (Albany NY).* 2022;14(13):5311.

32. Liu C, Wang Z, Hui Q, Goldberg J, Smith NL, Shah AJ, Murrah N, Shallenberger L, Diggers E, Bremner JD, Sun YV. Association between depression and epigenetic age acceleration: A co-twin control study. *Depress Anxiety.* 2022;39(12):741–750.

33. Ramnani N, Owen AM. Anterior prefrontal cortex: Insights into function from anatomy and neuroimaging. *Nat Rev Neurosci.* 2004;5(3):184–194.

34. Hamani C, Mayberg H, Stone S, Laxton A, Haber S, Lozano AM. The subcallosal cingulate gyrus in the context of major depression. *Biol Psychiatry.* 2011;69(4):301–308.

35. Wolf EJ, Logue MW, Morrison FG, Wilcox ES, Stone A, Schichman SA, McGlinchey RE, Milberg WP, Miller MW. Posttraumatic psychopathology and the pace of the epigenetic clock: A longitudinal investigation. *Psychol Med.* 2019;49(5):791–800.

36. Yang R, Wu GW, Verhoeven JE, Gautam A, Reus VI, Kang JI, Flory JD, Abu-Amara D, Hood L, Doyle FJ, Yehuda R. A DNA methylation clock associated with age-related

illnesses and mortality is accelerated in men with combat PTSD. *Mol Psychiatry.* 2021; 26(9):4999–5009.

37. Manczak EM, Scott SR, Millwood SN. Accelerated epigenetic aging at birth interacts with parenting hostility to predict child temperament and subsequent psychological symptoms. *Dev Psychopathol.* 2021;8:1–10.
38. McGill MG, Pokhvisneva I, Clappison AS, McEwen LM, Beijers R, Tollenaar MS, Pham H, Kee MZ, Garg E, de Mendonça Filho EJ, Karnani N. Maternal prenatal anxiety and the fetal origins of epigenetic aging. *Biol Psychiatry.* 2022;91(3):303–312.
39. Suarez A, Lahti J, Czamara D, Lahti-Pulkkinen M, Knight AK, Girchenko P, Hämäläinen E, Kajantie E, Lipsanen J, Laivuori H, Villa PM. The epigenetic clock at birth: Associations with maternal antenatal depression and child psychiatric problems. *J Am Acad Child Adolesc Psychiatry.* 2018;57(5):321–328.
40. Tollenaar MS, Beijers R, Garg E, Nguyen TT, Lin DT, MacIsaac JL, Shalev I, Kobor MS, Meaney MJ, O'Donnell KJ, de Weerth C. Internalizing symptoms associate with the pace of epigenetic aging in childhood. *Biol Psychol.* 2021;159:108021.
41. Appleton AA, Lin B, Kennedy EM, Holdsworth EA. Maternal depression and adverse neighbourhood conditions during pregnancy are associated with gestational epigenetic age deceleration. *Epigenetics.* 2022;17(13):1905–1919.
42. McKenna BG, Hendrix CL, Brennan PA, Smith AK, Stowe ZN, Newport DJ, Knight AK. Maternal prenatal depression and epigenetic age deceleration: Testing potentially confounding effects of prenatal stress and SSRI use. *Epigenetics.* 2021;16(3):327–337.
43. Blackburn EH. Telomeres and their synthesis. *Science.* 1990;249(4968):489–490.
44. Gilson E, Londoño-Vallejo JA. Telomere length profiles in humans: All ends are not equal. *Cell Cycle.* 2007 Oct 15;6(20):2486–2494.
45. Blackburn EH, Epel ES, Lin J. Human telomere biology: A contributory and interactive factor in aging, disease risks, and protection. *Science.* 2015;350(6265):1193–1198.
46. Lin J, Epel E. Stress and telomere shortening: Insights from cellular mechanisms. *Ageing Res Rev.* 2022;73:101507.
47. Epel ES, Blackburn EH, Lin J, Dhabhar FS, Adler NE, Morrow JD, Cawthon RM. Accelerated telomere shortening in response to life stress. *Proc Natl Acad Sci.* 2004; 101(49):17312–1735.
48. Andrews NP, Fujii H, Goronzy JJ, Weyand CM. Telomeres and immunological diseases of aging. *Gerontology.* 2010;56(4):390–403.
49. Haycock PC, Heydon EE, Kaptoge S, Butterworth AS, Thompson A, Willeit P. Leucocyte telomere length and risk of cardiovascular disease: Systematic review and meta-analysis. *BMJ.* 2014 Jul 8;349:g4227. doi: 10.1136/bmj.g4227.
50. Ma H, Zhou Z, Wei S, Liu Z, Pooley KA, Dunning AM, Svenson U, Roos G, Hosgood III HD, Shen M, Wei Q. Shortened telomere length is associated with increased risk of cancer: A meta-analysis. *PLoS One.* 2011 Jun 10;6(6):e20466.
51. Wang Q, Zhan Y, Pedersen NL, Fang F, Hägg S. Telomere length and all-cause mortality: A meta-analysis. *Ageing Res Rev.* 2018;48:11–20.
52. Darrow SM, Verhoeven JE, Révész D, Lindqvist D, Penninx BW, Delucchi KL, Wolkowitz OM, Mathews CA. The association between psychiatric disorders and telomere length: A meta-analysis involving 14,827 persons. *Psychosom Med.* 2016;78(7):776.
53. Pousa PA, Souza RM, Melo PH, Correa BH, Mendonça TS, Simões-e-Silva AC, Miranda DM. Telomere shortening and psychiatric disorders: A systematic review. *Cells.* 2021;10(6):1423.
54. Price LH, Kao HT, Burgers DE, Carpenter LL, Tyrka AR. Telomeres and early-life stress: An overview. *Biol Psychiatry.* 2013;73(1):15–23.
55. Zhang L, Hu XZ, Li X, Li H, Smerin S, Russell D, Ursano RJ. Telomere length–a cellular aging marker for depression and post-traumatic stress disorder. *Med Hypotheses.* 2014;83(2):182–185.

56. Carvalho CM, Coimbra BM, Xavier G, Bugiga AV, Fonseca T, Olff M, Polimanti R, Mello AF, Ota VK, Mello MF, Belangero SI. Shorter telomeres related to posttraumatic stress disorder re-experiencing symptoms in sexually assaulted civilian women. *Front Psychiatry.* 2022;13:1–9.

57. Ladwig KH, Brockhaus AC, Baumert J, Lukaschek K, Emeny RT, Kruse J, Codd V, Häfner S, Albrecht E, Illig T, Samani NJ. Posttraumatic stress disorder and not depression is associated with shorter leukocyte telomere length: Findings from 3,000 participants in the population-based KORA F4 study. *PLoS One.* 2013;8(7):e64762.

58. Lindqvist D, Epel ES, Mellon SH, Penninx BW, Révész D, Verhoeven JE, Reus VI, Lin J, Mahan L, Hough CM, Rosser R. Psychiatric disorders and leukocyte telomere length: Underlying mechanisms linking mental illness with cellular aging. *Neurosci Biobehav Rev.* 2015;55:333–364.

59. Schutte NS, Malouff JM. The association between depression and leukocyte telomere length: A meta-analysis. *Depress Anxiety.* 2015;32(4):229–238.

60. Verhoeven JE, Révész D, Epel ES, Lin J, Wolkowitz OM, Penninx BW. Major depressive disorder and accelerated cellular aging: Results from a large psychiatric cohort study. *Mol Psychiatry.* 2014;19(8):895–901.

61. Wolkowitz OM, Reus VI, Mellon SH. Of sound mind and body: depression, disease, and accelerated aging. *Dialogues Clin Neurosci.* 2011; 13(1):25–39.

62. Mendes-Silva AP, Vieira EL, Xavier G, Barroso LS, Bertola L, Martins EA, Brietzke EM, Belangero SI, Diniz BS. Telomere shortening in late-life depression: A potential marker of depression severity. *Brain Behav.* 2021;11(8):e2255.

63. Verhoeven JE, van Oppen P, Révész D, Wolkowitz OM, Penninx BW. Depressive and anxiety disorders showing robust, but non-dynamic, 6-year longitudinal association with short leukocyte telomere length. *Am J Psychiatry.* 2016;173(6):617–24.

64. Simon NM, Walton ZE, Bui E, Prescott J, Hoge E, Keshaviah A, Schwarz N, Dryman T, Ojserkis RA, Kovachy B, Mischoulon D. Telomere length and telomerase in a well-characterized sample of individuals with major depressive disorder compared to controls. *Psychoneuroendocrinology.* 2015;58:9–22.

65. Shalev I, Moffitt TE, Braithwaite AW, Danese A, Fleming NI, Goldman-Mellor S, Harrington H, Houts RM, Israel S, Poulton R, Robertson SP. Internalizing disorders and leukocyte telomere erosion: A prospective study of depression, generalized anxiety disorder and post-traumatic stress disorder. *Mol Psychiatry.* 2014;19(11):1163–70.

66. Gillis JC, Chang SC, Wang W, Simon NM, Normand SL, Rosner BA, Blacker D, DeVivo I, Okereke OI. The relation of telomere length at midlife to subsequent 20-year depression trajectories among women. *Depress Anxiety.* 2019;36(6):565–575.

67. Wade M, Fox NA, Zeanah CH, Nelson CA, Drury SS. Telomere length and psychopathology: Specificity and direction of effects within the Bucharest early intervention project. *J Am Acad Child Adolesc Psychiatry.* 2020;59(1):140–148.

68. Entringer S, Epel ES, Lin J, Buss C, Shahbaba B, Blackburn EH, Simhan HN, Wadhwa PD. Maternal psychosocial stress during pregnancy is associated with newborn leukocyte telomere length. *Am J Obstet Gynecol.* 2013;208(2):134–e1.

69. Stout-Oswald SA, Glynn LM, Bisoffi M, Demers CH, Davis EP. Prenatal exposure to maternal psychological distress and telomere length in childhood. *Dev Psychobiol.* 2022;64(1):e22238.

70. Entringer S, Epel ES, Kumsta R, Lin J, Hellhammer DH, Blackburn EH, Wüst S, Wadhwa PD. Stress exposure in intrauterine life is associated with shorter telomere length in young adulthood. *Proc Natl Acad Sci.* 2011 Aug 16;108(33):E513–E518.

71. Gotlib IH, LeMoult J, Colich NL, Foland-Ross LC, Hallmayer J, Joormann J, Lin J, Wolkowitz OM. Telomere length and cortisol reactivity in children of depressed mothers. *Mol Psychiatry.* 2015;20(5):615–620.

72. Epel ES. Can childhood adversity affect telomeres of the next generation? Possible mechanisms, implications, and next-generation research. *Am J Psychiatry.* 2020;177(1): 7–9.

73. Ornish D, Lin J, Daubenmier J, Weidner G, Epel E, Kemp C, Blackburn EH. Increased telomerase activity and comprehensive lifestyle changes: A pilot study. *Lancet Oncol.* 2008;9(11):1048–1057.

74. Barragán R, Ortega-Azorín C, Sorlí JV, Asensio EM, Coltell O, St-Onge MP, Portolés O, Corella D. Effect of physical activity, smoking, and sleep on telomere length: A systematic review of observational and intervention studies. *J Clin Med.* 2021 Dec 24;11(1):76.

75. Buttet M, Bagheri R, Ugbolue UC, Laporte C, Trousselard M, Benson A, Bouillon-Minois JB, Dutheil F. Effect of a lifestyle intervention on telomere length: A systematic review and meta-analysis. *Mech Ageing Dev.* 2022 Jun 26:111694. doi: 10.1016/j. mad.2022.111694

76. Schellnegger M, Lin AC, Hammer N, Kamolz LP. Physical activity on telomere length as a biomarker for aging: A systematic review. *Sports Med - Open.* 2022;8(1): 1–25.

77. Mason AE, Adler JM, Puterman E, Lakmazaheri A, Brucker M, Aschbacher K, Epel ES. Stress resilience: Narrative identity may buffer the longitudinal effects of chronic caregiving stress on mental health and telomere shortening. *Brain Behav Immun.* 2019; 77:101–109.

78. Puterman E, Weiss J, Lin J, Schilf S, Slusher AL, Johansen KL, Epel ES. Aerobic exercise lengthens telomeres and reduces stress in family caregivers: A randomized controlled trial. *Psychoneuroendocrinology.* 2018;98:245–252.

79. Fitzgerald KN, Hodges R, Hanes D, Stack E, Cheishvili D, Szyf M, Henkel J, Twedt MW, Giannopoulou D, Herdell J, Logan S. Potential reversal of epigenetic age using A diet and lifestyle intervention: A pilot randomized clinical trial. *Aging (Albany NY).* 2021 Apr 15;13(7):9419.

80. Fiorito G, Caini S, Palli D, Bendinelli B, Saieva C, Ermini I, Valentini V, Assedi M, Rizzolo P, Ambrogetti D, Ottini L. DNA methylation-based biomarkers of aging were slowed down in a two-year diet and physical activity intervention trial: The DAMA study. *Aging Cell.* 2021 Oct;20(10):e13439.

81. Bower JE, Irwin MR. Mind–body therapies and control of inflammatory biology: A descriptive review. *Brain Behav Immun.* 2016;51:1–1.

82. Black DS, Slavich GM. Mindfulness meditation and the immune system: A systematic review of randomized controlled trials. *Ann N Y Acad Sci.* 2016;1373(1):13–24.

83. Conklin QA, Crosswell AD, Saron CD, Epel ES. Meditation, stress processes, and telomere biology. *Curr Opin Psychol.* 2019;28:92–101.

84. Dasanayaka NN, Sirisena ND, Samaranayake N. The effects of meditation on length of telomeres in healthy individuals: A systematic review. *Syst Rev.* 2021;10(1):151.

85. Lavretsky H, Epel ES, Siddarth P, Nazarian N, Cyr NS, Khalsa DS, Lin J, Blackburn E, Irwin MR. A pilot study of yogic meditation for family dementia caregivers with depressive symptoms: Effects on mental health, cognition, and telomerase activity. *Int J Geriatr Psychiatry.* 2013;28(1):57–65.

86. Daubenmier J, Lin J, Blackburn E, Hecht FM, Kristeller J, Maninger N, Kuwata M, Bacchetti P, Havel PJ, Epel E. Changes in stress, eating, and metabolic factors are related to changes in telomerase activity in a randomized mindfulness intervention pilot study. *Psychoneuroendocrinology.* 2012;37(7):917–928.

87. Chaix R, Alvarez-López MJ, Fagny M, Lemee L, Regnault B, Davidson RJ, Lutz A, Kaliman P. Epigenetic clock analysis in long-term meditators. *Psychoneuroendocrinology.* 2017;85:210–214.

88. Elam KK, Johnson SL, Ruof A, Eisenberg DT, Rej PH, Sandler I, Wolchik S. Examining the influence of adversity, family contexts, and a family-based intervention on parent and child telomere length. *Eur J Psychotraumatol.* 2022 Jul 29;13(1):2088935.

89. Brody GH, Murry VM, Gerrard M, Gibbons FX, Molgaard V, McNair L, Brown AC, Wills TA, Spoth RL, Luo Z, Chen YF. The strong African American families program: Translating research into prevention programming. *Child Dev.* 2004;75(3):900–917.

90. Brody GH, Yu T, Chen YF, Kogan SM, Smith K. The adults in the making program: Long-term protective stabilizing effects on alcohol use and substance use problems for rural African American emerging adults. *J Consult Clin Psychol.* 2012;80(1):17.

91. Brody GH, Yu T, Beach SR, Philibert RA. Prevention effects ameliorate the prospective association between nonsupportive parenting and diminished telomere length. *Prev Sci.* 2015;16(2):171–180.

92. Brody GH, Yu T, Chen E, Beach SR, Miller GE. Family-centered prevention ameliorates the longitudinal association between risky family processes and epigenetic aging. *J Child Psychol Psychiatry.* 2016;57(5):566–574.

93. Månsson KN, Lindqvist D, Yang LL, Svanborg C, Isung J, Nilsonne G, Bergman-Nordgren L, EL Alaoui S, Hedman-Lagerlöf E, Kraepelien M, Högström J. Improvement in indices of cellular protection after psychological treatment for social anxiety disorder. *Transl Psychiatry.* 2019 Dec 19;9(1):340.

94. Hastings WJ, Shalev I, Belsky DW. Translating measures of biological aging to test effectiveness of geroprotective interventions: What can we learn from research on telomeres? *Front Genet.* 2017 Nov 22;8:164.

95. Puterman E, Gemmill A, Karasek D, Weir D, Adler NE, Prather AA, Epel ES. Lifespan adversity and later adulthood telomere length in the nationally representative US health and retirement study. *Proc Natl Acad Sci.* 2016;113(42):E6335–E6342.

96. O'Donovan A, Epel E, Lin J, Wolkowitz O, Cohen B, Maguen S, Neylan TC. Childhood trauma associated with short leukocyte telomere length in posttraumatic stress disorder. *Biol Psychiatry.* 2011;70(5):465–471.

97. Esteves KC, Jones CW, Wade M, Callerame K, Smith AK, Theall KP, Drury SS. Adverse childhood experiences: Implications for offspring telomere length and psychopathology. *Am J Psychiatry.* 2020;177(1):47–57.

98. Guidi J, Rafanelli C, Fava GA. The clinical role of well-being therapy. *Nord J Psychiatry.* 2018;72(6):447–453.

99. Erusalimsky JD. Oxidative stress, telomeres and cellular senescence: What non-drug interventions might break the link? *Free Radic Biol Med.* 2020;150:87–95.

100. Lorenzo EC, Kuchel GA, Kuo CL, Moffitt TE, Diniz BS. Major depression and the biological hallmarks of aging. *Ageing Res Rev.* 2022;21:101805.

14 Alzheimer's Disease and Related Dementias

Luis D. Medina, PhD,
Mirna L. Arroyo-Miranda, DrPH JD,
Joshua M. Garcia, BS, Michelle N. Martinez, MA,
and Andrea P. Ochoa Lopez, MA

KEY POINTS

- Dementia is a costly disease that affects multiple aspects of life and across various levels (e.g., individual, societal).
- There are multiple known factors that can increase or mitigate risk for dementia.
- Planning is essential for adequate treatment and caregiving.

14.1 DEFINITION, EPIDEMIOLOGY, AND TRENDS

Alzheimer's disease and related dementias (ADRDs) are a group of disorders characterized by a progressive decline in memory and other cognitive skills, such as language and attention. These declines lead to loss of autonomy and impaired ability to complete activities of daily living (ADLs), ultimately impacting health and quality of life. ADRDs represent a significant health risk for adults ages 65 and above; approximately 6.5 million adults in this age group live with dementia in the United States, where ADRDs are the fifth leading cause of death for this population.[1] ADRD mortality rates grew by 146% from 2000 to 2018; in 2019, dementia was considered the underlying cause of death for over 200,000 older adults.[2]

Biological, sociological, psychological, and cultural factors have been associated with the risk of developing dementia. Women represent nearly two-thirds of Americans living with Alzheimer's disease,[3] a trend that may be due to the greater longevity of women compared to men[4] and to the role of age as the greatest risk factor for dementia.[5] Beyond age and sex/gender, disparities have been identified in the prevalence and etiology of ADRDs concerning race/ethnicity; Hispanic/Latino and Black/African American older adults are at increased risk for ADRD, often develop dementia earlier in life, and show greater degrees of impairment than their non-Hispanic White counterparts, a trend that has remained stable over time.[6] Data suggest systemic barriers related to health care access and quality of services available for historically underserved groups contribute to these disparities.[7]

14.1.1   Cost

ADRDs represent a significant human and financial burden in the United States that impacts individuals living with these disorders, their families, and the health care system. Significant costs endured by persons living with dementia and their loved ones are related to quality of life, mental health, and finances during the years following dementia onset, when individuals experience severe impairment in their thinking abilities, physical strength, and overall autonomy.[8] Expenses associated with caring for a person living with dementia (PLWD) are equal to, and sometimes larger than, those for other serious chronic illnesses. This costliness is partly due to the unique needs of adults with cognitive impairment, and partly given the common comorbidity of ADRD with other conditions such as stroke and depression.[9] Managing the clinical symptoms of adults with dementia often involves pharmacological interventions, special services such as outpatient physical and/or occupational rehabilitation, surgeries, and stays of varying lengths at nursing homes and hospitals. As an individual's level of daily functioning declines, they may also require home health care or a change in residence (i.e., moving into assisted living communities) to ensure their safety and well-being. Based on data representative of the US population, the yearly monetary cost attributable to dementia was estimated to range between $30,000 and $70,000 per person.[10]

Caregivers of PLWDs often face significant demands, increasing their risk for stress, health complications, financial burden, social isolation, and other unfavorable outcomes.[11] In addition to expenses related to health care services, some caregivers personally provide home care for their loved ones, which can lead to financial burden in the form of lost work hours. Comprehensive care for persons living with dementia has reached a cost of as much as 305 billion dollars in hospice services and 244 billion dollars in hours of care labor by family members and unpaid caregivers.[12]

14.2   ETIOLOGY, COURSE, & PREVENTION

The clinical syndrome observed in ADRDs is associated with the neuroanatomical course of the pathology. Synaptic cleaving and necrosis due to pathological protein deposition leads to clinical symptoms across various cognitive domains, such as memory, language, and executive functioning (e.g., planning, decision-making). While Alzheimer's disease is the most common cause of dementia syndromes, other conditions associated with dementia syndromes include cerebrovascular disease, Lewy body disease, frontotemporal lobar degeneration, Parkinson's disease, hippocampal sclerosis, and mixed pathologies.[12] Understanding of ADRDs is constantly evolving as additional information is gleaned from scientific investigations. The currently accepted framework for defining the condition of Alzheimer's disease dementia is based on criteria proposed by the National Institutes on Aging – Alzheimer's Association (NIA-AA), which posits that the beta-amyloid plaques (Aβ) and neurofibrillary tau tangles are abnormal protein deposits that characterize the Alzheimer's disease diagnosis.[13]

ADRDs develop across a continuum, starting with the preclinical phase and progressing through a mild cognitive impairment (MCI) stage into the mild, moderate, and severe stages of dementia. The preclinical stage constitutes a period where pathological changes may be detected in the brain (e.g., accumulation of beta-amyloid or tau protein deposits) without evidence of clinically significant symptoms. It is possible during this preclinical stage that the individual reports subjective cognitive decline that is undetectable on objective cognitive testing (e.g., via neuropsychological evaluation).[14] In the MCI stage, very mild symptoms begin to manifest but these are not significant enough to impair everyday functioning. As disease severity progresses into the dementia stage, individuals often begin to experience noticeable interference in higher-level or instrumental ADLs, such as managing finances or medications, planning transportation, and other activities that require higher-level thinking abilities. In later stages of disease severity, more basic ADLs become impaired, including eating, toileting, and basic hygiene maintenance.[12,15–19] Notably, not all individuals who present with MCI advance to a dementia syndrome and about 18-24% of individuals with MCI cognitively revert to baseline functioning when tested at later dates.[20,21] Individuals with an amnestic form of MCI (i.e., predominantly characterized by deficits in memory abilities) are more likely to progress to ADRD diagnosis.[22]

14.2.1 Risk & Risk Reduction

The literature on ADRD has examined risk and protective factors associated with dementia etiologies. As noted earlier, age is the largest risk factor for ADRD; increasing age is associated with greater risk. Genetically, there is significant evidence of a relationship between ADRD and the apolipoprotein (APOE) ε4 allele in non-Hispanic White individuals. However, APOE ε4 may not be a consistent dementia risk factor in groups historically underrepresented and excluded from ADRD research.[23] Rare mutations in presenilin-1, presenilin-2, and amyloid precursor protein genes have been identified as pathogenic loci for ADRD that typically follow a fully penetrant, autosomal dominant pattern; however, these account for less than 1% of ADRD cases.[24] Down's Syndrome (trisomy 21) is associated with increased amyloidosis with advanced age, ultimately leading to a dementia syndrome.[25] Cardiovascular disease and related risk factors like hypertension and obesity have been shown to increase risk of cognitive decline,[26–29] possibly due to decreased vascular integrity of the blood-brain barrier.[30] Cholesterol levels from mid- to late-life may correlate with the development of AD pathology, but the reasons for this remain unclear.[31] Diabetes increases risk for global cognitive decline and is associated with increased prevalence of dementia.[32,33] Along these lines, management of these risk conditions may subsequently reduce risk for ADRD. However, lower socioeconomic resources, related stress, and reduced access to healthcare further contribute to ADRD risk profiles and aging-related health disparities.[34] Individuals who show early signs of ADRD but have limited health care access experience delayed diagnosis, treatment, and management, possibly accelerating the dementia process.

Several factors may help mitigate the risk for developing ADRD as well as possibly slow progression.[35] The APOE ε2 allele has been identified as a potentially protective variant[36] in ADRD. Behaviorally, higher levels of habitual physical activity have been associated with decreased amyloid accumulation and lower ADRD risk, regardless of

APOE ε4 status; however, physical activity tends to decline with age.[37–39] Long-term adherence to overall healthy dietary patterns as opposed to single nutrient supplements, such as the Mediterranean, DASH (Dietary Approach to Stop Hypertension), and MIND (Mediterranean-DASH Intervention for Neurodegenerative Delay) diets have been associated with decreased risk of cognitive impairments. These neuroprotective diets are characterized by high intake of plant-based foods, moderate intake of fish, and lower intake of red meat, sweets, cheese, high-fat dairy products, and pastries.[40] Stress also plays a role in disease resilience with early life stress and chronic stressful experiences demonstrating salient associations with dementia risk; therefore, stress reduction and improvements in stress management may lead to decreased dementia risk.[41] Abnormal sleeping patterns developed prior to dementia symptom onset play a role in amyloid accumulation and clearance.[42] Having good social support may contribute to resilience in ADRD; increasing and maintaining social networks may help prevent development of dementia via both direct (e.g., cognitive engagement) and indirect (social support) mechanisms, while evidence suggests social isolation may accelerate cognitive decline[43,44] Generally, these and other brain health strategies may help build resilience to decline, slowing progression of the disease and contributing to quality of life.

Cognitive reserve – the brain's ability to maintain normal cognitive performance despite processes related to aging or disease burden[45] – may contribute to resistance and resilience to ADRD, helping explain individual variability in disease presentation.[46] Greater cognitive reserve is also potentially associated with delayed onset of clinically significant disease. Intellectual enrichment and cognitive stimulation, such as through formal and informal educational experiences, both early and later in life seem to be associated with greater cognitive reserve.[47–49] While greater educational attainment has been predictive of lower rates of amyloid deposition,[35] findings have been mixed, especially in ethnoracially diverse samples.[50] One reason for this discrepancy may be related to differences between quality and quantity of education, given that historic and systemic issues have precluded equitable access to quality education in diverse communities. Indeed, quality of education has been shown to explain differences in age- and sex-adjusted memory scores between non-Hispanic Black/African American and non-Hispanic White individuals.[51] Cross-cultural relationships between education and cognitive abilities are further complicated by evidence of possible non-linear effects and diminishing returns of greater education in ethnoracially diverse groups compared to non-Hispanic Whites.[52] Despite equivocal findings related to educational attainment and cognition in historically underrepresented and excluded groups, there is growing evidence that factors such as biculturalism and bilingualism, which require cognitively switching between two or more cultural or linguistic frameworks, may contribute to reserve in some cultural groups.[53,54]

14.2.2 Screening and Diagnosis

The diagnosis of dementia requires cognitive impairment that is significant enough to affect independent living. Screening for early stages of ADRD (e.g., MCI) serves several purposes. First, it allows for the detection of reversible causes of cognitive decline, such as infections or hormonal conditions. Notably, managing health conditions related to cognitive decline may further help reduce risk of ADRD given the implications of these conditions on brain health and resilience to neurodegeneration. While no cure currently exists for ADRD, early diagnosis allows for access to pharmacological treatments that may be effective in the management of behavioral symptoms of dementia (e.g., insomnia, agitation, apathy)[55] as well as research opportunities that may contribute to finding a cure. Critically, early diagnosis also allows for a larger window of time for planning for a future with dementia considering its medical, financial, and legal implications.

14.3 MANAGEMENT

Care management for a person living with dementia can be both intimidating and burdening. Behavioral challenges, multiplicity of tasks, and social isolation can strain the caregiver, and even threaten safety and integrity for the PLWD. Effective organization of family, formal and informal caregivers, and integration of the interdisciplinary care team may help reduce burnout, facilitate management of potential complications, maximize resources, diminish obstacles to care, and improve quality of life for the PLWD and caregivers alike.[56-59]

Organization of caregiving can first begin with acceptance of the dementia diagnosis, given the level of stigma and avoidance often observed among families. Individuals, families, and caregivers may benefit from having a comprehensive view of what to expect along the disease spectrum rather than engaging in avoidant behaviors.[58] Identifying available resources within the family and elsewhere (e.g., community health agencies) may contribute to a reduced burden. The earlier the diagnosis, the larger the window of opportunity a PLWD will have to actively participate in this decision-making process, making it easier to respect their wishes throughout the disease span.[60]

The second step is to discuss a plan of action with the interdisciplinary care team, as they are integral to the caregiver system's well-being. While primary care physicians (PCPs) are not expected to lead all caregiving conversations or even have knowledge in all areas of expertise and support, they do play an essential role in fostering those discussions. At a minimum, PCPs are often familiar with support services for effective care.[61,62] Unfortunately, many PCPs do not engage in these conversations because many (1) lack the practical knowledge of these issues themselves,[63,64] (2) feel the patient needs to be shielded from what they perceive as difficult conversations,[65,66] or (3) because they lack time and have cost-effectiveness constraints.[59]

Caregiver burnout may negatively impact care of the person living with dementia and contribute to the caregiver's personal risk for poor health outcomes.[67,68] Burnout risk reduction may be achieved through the adequate distribution of tasks among all caregivers. Care partners may benefit from having clear roles and responsibilities. Even so, families may have to shift and adapt as the needs of the PLWD increase. Eventually, tasks may have to be divided among informal and formal caregivers, depending on financial resources. Lastly, individualized self-care for dementia caregivers involves activities that help the caregiver feel mentally and physically rested. However, caregivers may need help developing awareness to notice when help or respite might be needed as some may not be inclined to ask for help.[69]

14.3.1 PLANNING

Advance care planning (ACP) is generally defined as the process of discussing and documenting a person's wishes for the end of their life.[70] However, ACPs are often underutilized, with only one out of every three U.S. Americans reporting having a completed plan.[71] Moreover, most dementia ACPs focus on medical management during the final stages of life. Given the nature of the disease, end-of-life issues can extend over several years, and present unique challenges related to other factors such as finances, symptom management, long-term care and housing, and navigation of healthcare systems. These challenges vary with each successive stage of dementia (i.e., preclinical, mild, moderate, and severe stages). Therefore, adequate planning and coordination are key to successfully resolving those challenges along the disease spectrum. Below is a list of suggestions that can be incorporated into ACP:

- **Preclinical stage:** Financial allocation, medical directives/living will, homestead/asset protection, and family discussions regarding finances and legal affairs
- **Mild stage:** Durable Power of Attorney (DPoA), identification of additional financial resources, up-to-date bank signatures, fraud/financial scam prevention, discussion regarding home modifications, and other legal documents
- **Moderate stage:** Feasibility of home modifications, caregiving and medical care coordination, long-term care decision-making, and enforcement of DPoA
- **Severe stage:** Placement in long-term care, expanded medical/hospital care, hospice, and funeral arrangements

Notably, this list is not exhaustive, and cultural differences exist in the way people approach the end of life. Attitudes towards the healthcare system, cultural and religious beliefs about death, their prior experiences with the disease, and their view on autonomy and/or inter-dependent decision-making affect the family's approach to end-of-life decisions; these can be collaboratively discussed between the person living with dementia, families, and health care providers.[72] Persons and families living with dementia may wish to seek professional advice on how to protect assets and legal matters as well as how to prepare for care decision-making, treatment options, alternatives for respite care, home modifications, housing choices, and how to finance care costs.

REFERENCES

1. Center for Disease Control and Prevention. Underlying Cause of Death 1999–2020; 2022. Accessed June 8, 2022. https://wonder.cdc.gov/wonder/help/ucd.html
2. Kramarow EA, Tejada-Vera B. Dementia mortality in the United States, 2000–2017. *Natl Vital Stat Rep Cent Dis Control Prev Natl Cent Health Stat Natl Vital Stat Syst.* 2019;68(2):1–29.
3. Rajan KB, Weuve J, Barnes LL, McAninch EA, Wilson RS, Evans DA. Population estimate of people with clinical Alzheimer's disease and mild cognitive impairment in the

United States (2020–2060). *Alzheimers Dement.* 2021;17(12):1966–1975. doi:10.1002/alz.12362

4. Chêne G, Beiser A, Au R, et al. Gender and incidence of dementia in the Framingham Heart Study from mid-adult life. *Alzheimers Dement.* 2015;11(3):310–320. doi:10.1016/j.jalz.2013.10.005

5. Seshadri S, Wolf PA, Beiser A, et al. Lifetime risk of dementia and Alzheimer's disease: The impact of mortality on risk estimates in the Framingham Study. *Neurology.* 1997;49(6):1498–1504. doi:10.1212/WNL.49.6.1498

6. Dilworth-Anderson P, Hendrie HC, Manly JJ, Khachaturian AS, Fazio S. Diagnosis and assessment of Alzheimer's disease in diverse populations. *Alzheimers Dement.* 2008;4(4):305–309. doi:10.1016/j.jalz.2008.03.001

7. Lines LM, Wiener JM. Racial and Ethnic Disparities in Alzheimer's Disease: A Literature Review. US Department of Health and Human Services, Assistant Secretary for Planning and Evaluation; 2014. https://aspe.hhs.gov/reports/racial-ethnic-disparities-alzheimers-disease-literature-review-0

8. Etters L, Goodall D, Harrison BE. Caregiver burden among dementia patient caregivers: A review of the literature. *J Am Acad Nurse Pract.* 2008;20(8):423–428. doi:10.1111/j.1745-7599.2008.00342.x

9. Barnes DE, Yaffe K. The projected effect of risk factor reduction on Alzheimer's disease prevalence. *Lancet Neurol.* 2011;10(9):819–828. doi:10.1016/S1474-4422(11)70072-2

10. Hurd MD, Martorell P, Delavande A, Mullen KJ, Langa KM. Monetary costs of Dementia in the United States. *N Engl J Med.* 2013;368(14):1326–1334. doi:10.1056/NEJMsa1204629

11. Brodaty H, Donkin M. Family caregivers of people with dementia. *Dialogues Clin Neurosci.* 2009;11(2):217–228. doi:10.31887/DCNS.2009.11.2/hbrodaty

12. Alzheimer's Association. 2022 Alzheimer's disease facts and figures. *Alzheimers Dement.* 2022;18(4):700–789. doi:10.1002/alz.12638

13. Jack CR, Bennett DA, Blennow K, et al. NIA-AA research framework: Toward a biological definition of Alzheimer's disease. *Alzheimers Dement.* 2018;14(4):535–562. doi:10.1016/j.jalz.2018.02.018

14. Jessen F, Amariglio RE, Boxtel M, et al. A conceptual framework for research on subjective cognitive decline in preclinical Alzheimer's disease. *Alzheimers Dement.* 2014;10(6):844–852. doi:10.1016/j.jalz.2014.01.001

15. Albert MS, DeKosky ST, Dickson D, et al. The diagnosis of mild cognitive impairment due to Alzheimer's disease: Recommendations from the National Institute on Aging-Alzheimer's Association workgroups on diagnostic guidelines for Alzheimer's disease. *Alzheimers Dement.* 2011;7(3):270–279. doi:10.1016/j.jalz.2011.03.008

16. Jack CR, Albert MS, Knopman DS, et al. Introduction to the recommendations from the National Institute on Aging-Alzheimer's Association workgroups on diagnostic guidelines for Alzheimer's disease. *Alzheimers Dement.* 2011;7(3):257–262. doi:10.1016/j.jalz.2011.03.004

17. McKhann GM, Knopman DS, Chertkow H, et al. The diagnosis of dementia due to Alzheimer's disease: Recommendations from the National Institute on Aging-Alzheimer's Association workgroups on diagnostic guidelines for Alzheimer's disease. *Alzheimers Dement.* 2011;7(3):263–269. doi:10.1016/j.jalz.2011.03.005

18. Sperling RA, Aisen PS, Beckett LA, et al. Toward defining the preclinical stages of Alzheimer's disease: Recommendations from the National Institute on Aging-Alzheimer's Association workgroups on diagnostic guidelines for Alzheimer's disease. *Alzheimers Dement.* 2011;7(3):280–292. doi:10.1016/j.jalz.2011.03.003

19. Vermunt L, Sikkes SAM, Hout A, et al. Duration of preclinical, prodromal, and dementia stages of Alzheimer's disease in relation to age, sex, and *APOE* genotype. *Alzheimers Dement.* 2019;15(7):888–898. doi:10.1016/j.jalz.2019.04.001

20. Canevelli M, Grande G, Lacorte E, et al. Spontaneous reversion of mild cognitive impairment to normal cognition: A systematic review of literature and meta-analysis. *J Am Med Dir Assoc.* 2016;17(10):943–948. doi:10.1016/j.jamda.2016.06.020

21. Malek-Ahmadi M. Reversion from mild cognitive impairment to normal cognition: A meta-analysis. *Alzheimer Dis Assoc Disord.* 2016;30(4):324–330. doi:10.1097/WAD.0000000000000145

22. DeCarli C, Mungas D, Harvey D, et al. Memory impairment, but not cerebrovascular disease, predicts progression of MCI to dementia. *Neurology.* 2004;63(2):220. doi:10.1212/01.WNL.0000130531.90205.EF

23. González HM, Tarraf W, Schneiderman N, et al. Prevalence and correlates of mild cognitive impairment among diverse Hispanics/Latinos: Study of Latinos-investigation of neurocognitive aging results. *Alzheimers Dement.* 2019;15(12):1507–1515. doi:10.1016/j.jalz.2019.08.202

24. Van Cauwenberghe C, Van Broeckhoven C, Sleegers K. The genetic landscape of Alzheimer disease: Clinical implications and perspectives. *Genet Med.* 2016;18(5):421–430. doi:10.1038/gim.2015.117

25. Lott IT, Head E. Dementia in down syndrome: Unique insights for Alzheimer disease research. *Nat Rev Neurol.* 2019;15(3):135–147. doi:10.1038/s41582-018-0132-6

26. Gorelick PB, Scuteri A, Black SE, et al. Vascular contributions to cognitive impairment and dementia: A statement for healthcare professionals from the American Heart Association/American Stroke Association. *Stroke.* 2011;42(9):2672–2713. doi:10.1161/STR.0b013e3182299496

27. Gorelick PB, Furie KL, Iadecola C, et al. Defining optimal brain health in adults: A presidential advisory from the American Heart Association/American Stroke Association. *Stroke.* 2017;48(10). doi:10.1161/STR.0000000000000148

28. Frisoni GB, Molinuevo JL, Altomare D, et al. Precision prevention of Alzheimer's and other dementias: Anticipating future needs in the control of risk factors and implementation of disease-modifying therapies. *Alzheimers Dement.* 2020;16(10):1457–1468. doi:10.1002/alz.12132

29. Tarraf W, Kaplan R, Daviglus M, et al. Cardiovascular risk and cognitive function in middle-aged and older Hispanics/Latinos: Results from the Hispanic community health Study/Study of Latinos (HCHS/SOL). Calderón-Garcidueñas L, ed. *J Alzheimers Dis.* 2020;73(1):103–116. doi:10.3233/JAD-190830

30. Reitz C, Mayeux R. Alzheimer disease: Epidemiology, diagnostic criteria, risk factors and biomarkers. *Biochem Pharmacol.* 2014;88(4):640–651. doi:10.1016/j.bcp.2013.12.024

31. Hayden KM, Gaussoin SA, Hunter JC, et al. Cognitive resilience among *APOE* ε4 carriers in the oldest old. *Int J Geriatr Psychiatry.* 2019;34(12):1833–1844. doi:10.1002/gps.5199

32. Livingston G, Sommerlad A, Orgeta V, et al. Dementia prevention, intervention, and care. *Lancet.* 2017;390(10113):2673–2734. doi:10.1016/S0140-6736(17)31363-6

33. González HM, Tarraf W, González KA, et al. Diabetes, cognitive decline, and mild cognitive impairment among diverse Hispanics/Latinos: Study of Latinos–Investigation of neurocognitive aging results (HCHS/SOL). *Diabetes Care.* 2020;43(5):1111–1117. doi:10.2337/dc19-1676

34. Vega WA, Angel JL, Robledo LMFG, Markides KS. *Contextualizing Health and Aging in the Americas: Effects of Space, Time and Place.* 1st ed. Springer Cham; 2019. doi:10.1007/978-3-030-00584-9

35. Arenaza-Urquijo EM, Vemuri P. Resistance vs resilience to Alzheimer disease: Clarifying terminology for preclinical studies. *Neurology.* 2018;90(15):695–703. doi:10.1212/WNL.0000000000005303

36. James LM, Engdahl BE, Georgopoulos AP. Apolipoprotein E: The resilience gene. *Exp Brain Res*. 2017;235(6):1853–1859. doi:10.1007/s00221-017-4941-4

37. Arredondo EM, Sotres-Alvarez D, Stoutenberg M, et al. Physical activity levels in U.S. Latino/Hispanic adults: Results from the Hispanic Community Health Study/Study of Latinos. *Am J Prev Med*. 2016;50(4):500–508. doi:10.1016/j.amepre.2015.08.029

38. Farooq A, Martin A, Janssen X, et al. Longitudinal changes in moderate-to-vigorous-intensity physical activity in children and adolescents: A systematic review and meta-analysis. *Obes Rev*. 2020;21(1). doi:10.1111/obr.12953

39. Sallis JF. Age-related decline in physical activity: A synthesis of human and animal studies. *Med Sci Sports Exerc*. 2000;32(9):1598–1600. doi:10.1097/00005768-200009000-00012

40. Pistollato F, Iglesias RC, Ruiz R, et al. Nutritional patterns associated with the maintenance of neurocognitive functions and the risk of dementia and Alzheimer's disease: A focus on human studies. *Pharmacol Res*. 2018;131:32–43. doi:10.1016/j.phrs.2018.03.012

41. Luo J, Beam CR, Gatz M. Is stress an overlooked risk factor for dementia? A systematic review from a lifespan developmental perspective. *Prev Sci*. Published online May 27, 2022. doi:10.1007/s11121-022-01385-1

42. Mander BA, Winer JR, Jagust WJ, Walker MP. Sleep: A novel mechanistic pathway, biomarker, and treatment target in the pathology of Alzheimer's disease? *Trends Neurosci*. 2016;39(8):552–566. doi:10.1016/j.tins.2016.05.002

43. Fratiglioni L, Paillard-Borg S, Winblad B. An active and socially integrated lifestyle in late life might protect against dementia. *Lancet Neurol*. 2004;3(6):343–353. doi:10.1016/S1474-4422(04)00767-7

44. Pillai JA, Verghese J. Social networks and their role in preventing dementia. *Indian J Psychiatry*. 2009;51(Suppl1):S22–S28.

45. Stern Y. Cognitive reserve. *Neuropsychologia*. 2009;47(10):2015–2028. doi:10.1016/j.neuropsychologia.2009.03.004

46. Ossenkoppele R, Lyoo CH, Jester-Broms J, et al. Assessment of demographic, genetic, and imaging variables associated with brain resilience and cognitive resilience to pathological tau in patients with Alzheimer disease. *JAMA Neurol*. 2020;77(5):632. doi:10.1001/jamaneurol.2019.5154

47. Wada M, Noda Y, Shinagawa S, et al. Effect of education on Alzheimer's disease-related neuroimaging biomarkers in healthy controls, and participants with mild cognitive impairment and Alzheimer's disease: A cross-sectional study. *J Alzheimers Dis*. 2018;63(2):861–869. doi:10.3233/JAD-171168

48. Vemuri P, Lesnick TG, Przybelski SA, et al. Association of lifetime intellectual enrichment with cognitive decline in the older population. *JAMA Neurol*. 2014;71(8):1017. doi:10.1001/jamaneurol.2014.963

49. Wilson RS. Participation in cognitively stimulating activities and risk of incident Alzheimer disease. *JAMA*. 2002;287(6):742. doi:10.1001/jama.287.6.742

50. Avila JF, Rentería MA, Jones RN, et al. Education differentially contributes to cognitive reserve across racial/ethnic groups. *Alzheimers Dement*. 2021;17(1):70–80. doi:10.1002/alz.12176

51. Fyffe DC, Mukherjee S, Barnes LL, Manly JJ, Bennett DA, Crane PK. Explaining differences in episodic memory performance among older African Americans and Whites: The roles of factors related to cognitive reserve and test bias. *J Int Neuropsychol Soc*. 2011;17(4):625–638. doi:10.1017/S1355617711000476

52. Sims J, Coley RL. Variations in links between educational success and health: Implications for enduring health disparities. *Cultur Divers Ethnic Minor Psychol*. 2019;25(1):32–43. doi:10.1037/cdp0000239

53. Vallejo LG. *Biculturalism, Bilingualism, & Executive Function Among U.S. Latinos: Implications for Cognitive Reserve*. Dissertations (1934 -). Marquette University; 2017. https://epublications.marquette.edu/dissertations_mu/748

54. Arce Rentería M, Casalletto K, Tom S, et al. The contributions of active Spanish-English bilingualism to cognitive reserve among older Hispanic adults living in California. *Arch Clin Neuropsychol*. 2019;34(7):1235–1235. doi:10.1093/arclin/acz029.02

55. Cummings J. New approaches to symptomatic treatments for Alzheimer's disease. *Mol Neurodegener*. 2021;16(1):2. doi:10.1186/s13024-021-00424-9

56. Harris DP, Chodosh J, Vassar SD, Vickrey BG, Shapiro MF. Primary care providers' views of challenges and rewards of dementia care relative to other conditions. *J Am Geriatr Soc*. 2009;57(12):2209–2216. doi:10.1111/j.1532-5415.2009.02572.x

57. Gove D, Small N, Downs M, Vernooij-Dassen M. General practitioners' perceptions of the stigma of dementia and the role of reciprocity. *Dementia*. 2017;16(7):948–964. doi:10.1177/1471301215625657

58. Ashworth RM. Looking ahead to a future with Alzheimer's disease: Coping with the unknown. *Ageing Soc*. 2020;40(8):1647–1668. doi:10.1017/S0144686X19000151

59. Iliffe S, Manthorpe J, Eden A. Sooner or later? Issues in the early diagnosis of dementia in general practice: A qualitative study. *Fam Pract*. 2003;20(4):376–381. doi:10.1093/fampra/cmg407

60. de Vugt ME, Verhey FRJ. The impact of early dementia diagnosis and intervention on informal caregivers. *Neuroethics Neurodegener Dis*. 2013;110:54–62. doi:10.1016/j.pneurobio.2013.04.005

61. Murphy K, O'Connor DA, Browning CJ, et al. Understanding diagnosis and management of dementia and guideline implementation in general practice: A qualitative study using the theoretical domains framework. *Implement Sci*. 2014;9(1):31. doi:10.1186/1748-5908-9-31

62. Villars H, Oustric S, Andrieu S, et al. The primary care physician and Alzheimer's disease: An international position paper. *J Nutr*. 2010;14(2):11.

63. Harmand MGC, Meillon C, Rullier L, et al. Description of general practitioners' practices when suspecting cognitive impairment. Recourse to care in dementia (Recaredem) study. *Aging Ment Health*. 2018;22(8):1046–1055. doi:10.1080/13607863.2017.1330871

64. Somme D, Gautier A, Pin S, Corvol A. General practitioner's clinical practices, difficulties and educational needs to manage Alzheimer's disease in France: Analysis of national telephone-inquiry data. *BMC Fam Pract*. 2013;14(1):81. doi:10.1186/1471-2296-14-81

65. Lahjibi-Paulet H, Dauffy A, Minard A, Gaxatte C, Saint-Jean O, Somme D. Attitudes toward Alzheimer's disease: A qualitative study of the role played by social representation on a convenient sample of French general practitioners. *Aging Clin Exp Res*. 2012;24(4):384–390. doi:10.1007/BF03325270

66. Lahjibi-Paulet H, de Almedia A, Le Guen J, et al. Change on attitudes toward Alzheimer's disease: Four years after a qualitative study of the role played by social representation on French general practitioners. *9th Congr EUGMS Venice 2-4 Oct 2013*. 2013;4:S166. doi:10.1016/j.eurger.2013.07.554

67. Richardson TJ, Lee SJ, Berg-Weger M, Grossberg GT. Caregiver health: health of caregivers of Alzheimer's and other dementia patients. *Curr Psychiatry Rep*. 2013;15(7):367. doi:10.1007/s11920-013-0367-2

68. Alves LC de S, Monteiro DQ, Bento SR, Hayashi VD, Pelegrini LN de C, Vale FAC. Burnout syndrome in informal caregivers of older adults with dementia: A systematic review. *Dement Neuropsychol*. 2019;13(4):415–421. doi:10.1590/1980-57642018dn13-040008

69. Wang XR, Liu SX, Robinson KM, Shawler C, Zhou L. The impact of dementia caregiving on self-care management of caregivers and facilitators: A qualitative study:

Self-care of dementia caregivers. *Psychogeriatrics*. 2019;19(1):23–31. doi:10.1111/psyg. 12354

70. Nicholson B. Advanced care planning: The concept over time. *Nurs Forum (Auckl)*. 2021; 56(4):1024–1028. doi:10.1111/nuf.12631

71. Yadav KN, Gabler NB, Cooney E, et al. Approximately one in three US adults completes any type of advance directive for end-of-life care. *Health Aff (Millwood)*. 2017;36(7):1244–1251. doi:10.1377/hlthaff.2017.0175

72. Carr D. Racial differences in end-of-life planning: Why don't Blacks and Latinos prepare for the inevitable? *OMEGA - J Death Dying*. 2011;63(1):1–20. doi:10.2190/ OM.63.1.a

15 Biopsychosocial Perspective on Sleep

*Diana A. Chirinos, PhD, Julia Starkovsky, MA,
and Morgann West, BA*

KEY POINTS

- Sleep has an immediate impact on our state of mind upon waking, but it also has long-term effects on our body and mind.
- Both sleep dimensions and commonly occurring sleep disorders, such as insomnia and sleep-disordered breathing, are associated with risks for depression, anxiety, and post-traumatic stress disorder (PTSD).
- Sleep also affects our physical health, and established associations have been described with cardiometabolic diseases and cancer.

15.1 INTRODUCTION

Sleep is a seemingly passive state in which both our brain and our bodies are dormant. However, during sleep, the brain is actively engaged and carries out functions that are essential to every process in the body. Not only does sleep have an immediate impact on our state of mind and well-being upon waking, but it can also affect our long-term mental and physical health. In this chapter, we will discuss the importance of sleep as it relates to our body and mind by (1) defining sleep health, (2) outlining the most common sleep disorders and their respective current treatment regimens, and (3) describing associations between sleep and both mental and physical health outcomes in adult populations.

15.2 DEFINING SLEEP HEALTH

Sleep is essential to good health.[1] In spite of its importance, the field of sleep medicine, like with many other medical disciplines, has traditionally focused on educating patients about sleep, or the lack thereof, in the context of sleep deficiency. In doing so, previous approaches to sleep medicine largely outlined disorders/diseases in need of medical treatment to patients.[2] The health of populations, however, is increasingly being defined in terms of wellness, performance, and adaptation – not simply the absence of disease.[3] This shift in population science, coupled with the accumulation of research on the links between sleep and health, encouraged efforts to provide an explicit definition of optimal sleep health.

DOI: 10.1201/b22810-17

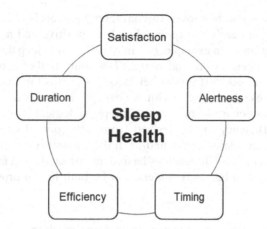

FIGURE 15.1 Five key dimensions of sleep that have consistently been associated with mental and physical health outcomes.

In 2014, a seminal paper proposed, for the first time, a definition of sleep health based on concepts derived from empirical data.[3] This manuscript described sleep health as follows:

> Sleep health is a multidimensional pattern of sleep-wakefulness, adapted to individual, social, and environmental demands, that promotes physical and mental well-being. Good sleep health is characterized by subjective satisfaction, appropriate timing, adequate duration, high efficiency, and sustained alertness during waking hours.

This definition did not include any specific sleep disorder, but rather provided attributes of sleep itself that can be measured in any individual with or without a sleep disorder. More importantly, it highlighted the multidimensional nature of sleep and outlined five key dimensions of sleep that have consistently been associated with (mental and physical) health outcomes (see Figure 15.1). The five key dimensions of sleep include:

Satisfaction with sleep. An individual's subjective assessment of the quality of their sleep (e.g., "poor", "good").

Sleep duration. The total amount of sleep an individual obtained in a period of 24 hours.

Alertness/Sleepiness. The degree to which an individual can maintain attentive wakefulness.

Sleep efficiency. The amount of time an individual was asleep while lying in bed with the intention to sleep. It is calculated using the total amount of actual sleep time divided by time spent in bed.

Timing of sleep. The placement of sleep within the 24-hour period (e.g., night vs. day).

These dimensions were chosen to characterize sleep health for several reasons.[3] First, they can each be expressed in both positive and negative terms. In taking sleep duration as an example, one may categorize sleep duration as "good" if it falls within a certain optimal range (7–9 hours is the recommended sleep time for adults)[4] or "poor" if it falls below or above this optimal range. Second, the majority of these dimensions (with the exception of satisfaction) can be measured via self-report or across behavioral and physiological levels of analyses. For instance, sleep efficiency can be derived from self-reported sleep diaries, actigraphy (wrist-worn accelerometers), and/or in the laboratory via polysomnography (PSG). Finally, all of these dimensions have demonstrated good face or ecological validity,[3] and they can be easily understood by both health providers and a lay audience.

15.3   SLEEP DISORDERS AND THEIR TREATMENT

Consistent disruptions in one (or all) of the dimensions of sleep health can lead to sleep disorders. In addition to a definition of sleep health, an international classification of sleep disorders is necessary to discriminate among symptoms, to understand their etiology, and most importantly, to deliver appropriate treatment.[5] Below, we review the most common sleep disorders and their treatments with a focus on evidence-based behavioral treatments.

15.3.1   INSOMNIA

The first most common sleep disorder that is unique to about one-third of adults is insomnia.[6] Insomnia is characterized by dissatisfaction with sleep (at sleep onset or sleep maintenance), as well as other daytime symptoms (e.g., sleepiness, impaired attention, mood disturbance). Although several insomnia subtypes have been identified (e.g., psychophysiological, paradoxical, idiopathic), diagnosis and treatment of each subtype are comparable to one another.

The American Academy of Sleep Medicine recommends the use of Cognitive-Behavioral Therapy for Insomnia (CBT-I) as the first line of treatment for insomnia.[7] CBT-I is an intervention that aims to change dysfunctional thought and behavior patterns in an effort to increase sleep time and improve sleep quality.[8] The effectiveness of CBT-I, the subject of several meta-analyses, has been documented across a variety of age ranges and patient populations.[9,10] In spite of the effectiveness of CBT-I, pharmacological treatment continues to be common either in addition to behavioral treatment or when access to CBT-I providers is limited.

15.3.2   SLEEP-DISORDERED BREATHING

Sleep apnea is a sleep disorder defined by pauses of breathing during sleep.[6] The three main types of sleep apnea are the following: obstructive (characterized by closure/reduction of airflow that occurs as a result of the collapse of the upper airway during sleep), central (lack of effort to breathe during sleep usually arising from the brain respiratory centers), and complex.[6] Sleep apnea is diagnosed with PSG, either at home or in the laboratory, by quantifying the number of respiratory events (cessations in breathing) per hour.[6] At least five events per hour are needed for a diagnosis of sleep apnea. Additional common symptoms of sleep apnea include loud snoring, choking/gasping, sleepiness and fatigue, and morning headaches. The primary treatment for obstructive sleep apnea is continuous positive airway pressure (CPAP) therapy, which provides an interpreted airway flow into the nose via a machine. This therapy has been able to lessen daytime sleepiness and enhance cognitive functioning, mood, and well-being.[11] Other treatments include positional therapy (for mild cases) or surgical treatments.

15.3.3 CIRCADIAN RHYTHM SLEEP DISORDERS

The sleep-wake cycle is regulated by two important factors: homeostatic sleep drive (usually described as "hunger" for sleep) and the circadian rhythm. The sleep phase of the circadian rhythm typically starts 2 hours after the onset of melatonin secretion.[6] Melatonin secretion taking place earlier or later than socially driven sleep times results in advanced or delayed circadian rhythm disorders, respectively. Usually, sleep length is normal and patients wake up refreshed when sleeping at their desired time. The treatment for circadian rhythm sleep disorders includes the use of a blue or bright light schedule, as well as melatonin prescribed approximately 1 hour before the desired sleep time.[6]

15.3.4 HYPERSOMNIA

Hypersomnia disorders are characterized by increased sleepiness in spite of adequate sleep opportunity and night-time sleep quality.[6] While rare, these types of sleep disorders include narcolepsy type 1 (with cataplexy [loss of muscle tone following intense, usually positive, emotions such as laughter]), narcolepsy type 2 (no cataplexy), idiopathic hypersomnia (with or without long sleep time), and periodic hypersomnia (such as Kleine-Levin syndrome). The diagnosis of narcolepsy is usually done in a clinic and is followed by a multiple sleep latency test (MSLT) to validate the sleepiness. This is usually performed following a night-time PSG and consists of five nap opportunities throughout the day (most narcolepsy patients fall asleep within minutes of being given a nap opportunity). The treatment of narcolepsy is usually pharmacological, although behavioral treatments with the aim of improving quality of life among narcolepsy patients are in development.[12]

15.3.5 PARASOMNIAS

Parasomnias are characterized by a wide range of behaviors occurring during sleep (e.g., walking).[6] They are commonly classified based on the time in which they occur in the sleep cycle (non-rapid eye movement [REM] or REM parasomnias). Therefore, the diagnosis of parasomnia is confirmed with nocturnal PSG. Treatment is usually pharmacological, although melatonin appears to be equally beneficial for some REM parasomnias.[13]

15.3.6 RESTLESS LEGS SYNDROME AND PERIODIC LIMB MOVEMENTS OF SLEEP

Restless legs syndrome is characterized by an uncomfortable urge to move the legs that occurs or worsens while at rest, occurs predominantly during the evening, and is partially relieved by physical activity.[6] One distinctive feature of restless legs syndrome is that its characteristic worsening during the late evening hours can affect sleep onset/quality. Restless legs syndrome can be idiopathic (no known cause) or secondary to another disorder (e.g., Parkinson's disease, multiple sclerosis, pregnancy, iron deficiency). Periodic limb movement disorder is described as repetitive limb movements that occur during sleep and cause sleep disruption.[6] Both of these conditions often co-occur. Treatment is usually pharmacological and includes iron supplementation when appropriate.[6]

The presence of sleep disorders or disruptions/disturbances to any or all of the five sleep health dimensions can affect the long-term mental and physical health of individuals. Below, we review the impact of sleep on mental and physical health.

15.4   THE IMPACT OF SLEEP ON MENTAL HEALTH

The association between sleep and mental health disorders in adults is often bi-directional, [14,15] with the most common comorbidities being depression, anxiety, and post-traumatic stress disorder. In this section, prevalence of these disorders in relation to sleep disturbances, causation, and treatments will be described.

15.4.1 SLEEP AND DEPRESSION

Sleep disturbance is one of the most prominent symptoms in adults with depression to the extent that sleep disturbance is sometimes regarded as a secondary manifestation of depression.[16] Depression is categorized as depressed mood, diminished pleasure, significant and unintentional weight loss, reduction of mental or physical movement, fatigue, feelings of worthlessness, inability to focus, and/or recurrent thoughts about death or suicide.[17] The lifetime prevalence of depression is 16%.[18,19]

Insomnia and depression often co-occur,[16] and the relationship is thought to be bi-directional. Common biological mechanisms include inflammatory factors, dysregulation of biochemical pathways, genetic correlations, and changes in circadian rhythm.[16] Insomnia has also been found to be associated with incident depression.[20] For example, a recent study showed that 71% of participants who endorsed having depression disclosed that insomnia symptoms occurred before the depressive symptoms.[21] Similarly, insomnia is a common secondary symptom of depression.[20] Current treatment regimens for depression typically do not address sleep disturbances. In fact, some antidepressant drugs have been linked to suppressed REM during sleep, leading to sleep disruption/poor quality that may result in insomnia.

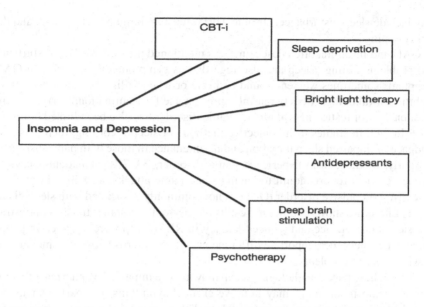

FIGURE 15.2 Describes the ways to treat insomnia and depression in conjunction.

Given the high comorbidity between insomnia and depression, recent research efforts have been devoted to the development of appropriate treatments that address both of these disorders. Treatments to date include antidepressants, cognitive CBT-I, sleep deprivation, bright light therapy, and deep brain stimulation.[16] Antidepressants help resolve depressive symptoms, but as mentioned earlier, may increase symptoms of insomnia. CBT-I is the gold standard for insomnia treatment, and modified versions of CBT-I have shown promise for patients with comorbid depression.[22] The combination of addressing sleep disturbance, barriers surrounding sleep, and reorganizing ruminating thoughts before bed appears to be advantageous for those who have comorbid insomnia and depression. Other lines of treatment like sleep deprivation, bright light therapy, deep brain stimulation, and psychotherapy can be used in conjunction with CBT-I and antidepressants to create an optimal outcome in the setting of both sleep and depressive symptoms (Figure 15.2).

15.4.2 SLEEP AND ANXIETY

Anxiety is defined as both a state and a trait.[23] Anxiety as a trait is a natural response to a threat. When anxiety is a state, our bodies turn on the sympathetic nervous system and can adapt to a risk. Anxiety as a trait, or psychiatric condition, describes a continuous experience that presents itself throughout life and may not serve as a necessity for survival.[23] Anxiety disorders like generalized anxiety disorder (GAD), panic disorder, post-traumatic stress disorder (PTSD), and obsessive-compulsive disorder (OCD) may disrupt the ability to function on a daily basis.[24] Anxiety symptoms may include sleep disturbance, chronic worry, tension, fatigue, restlessness, and difficulty coping.[24]

GAD and insomnia often co-occur.[25] As mentioned previously, sleep disturbance and problems falling asleep are also regarded as symptoms of anxiety.[24] In GAD, symptoms sometimes worsen around bedtime or when falling back to sleep after a nighttime awakening. Anxiety may also present itself as rumination, worry, negative emotionality, or restlessness at night.[15] Panic disorder has also been linked to insomnia.[25] In fact, in studies using objective methods of sleep recording, there has been evidence of impaired sleep initiation and maintenance in those with panic disorder.[26] Similarly, of those who experience panic disorder, 33–71% of patients surveyed through clinical reports admit to having sleep panic attacks, as well.[27] In contrast, obsessive-compulsive disorder (OCD) is not commonly associated with sleep disturbance. Literature shows conflicting results on this topic, as some studies demonstrate that sleep maintenance and reduced latency in REM sleep were reflected in people with OCD,[28] but others report no difference in sleep patterns between someone with or without sleep problems.[29]

Within these psychopathologies, sleep may also be impacted by pharmacotherapy. While certain medications may improve clinical symptoms of a particular mental disorder, adverse effects might include sleep disturbances.[24] However, some research notes that CBT-I may reduce anxiety symptoms in some patient populations.[30]

15.4.3 SLEEP AND PTSD

The comorbidity of sleep and trauma-induced conditions, specifically post-traumatic stress disorder (PTSD), is high.[31] About 7/100 people will develop PTSD in their lifetime. PTSD is defined by direct or indirect exposure to a traumatic event, intrusive symptoms (i.e., nightmares, flashbacks, emotional distress), avoidance of a stimuli, negative adaptations in cognition and mood, and alterations in arousal or reactivity.[17] Symptoms of PTSD must also last more than a month to be able to diagnose and cause functional impairment.[17] PTSD symptoms tend to wax and wane as different triggers may occur.

Given this change in mood, reactivity, and cognition, the relationship between PTSD and sleep disturbance is expected. In fact, sleep disturbance is one of the most prevalent symptoms of PTSD.[32] About 80-90% of people with PTSD experience insomnia symptoms and about 50–70% report experiencing nightmares.[33] Nightmare frequency averages to about five per week.[34] Insomnia is only one of the many sleep disturbances that people with PTSD may experience. Examples of sleep disturbances associated with PTSD include sleep-disordered breathing, periodic leg movement disorders, parasomnias, and disruptive nocturnal behaviors (i.e., night sweats, dysphoric dreams, dream reenactment).[35] Sleep helps emotional regulation. Thus, patients with PTSD may overconsolidate emotions attached to memories due to disruptions in their REM and sleep cycle. This may result in more intense symptoms and debilitation of PTSD.[36]

The treatments used for PTSD and sleep disturbance are similar to those mentioned for anxiety and depression. CBT-I, antidepressants, and psychotherapy tend to assist in the resolution of sleep disturbance and symptoms of PTSD.[36] Imagery rehearsal therapy (IRT) is also used to treat PTSD symptoms through mitigation of sleep disturbance.[37] IRT is a type of cognitive-behavioral treatment that helps rescript nightmares by creating a nightmare diary, addressing those nightmares, and adjusting the dream to pleasant imagery.

Overall, sleep and mental health problems often co-occur, and the comorbidity between sleep and psychiatric disorders is high, particularly for depression, anxiety disorders, and PTSD. Research on how best to address sleep disturbance in psychiatric disorders is imperative, and effective treatment options continue to be developed.

15.5 THE IMPACT OF SLEEP ON PHYSICAL HEALTH

Over the past two decades, epidemiological research has shown that disrupted sleep has a detrimental impact on our physical health. While research on sleep's association with various other conditions continues to emerge, established associations with highly prevalent chronic conditions, including cardio-metabolic disease and cancer, have been reported.

15.5.1 SLEEP AND CARDIO-METABOLIC DISEASE

Cardiovascular disease (CVD) is the leading cause of death in the United States.[38] There is increasing awareness of the fact that sleep disturbance is an important factor in CVD and also has established links to the development of cardio-metabolic risk factors such as obesity, diabetes, and hypertension.[39]

The strongest evidence of the link between sleep and cardio-metabolic disease can be derived from the study of sleep duration. The association between sleep duration and cardio-metabolic disease is well-established and has been the subject of several reviews.[40,41] Briefly, both short (<6 hrs. of sleep per night) and long sleep duration (>9 hrs.) have been linked with obesity-related outcomes,[42,43] with stronger associations in the context of short-sleep duration. Similarly, there is a strong link between short sleep duration and diabetes-related outcomes,[44] hypertension,[45] cholesterol levels,[46] and CVD endpoints such as heart attack[47] and stroke.[48]

In line with the findings from sleep duration studies, a growing number of data shows an association between insomnia and cardio-metabolic conditions. While a comprehensive assessment of insomnia disorder is challenging in epidemiological studies, a recent meta-analysis of prospective cohort studies illustrated a strong association between insomnia and increased risk of hypertension.[49] Other meta-analyses demonstrate associations between insomnia and type 2 diabetes (T2D), but not body mass index (BMI).[50] Some of these meta-analyses suggest that the cardio-metabolic risk associated with insomnia is particularly strong for those suffering from insomnia with short sleep duration.[50,51]

When it comes to circadian rhythm abnormalities, epidemiological studies have largely focused on the impact of unusual sleep timing, as in the case of individuals doing shift work, rather than circadian rhythm disorders *per se*. These studies show a significant detrimental effect of shift work on various cardio-metabolic conditions including incident obesity,[52] hypertension,[53] T2D, [54] and cholesterol.[55] It appears that eating behavior and timing may be at the root of the link between circadian rhythm abnormalities and cardio-metabolic conditions.[56] While reports are still equivocal, some studies suggest that night shift work was also associated with the consumption of unhealthy foods[57] (greater consumption of energy, fat, carbohydrates, saccharose, and lower consumption of fruits and vegetables) and increased snacking.[58] Similarly, shift work may have an impact on timing of food consumption, as some studies illustrate the prevalence of longer eating duration[59] and irregular eating timing among shift workers.[57]

Finally, the link between sleep-disordered breathing (specifically, obstructive sleep apnea [OSA]) and cardio-metabolic risk is well established.[60] OSA is significantly associated with obesity,[61] hypertension,[62] and T2D.[63] Most importantly, OSA has been linked to various CVD endpoints, including stroke,[64] coronary heart disease,[65] atrial fibrillation,[66] and heart failure.[65] Interestingly, regular CPAP use has been shown to significantly decrease cardiovascular risk among OSA patients. Unfortunately, the low rates of CPAP compliance is a challenge that warrants further attention.

In sum, various sleep domains (such as duration and timing) and some sleep disorders (such as insomnia and OSA) have a documented impact on CVD and cardio-metabolic risk. These associations have been so widely documented in recent years that the American Heart Association updated the list of factors that optimize and preserve cardiovascular health.[67] Previously known as "Life's Simple 7," past metrics for optimal cardiovascular health included smoking abstinence, healthy weight, eating healthy, exercising, and managing blood pressure, cholesterol, and blood sugar.[68] The updated list, labeled "Life's Essential 8," now includes sleep health as an important factor in both cardiovascular health promotion and the preservation of health across the life course.[67]

15.5.2 SLEEP AND CANCER

Cancer is the second leading cause of death in the US and one of the most common causes of death around the world.[38] The prevalence of cancer varies widely across cancer types. Although breast, lung, and prostate cancer are the most common cancers worldwide, lung, liver, and stomach cancer are associated with the highest rates of mortality.[69] Literature on the association between sleep and cancer suggests a bidirectional link.[70]

The largest and most conclusive evidence for a prospective association between sleep disorders and cancer onset comes from studies examining the role of insomnia. A recent review suggests that insomnia is a risk factor for a wide range of tumors,[70] including those of the breast, nose, trachea, liver, oral cavity, colon, thyroid, bladder, and kidney.[71]

Circadian rhythm disorders may also represent a risk factor for various types of cancer, including thyroid, gastrointestinal and breast cancer, as well as squamous cell carcinoma.[70] The link with breast cancer appears to be most conclusive given the role of melatonin in tumor genesis.[72] The literature on cancer and sleep disturbances related to shift work appears to be less conclusive,[70] with conflicting data limited to breast, thyroid, and gastrointestinal cancer.

Some recent studies have proposed an association between other sleep disorders and cancer, yet this is still an emerging area of research. A small body of literature suggests a link between narcolepsy and greater risk of head-neck and gastric cancers, particularly among women.[73] Furthermore, associations between OSA and prevalence of melanoma, breast, uterus, kidney, pancreas, colorectal, and central nervous system (CNS) cancer have also been reported.[74]

It is important to note that the onset of sleep disturbances and sleep disorders can also be a natural consequence of a cancer diagnosis.[70] General sleep disturbances have been documented in all major cancer types.[75] Unfortunately, sleep disturbances appear to linger beyond treatment and recovery, particularly among breast cancer survivors.[76] Insomnia is perhaps the most common complaint in cancer patients and has been documented in all cancer types, especially those of head, neck, breast, and lung, with a prevalence ranging from 16% to 63%.[70] Similarly, the onset of circadian rhythm disorders has been identified among patients with brain, lung, and breast cancer.[77] Furthermore, a recent review has documented the onset of narcolepsy in the context of brain cancer,[78] as well as a link between cancer diagnosis and the worsening of OSA symptoms, particularly in lung cancer.[79]

Overall, sleep disturbance and some sleep disorders have been shown to have a prospective association with cancer onset across various cancer types. Similarly, sleep disturbance is a common experience following a cancer diagnosis. While research on the link between cancer and sleep disturbances continues to expand, there is a need for the development of interventions aimed at reducing sleep disturbance among cancer patients.

15.5.3 SLEEP AND OTHER HEALTH CONDITIONS

The effect of sleep on the risk for cardio-metabolic conditions and cancers has been widely documented over the past couple of decades. However, emerging research is also linking sleep to other physical conditions, including Alzheimer disease and other dementias,[80] gastrointestinal disorders,[81] and polycystic ovary syndrome,[82] among others. Similarly, a significant association between sleep and pain has been widely documented.[83]

15.6 CONCLUSIONS

Sleep is essential to optimal functioning in everyday life at an individual level, and its relationship to our mind and body is extensively documented. A close bi-directional link between sleep and psychiatric disorders exists, in particular, for depression, anxiety, and PTSD. The effects of sleep, or lack thereof, on physical health are most widely documented for chronic diseases such as CVD and cancer. Future studies should focus on improving sleep and preventing the adverse effects of sleep on mental and physical health.

REFERENCES

1. Zee PC, Turek FW. Sleep and health: Everywhere and in both directions. *Arch Intern Med.* 2006;166(16):1686–1688.
2. Sateia MJ. International classification of sleep disorders-third edition. *Chest.* 2014;1 46(5):1387–1394.
3. Buysse DJ. Sleep health: Can we define it? Does it matter? *Sleep.* 2014;37(1):9–17.
4. Watson NF, Badr MS, Belenky G, et al. Recommended amount of sleep for a healthy adult: A joint consensus statement of the American academy of sleep medicine and sleep research society. *J Clin Sleep Med.* 2015;11(06):591–592.
5. Thorpy MJ. Classification of sleep disorders. *Neurotherapeutics.* 2012;9(4):687–701.
6. K. Pavlova M, Latreille V. Sleep disorders. *Am J Med.* 2019;132(3):292–299.
7. Report AAAoSM. Practice parameters for the psychological and behavioral treatment of insomnia: An update. An American academy of sleep medicine report. *Sleep.* 2006;29(11):1415–1419.
8. Edinger JD, Wohlgemuth WK, Radtke RA, Marsh GR, Quillian RE. Cognitive behavioral therapy for treatment of chronic primary insomnia: A randomized controlled trial. *JAMA.* 2001;285(14):1856–1864.
9. Koffel EA, Koffel JB, Gehrman PR. A meta-analysis of group cognitive behavioral therapy for insomnia. *Sleep Med Rev.* 2015;19:6–16.
10. Trauer JM, Qian MY, Doyle JS, Rajaratnam SM, Cunnington D. Cognitive behavioral therapy for chronic insomnia. *Ann Intern Med.* 2015;163(3):191–204.
11. Lloberes P, Durán-Cantolla J, Martínez-García M, et al. Diagnosis and treatment of sleep apnea-hypopnea syndrome. *Archivos de Bronconeumología ((English Edition)).* 2011;47(3):143–156.
12. Ong JC, Dawson SC, Mundt JM, Moore C. Developing a cognitive behavioral therapy for hypersomnia using telehealth: A feasibility study. *J Clin Sleep Med.* 2020;16(12): 2047–2062.
13. McGrane IR, Leung JG, St. Louis EK, Boeve BF. Melatonin therapy for REM sleep behavior disorder: A critical review of evidence. *Sleep Med.* 2015;16(1):19–26.
14. Clement-Carbonell V, Portilla-Tamarit I, Rubio-Aparicio M, Madrid-Valero JJ. Sleep quality, mental and physical health: A differential relationship. *IJERPH.* 2021; 18(2):460.
15. Magee JC, Carmin CN. The relationship between sleep and anxiety in older adults. *Curr Psychiatry Rep.* 2010;12(1):13–19.
16. Fang H, Tu S, Sheng J, Shao A. Depression in sleep disturbance: A review on a bidirectional relationship, mechanisms and treatment. *J Cellular Molecular Medi.* 2019; 23(4):2324–2332.
17. Association AP. *Diagnostic and Statistical Manual of Mental Disorder* (Vol. 5th). Washington DC2013.
18. Morin CM, LeBlanc M, Fau - Daley M, Daley M, Fau - Gregoire JP, Gregoire JP, Fau - Mérette C, Mérette C. Epidemiology of insomnia: Prevalence, self-help treatments, consultations, and determinants of help-seeking behaviors. *Sleep Med.* 2006 Mar;7(2):123–30. doi: 10.1016/j.sleep.2005.08.008.
19. Ohayon MM. Epidemiology of insomnia: What we know and what we still need to learn. *Sleep Med Rev.* 2002 Apr;6(2):97–111. doi: 10.1053/smrv.2002.0186.
20. Staner L. Comorbidity of insomnia and depression. *Sleep Med Rev.* 2010;14(1):35–46.
21. Ohayon MM, Roth T. Place of chronic insomnia in the course of depressive and anxiety disorders. *J Psychiatr Res.* 2003;37(1):9–15.
22. Feng G, Han M, Li X, Geng L, Miao Y. The clinical effectiveness of cognitive behavioral therapy for patients with insomnia and depression: A systematic review and meta-analysis. *Evid Based Complementary Altern Med.* 2020;2020:8071821.

23. Staner L. Sleep and anxiety disorders. *Dialogues Clin Neurosci.* 2003;5(3):249–258.

24. Mellman TA. Sleep and anxiety disorders. *Sleep Med Clin.* 2008;3(2):261–268.

25. Ohayon MM, Caulet M, Lemoine P. Comorbidity of mental and insomnia disorders in the general population. *Compr Psychiatry.* 1998;39(4):185–197.

26. Sloan EP, Natarajan M, Baker B, et al. Nocturnal and daytime panic attacks—Comparison of sleep architecture, heart rate variability, and response to sodium lactate challenge. *Biol Psychiatry.* 1999;45(10):1313–1320.

27. Craske MG, Lang AJ, Rowe M, et al. Presleep attributions about arousal during sleep: Nocturnal panic. *J Abnorm Psychol.* 2002;111(1):53–62.

28. Insel TR, Gillin JC, Moore A, Mendelson WB, Loewenstein RJ, Murphy DL. The sleep of patients with obsessive-compulsive disorder. *Arch Gen Psychiatry.* 1982;39(12):1372–1377.

29. Robinson D, Walsleben J, Fau - Pollack S, Pollack S, Fau - Lerner G, Lerner G. Nocturnal polysomnography in obsessive-compulsive disorder. *Psychiatry Res.* 1998; Sep 21;80(3):257–63. doi: 10.1016/s0165-1781(98)00068-7.

30. Luik AI, Bostock S, Chisnall L, et al. Treating depression and anxiety with digital cognitive behavioural therapy for insomnia: A real world NHS evaluation using standardized outcome measures. *Behav Cogn Psychother.* 2017;45(1):91–96.

31. Miller KE, Brownlow JA, Gehrman PR. Sleep in PTSD: Treatment approaches and outcomes. *Curr Opin Psychol.* 2020;34:12–17.

32. Green BL, Lindy JD, Grace MC. Posttraumatic stress disorder: Toward DSM-IV. *J Nerv Ment Dis.* 1985;173(7):406–411.

33. Leskin GA, Woodward SH, Fau - Young HE, Young HE, Fau - Sheikh JI, Sheikh JI. Effects of comorbid diagnoses on sleep disturbance in PTSD. *J Psychiatr Res.* 2002 Nov-Dec;36(6):449–52. doi: 10.1016/s0022-3956(02)00025-0.

34. Krakow B, Schrader R, Fau - Tandberg D, Tandberg D, Fau - Hollifield M, et al. Nightmare frequency in sexual assault survivors with PTSD. *J Anxiety Disord.* 2002;16(2):175–190. doi:10.1016/s0887-6185(02)00093-2.

35. Krakow BJ, Ulibarri VA, Moore BA, McIver ND. Posttraumatic stress disorder and sleep-disordered breathing: A review of comorbidity research. *Sleep Med Rev.* 2015 Dec;24:37–45. doi: 10.1016/j.smrv.2014.11.001.

36. Koffel E, Khawaja IS, Germain A. Sleep disturbances in posttraumatic stress disorder: Updated review and implications for treatment. *Psychiatr Ann.* 2016;46(3): 173–176.

37. Aurora RN, Zak RS, Fau - Auerbach SH, Auerbach SH, Fau - Casey KR, et al. Best practice guide for the treatment of nightmare disorder in adults. *J Clin Sleep Med.* 2010 Aug 15;6(4):389–401.

38. Ahmad FB, Anderson RN. The leading causes of death in the US for 2020. *JAMA.* 2021;325(18):1829–1830.

39. Grandner MA. Addressing sleep disturbances: An opportunity to prevent cardiometabolic disease? *Int Rev Psychiatry.* 2014;26(2):155–176.

40. Knutson KL. Sleep duration and cardiometabolic risk: A review of the epidemiologic evidence. *Best Pract Res Clin Endocrinol Metab.* 2010;24(5):731–743.

41. Cappuccio FP, Miller MA. Sleep and cardio-metabolic disease. *Curr Cardiol Rep.* 2017;19(11):1–9.

42. Chaput J-P, Tremblay A. Insufficient sleep as a contributor to weight gain: An update. *Curr Obes Rep.* 2012;1(4):245–256.

43. Zhou Q, Zhang M, Hu D. Dose-response association between sleep duration and obesity risk: A systematic review and meta-analysis of prospective cohort studies. *Sleep Breath.* 2019;23(4):1035–1045.

44. Ogilvie RP, Patel SR. The epidemiology of sleep and diabetes. *Curr Diabetes Rep.* 2018;18(10):1–11.

45. Makarem N, Alcántara C, Williams N, Bello NA, Abdalla M. Effect of sleep disturbances on blood pressure. *Hypertension*. 2021;77(4):1036–1046.
46. Zhang J, Zhang J, Wu H, Wang R. Sleep duration and risk of hyperlipidemia: A systematic review and meta-analysis of prospective studies. *Sleep Breath*. 2021:1–14.
47. Madsen MT, Huang C, Zangger G, Zwisler ADO, Gögenur I. Sleep disturbances in patients with coronary heart disease: A systematic review. *J Clin Sleep Med*. 2019;15(3): 489–504.
48. Khot SP, Morgenstern LB. Sleep and stroke. *Stroke*. 2019;50(6):1612–1617.
49. Li L, Gan Y, Zhou X, et al. Insomnia and the risk of hypertension: A meta-analysis of prospective cohort studies. *Sleep Med Rev*. 2021;56:101403.
50. Johnson KA, Gordon CJ, Chapman JL, et al. The association of insomnia disorder characterised by objective short sleep duration with hypertension, diabetes and body mass index: A systematic review and meta-analysis. *Sleep Med Rev*. 2021;59:101456.
51. Sands-Lincoln M, Loucks EB, Lu B, et al. Sleep duration, insomnia, and coronary heart disease among postmenopausal women in the Women's health initiative. *J Womens Health (Larchmt)*. 2013;22(6):477–486.
52. Sun M, Feng W, Wang F, et al. Meta-analysis on shift work and risks of specific obesity types. *Obes Rev*. 2018;19(1):28–40.
53. Manohar S, Thongprayoon C, Cheungpasitporn W, Mao MA, Herrmann SM. Associations of rotational shift work and night shift status with hypertension: A systematic review and meta-analysis. *J Hypertens*. 2017;35(10):1929–1937.
54. Li W, Chen Z, Ruan W, Yi G, Wang D, Lu Z. A meta-analysis of cohort studies including dose-response relationship between shift work and the risk of diabetes mellitus. *Eur J Epidemiol*. 2019;34(11):1013–1024.
55. Dutheil F, Baker JS, Mermillod M, et al. Shift work, and particularly permanent night shifts, promote dyslipidaemia: A systematic review and meta-analysis. *Atherosclerosis*. 2020;313:156–169.
56. Hemmer A, Mareschal J, Dibner C, et al. The effects of shift work on cardio-metabolic diseases and eating patterns. *Nutrients*. 2021;13(11):4178.
57. Peplonska B, Kaluzny P, Trafalska E. Rotating night shift work and nutrition of nurses and midwives. *Chronobiol Int*. 2019;36(7):945–954.
58. Chen C, ValizadehAslani T, Rosen GL, Anderson LM, Jungquist CR. Healthcare shift workers' temporal habits for eating, sleeping, and light exposure: A multi-instrument pilot study. *J Circadian Rhythms*. 2020;18:6.
59. Shaw E, Dorrian J, Coates AM, et al. Temporal pattern of eating in night shift workers. *Chronobiol Int*. 2019;36(12):1613–1625.
60. Bauters F, Rietzschel ER, Hertegonne KBC, Chirinos JA. The link between obstructive sleep apnea and cardiovascular disease. *Curr Atheroscler Rep*. 2015;18(1):1.
61. Jehan S, Zizi F, Pandi-Perumal SR, et al. Obstructive sleep apnea and obesity: Implications for public health. *Sleep Med Dis Int J*. 2017;1(4):1–15.
62. Hou H, Zhao Y, Yu W, et al. Association of obstructive sleep apnea with hypertension: A systematic review and meta-analysis. *J Glob Health*. 2018;8(1):010405. doi: 10.7189/jogh.08.010405.
63. Jehan S, Myers AK, Zizi F, Pandi-Perumal SR, Jean-Louis G, McFarlane SI. Obesity, obstructive sleep apnea and type 2 diabetes mellitus: Epidemiology and pathophysiologic insights. *Sleep Med Dis Int J*. 2018;2(3):52.
64. Yaggi HK, Concato J, Kernan WN, Lichtman JH, Brass LM, Mohsenin V. Obstructive sleep apnea as a risk factor for stroke and death. *N Engl J Med*. 2005;353(19):2034–2041.
65. Gottlieb DJ, Yenokyan G, Newman AB, et al. Prospective study of obstructive sleep apnea and incident coronary heart disease and heart failure. *Circulation*. 2010;122(4): 352–360.

66. Mehra R, Benjamin EJ, Shahar E, et al. Association of nocturnal arrhythmias with sleep-disordered breathing: The sleep heart health study. *Am J Respir Crit Care Med.* 2006;173(8):910–916.

67. Lloyd-Jones DM, Allen NB, Anderson CAM, et al. Life's essential 8: Updating and enhancing the American Heart Association's construct of cardiovascular health: A presidential advisory from the American Heart Association. *Circulation.* 146(5). doi:10.1161/CIR.0000000000001078

68. Lloyd-Jones DM, Hong Y, Labarthe D, et al. Defining and setting national goals for cardiovascular health promotion and disease reduction: The American Heart Association's strategic impact goal through 2020 and beyond. *Circulation.* 2010;121(4):586–613.

69. Ferlay J, Colombet M, Soerjomataram I, et al. Cancer statistics for the year 2020: An overview. *Int J Cancer.* 2021;149(4):778–789.

70. Mogavero MP, DelRosso LM, Fanfulla F, Bruni O, Ferri R. Sleep disorders and cancer: State of the art and future perspectives. *Sleep Med Rev.* 2021;56:101409.

71. Fang H-F, Miao N-F, Chen C-D, Sithole T, Chung M-H. Risk of cancer in patients with insomnia, parasomnia, and obstructive sleep apnea: A nationwide nested case-control study. *J Cancer.* 2015;6(11):1140–1147.

72. He C, Anand ST, Ebell MH, Vena JE, Robb SW. Circadian disrupting exposures and breast cancer risk: A meta-analysis. *Int Arch Occup Environ Health.* 2015;88(5):533–547.

73. Tseng C-M, Chen Y-T, Tao C-W, et al. Adult narcoleptic patients have increased risk of cancer: A nationwide population-based study. *Cancer Epidemiol.* 2015;39(6):793–797.

74. Gozal D, Farré R, Nieto FJ. Obstructive sleep apnea and cancer: Epidemiologic links and theoretical biological constructs. *Sleep Med Rev.* 2016;27:43–55.

75. Ancoli-Israel S. Sleep disturbances in cancer: A review. *Sleep Med Res.* 2015;6(2):45–49.

76. Otte JL, Carpenter JS, Russell KM, Bigatti S, Champion VL. Prevalence, severity, and correlates of sleep-wake disturbances in long-term breast cancer survivors. *J Pain Symptom Manag.* 2010;39(3):535–547.

77. Tell D, Mathews HL, Janusek LW. Day-to-day dynamics of associations between sleep, napping, fatigue, and the cortisol diurnal rhythm in women diagnosed as having breast cancer. *Psychosom Med.* 2014;76(7):519–528.

78. Weil AG, Muir K, Hukin J, Desautels A, Martel V, Perreault S. Narcolepsy and hypothalamic region tumors: Presentation and evolution. *Pediatr Neurol.* 2018;84:27–31.

79. Dreher M, Krüger S, Schulze-Olden S, et al. Sleep-disordered breathing in patients with newly diagnosed lung cancer. *BMC Pulm Med.* 2018;18(1):72. Published 2018 May 16. doi:10.1186/s12890-018-0645-1.

80. Vaou OE, Lin SH, Branson C, Auerbach S. Sleep and dementia. *Curr Sleep Med Rep.* 2018;4(2):134–142.

81. Orr WC, Fass R, Sundaram SS, Scheimann AO. The effect of sleep on gastrointestinal functioning in common digestive diseases. *Lancet Gastroenterol Hepatol.* 2020;5(6):616–624.

82. Teo P, Henry BA, Moran LJ, Cowan S, Bennett C. The role of sleep in PCOS: What we know and What to consider in the future. *Expert Rev Endocrinol Metab.* 2022;17(4):305–318.

83. Husak AJ, Bair MJ. Chronic pain and sleep disturbances: A pragmatic review of their relationships, comorbidities, and treatments. *Pain Med.* 2020;21(6):1142–1152.

16 Exercise for Mental Health

Emily C. LaVoy, PhD and Charles F. Hodgman, MS

KEY POINTS

- Regular physical activity or exercise training is negatively associated with risk for mental illness and neurological disease, and exercise interventions may diminish disease burden.
- The mechanisms through which exercise mitigates the burden of mental illness and neurological disease are likely multi-factorial, including both physiological and psychosocial effects.
- Despite the potential protective and therapeutic effects of exercise, the etiology and disease presentation must be considered as a part of programming. Though generally beneficial, optimal exercise programming strategies may necessarily vary between diseases and individuals.

16.1 INTRODUCTION

Consistent, lifelong exercise is almost universally recommended due to many diseases and conditions that it can prevent and manage. Exercise is known to provide benefits against cardiovascular disease, certain cancers, insulin insensitivity, and all-cause mortality. It also improves bone health and increases muscle mass, thus decreasing the risk for functional impairments and disability, such as the age-related conditions of osteoporosis and sarcopenia. Additionally, along with a balanced diet, exercise helps maintain a healthy body weight, thereby lowering the risk for metabolic syndrome and obesity. Finally, regular physical exercise is associated with reduced risk for mental illness and neurological disease and may lessen the symptoms of those afflicted. Exercise reduces risk for and may improve symptoms of anxiety, depression, Alzheimer's disease and related dementias, schizophrenia, and bipolar disorder.[1-3]

Exercise is classified as a subtype of physical activity: the movement of the body produced by skeletal muscles that results in increased energy expenditure. Specifically, exercise is planned, structured, and repeated physical activity performed for the purpose of physical conditioning.[4] Exercise has broad physiological impacts across many systems of the body; consequently, exercise may reduce disease risk and maintain health through various potential mechanisms.[5] This chapter discusses the effects of exercise on mental health and potential mechanisms mediating these effects. We conclude with implications of these effects on the role of exercise in maintaining or improving mental health.

DOI: 10.1201/b22810-18

16.2   EXERCISE AND MENTAL HEALTH

Exercise training may promote health through its ability to buffer responses to psychological stress. Long-lasting psychological stress can contribute to disease by inducing a state of chronic inflammation, a known risk factor for many health conditions, such as cardiovascular and metabolic diseases.[6,7] Psychological stress is also a risk factor for mental illnesses, including depression.[8] Both moderate and high-intensity exercise can reduce general stress, and aerobic exercise training reduces work-related stress.[1] Individuals with greater aerobic fitness, suggesting regular participation in exercise, typically demonstrate lower physiological activation in response to psychological stress, such as smaller elevations in blood pressure, cortisol, and heart rate.[9]

Exercise training has shown benefits for reducing symptoms and/or improving quality of life in a range of mental illnesses and chronic neurological diseases. Discussed below are mental illnesses and neurological diseases that have been most frequently studied in the context of exercise training. However, the specific needs of each affliction may require unique programming considerations to elicit beneficial effects, and optimal exercise prescriptions may necessarily vary between illnesses and individuals. These caveats are emphasized to provide context for interpreting the following data. See Table 16.1 for abbreviated review.

16.2.1   ANXIETY

Exercise training is consistently associated with a small but significant decrease in anxiety among non-clinically afflicted adults.[10] Although exercise has been demonstrated to diminish comorbid anxiety, patients with clinical manifestations of anxiety disorders less consistently demonstrate symptom improvements with exercise.[10,11] This discrepancy may be due to the heterogeneous etiology and symptom triggers among anxiety disorders and reinforces the importance of individualized exercise prescriptions among clinically afflicted individuals.[12]

16.2.2   DEPRESSION

Individuals who are more physically active are at lower risk of developing depressive symptoms compared to less active individuals.[13] Exercise may also be an important intervention in the treatment of depression. Exercise training is associated with a moderate reduction in depressive symptoms among non-clinically afflicted individuals and a moderate to large reduction among those diagnosed with clinical depression.[2,10,11,14] The latter effects may be equal or superior to traditional therapies and suggest exercise as an important intervention in the treatment of depression.[11] Generally, interventions that prescribe more frequent and/or intense exercise demonstrate larger reductions in depressive symptoms.[1] Exercise may also be useful in addressing cognitive deficits that frequently accompany clinical depression.[2,11]

16.2.3 Dementia and Alzheimer's Disease

Exercise training, especially aerobic exercise, can limit age-related declines in cognition and the incidence of dementia and Alzheimer's disease.[15] For example, adults aged 65 years and older who engaged in moderate-intensity exercise such as walking had lower cognitive impairment risk than sedentary older adults. There is also evidence that exercise training a few hours per week can improve physical function and ability for activities of daily living, and memory and cognition in people with dementia.[15] Even among older adults without dementia, exercise training can improve cognitive processes, particularly executive function.[1,16] This benefit may remain for some time even after cessation of exercise training.

16.2.4 Schizophrenia and Bipolar Disorder

Exercise training has also shown benefit for individuals with schizophrenia and bipolar disorder, although the effects of exercise in the latter condition have been less frequently examined. Those with schizophrenia are frequently at higher risk of developing cardiometabolic disease, likely due to low activity.[1,2] Routine physical activity (e.g., 90 minutes per week of moderate-to-vigorous exercise) can ameliorate both cardiometabolic risk factors and schizophrenia symptoms, including reduced frequency and severity of auditory hallucinations.[1,2] Exercise training may also improve cognition among patients with schizophrenia and bipolar disorder. People with schizophrenia or bipolar disorder who performed physical activity at least 90 minutes each week had greater global function, working memory, and executive function compared to those who were less physically active[2,3] Aerobic exercise interventions have also demonstrated improvements in global and social cognition, working memory, processing speed, and attention among those with schizophrenia.[2]

16.3 MECHANISMS TO EXPLAIN THE EFFECTS OF EXERCISE ON MENTAL HEALTH

16.3.1 Inflammation

Inflammation begins with the detection of a physiological insult, such as a pathogen, by innate immune cells. In response, activated innate immune cells release inflammatory mediators that act locally and systemically, leading to swelling, redness, pain, and recruitment of other immune cells. Acute inflammation may last for hours to days and resolves after the insult is removed. In contrast, chronic inflammation is generally of lower magnitude (i.e., low-grade) and may last for weeks to years, fueled by persistent infection, collateral tissue damage, and/or dysregulated inflammatory responses. The causes of chronic, low-grade inflammation are almost certainly multi-factorial, with genetic and environmental factors contributing individually and interacting to perpetuate inflammation. Adipose tissue is a large source of the inflammatory mediator tumor necrosis factor (TNF)-α, the secretion of which stimulates interleukin (IL)-6 production, which in turn increases levels of IL-1 and C-reactive protein (CRP) systemically. Thus, obesity is associated with chronic low-grade inflammation.[17] Aging is also associated with chronic inflammation, leading to the coin of the term "inflammaging" to describe the age-associated increase in inflammatory-related conditions.[18]

Systemic inflammation and neuroinflammation are implicated in the onset and progression of mental illness.[19] Induction of systemic inflammation reliably produces depressive symptoms including social withdrawal and anhedonia. Further, individuals diagnosed with depression frequently display elevated plasma or serum levels of pro-inflammatory cytokines.[20] Acute inflammatory events, such as the response to infection, injury, or surgery, have been linked to rapid cognitive decline in previously high-functioning older adults.[21] Inflammation in the periphery can be communicated across the blood-brain barrier through several mechanisms, including stimulation of afferent nerves, the active transport of pro-inflammatory cytokines and proteins through the blood-brain barrier, and other signaling pathways.[22,23] For example, activated macrophages may reduce the synthesis of dopamine, norepinephrine, and serotonin.[24] Inflammation also activates enzymes which convert the serotonin precursor tryptophan into kynurenine. Beyond decreasing serotonin availability, kynurenine can be degraded into neurotoxic metabolites and is implicated in several mental health disorders.[25] Within the brain, inflammation-activated microglia and astrocytes release additional inflammatory cytokines. These cytokines negatively affect neurotransmitter signaling by decreasing precursor molecules availability, inhibiting neurotransmitter transmission, and increasing neurotransmitter reuptake. These changes promote anxiety, cognitive dysfunction, dementia, and depression.[26-28]

Exercise training is inversely associated with chronic inflammation.[29] This may be explained in part through reductions in adipose tissue. For example, declines in circulating CRP among adults with obesity relate to fat mass reductions following exercise interventions.[30] However, reductions in circulating TNF-α and IL-6 following exercise training have been reported independently of fat mass change, indicating exercise may decrease inflammation via mechanisms additional to reduced adiposity. Such mechanisms may include the release of anti-inflammatory myokines from contracting skeletal muscle, and reduced toll-like receptor expression on monocytes, thereby lowering inflammatory responses.[31] Exercise training appears to reduce the number of circulating immune cells, thus decreasing the probability of potentially inflammatory immune cells.[32] Further, physically active adults demonstrate fewer exhausted and highly differentiated T cells (cells typically exhibiting a pro-inflammatory phenotype) relative to those who are less active.[33] The mechanisms underlying these effects are still being elucidated. Leptin, heat shock proteins, adrenergic, and myokine signaling all appear to play a role.[32-34] Finally, exercise training is also associated with reductions in sympathetic nervous system and hypothalamic-pituitary-adrenal axis activity, and these reductions may contribute to improvements in both systemic inflammation and maladaptive responses to acute stress.[11].

Given the relationship between peripheral inflammation and mental illness described above, exercise-induced reductions in inflammation may be expected to improve mental health. Promisingly, exercise-induced reductions in neuroinflammation have been demonstrated in animal models.[28] Further, increased expression of peroxisome proliferator-activated receptor-gamma co-activator (PGC)-1α in skeletal muscle, frequently observed with endurance exercise training, elicits the expression of enzymes to detoxify kynurenine and prevent its neurotoxic effects.[35]

16.3.2 BRAIN PLASTICITY

Structural changes within the hippocampus, amygdala, striatum, and frontal cortex have been observed across several neurological and mental illnesses, including Alzheimer's and dementia, depression, and schizophrenia.[1,2,28] Exercise training has shown the potential to counter such changes, particularly within the hippocampus. As reductions in hippocampal volume are frequently observed in patients with mental illness and neurological disease, exercise-induced improvements in hippocampal volume may directly antagonize this aspect of the disease process. As can be achieved through regular exercise, cardiorespiratory fitness has been positively related to hippocampal volume in the general population, and improvements in cardiorespiratory fitness have been related to increases in hippocampal volume.[1,11,28] Additionally, exercise training among patients with schizophrenia may improve neuronal viability in the prefrontal cortex.[2]

Mechanistically, physical exercise modulates the release of a variety of hormones and signaling factors including the following: adiponectin, brain-derived neurotrophic factor (BDNF), dopamine, epinephrine, endocannabinoids, insulin-like growth factor 1, irisin, nerve growth factor, serotonin, and vascular endothelial growth factor. Each of these may participate in exercise-induced neurological effects.[28] As an example, increases in BDNF levels with exercise have been reported both centrally and in the periphery.[1,28,36] As BDNF acts as a growth factor in the hippocampus, elevations in BDNF with acute exercise may improve brain architecture and symptom severity among individuals with mental illness or neurological disease.[2,11,28,37] Exercise also increases adiponectin, a hormone with anti-inflammatory and insulin-sensitizing properties. Adiponectin decreases risk for type 2 diabetes and insulin resistance, which are risk factors for dementia. Adiponectin also limits neuroinflammation and may enhance hippocampal neurogenesis.[28] Although less studied, exercise-induced elevations in endocannabinoids appear to facilitate improvements in mood and reductions in pain perception.[11]

16.3.3 OXIDATIVE STRESS

Oxidative stress occurs when the production of free radicals (unbalanced, highly reactive chemical species) is not managed by antioxidant defenses. Oxidative stress impairs normal cellular activity and can trigger inflammation, which in turn results in the production of free radicals and perpetuates a cycle of oxidative stress. Oxidative stress is implicated in microglial and astrocyte activation within the brain, leading to neuroinflammation, and the neurotoxicity of plaques and tau proteins in Alzheimer's disease.[11,28] Exercise training increases endogenous antioxidant enzymes such as glutathione peroxidase and superoxide dismutase, which downregulate inflammatory signals within glial cells.[38] Exercise also increases levels of irisin throughout the body, which may protect neurons from oxidative stress via attenuation of inflamma-tion.[28] Thus, exercise training may protect against oxidative stress-induced neuroin-flammation and neurotoxicity, and thereby offer protection against associated mental illnesses.

16.3.4 PSYCHOSOCIAL FACTORS

Downstream of or parallel to its physiological effects, exercise training may diminish the burden of mental illness through its behavioral and perceptual impacts. Exercise training can improve sleep quality, and decrease mood disturbances.[2] The regular practice of exercise may provide structure and a sense of normal societal integra-tion for individuals with mental illness, particularly when practiced in a group set-ting. This feedback counteracts tendencies towards social withdrawal and anxiety, which are common features of mental illness.[1] Additionally, physiological arousal experienced during structured exercise (i.e., in a non-threatening setting) has the potential to distract from psychological distress. This distraction from other sensory input during exercise may provide episodic relief from distress and be of significant magnitude when practiced regularly.[11] The physiological arousal of exercise can also demonstrate that certain illness symptoms (i.e., sweating, elevated heart and breath-ing rate) are not signs of danger.[1]

Exercise training may also counteract negative self-conception consequent to mental illness or neurological disease via its potential to strengthen self-efficacy. Recognition of one's ability to complete a daunting workout or exercise program, with or without quantifiable improvements in fitness, can improve the individual's estimation of their capacity to confront challenges (i.e., self-efficacy). Such con-fidence may improve self-esteem and mood and has the potential to decrease the severity of mental illness symptoms.[11] Collectively, physical exercise may provide therapeutic benefit to individuals with mental illness or neurological disease through both short and long-term psychological mechanisms.

16.4 INTERACTION BETWEEN EXERCISE AND DIET

Exercise and diet (referring to caloric intake and diet quality) may interact to influence neuroplasticity and mental health.[36,37] As discussed above, exercise increases levels of BDNF in the hippocampus, which has important implications for neuroplasticity and protecting neural function. Hippocampal BDNF is also sensitive to diet; it is increased by consumption of omega-3-fatty acids and by calorie restriction, whereas a diet high in sucrose and saturated fats decreases hippocampal BDNF in animal models.[36,37] Exercise training can reduce the negative effects of a high sucrose/high saturated fat diet on cognition and synaptic plasticity, at least in animal models.[39] The omega-3 fatty acid docosahexaenoic acid (DHA) is of particular importance in supporting brain health, as it reduces oxidative stress and inflammation and pro-motes synaptic signaling.[36,39] The combinations of exercise with caloric restriction and exercise with DHA supplementation yields greater increases in BDNF in animal models than either exercise or diet-intervention alone.[36,39] As predicted from these effects on BDNF, interventions combining exercise and healthy diet (high in fruits, vegetables, and fish) have also demonstrated greater cognitive benefit to middle-aged and older adults than diet-interventions alone.[36] Thus, although more frequently examined separately, exercise and diet may interact synergistically to benefit mental health.

16.5 IMPLICATIONS

Higher levels of aerobic fitness, as provided by regular exercise training, are associated with lower physiological activation during stress, less depressive symptoms, and superior self-reported well-being. Exercise training also appears to improve memory and cognition and may alleviate symptoms of schizophrenia. Conversely, low aerobic fitness is a common consequence of mental illness due to low activity and is a risk factor for dementia. Lack of physical activity likewise contributes to the development of comorbidities among those with mental illness or neurological disorders that adds to excess mortality in these populations.[1,2] As is true in the general population, exercise training can improve cardiometabolic risk biomarkers (e.g., inflammation, blood lipids) and vascular health among those affected by mental illness. In addition to potential direct involvement with symptom severity, improvements in the latter risk factors may be important to ameliorate the risk or burden of comorbid conditions and death.[1] A properly designed exercise training program is also likely to improve cardiorespiratory fitness and strength. These effects may provide a range of benefits in mental illnesses as low fitness and fatigue are common consequences of illness and are generally associated with more severe disease.[10]

Collectively, data demonstrate regular physical activity is a preventative factor against the development of mental illness and some neurological conditions. Low physical activity is associated with worse outcomes. This suggests that physiological adaptations to exercise (e.g., improved aerobic fitness) may play a critical role in mitigating the risk for and burden of mental and neurological illnesses. Thus, exercise interventions ought to be a routine part of addressing health challenges in those with mental illness. The evidence for a protective effect of exercise appears strongest for aerobic exercise training, although benefits from resistance training, combined aerobic and resistance training, and yoga have also been noted in people with depression and schizophrenia.[2] There is also evidence that more frequent and/or intense interventions may elicit more robust responses. However, such programming may need to be balanced against the low energy or motivation for physical activity among ill individuals to facilitate the accessibility of exercise for patients. Importantly, improvements in fitness or strength may not be necessary for symptom improvement.[10] Interventionists must also be mindful that some patients with mental illness may be taking medications that impact their response to exercise, such as beta-blockers. Thus, prescribing exercise intensity via heart rate zones will not apply; these individuals may instead be instructed to monitor exercise intensity via perceived effort scales. Finally, safety concerns may exist for exercise among people with dementia and Alzheimer's disease, and these individuals may see the greatest benefit from supervised exercise. Table 16.1 summarizes these key points.

TABLE 16.1
Summary Table

Condition	Effects of Exercise	Additional Considerations	Key References
Stress and Anxiety	• Reduces stress and acute stress response • Small and moderate anxiolytic effects for non-clinical and clinically affected adults, respectively	• Less consistent benefits against clinical anxiety. Benefits of exercise should be weighed against its potential to provoke symptoms.	1,10–12
Depression	• Lowers risk for depressive symptoms • Moderate and moderate-to-large anti-depressive effect for non-clinical and clinically affected adults, respectively • May increase hippocampal volume and mitigate cognitive deficits associated with depression	• Higher frequency and/or intensity yields larger benefits, where tolerated	2,10,11,13,14
Dementia & Alzheimer's Disease	• Lowers risk for age-related cognitive impairment, dementia, Alzheimer's disease • Training benefits both physical and cognitive function in older adults, with or without dementia	• Supervised training advised	1,15,16
Schizophrenia and Bipolar Disorder	• Lowers levels of cardiometabolic risk factors • May diminish schizophrenia symptom frequency and severity • May improve various measures of cognitive function	• Supervised and/or group-based training may provide beneficial structure	1–3

REFERENCES

1. Pedersen BK, Saltin B. Exercise as medicine - evidence for prescribing exercise as therapy in 26 different chronic diseases. *Scand J Med Sci Sports*. 2015;3(Suppl 25):1–72. doi:10.1111/sms.12581
2. Falkai P, Schmitt A, Rosenbeiger CP, et al. Aerobic exercise in severe mental illness: Requirements from the perspective of sports medicine. *Eur Arch Psychiatry Clin Neurosci*. December 2021. doi:10.1007/s00406-021-01360-x
3. Caponnetto P, Casu M, Amato M, et al. The effects of physical exercise on mental health: From cognitive improvements to risk of addiction. *Int J Environ Res Public Health*. 2021;18(24). doi:10.3390/ijerph182413384
4. Caspersen CJ, Powell KE, Christenson GM. Physical activity, exercise, and physical fitness: Definitions and distinctions for health-related research. *Public Health Rep*. 1985;100(2):126–131.
5. Hawley JA, Hargreaves M, Joyner MJ, Zierath JR. Integrative biology of exercise. *Cell*. 2014;159(4):738–749. doi:10.1016/j.cell.2014.10.029
6. Rohleder N. Stimulation of systemic low-grade inflammation by psychosocial stress. *Psychosom Med*. 2014;76(3):181–189. doi:10.1097/PSY.0000000000000049

7. Mooy JM, de Vries H, Grootenhuis PA, Bouter LM, Heine RJ. Major stressful life events in relation to prevalence of undetected type 2 diabetes: The Hoorn study. *Diabetes Care.* 2000;23(2):197–201. doi:10.2337/diacare.23.2.197

8. Cohen S, Janicki-Deverts D, Miller GE. Psychological stress and disease. *JAMA.* 2007;298(14):1685–1687. doi:10.1001/jama.298.14.1685

9. Silverman MN, Deuster PA. Biological mechanisms underlying the role of physical fitness in health and resilience. *Interface Focus.* 2014;4(5):20140040. doi:10.1098/rsfs.2014.0040

10. Rebar AL, Stanton R, Geard D, Short C, Duncan MJ, Vandelanotte C. A meta-meta-analysis of the effect of physical activity on depression and anxiety in non-clinical adult populations. *Health Psychol Rev.* 2015;9(3):366–378. doi:10.1080/17437199.2015.1022901

11. Chen Z, Lan W, Yang G, et al. Exercise intervention in treatment of neuropsychological diseases: A review. *Front Psychol.* 2020;11:569206. doi:10.3389/fpsyg.2020.569206

12. Kandola A, Vancampfort D, Herring M, et al. Moving to beat anxiety: Epidemiology and therapeutic issues with physical activity for anxiety. *Curr Psychiatry Rep.* 2018;20(8):63. doi:10.1007/s11920-018-0923-x

13. Farmer ME, Locke BZ, Mościcki EK, Dannenberg AL, Larson DB, Radloff LS. Physical activity and depressive symptoms: The NHANES I epidemiologic follow-up study. *Am J Epidemiol.* 1988;128(6):1340–1351. doi:10.1093/oxfordjournals.aje.a115087

14. Cooney GM, Dwan K, Greig CA, et al. Exercise for depression. *Cochrane Database Syst Rev.* 2013;9:CD004366. doi:10.1002/14651858.CD004366.pub6

15. Kramer AF, Erickson KI, Colcombe SJ. Exercise, cognition, and the aging brain. *J Appl Physiol.* 2006;101(4):1237–1242. doi:10.1152/japplphysiol.00500.2006

16. Colcombe S, Kramer AF. Fitness effects on the cognitive function of older adults: A meta-analytic study. *Psychol Sci.* 2003;14(2):125–130. doi:10.1111/1467-9280.t01-1-01430

17. Phillips CL, Grayson BE. The immune remodel: Weight loss-mediated inflammatory changes to obesity. *Exp Biol Med (Maywood).* 2020;245(2):109–121. doi:10.1177/1535370219900185

18. Franceschi C, Bonafè M, Valensin S, et al. Inflamm-aging. An evolutionary perspective on immunosenescence. *Ann N Y Acad Sci.* 2000;908:244–254. doi:10.1111/j.1749-6632.2000.tb06651.x

19. Najjar S, Pearlman DM, Alper K, Najjar A, Devinsky O. Neuroinflammation and psychiatric illness. *J Neuroinflammation.* 2013;10:43. doi:10.1186/1742-2094-10-43

20. Chan KL, Cathomas F, Russo SJ. Central And peripheral inflammation link metabolic syndrome and major depressive disorder. *Physiology (Bethesda).* 2019;34(2):123–133. doi:10.1152/physiol.00047.2018

21. Fong TG, Tulebaev SR, Inouye SK. Delirium in elderly adults: Diagnosis, prevention and treatment. *Nat Rev Neurol.* 2009;5(4):210–220. doi:10.1038/nrneurol.2009.24

22. Dantzer R, O'Connor JC, Freund GG, Johnson RW, Kelley KW. From inflammation to sickness and depression: When the immune system subjugates the brain. *Nat Rev Neurosci.* 2008;9(1):46–56. doi:10.1038/nrn2297

23. McCusker RH, Kelley KW. Immune-neural connections: How the immune system's response to infectious agents influences behavior. *J Exp Biol.* 2013;216(Pt 1):84–98. doi:10.1242/jeb.073411

24. Neurauter G, Schröcksnadel K, Scholl-Bürgi S, et al. Chronic immune stimulation correlates with reduced phenylalanine turnover. *Curr Drug Metab.* 2008;9(7):622–627. doi:10.2174/138920008785821738

25. Cervenka I, Agudelo LZ, Ruas JL. Kynurenines: Tryptophan's metabolites in exercise, inflammation, and mental health. *Science.* 2017;357(6349). doi:10.1126/science.aaf9794

26. Felger JC. Imaging the role of inflammation in mood and anxiety-related disorders. *Curr Neuropharmacol.* 2018;16(5):533–558. doi:10.2174/1570159X15666171123201142

27. Patterson SL. Immune dysregulation and cognitive vulnerability in the aging brain: Interactions of microglia, IL-1β, BDNF and synaptic plasticity. *Neuropharmacology.* 2015;96(Pt A):11–18. doi:10.1016/j.neuropharm.2014.12.020

28. Liang Y-Y, Zhang L-D, Luo X, et al. All roads lead to Rome - a review of the potential mechanisms by which exerkines exhibit neuroprotective effects in Alzheimer's disease. *Neural Regen Res.* 2022;17(6):1210–1227. doi:10.4103/1673-5374.325012

29. Lavie CJ, Church TS, Milani RV, Earnest CP. Impact of physical activity, cardiorespiratory fitness, and exercise training on markers of inflammation. *J Cardiopulm Rehabil Prev.* 2011;31(3):137–145. doi:10.1097/HCR.0b013e3182122827

30. Gonzalo-Encabo P, Maldonado G, Valadés D, Ferragut C, Pérez-López A. The role of exercise training on low-grade systemic inflammation in adults with overweight and obesity: A systematic review. *Int J Environ Res Public Health.* 2021;18(24). doi:10.3390/ijerph182413258

31. Gleeson M, Bishop NC, Stensel DJ, Lindley MR, Mastana SS, Nimmo MA. The anti-inflammatory effects of exercise: Mechanisms and implications for the prevention and treatment of disease. *Nat Rev Immunol.* 2011;11(9):607–615. doi:10.1038/nri3041

32. Frodermann V, Rohde D, Courties G, et al. Exercise reduces inflammatory cell production and cardiovascular inflammation via instruction of hematopoietic progenitor cells. *Nat Med.* 2019;25(11):1761–1771. doi:10.1038/s41591-019-0633-x

33. Duggal NA, Niemiro G, Harridge SDR, Simpson RJ, Lord JM. Can physical activity ameliorate immunosenescence and thereby reduce age-related multi-morbidity? *Nat Rev Immunol.* 2019;19(9):563–572. doi:10.1038/s41577-019-0177-9

34. Krüger K, Reichel T, Zeilinger C. Role of heat shock proteins 70/90 in exercise physiology and exercise immunology and their diagnostic potential in sports. *J Appl Physiol.* 2019;126(4):916–927. doi:10.1152/japplphysiol.01052.2018

35. Agudelo LZ, Femenía T, Orhan F, et al. Skeletal muscle PGC-1α1 modulates kynurenine metabolism and mediates resilience to stress-induced depression. *Cell.* 2014;159(1): 33–45. doi:10.1016/j.cell.2014.07.051

36. Pickersgill JW, Turco CV, Ramdeo K, Rehsi RS, Foglia SD, Nelson AJ. The combined influences of exercise, diet and sleep on neuroplasticity. *Front Psychol.* 2022;13:831819. doi:10.3389/fpsyg.2022.831819

37. Gomez-Pinilla F. The influences of diet and exercise on mental health through hormesis. *Ageing Res Rev.* 2008;7(1):49–62. doi:10.1016/j.arr.2007.04.003

38. Mee-Inta O, Zhao Z-W, Kuo Y-M. Physical exercise inhibits inflammation and microglial activation. *Cells.* 2019;8(7). doi:10.3390/cells8070691

39. Gomez-Pinilla F. The combined effects of exercise and foods in preventing neurological and cognitive disorders. *Prev Med (Baltim).* 2011;52(Suppl 1):S75–80. doi:10.1016/j.ypmed.2011.01.023

Section III

Risk and Protective Lifestyle Factors for Mental Health and Psychological Well-Being

17 Sleep-Related Disorders

Matthew R. Cribbet, PhD, Andrea N. Decker, MA,
Francisco D. Marquez, ScM, MA, and
Emily A. Halvorson, MA

KEY POINTS

- Insomnia disorder is associated with short-term and long-term deficits in functioning, including co-morbid medical and psychiatric complaints.
- Cognitive Behavioral Therapy for Insomnia is an evidence-based treatment with demonstrated efficacy and effectiveness.
- Scaling up insomnia treatments will address growing demands for patient care.

17.1 INTRODUCTION

Insomnia disorder is characterized by difficulties falling asleep, staying asleep, or non-restorative sleep that occurs despite the opportunity for adequate sleep. Insomnia disorder is associated with significant distress or impairment in functioning, along with daytime symptoms, including mood disturbances, fatigue, daytime sleepiness, and impairments in cognitive functioning.[1] While nearly one-third to one-fourth of individuals in industrialized countries report disrupted sleep at some point during their lives, approximately 10% to 25% of the population meets the diagnostic threshold for insomnia disorder.[2] Insomnia is a chronic problem in one-third to three-fourths of patients,[3,4] with more than two-thirds of patients reporting symptoms for at least 1 year.[5] Without intervention, chronic insomnia is unremitting, disabling, costly, and may pose a risk for additional morbidity and potentially mortality.[6,7] Given the scope and significance of this problem the identification and implementation of efficacious and effective forms of treatment is necessary. Cognitive behavioral therapy for insomnia (CBT-I) is not only efficacious and effective, it is now considered the standard of treatment for chronic insomnia[8] and is recommended as the initial treatment by the American College of Physicians.[9] First, a theoretical overview of insomnia and CBT-I will be discussed, followed by a review of the efficacy and effectiveness of CBT-I, including a consideration of key demographic factors such as race, sex, and age. Finally, alternatives to CBT-I for the treatment of insomnia will be discussed, followed by a discussion of approaches to scale-up insomnia interventions.

17.2 THEORETICAL FOUNDATION OF COGNITIVE BEHAVIORAL THERAPY FOR INSOMNIA

Insomnia can be broadly conceptualized within a diathesis-stress framework. Within this diathesis-stress framework, an influential theoretical model, known as

DOI: 10.1201/b22810-20

the 3-P Model[10] suggests that individual vulnerabilities or predisposing characteristics (e.g., various forms of hyperarousal and/or tendency to worry or ruminate), when paired with precipitating factors (e.g., stressful life events, daily hassles, and/or illness), result in acute insomnia. Negative thoughts and maladaptive coping behaviors (e.g., anticipatory anxiety about one's ability to initiate or maintain sleep, remaining in bed without sleeping) result in conditioned arousal that when repeated over time, is learned and leads to chronic insomnia. This heuristic model captures, in a way that can be used as treatment rationale for patients, the dynamic course of insomnia; readers interested in a more in-depth review of insomnia pathophysiology models are referred elsewhere.[11,12]

17.3   COMPONENTS OF COGNITIVE BEHAVIORAL THERAPY FOR INSOMNIA

CBT-I has demonstrated empirical support for its efficacy[13–18] and growing support for its effectiveness.[19] CBT-I is a multi-component therapeutic approach that includes psycho-education, in addition to behavioral strategies and cognitive therapy. Specifically, CBT-I includes three behavioral strategies (e.g., stimulus control, sleep restriction therapy, and sleep hygiene), cognitive therapy, and relaxation training. CBT-I targets the factors that interfere with sleep initiation and maintenance by utilizing operant and classical conditioning principles in the form of stimulus control, promoting sleep hygiene to limit behaviors that interfere with sleep, reducing cognitive and physiological hyperarousal, and regulating the homeostatic and circadian influences on sleep through sleep scheduling and sleep restriction.

Stimulus control is an intervention that rests on behavioral principles designed to extinguish learned associations between the bed and negative states such as worry, wakefulness, or frustration.[20] Wakefulness and its associated negative emotions are conditioned by frequent and prolonged periods of time spent awake in bed. The goals of stimulus control therapy are to establish a stable sleep-wake schedule and for the patient to maintain a positive association between the bed and sleep. The goal of stimulus control is to re-associate the bed/bedroom with sleep. This includes telling patients to get into bed when they feel sleepy, to maintain a consistent wake time, to avoid naps, to use the bed only for sleep and intimacy, and if they are unable to fall asleep (or fall back to sleep following awakenings) within 20 minutes, to get out of bed and engage in a relaxing activity until drowsy, and to then return to sleep.

Sleep restriction therapy[21] attempts to align the time in bed and total sleep time (TST) based on data from at-home sleep dairies. This intervention is designed to improve sleep consolidation by restricting TST to enhance sleep drive, or "readiness" for sleep by prolonging wakefulness. As the drive for sleep increases and the opportunity for sleep remains, restricted sleep becomes consolidated (i.e., patients fall asleep more quickly and remain asleep for longer periods of time). Sleep restriction instructions include using an at-home sleep log or sleep diary to determine average TST for a baseline period of 1 to 2 weeks. Next, bedtimes are delayed and wake times are set at a consistent time so that time in bed approximates mean TST. As an intervention, this controlled form of mild to moderate sleep deprivation usually decreases the amount of time it takes to fall asleep or return to sleep. Initially, patients get less sleep, but tend to produce sleep that is consolidated. As sleep efficiency (TST divided by time in bed x 100%) increases, weekly adjustments to the sleep schedule may be made. With sustained sleep efficiencies (7 days or more) above 85%, time in bed can be increased by 15 to 20 minutes. This adjustment provides the opportunity for increased TST while maintaining consolidated sleep.

Sleep hygiene[22] involves educating the patient about health practices (e.g., avoiding tobacco, alcohol, large meals, and vigorous exercise for several hours before bed) and environmental factors (e.g., light, noise, temperature) that are either conducive or detrimental to sleep. Sleep hygiene is not effective when delivered as a monotherapy but may be useful in combination with cognitive therapy or other behavioral strategies (e.g., sleep restriction, stimulus control therapy) aimed at improving sleep.

Cognitive therapy for insomnia[23] addresses the preoccupations and potential consequences of the patient's sleep disruption. While specific cognitive interventions differ in their approach, all rest on the notion that insomniacs have negative beliefs and attitudes about their sleep. Helping patients challenge the usefulness and validity of their negative beliefs and thoughts is believed to reduce the anxiety and arousal associated with nighttime worry and daytime concerns.

Relaxation training targets cognitive and physiological hyperarousal that interferes with sleep and is often utilized with CBT-I. A variety of relaxation techniques may be utilized (e.g., progressive muscle relaxation, diaphragmatic breathing, autogenics, mindfulness meditation), but the optimal method is the one that is most suitable or easiest for the patient to learn. The goal of relaxation training is not to induce sleep, but rather a reduction in basal levels of arousal.

17.4 EFFICACY OF COGNITIVE BEHAVIORAL THERAPY FOR INSOMNIA

A recent meta-analysis shows that randomized controlled trials of CBT-I have significant positive effects on all reported sleep outcomes, with the smallest effects on total sleep time.[24] Across all studies reviewed in this meta-analysis, the largest effects were for reductions in insomnia severity, with large effects also obtained for sleep efficiency, wake after sleep onset, and sleep onset latency.[24] For example, in a randomized, placebo-controlled trial, 78 adults with chronic insomnia were randomly assigned to CBT-I, pharmacotherapy, or both. These three active treatment conditions were compared to a placebo group. All 3 active treatments were more effective than the placebo immediately post-treatment. However, over the long-term, CBT-I alone was associated with sustained improvements in sleep outcomes.[25] Moreover, CBT-I is as effective as sedative-hypnotics during acute treatment (4 to 8 weeks)[15,17,18,26] and is more effective than sedative-hypnotics in the long-term (more than 3 months after treatment).[27]

17.5 CBT-I OUTCOMES BY DEMOGRAPHIC CHARACTERISTICS

17.5.1 RACE

Patients enrolled in CBT-I treatment studies are predominantly White, with some notable exceptions.[28,29] When minorities are included, the group size is too small to conduct meaningful post-hoc analyses of race or ethnicity differences.[28] In an efficacy study of a six-session, internet-based study of CBT-I of 658 participants (21% African American), secondary analyses revealed no differences in treatment outcomes or attrition based on race.[29] Clearly, future studies need to be planned and conducted to test race and/or ethnicity as an important factor.

17.5.2 SEX

Efficacy studies of insomnia show comorbidities with women's reproductive health, including in pregnancy, the post-partum period, menopause, and pre-menstrual dysphoric disorder.[30-37] For example, in a randomized, unmasked, 3-site controlled trial where pregnant women were randomly allocated to CBT-I or to an active control condition, those in the CBT-I condition had a significantly greater reduction in self-reported total wake time. Importantly, a larger percentage of women in the CBT-I condition experienced remission of their insomnia compared to those in the control condition (64% compared to 52%). This study not only demonstrated the effectiveness of CBT-I during pregnancy but offers a safe, non-pharmacological approach for treating insomnia during pregnancy.[35]

In a single-site randomized controlled trial of 150 postmenopausal women with chronic insomnia disorder, women were randomized to one of three conditions: sleep hygiene education, multi-component CBT-I, or sleep restriction therapy.[31] While average sleep duration increased in all 3 groups at 6 months, women in the CBT-I group obtained almost 45 more minutes of sleep per night compared to those in the sleep hygiene education or sleep restriction conditions. Remission rates were higher in the sleep restriction and the CBT-I groups compared to the sleep hygiene education group.

17.5.3 AGE

CBT-I is effective for treating insomnia across the lifespan, including well into late life.[16,25] In a meta-analysis of randomized controlled trials conducted on middle-aged and older adults with insomnia,[16] the authors evaluated the relative efficacy of three different treatment modalities (cognitive-behavioral treatment, behavioral only, and relaxation) on five different sleep outcomes (sleep quality, total sleep time, sleep latency, sleep efficiency, and wake after sleep onset). This meta-analysis supported the efficacy of behavioral interventions across all sleep outcomes, except for total sleep time. The authors hypothesized that these behavioral treatments may be operating through common mechanisms that led to general improvements in sleep outcomes. Moreover, they suggested that total sleep time may be influenced by factors such as work schedules and nighttime activities that were not addressed by the behavioral interventions examined in this meta-analysis. Behavioral interventions produced medium effects for sleep latency and wake after sleep onset. Large effects were observed for sleep quality and sleep efficiency. This meta-analysis did not reveal differences between behavioral intervention modalities, with one exception. Namely, CBT proved to be substantially more effective than relaxation training for improving sleep efficiency. Moreover, when age was tested as a moderator of the effectiveness of behavioral interventions for insomnia, there were notable differences between those younger than 55 years old and those older than 55 years old. Behavioral interventions were more effective for total sleep time and efficiency in those under 55 years old. Moreover, older adults did not differ from the control group on total sleep time following behavioral interventions for insomnia.

17.6   DO THE TREATMENT EFFECTS OF CBT-I LAST?

There are proven clinical gains that are maintained months to years after CBT-I has ended. In long-term randomized controlled trials of CBT-I, it was found that sleep latency and wake after sleep onset effects are stable for time periods up to 2 years.[25,38] While effects for total sleep time are marginal in the short term, they appear to accrue with time. For example, when followed over time, patients had an average increase in total sleep time of 50 minutes after 2 years. This improvement in total sleep time appears to be due to increased time in bed while maintaining good sleep efficiency. In contrast to these findings, results from recent meta-analysis showed that CBT-I continues to be effective at 3, 6, and 12 months compared to non-active controls, but the clinical gains for sleep onset latency, sleep efficiency, and wake after sleep onset, in the treatment condition wane over time.[25,38,39] It is likely that the discrepancy between the results of individual studies and the findings of the recent meta-analysis may be due to several factors, including the between-study differences in the administration of CBT-I, variability in effect size estimates, and the inclusion of small studies in the meta-analysis.

17.7   IS THERE AN ESSENTIAL COMPONENT OF CBT-I?

Comparative efficacy studies, or dismantling studies are one approach for determining which components of a therapy are essential or carry the majority of the outcome variance. To date, there have been two CBT-I dismantling studies.[40,41] In an initial dismantling study,[40] patients with primary insomnia were randomly assigned to one of four conditions: stimulus control therapy, sleep restriction therapy, a combination of stimulus control therapy and sleep restriction, or a waitlist control condition. Compared to those in the control condition, patients in intervention conditions experienced improvements in sleep onset latency (SOL), wake after sleep onset, total sleep time, and sleep efficiency. Patients also reported reductions in negative thoughts and beliefs about sleep. The largest effects and greatest remission of symptoms were observed for patients in the combined sleep restriction/stimulus control therapy condition. The findings from this dismantling study align with recommendations from the American Academy of Sleep Medicine (AASM) in that they support stimulus control therapy and sleep restriction therapy as standards of practice for the treatment of primary insomnia.[1]

However, this study did not directly compare behavioral interventions to cognitive therapy for insomnia or clearly distinguish whether any of the interventions are uniquely targeting underlying mechanisms of insomnia. A second dismantling study[41] addressed a limitation of the prior dismantling study by directly comparing the behavior therapy, cognitive therapy, and full multi-component CBT-I in a sample of mid-life patients with persistent insomnia. Behavior therapy led to faster treatment responses, but those treatment gains were not maintained over time, in the absence of cognitive therapy. Cognitive therapy led to slower but more sustained treatment gains. Ultimately multi-component CBT-I was found to be the optimal treatment, with both behavioral and cognitive therapy components contributing uniquely to short and long-term efficacy. The authors concluded that the different trajectories of change may provide some insight into the process of behavior change through cognitive compared to behavioral pathways.

17.8 EFFECTIVENESS OF CBT-I

Moreover, there is mounting evidence to suggest that treating insomnia may actually improve other mental and physical health conditions. Randomized controlled trials have demonstrated that CBT-I is effective for patients with comorbid insomnia with a host of mental health conditions, such as depression,[42,43] post-traumatic stress disorder,[44,45] generalized anxiety disorder,[46] and schizophrenia.[47] CBT-I has also proven effective for patients with a wide range of comorbid medical conditions, including heart failure,[48] cancer,[49] chronic pain,[50] Alzheimer's disease,[51] alcohol misuse disorder,[52] obstructive sleep apnea,[53] and chronic obstructive pulmonary disease.[54] Randomized controlled trials conducted in these patient populations have found treatment outcomes similar to those observed in patients with insomnia disorder only, and some have demonstrated even better treatment outcomes.[43–45] For example, individuals with major depression and insomnia disorder had better depression remission rates when their treatment included CBT-I in addition to pharmaceutical treatment for depression.[55] CBT-I, in comparison to an attention control group, significantly improved sleep and reduced pain in a sample of 23 patients with osteoarthritis randomly assigned to CBT-I.[56] At a one-year follow-up, improved sleep and reduced pain were maintained for those enrolled in CBT-I.

17.9 ALTERNATIVES TO CBT-I

Alternatives to CBT-I include intensive sleep retraining (ISR), a brief 25-hour treatment that relies on acute sleep deprivation to facilitate rapid sleep onsets across a series of 50 half-hourly sleep onset opportunities to counteract conditioned insomnia.[57] The ISR intervention has been associated with significant improvements in sleep onset latency, total sleep time, and sleep efficiency that are comparable to other behavioral treatments for insomnia (e.g., stimulus control therapy). However, the greatest improvements in sleep outcomes (e.g., total sleep time, wake after sleep onset, sleep efficiency) are found when ISR is combined with more traditional behavioral interventions, such as stimulus control therapy. Benefits from ISR (either alone or in combination with stimulus control) often emerge within one week and are maintained for 6 months.

Additional treatment approaches include brief behavioral treatment for insomnia (BBTI).[58,59] The goals of BBTI are similar to other treatment approaches for insomnia: (1) to improve sleep quantity and quality and (2) to reduce daytime impairment associated with insomnia. This intervention is delivered as a single 45- to 75-minute session focused on sleep education, stimulus control, and sleep restriction with a booster session at two weeks. Two follow-up phone calls, occurring after the first session and following the third session, lasting less than 20 minutes each, address the patient's current sleep and daytime functioning, discuss treatment challenges, increase time in bed as needed, and review relapse prevention. Preliminary empirical support from a handful of studies on BBTI demonstrates that it is acceptable and efficacious in improving insomnia symptoms.[59–64] These studies found better remission and response rates in BBTI groups compared to control groups.[59–64] For example, in a randomized controlled trial of 79 older adults, those in the BBTI group showed improvements in sleep onset latency, wake after sleep onset, and sleep efficiency, compared to an information control group. Moreover, over half of the participants in the BBTI group no longer met criteria for insomnia disorder, compared to only 13% in the control group.[59] While much of what is known about the efficacy of BBTI has been observed in older adult populations, BBTI has also proven useful for treating insomnia among patients with human immunodeficiency virus (HIV)[62] and cancer survivors.[63] In a one-group quasi-experimental pilot study of 12 men with HIV, there were significant improvements in sleep onset latency, wake after sleep onset, and sleep quality.[62] Taken together, these findings suggest that BBTI is acceptable and efficacious in improving both global and specific symptoms of insomnia, with some participants no longer meeting criteria for insomnia. Further, it appears, based on the existing literature, that BBTI is efficacious among older adults with diverse medical histories, but that treatment responses may differ based on medical and psychological comorbidities.

17.10   SCALING-UP OF INSOMNIA TREATMENTS

Despite the favorable results of CBT-I, there is, unfortunately, a gap between evidence-based practice guidelines and current clinical practices. In many parts of the country, CBT-I is rarely available, and few patients have access to this treatment modality. That is, there is a discrepancy between the needs of patients and the supply of practitioners who are adequately trained to provide high-quality CBT-I.[65]

17.10.1   TELEHEALTH AND ONLINE MODES OF DELIVERY

One option for addressing this discrepancy is to utilize technology such as video conferencing and online applications. For example, in a study comparing CBT-I delivered in-person to CBT-I delivered via videoconference, 65 adults with chronic insomnia were randomly assigned to six sessions of telemedicine or six sessions of in-person CBT-I.[66] Across sleep outcomes, CBT-I delivered via video conference performed as well as in-person CBT-I for reducing sleep latency and wake after sleep onset. There were also increases in sleep efficiency, but total sleep time did not differ for either group following intervention.

In a study using an online CBT-I application, 45 adults were randomly assigned to an internet condition or to a wait-list control.[67] Compared to those in the waitlist control, participants in the treatment condition had significantly shorter sleep latency and wake after sleep onset times. There were also improvements in total sleep time and sleep continuity for participants in the treatment condition.

Online CBT-I applications have also been used to address sleep complaints among US service members. For example, in a randomized controlled trial of 100 active-duty soldiers, both internet and in-person CBT-I performed significantly better than waitlist control. Specifically, sleep latency decreased by 10 minutes for the internet group and 15 minutes for the in-person group. There were also increases in total sleep time in both the internet group and the in-person CBT-I group. Of note, the overall effect size for in-person CBT-I was larger than the internet treatment.[68] Overall, taken together, these findings suggest the internet-based delivery of CBT-I may be an adequate mode of delivery when in-person CBT-I is not available.

17.10.2 STEPPED CARE

A second option is to utilize a stepped-care approach for the treatment of insomnia. In this approach, the least intensive therapy that is the most readily accessible, lowest cost, least personal inconvenience, and least specialist time is the entry step. Next, progressively smaller numbers of patients move into more intensive treatment as needed.[69,70] When applied to insomnia treatment, patient needs, including insomnia comorbid with other mental health or physical health conditions would be taken into account along with the method of treatment delivery and provider expertise. For example, one proposed approach starts with patient-administered CBT-I using booklets or the internet and ends with a certified behavioral sleep medicine specialist delivering in-person CBT-I.[69]

17.10.3 SLEEP HEALTH PROMOTION

One final option could include leveraging health behavior theories to improve sleep hygiene at a community or population level.[71] Many studies have utilized the theory of planned behavior[72,73] as a framework for promoting or modifying sleep hygiene.[71] Applied to sleep hygiene, the theory of planned behavior would focus on sleep-related decision making. In fact, several studies have demonstrated that the theory of planned behavior predicted behavioral intentions to sleep between 7 and 8 hours per night and actual behavior both in the short-term[74-76] and up to 6 months later.[77] Integrating traditional health behavior models in order to promote sleep is a promising future direction and should be applied to other aspects of CBT-I, such as sleep restriction and stimulus control therapy, that have greater demonstrated efficacy compared to sleep hygiene.

17.11 SUMMARY AND CONCLUSIONS

Insomnia is one of the most common sleep complaints. In the short-term, the impact of insomnia includes fatigue, mood disturbances, poor cognitive functioning, and impairments in daily living. If untreated, insomnia is associated with substantial societal costs and may pose a risk for additional medical and psychiatric comorbidities. Given that many different factors contribute to the development and maintenance of insomnia, a multifaceted treatment approach such as CBT-I is a preferred treatment of chronic insomnia in adults. As an AASM standard of practice, CBT-I produces treatment gains that are long-lasting and efficacious, with some demonstrated effectiveness. Future treatment considerations include adapting the delivery of CBT-I into brief modules and examining the utility of CBT-I for conditions that commonly co-occur with insomnia, such as depression, chronic pain, cancer, and post-traumatic stress disorder. Opportunities to scale up the treatment of insomnia to increase patient access include the delivery of CBT-I through internet applications and public sleep health promotion efforts.

REFERENCES

1. Schutte-Rodin S, Broch L, Buysse D, Dorsey C, Sateia M. Clinical guideline for the evaluation and management of chronic insomnia in adults. *J Clin Sleep Med*. 2008;4(5): 487–504.
2. Ohayon MM. Epidemiology of insomnia: What we know and What we still need to learn. *Sleep Med Rev*. 2002;6(2):97–111.
3. Morin CM, LeBlanc M, Bélanger L, Ivers H, Mérette C, Savard J. Prevalence of insomnia and its treatment in Canada. *Can J Psychiatry*. 2011;56:540–548.
4. Morin CM, Jarrin DC. Epidemiology of insomnia: Prevalence, course, risk factors, and public health burden. *Sleep Med Clin*. 2013;8:281–297.
5. Morin CM, Bélanger L, LeBlanc M, et al. The natural history of insomnia: A population-based 3-year longitudinal study. *Arch Intern Med*. 2009;169:447–453.
6. Léger D, Morin CM, Uchiyama M, Hakimi Z, Cure S, Walsh JK. Chronic insomnia, quality-of-life, and utility scores: Comparison with good sleepers in a cross-sectional international survey. *Sleep Med*. 2012;13(1):43–51. doi:10.1016/j.sleep.2011.03.020.
7. Rosekind MR, Gregory KB. Insomnia risks and costs: Health, safety, and quality of life. *Am J Manag Care*. 2010;16(8):617–626.
8. Sateia MJ, Buysse DJ, Krystal AD, Neubauer DN, Heald JL. Clinical practice guideline for the pharmacologic treatment of chronic insomnia in adults: An American academy of sleep medicine clinical practice guideline. *J Clin Sleep Med*. 2017;13(2):307–349. doi:10.5664/jcsm.6470
9. Qaseem A, Kansagara D, Forciea MA, Cooke M, Denberg TD, Clinical Guidelines Committee of the American College of Physicians. Management of chronic insomnia disorder in adults: A clinical practice guideline from the American college of physicians. *Ann Intern Med*. 2016;165(2):125–133.
10. Spielman A, Caruso LS, Glovinsky P. A behavioral perspective on insomnia treatment. *Psychiatr Clin North Am*. 1987;10:541–553.
11. Pigeon WR, Cribbet MR. The pathophysiology of insomnia: From models to molecules (and back). *Curr Opin Pulm Med*. 2012;18(6):546–553. doi:10.1097/MCP. 0b013e328358be41. PMID: 22990658.
12. Levenson JC, Kay DB, Buysse DJ. The pathophysiology of insomnia. *Chest*. 2015; 147(4):1179–1192. doi:10.1378/chest.14-1617.
13. Morin CM, Culbert JP, Schwartz SM. Nonpharmacological interventions for insomnia: A meta-analysis of treatment efficacy. *Am J Psychiatry*. 1994;151(8):1172–1180.
14. Murtagh DR, Greenwood KM. Identifying effective psychological treatments for insomnia: A meta-analysis. *J Consult Clin Psychol*. 1995;63(1):79–89.
15. Smith MT, Perlis ML, Park A, et al. Comparative meta-analysis of pharmacotherapy and behavior therapy for persistent insomnia. *Am J Psychiatry*. 2002;159(1):5–11.
16. Irwin MR, Cole JC, Nicassio PM. Comparative meta-analysis of behavioral interventions for insomnia and their efficacy in middle-aged adults and in older adults 55+ years of age. *Health Psychol*. 2006;25(1):3–14.

17. Mitchell MD, Gehrman P, Perlis M, et al. Comparative effectiveness of cognitive behavioral therapy for insomnia: A systematic review. *BMC Fam Pract*. 2012;13:40.
18. Pallesen S, Nordhus IH, Kvale G. Nonpharmacological interventions for insomnia in older adults: A meta-analysis of treatment efficacy. *Psychotherapy*. 1998;35(4):472–482.
19. Leshner A. NIH state-of-the-science conference statement on manifestations and management of chronic insomnia in adults. *NIH Consens State Sci Statements*. 2005;22:1–30.
20. Bootzin RR, Nicassio P. "Behavioral treatments for insomnia." In Hersen M, Eisler RM, & Miller PM, eds. *Progress in Behavior Modification*. Academic Press; 1978:1–47.
21. Spielman A, Saskin P, Thorpy MT. Treatment of chronic insomnia by restriction of time in bed. *Sleep*. 1987;10:45–56.
22. Hauri P. *Sleep Disorders: Current Concepts*, 2nd ed. Kalamazoo, MI: Upjohn Company; 1982.
23. Morin CM, Azrin NH. Behavioral and cognitive treatments of geriatric insomnia. *J Consult Clin Psychol*. 1988;56:748–753.
24. Van Straten A, van der Zweerde T, Kleiboer A, Cuijpers P, Morin CM, Lancee J. Cognitive and behavioral therapies in the treatment of insomnia: A meta-analysis. *Sleep Med Revs*. 2018;38:1–14.
25. Morin CM, Colecchi C, Stone J, et al. Behavioral and pharmacological therapies for late-life insomnia: A randomized controlled trial. *JAMA*. 1999;281(11):991–999.
26. Rios P, Cardoso R, Morra D, et al. Comparative effectiveness and safety of pharmacological and non-pharmacological interventions for insomnia: An overview of reviews. *Syst Rev*. 2019;8(1):281.
27. Okajima I, Komada Y, Inoue Y. A meta-analysis on the treatment effectiveness of cognitive behavioral therapy for primary insomnia. *Sleep Biol Rhythms*. 2011;9(1): 24–34.
28. Williams NJ, He Z, Langford A, et al. 1187 racial and ethnic participation in obstructive sleep apnea and insomnia clinical trials. *Sleep*. 2017;40(suppl_1):A443
29. Cheng P, Luik AI, Fellman-Couture C, et al. Efficacy of digital CBT for insomnia to reduce depression across demographic groups: A randomized trial. *Psychol Med*. 2019;49(3):491–500.
30. McCurry SM, Guthrie KA, Morin CM, et al. Telephone-based cognitive behavioral therapy for insomnia in perimenopausal and postmenopausal women with vasomotor symptoms: A MsFLASH randomized clinical trial. *JAMA Intern Med*. 2016;176(7): 913–920.
31. Drake CL, Kalmbach DA, Arnedt JT, et al. Treating chronic insomnia in postmenopausal women: A randomized clinical trial comparing cognitive behavioral therapy for insomnia, sleep restriction therapy, and sleep hygiene education. *Sleep*. 2019;42(2): zsy217.
32. Kalmbach DA, Cheng P, Arnedt JT, et al. Treating insomnia improves depression, maladaptive thinking, and hyperarousal in postmenopausal women: Comparing cognitive-behavioral therapy for insomnia (CBTI), sleep restriction therapy, and sleep hygiene education. *Sleep Med*. 2019;55:124–134
33. Kalmbach DA, Cheng P, Roth T, et al. Objective sleep disturbance is associated with poor response to cognitive and behavioral treatments for insomnia in postmenopausal women. *Sleep Med*. 2020;73:82–92
34. Kalmbach DA, Cheng P, Roth T, et al. Examining patient feedback and the role of cognitive arousal in treatment non-response to digital cognitive-behavioral therapy for insomnia during pregnancy. *Behav Sleep Med*. 2021;20;1–20.
35. Manber R, Bei B, Simpson N, et al. Cognitive behavioral therapy for prenatal insomnia: A randomized controlled trial. *Obstet Gynecol*. 2019;133(5):911–919
36. Tomfohr-Madsen LM, Clayborne ZM, Rouleau CR, et al. Sleeping for two: An open-pilot study of cognitive behavioral therapy for insomnia in pregnancy. *Behav Sleep Med*. 2017;15(5):377–393

37. Swanson LM, Flynn H, Adams-Mundy JD, et al. An open pilot of cognitive behavioral therapy for insomnia in women with postpartum depression. *Behav Sleep Med.* 2013;11(4):297–307.

38. Beaulieu-Bonneau S, Ivers H, Guay B, et al. Long-term maintenance of therapeutic gains associated with cognitive-behavioral therapy for insomnia delivered alone or combined with zolpidem. *Sleep.* 2017;40(3):zsx002.

39. Morin CM, Benca R. Chronic insomnia. *Lancet.* 2012;379(9821):1129–1141.

40. Epstein DR, Sidani S, Bootzin RR, Belyea MJ. Dismantling multi-component behavioral treatment for insomnia in older adults a randomized controlled trial. *Sleep.* 2012: 35:797–805. doi:10.5665/sleep.1878

41. Harvey AG, Bélanger L, Talbot L, Eidelman P, Beaulieu-Bonneau S, Fortier-Brochu É, Ivers H, Lamy M, Hein K, Soehner AM, Mérette C, Morin CM. Comparative efficacy of behavior therapy, cognitive therapy, and cognitive behavior therapy for chronic insomnia: A randomized controlled trial. *J Consult Clin Psychol.* 2014;82(4):670–683. doi:10.1037/a0036606

42. Carney CE, Edinger JD, Kuchibhatla M, et al. Cognitive behavioral insomnia therapy for those with insomnia and depression: A randomized controlled clinical trial. *Sleep.* 2017;40(4):zsx019.

43. Cunningham JEA, Shapiro CM. Cognitive behavioural therapy for insomnia (CBT-I) to treat depression: A systematic review. *J Psychosom Res.* 2018;106:1–12.

44. Harvey AG, Soehner AM, Kaplan KA, et al. Treating insomnia improves mood state, sleep, and functioning in bipolar disorder: A pilot randomized controlled trial. *J Consult Clin Psychol.* 2015;83(3):564–577.

45. Simon N, McGillivray L, Roberts NP, et al. Acceptability of internet-based cognitive behavioural therapy (i-CBT) for post-traumatic stress disorder (PTSD): A systematic review. *Eur J Psychotraumatol.* 2019;10(1):1646092.

46. Ye YY, Zhang YF, Chen J, et al. Internet-based cognitive behavioral therapy for insomnia (ICBT-i) improves co-morbid anxiety and depression-a meta-analysis of randomized controlled trials. *PLoS ONE.* 2015;10(11):e0142258.

47. Hwang DK, Nam M, Lee YG. The effect of cognitive behavioral therapy for insomnia in schizophrenia patients with sleep disturbance: A nonrandomized, assessor-blind trial. *Psychiatry Res.* 2019;274:182–188.

48. Redeker NS, Conley S, Anderson G, et al. Effects of cognitive behavioral therapy for insomnia on sleep, symptoms, stress, and autonomic function among patients with heart failure. *Behav Sleep Med.* 2020;18(2):190–202.

49. Ma Y, Hall DL, Ngo LH, et al. Efficacy of cognitive behavioral therapy for insomnia in breast cancer: A meta-analysis. *Sleep Med Rev.* 2021;55:101376.

50. McCrae CS, Williams J, Roditi D, et al. Cognitive behavioral treatments for insomnia and pain in adults with co-morbid chronic insomnia and fibromyalgia: Clinical outcomes from the SPIN randomized controlled trial. *Sleep.* 2019;42(2):zsy234.

51. Siengsukon CF, Nelson E, Williams-Cooke C, et al. Cognitive behavioral therapy for insomnia to enhance cognitive function and reduce the rate of Aβ deposition in older adults with symptoms of insomnia: A single-site randomized pilot clinical trial protocol. *Contemp Clin Trials.* 2020;99:106190.

52. Chakravorty S, Morales KH, Arnedt JT, et al. Cognitive behavioral therapy for insomnia in alcohol-dependent veterans: A randomized, controlled pilot study. *Alcohol Clin Exp Res.* 2019;43(6):1244–1253.

53. Ong JC, Crawford MR, Dawson SC, et al. A randomized controlled trial of CBT-I and PAP for obstructive sleep apnea and co-morbid insomnia: Main outcomes from the MATRICS study. *Sleep.* 2020;43(9):zsaa041.

54. Kapella MC, Herdegen JJ, Perlis ML, et al. Cognitive behavioral therapy for insomnia co-morbid with COPD is feasible with preliminary evidence of positive sleep and fatigue effects. *Int J Chron Obstruct Pulmon Dis.* 2011;6:625–635.

55. Manber R, Edinger JD, Gress JL, San Pedro-Salcedo MG, Kuo TF, Kalista T. Cognitive behavioral therapy for insomnia enhances depression outcome in patients with co-morbid major depressive disorder and insomnia. *Sleep.* 2008;31(4):489–495. doi:10.1093/sleep/31.4.489.

56. Vitiello MV, Rybarczyk B, Von Korff M, Stepanski EJ. Cognitive behavioral therapy for insomnia improves sleep and decreases pain in older adults with co-morbid insomnia and osteoarthritis. *J Clin Sleep Med.* 2009;5(4):355–362.

57. Harris J, Lack L, Kemp K, Wright H, Bootzin RR. A randomized controlled trial of intensive sleep retraining (ISR): A brief conditioning treatment for chronic insomnia. *Sleep.* 2012;35:49–60.

58. Troxel WM, Germain A, Buysse DJ. Clinical management of insomnia with brief behavioral treatment (BBTI). *Behav Sleep Med.* 2012;10(4):266–279.

59. Buysse DJ, Germain A, Moul DE, et al. Efficacy of brief behavioral treatment for chronic insomnia in older adults. *Arch Intern Med.* 2011;171(10):887–895.

60. Germain A, Moul DE, Franzen PL, et al. Effects of a brief behavioral treatment for late-life insomnia: Preliminary findings. *J Clin Sleep Med.* 2006;2(4):403–406.

61. McCrae CS, Curtis AF, Williams JM, et al. Efficacy of brief behavioral treatment for insomnia in older adults: Examination of sleep, mood, and cognitive outcomes. *Sleep Med.* 2018;51:153–166.

62. Buchanan DT, McCurry SM, Eilers K, et al. Brief behavioral treatment for insomnia in persons living with HIV. *Behav Sleep Med.* 2018;16(3):244–258.

63. Zhou ES, Vrooman LM, Manley PE, et al. Adapted delivery of cognitive-behavioral treatment for insomnia in adolescent and young adult cancer survivors: A pilot study. *Behav Sleep Med* 2017;15(4):288–301.

64. Wang J, Wei Q, Wu X, et al. Brief behavioral treatment for patients with treatment-resistant insomnia. *Neuropsychiatr Dis Treat.* 2016;12:1967–1975.

65. Morin CM. Cognitive behavioural therapy for insomnia (CBTi): From randomized controlled trials to practice guidelines to implementation in clinical practice. *J Sleep Res.* 2020;29(2):e13017. doi:10.1111/jsr.13017.

66. Arnedt JT, Conroy DA, Mooney A, et al. Telemedicine versus face-to-face delivery of cognitive behavioral therapy for insomnia: A randomized controlled noninferiority trial. *Sleep.* 2021;44(1):zsaa136.

67. Ritterband LM, Thorndike FP, Gonder-Frederick LA, et al. Efficacy of an internet-based behavioral intervention for adults with insomnia. *Arch Gen Psychiatry.* 2009;66(7):692–698.

68. Taylor DJ, Peterson A, Pruiksma KE, et al. Internet and in-person cognitive behavioral therapy for insomnia in military personnel: A randomized clinical trial. *Sleep.* 2017;40(6):zsx075.

69. Espie CA. "Stepped care": A health technology solution for delivering cognitive behavioral therapy as a first line insomnia treatment. *Sleep.* 2009;32(12):1549–1558. doi:10.1093/sleep/32.12.1549.

70. Edinger JD. Is it time to step up to stepped care with our cognitive-behavioral insomnia therapies? *Sleep.* 2009;32(12):1539–1541. doi:10.1093/sleep/32.12.1539.

71. Mead MP, Irish LA. Application of health behaviour theory to sleep health improvement. *J Sleep Res.* 2020;29:e12950.

72. Ajzen I. From intentions to actions: A theory of planned behavior. In *Action Control.* Berlin, Germany: Springer; 1985:11–39.

73. Fishbein M, Ajzen I. *Predicting and Changing Behavior: The Reasoned Action Approach.* New York, NY: Psychology Press; 2011.

74. Knowlden AP, Sharma M, Bernard AL. A theory of planned behavior research model for predicting the sleep intentions and behaviors of undergraduate college students. *J Prim Prev.* 2012;33(1):19–31. doi:10.1007/s10935-012-0263-2.

75. Tagler MJ, Stanko KA, Forbey JD. Predicting sleep hygiene: A reasoned action approach. *J Applied Soc Psychol.* 2017;47(1):3–12.
76. Lao HC, Tao VYK, Wu AMS. Theory of planned behaviour and healthy sleep of college students. *Aus J Psychol.* 2016;68(1):20–28.
77. Strong C, Lin CY, Jalilolghadr S, Updegraff JA, Broström A, Pakpour AH. Sleep hygiene behaviours in Iranian adolescents: An application of the theory of planned behavior. *J Sleep Res.* 2018;27(1):23–31. doi:10.1111/jsr.12566.

18 Physical Activity

Khadija Ziauddin, MBBS, MPH and
Christopher P. Fagundes, PhD

KEY POINTS

- Physical activity has manifold benefits for physical and mental health. Federal agencies and health departments issue guidelines for physical activity to help attain and maintain health, prevent disease, and improve quality of life.
- Theories of behavioral change are operationalized at multiple levels of influence to help increase physical activity.
- Empirically valid interventions that utilize the latest technology are being developed and implemented to help individuals and groups increase physical activity and, in turn, to improve health and well-being.

18.1 DEFINITIONS, BENEFITS, AND GUIDELINES BY AGE

Regular physical activity represents one of the pillars of lifestyle medicine. As one of the most potent predictors of good physical health, regular physical activity reduces the risk of chronic diseases of older adulthood, including cancer, type 2 diabetes, cardiovascular disease, and dementia. Not only does exercise foster physical health, it also has a substantial effect on mental health.[1] Those who report low levels of fitness have a 47% greater likelihood of developing depression than those with high levels of fitness.[2] In this chapter, we briefly describe the health benefits of exercise. Then, we summarize current exercise guidelines by age. Finally, we describe current theories of health behaviors, emphasizing the importance of considering multiple levels of influence to design effective interventions. In so doing, we provide an example of an exercise intervention designed based on the principles and theories outlined in this chapter.

Physical activity can be defined as any bodily movement produced by skeletal muscles that causes energy expenditure, measured in kilocalories.[3] Physical activity encompasses many activities, including, but not limited to, recreational activity, household activity, occupational activity, etc. Exercise is a physical activity that is planned, structured, intentional, and repetitive and aims to improve or maintain physical fitness.[3]

According to the U.S. Department of Health and Human Services, engaging in regular physical activity, being less sedentary, and moving more helps maintain and improve health.[4] Being physically active has many beneficial effects on mental and physical health[4,5], details of which are provided in Table 18.1.

DOI: 10.1201/b22810-21

TABLE 18.1
Benefits of Physical Activity for Physical & Mental Health[4,5]

All-Cause Mortality	**Reduces Risk of All-Cause Mortality by 33 Percent**
Cancer	Regular physical activity reduces risk for the following malignancies:
	• Bladder
	• Breast
	• Colon
	• Endometrium
	• Esophagus (adenocarcinoma)
	• Kidney
	• Lung
	• Stomach
Musculoskeletal system	• Improves bone health
	• Reduces risk of osteoporosis
	• Reduces risk of fractures.
	• Muscle-strengthening activity helps maintain and improve muscle mass and strength.
Cardiovascular system	Reduces risk of
	• Hypertension
	• Coronary heart disease
	• Heart failure
	• Stroke
Metabolic system	Reduces risk of, and helps control
	• Type 2 diabetes
	• Obesity
	• Adverse blood lipid profile
Neurological system	• Improves cognition
	• Reduces risk of Alzheimer's disease
	• Delays age-associated cognitive decline
Mental health	Reduces risk of
	• Symptoms of depression and Major Depressive Disorder
	• Anxiety symptoms and disorders
	• Chronic fatigue and low energy
General health	• Helps improve sleep quality
	• Helps reduce feelings of distress
	• Helps enhance sense of well-being
	• Helps lower risk of falls in older adults

Several of the most common chronic diseases in the U.S., such as heart disease, cancer, diabetes, etc., are benefited from regular physical activity.[4] A lack of physical activity is associated with approximately $117 billion in annual healthcare costs.[4] Federal agencies, thus, provide recommendations for physical activity to help improve the population's health and quality of life and mitigate preventable healthcare costs. Table 18.2 provides physical activity guidelines by age, modified from the

TABLE 18.2
Physical Activity Guidelines by Age[4]

Age	Guidelines
3 years to 5 years (preschool)	Children, between the age of 3 and 5 years should be physically active through the course of the day, and should be encouraged to engage in active play.
6 years to 17 years (children and adolescents)	Children and adolescents should do at least 60 minutes of moderate-to-vigorous physical activity daily. This should include the following: • Aerobic: Most of the daily physical activity should be either moderate- or vigorous-intensity aerobic activity and should include vigorous-intensity physical activity on at least 3 days a week. • Muscle-strengthening: Muscle-strengthening physical activity should be included at least 3 days a week. • Bone-strengthening: Bone-strengthening physical activity should be included at least 3 days a week.
18 years to 59 years	Adults should do, at least the following: • 150 minutes (2.5 hours) to 300 minutes (5 hours) a week of moderate-intensity, or • 75 minutes (1.25 hours) to 150 minutes (2.5 hours) a week of vigorous-intensity aerobic physical activity, or • an equivalent combination of moderate- and vigorous-intensity aerobic activity
>60 years	Older adults should do at least • 150 minutes (2.5 hours) to 300 minutes (5 hours) a week of moderate-intensity, or • 75 minutes (1.25 hours) to 150 minutes (2.5 hours) a week of vigorous-intensity aerobic physical activity, or • an equivalent combination of moderate- and vigorous-intensity aerobic activity Additionally, older adults should include balance training in their weekly physical activity Older adults with chronic conditions should assess their ability to do regular physical activity safely. If unable to do 150 minutes of moderate-intensity aerobic activity a week, they should be as physically active as their abilities and conditions allow.

Physical Activity Guidelines for Americans based on the recommendations of the 2018 Physical Activity Guidelines Advisory Committee.

18.2 DETERMINANTS OF PHYSICAL ACTIVITY

A large fraction of the population does not engage in adequate physical activity.[4] This is despite information regarding benefits of physical activity and guidelines being widely disseminated. Understanding the underlying reasons behind this lack of activity is essential in developing targeted interventions to improve physical activity levels.

Human behavior results from multiple factors and influences.[6] Individual and interpersonal factors, along with social determinants are extremely important in understanding and changing behavior. Individual determinants include knowledge, self-efficacy, attitudes, etc. toward physical activity.[6] Examples of interpersonal factors could be social support from peers, friends, and family.[7] Social determinants are subjective social norms and other social influences[8] on behavior which include socioeconomic position, safety, crime rates, etc.[6] Additionally, environmental factors such as built environment, access to green spaces/walking paths, etc. are closely related to, and overlap with, social determinants.[6]

Like individual factors, social and environmental determinants vary significantly for individuals and groups. It is essential to keep this variance in mind while assessing determinants to tailor interventions to target populations at multiple levels.

18.3   THEORIES OF HEALTH BEHAVIOR FOR PHYSICAL ACTIVITY

Theory-based interventions and programs can help identify the influences on health behavior and targets for behavior change.[9] A theory is a set of interrelated concepts (or constructs) that specifies relationships among variables to explain events and behaviors.[9] Theory-based research helps determine why individuals are not physically active, what factors must be changed, and how to implement effective change.

Table 18.3 provides a brief overview of a few theories and models that have been used for physical activity behavior change.[10] For example, the Health Belief Model (HBM) was developed to understand why individuals do not engage in preventive and health-promoting behavior despite the availability of resources.[9,11] Since this model was found to be more beneficial for occasional behaviors, the stage-based model (Transtheoretical Model) and cognitive-based theories were operationalized for physical activity behaviors.[12]

Cognitive-based theories propose that complex behaviors are controlled by rational cognitive activity.[10,13–15] The Transtheoretical Model assumes that individuals undergo stages while adopting or maintaining complex behaviors such as physical activity.[10,16] Implementing theory-based research elucidates factors that impact physical activity behavior. No one specific theory, however, can be used to target behavior change.[9] Rather, the choice of a theory and constructs should begin with identifying the level of influence, problem, and aim of the intervention.[9,17]

18.4   INTERVENTIONS

18.4.1   LEVELS OF INFLUENCE

Multiple factors influence physical activity behavior.[9,10] As a result, a multi-level approach is recommended for interventionists targeting physical activity behavior change.[9,19]

The Socio-Ecological model considers factors at many levels, all of which influence behavior. These factors also tend to interact across the following levels of influence: Intrapersonal, Interpersonal, Organizational, Community, and Policy[9] (as seen in Figure 18.1). For example, educational interventions designed to improve knowledge

TABLE 18.3
Theories of Health Behavior[9,10,12]

Theory/Model	Overview	Constructs
Health Belief Model[11]	HBM was developed to predict health-related behaviors. Belief in a personal threat of disease along with belief in the effectiveness of the recommended health behavior predicts the likelihood of health behavior	• Perceived susceptibility • Perceived severity • Perceived benefits • Perceived barriers • Cues to action • Self-efficacy
Transtheoretical Model[16]	Assumes that individuals do not change behaviors quickly and decisively, but rather, through a cyclical process of change Also referred to as the 'Stages of Change' Model	• Precontemplation (unaware of problem & behavior) • Contemplation (aware of problem and behavior) • Preparation (intent to act) • Action (practices behavior) • Maintenance (sustains behavior change) • Self-efficacy • Decisional balance

Theory of Planned Behavior[14]	Attitude toward the behavior is a stronger predictor of the behavior being adopted rather than attitude toward the target or outcome.
	Behavioral intention is a function of the attitude toward the behavior, subjective norms, and perceived behavioral control.
		• Attitudes
		  • Behavioral beliefs
		  • Evaluation of outcome
		• Subjective norms
		  • Normative beliefs
		  • Motivation to comply
		• Perceived behavioral control
		  • Control beliefs
		  • Perceived power

Social Cognitive Theory[13,18]	Human behavior results from the interaction between personal, behavioral, and environmental influences. Health and behavior are the result of multiple factors.	• Reciprocal determinism • Observational learning • Outcome expectations • Self-efficacy • Collective efficacy • Incentive motivation • Facilitation • Self-regulation • Moral disengagement
Self Determination Theory[15]	Behavioral regulation varies in the extent to which it is self-determined or controlling.	• Autonomy • Competence • Relatedness

about physical activity (Individual/Intrapersonal level) may be more effective when motivation from peers is incorporated into the study design[20] (Interpersonal level). Additionally, to attain and sustain such complex behaviors, more up-stream factors such as access to safe neighborhoods, green spaces, sidewalks (Organizational/Community level), and policies such as insurance discounts for regular exercise, further help improve physical activity levels.[9] Health psychologists even suggest that

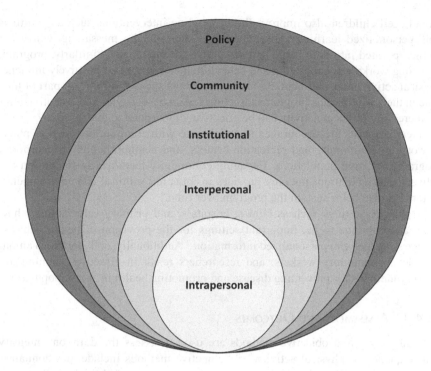

FIGURE 18.1   The Socio-Ecological model.[22]

rather than individual characteristics, the situations people experience may be better predictors of complex behaviors.[9,21]

Changing higher levels of influence may be beyond the scope of many interventions. Despite this, considering multiple influences on behavior across levels is beneficial as it aids interventionists to personalize and target their interventions.

18.4.2   Settings and Modes of Delivery

Homes, schools, communities, places of work, and healthcare sites are common settings for interventions designed to improve physical activity behavior.[23]

Within these settings, interventions can be delivered in residences through in-person home visits or remotely conducted phone/internet calls, text messages, mail, smartphone applications, and email. Such interventions provide personalized physical activity-enhancing strategies.[9] Additionally, remote access can help reduce costs and allow interventionists to reach more significant and more vulnerable populations.[9,24]

School-based physical activity programs increase the duration of physical activity, reduce television viewing, and decrease blood cholesterol levels.[25] These outcomes are achieved through changes in school curriculum and interactive education provided by teachers.[25] Compulsory PE classes, longer recess, and incentivized exercise performance can mitigate increasingly sedentary lifestyles of children and reduce the risk of childhood obesity and diabetes.[25] Physical activity behaviors in

school-aged children also improve through online interventions such as gamifica-
tion, personalized learning applications, and social media messaging, which can
be incorporated into both home and school-based programs.[26] Similarly, programs
providing workplace counseling and behavior change strategies positively influence
physical activity and well-being.[27,28] As many adults spend a significant part of their
time in their workplaces, programs targeting sedentary behavior and incentivization
for increasing physical activity can be effectively incorporated at worksites.[9]

Interventionists are encouraged to collaborate with communities such as places
of worship, community and recreation centers, and neighborhoods to incorporate
programs for large populations. Engaging community members in the design and
delivery of interventions not only provides insights into cultural and environmental
factors but also helps sustain the program over time.[9]

Healthcare settings such as clinics, hospitals, and primary care facilities have
been, and continue to be, important settings for the provision of health behavior
change strategies and personalized information.[9] Additionally, collaborations among
providers, community workers, and researchers result in effective planning and
delivery methods for preventing disease and promoting health in at-risk populations.

18.4.3 ASSESSMENT AND OUTCOMES

Both subjective and objective methods are used to assess the duration, intensity,
and frequency of physical activity.[29,30] Subjective methods include questionnaires,
diaries, and logs. Objective methods include measurement of physiological markers
such as heart rate, calorimetry, and data from motion sensors.[29,31]

The International Physical Activity Questionnaire (I-PAQ),[32] Global Physical
Activity Questionnaire (GPAQ),[33] and the European Health Interview Survey -
Physical Activity Questionnaire (EHIS-PAQ)[34] are some commonly used surveys
to assess physical activity. Despite being cost-effective and associated with low
researcher and patient burden,[29] questionnaires tend to have low reliability and validity and are subject to biases.[29,31] As such, combined monitoring strategies can better
assess physical activity behavior.[35]

Wearable devices are being continuously developed and updated. These devices
measure body motion, assess physical activity, and estimate energy expenditure.
For example, accelerometers estimate the level of movement, pedometers calculate
steps and distance walked,[29] and calorimeters assess oxygen consumption.[35] Using
a combination of assessments, self-report data can be cross-checked with activity
and physiological data.[29] More recently, major corporations have developed devices
that allow simultaneous monitoring of accelerations, heart rate, energy expenditure,
sleep, etc. with the ability to collect data on computers and smartphones. This simultaneous monitoring, and the recorded data, provide an unprecedented amount of
health information.[30,36]

Monitoring biomarkers and biological mediators helps researchers establish associations between physical activity and health.[31] Measurement of changes in weight,
waistline, BMI, cholesterol, blood glucose, and inflammatory blood markers can
be used to investigate the impact of interventions on health and the outcomes of
physical activity.[37] By assessing health indicators at multiple levels of analysis (e.g.,

behavioral, biological, psychosocial), researchers are able to ascertain a comprehensive profile of how physical health interventions impact health outcomes.

18.5   EXAMPLE OF INTERVENTION DEVELOPMENT USING THEORIES & INTERVENTION APPROACHES

We provide an example of an ongoing intervention and explain the decisional and planning aspects for selecting levels of influence, setting, mode of delivery, and assessment. The COVID-19 pandemic increased the need to improve physical activity[38] and address the loneliness resulting from social distancing and isolation guidelines. A dyadic study was designed incorporating the principles of Motivational Interviewing (MI) to increase physical activity levels in an at-risk population (Alzheimer's disease and related dementia caregivers). On average, caregivers experience higher levels of loneliness than non-caregivers[39,40]; significantly, social isolation guidelines during the COVID-19 pandemic further enhanced feelings of loneliness and isolation in this population.[41] This intervention aimed to assess whether attempts to increase physical activity levels with a friend/family member while maintaining social distancing lead to sustained increases in exercise time and quality, intrinsic motivation, and reduction in stress levels.

18.5.1   LEVEL OF INFLUENCE

Dyadic partnerships were encouraged to facilitate emotional bonds, reduce loneliness, and enable productive interpersonal interactions. Motivational interviewing-based methods aimed to build intrapersonal self-efficacy and optimism through reflective listening and developing discrepancy between goals and current behavior.[42] These methods also enabled the research team to tailor the intervention to the participants' needs and address behavioral barriers at multiple levels of influence.

18.5.2   SETTING, MODE, AND ASSESSMENT

The pandemic made it necessary to deliver the intervention remotely. The sessions were conducted through Zoom or via phone calls with both dyad partners. The educational components, which consisted of a physical activity guidebook and motivational messages, were sent via email and text respectively. Physical activity levels, psychological stress levels, and motivation were assessed before and after the intervention, using online questionnaires. Only self-report assessments were used due to the preliminary nature of the study and pandemic-related constraints. In the next stage of feasibility and acceptability testing, we will include objective measures of activity levels and autonomic physiology for Alzheimer's disease and related dementia caregivers.

18.5.3   THEORY

This study used a combination of MI and TTM (Transtheoretical Model) strategies which are recommended as an approach to improve the likelihood of increasing physical activity.[43] After verification that the participants were in the preparation stage (intent to act), the three calls were scheduled during the preparation and early action stages to focus on strategies such as development of realistic goals and a time-line for change, positive reinforcement, and self-liberation (choosing and making a commitment to change).[44] The calls consisted of material from the physical activity booklet which we designed using material from (1) The Centers for Disease Control and Prevention, Division of Nutrition, Physical Activity and Obesity fact-sheets,[45], and (2) Daughters and Mothers Against Breast Cancer (DAMES): Main Outcomes of a Randomized Controlled Trial of Weight Loss in Overweight Mothers With Breast Cancer and Their Overweight Daughters.[46]

We randomized participants into experimental and control groups to ensure an unbiased assignment to intervention conditions. Both groups were offered the intervention for ethical purposes. Participants in the experimental group received the intervention before those in the control group. The experimental approach also allowed a time-effective and cost-effective means of testing whether a larger inter-vention can work in a similar population and setting.[47]

18.6 FUTURE DIRECTIONS & CONCLUSION

Lifestyles have become increasingly sedentary in the US and some developed coun-tries worldwide.[48] Accordingly, interventions designed to increase physical activity and reduce sedentary habits are critically needed.[49] There is a crucial need for more theory-based randomized controlled trials that capitalize on mobile technology to assess and intervene on physical activity and sedentary behaviors.[49] To improve the adoption and efficacy of sustainable community-based interventions, we propose that researchers should account for multiple levels of influence and tailor interventions to target populations. Toward this end, it will be imperative for researchers to investigate why disparities in physical activity exist (e.g., gender, race/ethnicity, environment).[50] Finally, to maximize the impact of evidence-based interventions, an interdisciplin-ary team of stakeholders should be included at every intervention development and dissemination stage.[9]

Physical activity is a critical component of Lifestyle Medicine.[51] The health ben-efits of physical activity are well established.[52] Although patients report a desire to exercise regularly, the majority have difficulty adopting a regular exercise practice that can be maintained. Given the importance of exercise for preventing and treat-ing chronic disease and mental health, it will be critical for intervention scientists to design and test evidence-based interventions that lifestyle medicine practitioners can prescribe. For these interventions to be disseminated broadly, it will be essential to tailor them to the individual patient, based on his/her needs and limitations.

REFERENCES

1. Chekroud SR, Gueorguieva R, Zheutlin AB, Paulus M, Krumholz HM, Krystal JH, et al. Association between physical exercise and mental health in 1·2 million individu-als in the USA between 2011 and 2015: A cross-sectional study. *Lancet Psychiatry* 2018;5:739–746. https://doi.org/10.1016/S2215-0366(18)30227-X

2. Schuch FB, Vancampfort D, Firth J, Rosenbaum S, Ward PB, Silva ES, et al. Physical activity and incident depression: A meta-analysis of prospective cohort studies. *Am J Psychiatry* 2018;175:631–648. https://doi.org/10.1176/appi.ajp.2018.17111194

3. Caspersen CJ, Powell KE, Christenson GM. Physical activity, exercise, and physical fitness: Definitions and distinctions for health-related research. *Public Health Rep.* 1985;100:126–131.

4. U.S. Department of Health and Human Services. *Physical Activity Guidelines for Americans, 2nd edition - Healthy People 2030 | health.gov.* Https://Health.Gov/ Paguidelines/Second-Edition/Pdf/Physical_Activity_Guidelines_2nd_edition.Pdf n.d. URL: https://health.gov/healthypeople/tools-action/browse-evidence-based-resources/ physical-activity-guidelines-americans-2nd-edition (Accessed 30 August 2022).

5. CDC. *Benefits of Physical Activity.* Centers for Disease Control and Prevention. 2022. URL: https://www.cdc.gov/physicalactivity/basics/pa-health/index.htm (Accessed 6 September 2022).

6. Cleland VJ, Ball K, Crawford D. Social and environmental determinants of health behaviors. In Steptoe A, ed. *Handbook of Behavioral Medicine: Methods and Applications.* New York, NY: Springer; 2010:3–17.

7. Wilk P, Clark AF, Maltby A, Smith C, Tucker P, Gilliland JA. Examining individual, interpersonal, and environmental influences on children's physical activity levels. *SSM Popul Health.* 2017;4:76–85. https://doi.org/10.1016/j.ssmph.2017.11.004

8. Brug J, Kremers SP, Lenthe F, Ball K, Crawford D. Environmental determinants of healthy eating: In need of theory and evidence. *Proc Nutr Soc.* 2008;67:307–316. https://doi.org/10.1017/S0029665108008616

9. Glanz K, Rimer BK, Viswanath K, eds. *Health Behavior: Theory, Research, and Practice,* 5th ed. Jossey-Bass; 2015.

10. Buchan DS, Ollis S, Thomas NE, Baker JS. Physical activity behaviour: An overview of current and emergent theoretical practices. *J Obes.* 2012;2012:546459. doi:10.1155/ 2012/546459

11. Skinner CS, Tiro J, Champion VL. The health belief model. In *Health Behavior: Theory, Research, and Practice,* 5th ed. Hoboken, NJ, US: Jossey-Bass/Wiley; 2015:75–94.

12. Marcus B, King T, Clark M, Pinto B, Bock B. Theories and techniques for promoting physical activity behaviours. *Sports Med.* 1996;22:321–331. doi:10.2165/00007256-199622050-00005

13. Bandura A. *Social Cognitive Theory: An Agentic Perspective* on Human Nature. John Wiley & Sons; 2023:29.

14. Ajzen I. The theory of planned behavior. *Organ Behav Hum Decis Process.* 1991; 50:179–211. doi:10.1016/0749-5978(91)90020-T

15. Deci EL, Ryan RM. Self-determination theory. *Handbook of Theories of Social Psychology,* Vol. 1. Thousand Oaks, CA: Sage Publications Ltd.; 2012:416–436.

16. Prochaska JO. Transtheoretical model of behavior change. In: Gellman MD, ed. *Encyclopedia of Behavioral Medicine.* Cham: Springer International Publishing; 2020:2266–2270.

17. van Ryn M, Heaney CA. What's the use of theory? *Health Educ Q.* 1992;19:315–330. doi:10.1177/109019819201900304

18. Bandura A. Self-efficacy: Toward a unifying theory of behavioral change. *Psychol Rev.* 1977;84:191–215. doi:10.1037/0033-295X.84.2.191

19. Bauman AE, Reis RS, Sallis JF, Wells JC, Loos RJF, Martin BW, et al. Correlates of physical activity: Why are some people physically active and others not? *Lancet.* 2012;380:258–271. doi:10.1016/S0140-6736(12)60735-1

20. Haidar A, Ranjit N, Archer N, Hoelscher DM. Parental and peer social support is associated with healthier physical activity behaviors in adolescents: A cross-sectional analysis of Texas school physical activity and nutrition (TX SPAN) data. *BMC Public Health.* 2019;19:640. doi:10.1186/s12889-019-7001-0

21. Wicker AW. Ecological psychology: Some recent and prospective developments. *American Psychologist.* 1979;34:755–765. doi:10.1037/0003-066X.34.9.755

22. Ma P, Chan Z, Loke A. The socio-ecological model approach to understanding barriers and facilitators to the accessing of health services by sex workers: A systematic review. *AIDS and Behavior.* 2017;21. doi:10.1007/s10461-017-1818-2

23. Revenson TA, Gurung RAR. Health psychology rising: The current status and future directions of health psychology. *Handbook Health Psychol.* 2018; 3–14.

24. McBride CM, Rimer BK. Using the telephone to improve health behavior and health service delivery. *Patient Educ Couns.* 1999;37:3–18. doi:10.1016/S0738-3991(98)00098-6

25. Dobbins M, Husson H, DeCorby K, LaRocca RL. School-based physical activity programs for promoting physical activity and fitness in children and adolescents aged 6 to 18. *Cochrane Database Syst Rev.* 2013;2013:CD007651. doi:10.1002/14651858. CD007651.pub2

26. Goodyear VA, Skinner B, McKeever J, Griffiths M. The influence of online physical activity interventions on children and young people's engagement with physical activity: A systematic review. *Phys Educ Sport Pedagogy.* 2021;28:1–15. doi:10.1080/17408989. 2021.1953459

27. Dugdill L, Brettle A, Hulme C, Bartys S, Long A. Workplace physical activity interventions: A systematic review. *Int J Workplace Health Manag.* 2008;1. doi:10.1108/ 17538350810865578

28. Abdin S, Welch RK, Byron-Daniel J, Meyrick J. The effectiveness of physical activity interventions in improving well-being across office-based workplace settings: A systematic review. *Public Health.* 2018;160:70–76. doi:10.1016/j.puhe.2018.03.029

29. Strath SJ, Kaminsky LA, Ainsworth BE, Ekelund U, Freedson PS, Gary RA, et al. Guide to the assessment of physical activity: Clinical and research applications: A scientific statement from the American Heart Association. *Circulation.* 2013;128:2259–2279. doi:10.1161/01.cir.0000435708.67487.da

30. McClung HL, Ptomey LT, Shook RP, Aggarwal A, Gorczyca AM, Sazonov ES, et al. Dietary intake and physical activity assessment: Current tools, techniques, and technologies for use in adult populations. *Am J Prev Med.* 2018;55:e93–e104. doi:10.1016/j. amepre.2018.06.011

31. Westerterp KR. Assessment of physical activity: A critical appraisal. *Eur J Appl Physiol.* 2009;105:823–828. doi:10.1007/s00421-009-1000-2

32. Craig CL, Marshall AL, Sjöström M, Bauman AE, Booth ML, Ainsworth BE, et al. International physical activity questionnaire: 12-country reliability and validity. *Med Sci Sports Exerc.* 2003;35:1381–1395. doi:10.1249/01.MSS.0000078924.61453.FB

33. Cleland CL, Hunter RF, Kee F, Cupples ME, Sallis JF, Tully MA. Validity of the global physical activity questionnaire (GPAQ) in assessing levels and change in moderate-vigorous physical activity and sedentary behaviour. *BMC Public Health.* 2014;14:1255. doi:10.1186/1471-2458-14-1255

34. Finger JD, Tafforeau J, Gisle L, Oja L, Ziese T, Thelen J, et al. Development of the European health interview survey - physical activity questionnaire (EHIS-PAQ) to monitor physical activity in the European union. *Arch Public Health.* 2015;73:59. doi: 10.1186/s13690-015-0110-z

35. Ong L, Blumenthal JA. Assessment of physical activity in research and clinical practice. In: Steptoe A, ed. *Handbook of Behavioral Medicine: Methods and Applications.* New York, NY: Springer; 2010:31–48.

36. Morabito V. Wearable technologies. In: Morabito V, ed. *The Future of Digital Business Innovation: Trends and Practices.* Cham: Springer International Publishing; 2016:23–42.

37. Mulchandani R, Chandrasekaran AM, Shivashankar R, Kondal D, Agrawal A, Panniyammakal J, et al. Effect of workplace physical activity interventions on the cardio-metabolic health of working adults: Systematic review and meta-analysis. *Int J Behav Nutr Phys Act.* 2019;16:134. doi:10.1186/s12966-019-0896-0

38. Simpson RJ, Katsanis E. The immunological case for staying active during the COVID-19 pandemic. *Brain Behav Immun.* 2020;87:6–7. doi:10.1016/j.bbi.2020.04.041
39. Beeson RA. Loneliness and depression in spousal caregivers of those with Alzheimer's disease versus non-caregiving spouses. *Arch Psychiatr Nurs.* 2003;17:135–143. doi:10.1016/s0883-9417(03)00057-8
40. Beeson R, Horton-Deutsch S, Farran C, Neundorfer M. Loneliness and depression in caregivers of persons with Alzheimer's disease or related disorders. *Issues Ment Health Nurs.* 2000;21:779–806. doi:10.1080/016128400750044279
41. Kilaberia T, Bell J, Bettega K, Mongoven J, Kelly K, Young H. Impact of the COVID-19 pandemic on family caregivers. *Innov Aging.* 2020;4:950. doi:10.1093/geroni/igaa057.3475
42. Miller WR, Rollnick S. *Motivational Interviewing: Preparing People for Change,* 2nd ed. New York, NY, US: The Guilford Press; 2002.
43. Stonerock GL, Blumenthal JA. Role of counseling to promote adherence in healthy lifestyle medicine: Strategies to improve exercise adherence and enhance physical activity. *Prog Cardiovasc Dis.* 2017;59:455–462. doi:10.1016/j.pcad.2016.09.003.
44. Prochaska JO, DiClemente CC. Stages and processes of self-change of smoking: Toward an integrative model of change. *J Consult Clin Psychol.* 1983;51:390–395. doi:10.1037//0022-006x.51.3.390
45. CDC. *Physical Activity.* Centers for Disease Control and Prevention. 2022. URL: https://www.cdc.gov/physicalactivity/index.html (Accessed 26 September 2022).
46. Demark-Wahnefried W, Jones LW, Snyder DC, Sloane RJ, Kimmick GG, Hughes DC, *et al.* Daughters and mothers against breast cancer (DAMES): Main outcomes of a randomized controlled trial of weight loss in overweight mothers with breast cancer and their overweight daughters. *Cancer.* 2014;120:2522–2534. doi:10.1002/cncr.28761
47. Bowen DJ, Kreuter M, Spring B, Cofta-Woerpel L, Linnan L, Weiner D, et al. How we design feasibility studies. *Am J Prev Med.* 2009;36:452–457. doi:10.1016/j.amepre.2009.02.002
48. Owen N, Sparling PB, Healy GN, Dunstan DW, Matthews CE. Sedentary behavior: Emerging evidence for a new health risk. *Mayo Clin Proc.* 2010;85:1138–1141. doi:10.4065/mcp.2010.0444
49. Lewis B, Napolitano M, Buman M, Williams D, Nigg C. Future directions in physical activity intervention research: Expanding our focus to sedentary behaviors, technology, and dissemination. *J Behav Med.* 2017;40. https://doi.org/10.1007/s10865-016-9797-8
50. Griffith DM, Bergner EM, Cornish EK, McQueen CM. Physical activity interventions with African American or Latino men: A systematic review. *Am J Mens Health* 2018;12:1102–1117. https://doi.org/10.1177/1557988318763647
51. American College of Lifestyle Medicine. 6 Pillars of Lifestyle Medicine. American College of Lifestyle Medicine. n.d. URL: https://lifestylemedicine.org/ (Accessed 18 January 2023).
52. Woolf SH, Schoomaker H. Life expectancy and mortality rates in the United States, 1959–2017. *JAMA* 2019;322:1996–2016. doi:10.1001/jama.2019.16932

19 Nutrition in Lifestyle Psychiatry

Gia Merlo, MD, MBA, MEd
and Gabrielle Bachtel, BS

KEY POINTS

- Research has shown that dietary interventions can play an important role in preventing and treating mental health problems and reducing mortality, morbidity, and health inequalities associated with mental illnesses.
- Eating patterns can impact brain function, mood, and cognitive performance.
- Whole food, nutrient-dense, plant-predominant dietary interventions may be considered an essential component of mental health care because they provide important nutrients for brain function, support the brain-gut-microbiota axis, reduce inflammation and oxidative stress, and can have specific effects on neurotransmitter production and mental health outcomes.

19.1 INTRODUCTION

Consideration of nutritional interventions within the mental health care space may have major clinical implications for improving mental health, physical health, and brain health outcomes. Poor diet, defined as low consumption of fruits, vegetables, legumes, whole grains, and nuts and seeds, as well as high consumption of red meat, processed meat, and sugar-sweetened beverages, has been identified as a leading contributor to the global burden of disease.[1] According to the World Health Organization (WHO), a healthy diet includes fruits, vegetables, legumes, nuts, and whole grains, limited refined sugar and sodium, and polyunsaturated fats in replacement of saturated fats and trans-fats.[2] Data indicate that adherence to the minimum WHO dietary recommendations would necessitate at least a twofold increase in the consumption of fruits and vegetables by most adults worldwide.[3] One in ten Americans consume enough fruits or vegetables to meet daily recommendations, nine in ten Americans consume too much sodium, and at least five in ten Americans consume at least one sugar-sweetened beverage per day.[4] Dietary factors contribute to almost 20% of all US healthcare costs related to chronic disease.[5] Almost one in three people affected by a long-term physical health condition are also affected by a mental health condition.[6] Dietary patterns can significantly impact overall health and well-being, thereby establishing nutrition as a critical interventional target and key physical and mental health for healthcare professionals, as well as a key risk factor for chronic disease onset and progression.[7]

DOI: 10.1201/b22810-22

There is emerging data demonstrating that there may be a link between chronic conditions (e.g., diabetes, cardiovascular disease) and mental health conditions (e.g., depression, anxiety).[8] A bidirectional relationship between diet and mental health has also been established by both epidemiological studies and intervention studies.[9,10] The possible entanglement of the associations between chronic diseases, mental health, and nutrition may provide insight into the global trends in mental health, burden of disease, and unhealthy dietary patterns. In light of evidence clustering psychiatric disorders, cardiometabolic diseases, and lifestyle factors, such as daily food choices, mental healthcare professionals have the unique opportunity to utilize nutritional interventions from a lifestyle psychiatry perspective as a patient-centered tool to address both individual health concerns and the global need for attenuation of mental illness and chronic disease on a population-level scale. This chapter will discuss nutrition as an integral component of lifestyle psychiatry, as well as a key determinant and factor in mental health outcomes and outcomes for those with mental health illness.

19.2 THE SYNERGY OF MENTAL HEALTH CARE AND NUTRITIONAL INTERVENTIONS

Those suffering from subsyndromal or syndromal psychiatric symptoms are at increased risk for inadequate nutrition, which may further exacerbate mental, physical, and brain health issues.[11] The World Health Organization has reported that mental health disorders are the leading cause of years lived with disability.[12] Mental health care, in conjunction with healthy dietary interventions, can significantly improve health outcomes in psychiatric patients.[13] However, individuals with mental health disorders are more likely to encounter obstacles to attaining adequate mental health care and adhering to healthy dietary patterns than those without mental health disorders.[9] Multiple factors can affect the ability of people living with mental illnesses to receive proper mental health treatment and make healthy food choices, including financial obstacles, geographic barriers, inadequate social support, and availability of and access to healthy food and mental health providers, as well as healthcare professionals equipped with dietary information and resources in the setting of mental health conditions.[14–16] Data suggest that only half of all individuals with mental disorders receive appropriate mental health treatment.[17] One in four Americans must decide between paying for daily necessities and receiving mental health treatment.[18] Moreover, 37% of the U.S. population live in areas with a shortage of mental health practitioners as of 2021.[19]

Insufficient mental health treatment for people living with mental health disorders can compound barriers to healthy eating. Cognitive impairments; decreased attention, motivation, and information processing; limited nutrition knowledge and skills essential to making informed and healthy dietary decisions; increased appetite due to psychotropic medications; and certain personality traits (e.g., neuroticism) are barriers to healthy eating associated with mental health conditions that can impact lifestyle decision-making, shopping, and food preparation capabilities.[15,20–22] Individuals affected by severe mental illness have a higher risk of food insecurity, which further hinders ability to adhere to healthy eating behaviors.[21,23] Awareness and prioritization of mental health and the implications of lifestyle factors, such as nutrition, on mental and physical health alike is increasing. However, the average governmental health budget worldwide spends only slightly more than two percent on mental health services.[12] The statistics surrounding mental health care and nutrition in those at risk for or affected by mental health conditions indicate that further integration of dietary components may be an effective strategy to provide patients with crucial tools and support to make healthy lifestyle choices and achieve improved health outcomes.[24]

19.3   THE EFFECTS OF PSYCHIATRIC MEDICATIONS ON MENTAL HEALTH THROUGH THE LENS OF NUTRITION

Pharmacotherapy and psychotherapy have been historically recommended as the first line of treatment for those with mental disorders.[25] Emerging evidence indicates that traditional treatment regimens for mental disorders may be less effective than established literature suggests.[26] Psychopharmacological interventions for mental conditions may attenuate individual disability and suffering. However, pharmacotherapy may have limited influence on the burden associated with mental disorders at the population level.[27–29] Research has shown that about half of those diagnosed with a psychiatric disorder do not appropriately adhere to their medication regimen.[30] An average of one in five patients assigned to pharmacotherapy and psychotherapy prematurely terminate their treatment.[31] Of note, patients with mental health conditions who are treated with pharmacotherapy alone are more likely to prematurely terminate or refuse treatment than those treated with psychotherapy.[31] There is a current paucity of evidence analyzing adherence to lifestyle interventions, such as dietary interventions, in patients with poor mental health and mental health illnesses.

19.3.1   ADVERSE EFFECTS OF PSYCHOTROPIC MEDICATIONS

There are differences between and within drug classes regarding the effects of psychotropic medications on bodyweight, metabolic status, and appetite. Weight gain is recognized as a common adverse effect of antidepressant, antipsychotic, mood-stabilizing, and other classes of pharmacotherapeutic agents used in the treatment and management of psychiatric disorders.[32–34] The association between psychotropic drugs and weight gain may be mediated by increased appetite via drug-induced metabolic effects.[35] Some medications used in patients with mental health conditions can also have sedative effects, including decreased mental alertness, attenuated cognitive and psychomotor function, and increased fatigue.[36] These adverse effects may impact lifestyle-related decision-making abilities, as well as exercise habits in patients taking psychotropic medications, which may lead to insufficient physical activity necessary to balance caloric consumption and weight gain. However, further research is needed to elucidate the mechanisms by which appetite is increased via psychotropic medications.

19.3.2 Psychiatric Medications

Most of the most commonly prescribed psychiatric medications (i.e., selective serotonin reuptake inhibitors) are antidepressants which target the serotonin network.[37] Almost every aspect of human behavior is modulated by serotonin, including but not limited to attention, mood, perception, memory, reward, sexuality, and appetite.[38] Data indicate that a serotonergic antidepressant administered alone results in remission in less than a third of patients.[39] Of note, remission is achieved in only half of patients taking a second medication in addition to a traditional antidepressant. The use of a third medication targeting the serotonin pathway rarely results in remission for patients who do not adequately respond to two different monoaminergic antidepressants.[40] Systemic inflammation, neuroinflammation, and chronic stress, which may be at least partially mediated by diet, can interfere with the efficacy of medications used to treat mental and brain health disorders, as well as treatment resistance.[41] Research suggests that there is a bidirectional link between inflammation, health status, and mental conditions.[42] Data have revealed that negative outcomes of first-line antidepressant therapy are associated with the presence of inflammation in patients with major depressive disorder.[43] Pro-inflammatory processes and overactivation of the immune system have also been correlated with the attenuated clinical therapeutic benefit of antidepressants and pharmacotherapeutic agents used in the management of mental health illnesses.[44]

19.3.3 Anti-inflammatory Effects

Dietary intake of anti-inflammatory compounds, including vitamins, minerals, omega-3 fatty acids, polyphenol, and probiotics through fruits, vegetables, legumes, nuts, seeds, spices, and herbs, in conjunction with avoidance of foodstuffs that promote inflammation may facilitate regulation of metabolic, oxidative, and inflammatory processes, as well as enhance production of neurotransmitters and integrity of the blood-brain barrier.[45] These diet-induced effects on the brain-gut-microbiota (BGM) axis are linked to lower risk of neurological and psychiatric conditions and may enhance health outcomes and effectiveness of pharmaceutical agents that target neurotransmitter systems in patients with mental illnesses.[13] According to a blueprint for protecting physical health in individuals living with mental illness, the combination of dietary interventions with best-practice prescription of psychotropic medications, physical activity, smoking cessation, and metformin use are key strategies that ought to be implemented in the healthcare field in order to improve health outcomes, as well as reduce health inequalities and increased risk of mortality in psychiatric patients.[46]

19.4 WEIGHT, METABOLIC STATUS, AND MENTAL HEALTH

Metabolic mechanisms may play a crucial mediatory role in the link between mental illness, chronic disease, and nutrition. An emerging body of evidence suggests a potential positive bidirectional relationship between metabolic status, body mass index (BMI), and mental health.[47] Individuals with overweight and obesity have an increased risk of psychiatric conditions, including mood disorders, anxiety disorders, and substance use disorders, that are independent of physical health conditions.[48,49] Those with BMIs in the overweight or obese ranges also have an increased risk of physical health issues, decreased life expectancy, and worsened quality of life compared to those with a normal BMI.[50,51] The prevalence of overweight, obesity, metabolic syndrome, diabetes, hypertension, hypertriglyceridemia, and low HDL is higher among individuals with severe mental illness in comparison to the general population.[52] Data have shown that individuals with mental conditions have more years of potential life loss than the general population.[53] Indeed, physical comorbidities (e.g., cardiovascular diseases) account for approximately 60% of the increased mortality in psychiatric patients.[52]

Dietary interventions, in conjunction with other lifestyle interventions (e.g., physical activity, substance use harm reduction), appropriate psychotropic pharmacotherapy, and metformin, may be key strategies to reduce health inequities, attenuate adverse effects of drugs, and decrease the mortality gap and common comorbid physical conditions, such as overweight or obesity, in people with mental illness.[46] Lifestyle interventions have been found to attenuate medication-induced weight gain in individuals with mental health disorders and may reduce risk of comorbidity and reduce the life expectancy gap for people living with poor mental health or mental health conditions.[54,55] Multiple variables, including lifestyle and behavioral factors, quality of healthcare, and social determinants of health (e.g. social connectivity, socioeconomic status), as well as availability of and access to healthcare, contribute to the increased mortality observed among individuals with mental health conditions.[56] It is important to note that those with mental disorders are often not provided with preventive services or consultation, which may further increase their risk of multimorbidity and poorer health outcomes and mental health symptoms.[57]

19.5 INSULIN RESISTANCE AND MENTAL HEALTH

Growing evidence suggests that insulin resistance may be linked to mental health conditions.[58] Insulin receptors are expressed ubiquitously throughout the brain. There is a higher expression of insulin receptors in specific brain regions, such as the hypothalamus, cerebellum, and cortex.[59] Glucose uptake in the brain is primarily insulin-independent. However, insulin activity modulates mitochondrial and cellular metabolism in both the periphery and the brain.[59] Several higher-order cognitive functions, such as learning and memory, are regulated by insulin through modulation of neural stem cell fate and neural network function.[60] Insulin has been shown to exert neurotrophic effects and promote metabolic and central nervous system homeostasis that facilitates neuroplasticity.[61] Insulin may alter mitochondrial function and turnover of neurotransmitters, thereby indicating a potential link between insulin resistance and mental health conditions.[27,62]

It has been noted that high-fat diets and excess daily calorie intake can result in insulin resistance and impaired signaling throughout the BGM axis via mechanisms such as inflammation, mitochondrial dysfunction, and endoplasmic reticulum stress in the hypothalamus.[63] Research has indicated an association between insulin resistance, impaired executive function, and memory, decreased hippocampal volume, abnormal neural connectivity between the hippocampus and medial prefrontal cortex, and altered metabolism in the medial prefrontal cortex.[64] Higher levels of insulin resistance are associated with more severe neuropsychiatric symptoms.[65] Moreover, data that consider confounding variables (e.g., body mass index) suggest that psychological factors may be linked to the development and progression of insulin resistance and type 2 diabetes.[66,67] Therefore, there may be a bidirectional relationship between depressive and affective symptomatology and insulin resistance due to altered insulin signaling, increased pro-inflammatory compounds, upregulated distress-related signals in the hypothalamic-pituitary-adrenal (HPA) axis, and enhanced activation of the sympathetic nervous system.[68]

Insulin resistance can be appropriately addressed through lifestyle interventions, such as diet, exercise, and behavioral therapies.[69] There is a well-established link between lower insulin resistance and diets high in plant-based foods and low in animal-based foods. A whole food, plant-predominant eating pattern can reduce the risk of insulin resistance by over 30%.[70] Of note, a plant-predominant eating pattern with reduced quality and increased processed foods has been correlated to an increased risk of insulin resistance.[71] Therefore, dietary interventions in clinical practices that aim to promote mental health, physical health, and overall well-being through insulin and blood sugar regulation should emphasize the importance of dietary quality and whole foods in healthy plant-based diets.

19.6 TRYPTOPHAN-KYNURENINE METABOLISM

Psychiatric disorders, neurodegenerative diseases, cancer, and immune diseases have been linked to disruptions in the tryptophan-kynurenine metabolic pathway.[72,73] There is an emerging area of research in psychiatry related to the metabolism of tryptophan along the kynurenine pathway and how it may influence mental health issues. It has been hypothesized that a serotonin deficiency or excess of kynurenine metabolites may affect the onset, progression, and outcomes of depression, mood disorders, and other mental health conditions.[74-76] The tryptophan-kynurenine metabolic pathway converts the essential amino acid tryptophan, a precursor for neurotransmitters and hormones, into various metabolites, including serotonin and kynurenine. Both neurotoxic metabolites (e.g., quinolinic acid) and neuroprotective metabolites (e.g., kynurenic acid) are involved in the tryptophan-kynurenine metabolic pathway. The tryptophan-kynurenine metabolic pathway is activated in the setting of acute or chronic inflammation and is regulated by a variety of factors, such as oxidative stress, inflammation, and availability of tryptophan. Evidence suggests that there is a strong correlation between dietary intake and tryptophan availability.[77] Gut microbiota directly and indirectly modulate the tryptophan metabolism.[78-80] Therefore, tryptophan and its related metabolic pathways play an important role in maintaining the proper function of the BGM and the immune system.[81]

Many pharmacotherapeutic agents prescribed for the treatment of mental health conditions, such as depression and anxiety disorders, involve neuroactive compounds that are derived from tryptophan.[82] Serotonergic neurotransmission is enhanced by a diet rich in tryptophan.[83] Dietary tryptophan intake is correlated to attenuated depressive symptoms, decreased anxiety, reduced stress, improved mood, and enhanced cognitive functioning.[84-88] The gut microbiota produces indole byproducts of tryptophan metabolism that play a critical role in transmitting signals along the BGM axis.[89] Clinical interventions promoting a balanced diet that incorporates foods with anti-inflammatory and antioxidant benefits, as well as adequate levels of dietary tryptophan, may be beneficial for optimal mental and physical health through mechanisms related to the tryptophan-kynurenine metabolic pathway, enhanced production of neurotransmitters, and increased diversity of gut microbiota.

19.7   THE BRAIN-GUT-MICROBIOTA AXIS AND MENTAL HEALTH

Dietary factors may regulate a multitude of pathways along the BGM axis that can have implications on mental health.[90] The BGM axis involves bidirectional communication between the central nervous system (CNS) and gut microbiota. Microorganisms living in the gastrointestinal tract, including bacteria, fungi, viruses, and protozoa, compose the gut microbiota. The gut microbiota plays a key role in overall health across the lifespan.[91] The gut microbiota aid digestion and absorption of nutrients, regulation of the immune system, production of substances involved in various metabolic and endocrine pathways in the body, and communication with the central nervous system to influence behavior, mood, and cognitive function.[92] Neural, endocrine, and immune signaling channels transmit information from gut flora to the CNS. The CNS is capable of directly communicating with gut microbiota by altering the expression of virulence genes through stress-related mediators, such as through the HPA axis, and indirectly communicating with gut microbiota by influencing gut function through the autonomic nervous system.[93,94]

Human gut microbiota colonization begins at the time of birth.[95] Diet, genetics, metabolic status, body mass index, age, epigenetics, psychological and physical stress, and other environmental factors can affect the gut microbiome and thereby alter communication along the BGM axis and the vast array of bodily mechanisms mediated by the BGM axis.[96] Diet is the most significant determinant of microbiota composition in adults over the course of the lifespan.[97] Structure and function of the gut microbiome, the collective genetic material within the gut microbiota, can be influenced by a variety of dietary factors, such as quantity and quality of carbohydrates, proteins, fats, vitamins, and minerals, as well as food processing and food additives.[98] Gut dysbiosis is characterized by decreased diversity of gut microbiota, reduced beneficial microbiota, and increased harmful microbiota.[99] Studies have shown that gut dysbiosis may be associated with mental illnesses, neurodevelopmental disorders, and other conditions, such as cancer, neurodegenerative disorders, and cardiovascular, metabolic, skin, and infectious diseases.[100-102]

19.8   HPA AXIS

A growing body of data suggests that dysregulation or alterations of the hypothalamic-pituitary-adrenal (HPA) axis may affect psychoneuroendoimmunological functions in the body (i.e., behavioral, metabolic, autonomic, and neuroendocrine activities).[103] The HPA axis is a major component of the BGM axis that plays a central role in maintaining homeostasis in the setting of stress by modulating immune responses, metabolism, and autonomic nervous system processes through neuroendocrine mechanisms. Stress-mediated activation of the HPA axis facilitates communication along the BGM axis. Activation of the HPA axis triggers immune responses that can lead to dysbiosis. Bacteria produce substances that stimulate the enteric nervous system and vagal afferents in the setting of reduced diversity of the gut microbiota diversity, which results in enhanced activation of the HPA axis.[104] Research has revealed that several environmental factors influence HPA axis functioning, including insulin regulation, metabolic status, and composition of gut microbiota.[105] There is evidence that the high comorbidity of mental disorders and obesity may be linked to altered insulin receptor signaling in neurons responsible for the integration of psychiatric and metabolic information.[106,107] Research indicates that diet may be a key common modulatory factor among the mechanisms that contribute to worsened mental and physical health outcomes, including metabolic abnormalities, gut dysbiosis, HPA axis dysfunction, and inflammation.

19.9 INFLAMMATION

The role of nutrition in mental health status and mental health disorders may be largely modulated by inflammation, including neuroinflammation. Numerous factors can contribute to inflammation, such as diet, dysbiosis of the gut microbiome, leaky gut syndrome, epigenetics, biopsychosocial factors, genetics, metabolic status, and early life adversity (Haroon et al., 2012).[108] Research has demonstrated that diets high in pro-inflammatory foodstuffs, such as saturated fats, trans-fats, simple carbohydrates, refined sugars, and processed food products increase levels of inflammation in the body.[109–113] Excess caloric intake and unhealthy dietary patterns can damage the blood-brain barrier and allow proinflammatory substances to enter the CNS.[114] The microorganisms and immune cells involved in the BGM axis play a critical role in maintaining overall health and protecting the body against harmful stimuli. Excessive or prolonged levels of inflammation can eventually lead to chronic inflammation through tissue and organ damage, which has been linked to poor mental health and severe mental illnesses, as well as chronic disease.[46]

Diet plays a significant role in the mediation of inflammation, oxidative stress, and mitochondrial function.[115] Inflammation is closely linked to oxidative stress and mitochondrial dysfunction. Inflammatory cells produce reactive oxygen species in immunological pathways, which can lead to oxidative stress and mitochondrial dysfunction. Oxidative stress can be induced by inflammation, exposure to toxins or infection, and unhealthy dietary habits. Increasing evidence indicates that neuropsychiatric disorders are mediated by impaired antioxidant capacity, inflammation, neurotoxicity, and free radicals.[116] It is important to note that nutritionally-induced oxidative stress can occur even in the setting of normal physiological conditions.[117] Evidence has also indicated that there may be a link between poor diet and mitochondrial dysfunction.[118] Excessive long-term exposure to pro-oxidant and proinflammatory factors can lead to abnormal mitochondrial biogenesis, which leads to an increase in free radical production, inflammation, and insulin resistance.[119] Notably, the saturated fats, heme iron, and other compounds found in many animal products can cause oxidative stress, inflammation, and damage to mitochondrial

DNA when consumed in excess. Plant-predominant eating patterns are linked to attenuated inflammation and oxidative damage.[120] Dietary patterns that emphasize plant-based foods may be useful for lifestyle interventions in the mental health care space for individuals who are at risk of or affected by mental illness to reduce inflammation and oxidative damage, improve gut health, and enhance overall health in patients whose mental health conditions may be directly and indirectly affected by food choices.

19.10 EPIGENETIC CHANGE

Epigenetic nutrition-gene interactions have implications for mental health and well-being, mental disorders, and neurological (e.g., neurodegenerative, neurodevelopmental) disorders.[121] Epigenetics is the study of changes in gene expression that do not involve alterations to the underlying DNA sequence. Epigenetic changes in gene expression can be influenced by a variety of factors, including environmental and lifestyle factors (e.g., diet). The chemical modification of DNA appears to be one of the most important epigenetic mechanisms underpinning the interaction between lifestyle and environmental factors. There are biochemical links between nutritional quality and mental health that may be partially explained by the influence of many dietary components on genomic pathways that methylate DNA.[122] It is becoming increasingly evident that epigenetic changes contribute to many diseases, such as mental illnesses, cognitive dysfunction, autoimmune disorders, and cancer.[123,124] There is evidence that diets rich in fruits and vegetables may have similar effects on DNA compared to those of epigenetic drugs.[125] Advances in nutritional epigenomics and genomics have led to a greater understanding of the mechanisms by which nutrition interacts with genes. Research has shown that cell structure and function in the brain are significantly influenced by nutrition-gene interactions.[126] Therefore, nutrition-gene interactions can impart significant effects on brain health, dysfunction, and disease. Changing gene expression is one of the primary mechanisms by which nutrition impacts the functioning of the central nervous system. These diet-induced genetic alterations may be transient, dynamic, stable, long-term, or heritable and can have significant impacts on mental health, physical health, and overall health.[127] However, more studies in clinical settings are needed to gain deeper insight into the impact of nutritional interventions on epigenetics and their potential therapeutic applications, as well as effects in the setting of specific psychiatric conditions.

19.11 ULTRA-PROCESSED FOODS

There is growing evidence to suggest that there may be a link between ultra-processed foods and mental health.[128] The Food and Agriculture Organization of the United Nations defines ultra-processed foods as "formulations of ingredients, mostly of exclusive industrial use, typically created by series of industrial techniques and processes...some common ultra-processed products are carbonated soft drinks; sweet, fatty or salty packaged snacks; candies (confectionery); mass-produced packaged breads and buns, cookies (biscuits), pastries, cakes and cake mixes; margarine and other spreads; sweetened breakfast 'cereals' and fruit yogurt and 'energy' drinks; pre-prepared meat, cheese, pasta and pizza dishes; poultry and fish 'nuggets' and 'sticks'; sausages, burgers, hot dogs and other reconstituted meat products; powdered and packaged 'instant' soups, noodles, and desserts; baby formula; and many other types of product".[129] Ultra-processed food intake has continuously increased in the majority of the US population in the past two decades. Consumption of ultra-processed foods in the US increased from 53.5% of daily calorie intake to 57% of daily calorie intake between 2001 and 2018.[130] Data have demonstrated that there is a 25% higher risk of dementia for every 10% increase in daily intake of ultra-processed foods after adjusting for factors such as age, gender, and family history of disease.[131]

Research has also shown that the consumption of ultra-processed foods is associated with a higher risk of developing depression and anxiety.[132,133] There is a statistically significant increase in mild depression, poor mental health, and anxious days among individuals who report eating ultra-processed foods.[134] Consumption of ultra-processed foods has also been associated with an increased risk of chronic metabolic diseases.[135] Data suggest that ultra-processed foods negatively impact the gut microbiota and promote inflammation, which play a crucial role in mental health status.[136] Of note, gut microbiome dysbiosis has been linked to the development of neurodegenerative diseases and mental illnesses, as well as an increased risk of poor mental health. The consumption of ultra-processed foods can have negative effects on mental health and increase the risk of mental illness, as well as adverse health consequences such as multimorbidity and inflammation, that may result in poorer health outcomes.

19.12 NEUROTRANSMITTERS, DIET, AND MENTAL HEALTH

Altered levels of neurotransmitters, including serotonin, dopamine, norepinephrine, histamine, acetylcholine, glutamate, and gamma-aminobutyric acid (GABA), contribute to the pathophysiology of numerous diseases, such as depression, substance use disorders, Alzheimer's disease, Parkinson's disease, autism spectrum disorders, schizophrenia, multiple sclerosis, sleep disorders, amyotrophic lateral sclerosis, epilepsy, and Huntington's disease.[137–141] The composition of microbiota in the gut can alter neurotransmitter levels via both direct production of neurotransmitters or indirect regulation of pathways related to neurotransmitter metabolism.[142] Gut microbiota release various molecules, metabolites, and toxins that can significantly impact neurotransmitter production, metabolism, and signaling.[143,144] Interactions within the BGM system can alter the expression of neurotransmitters, precursors to neurotransmitters, and neurotransmitter receptors in the central nervous system through the bloodstream or vagus nerve pathways, thereby influencing brain function, cognitive behavior, and a wide range of physiological and psychological processes.[145]

Over 90% of serotonin is synthesized in the gastrointestinal tract.[146,147] About half of all dopamine in the body is produced and stored in the gut.[148,149] Increasing evidence suggests that gut microbiota also synthesize or play a role in metabolizing other neurotransmitters, such as norepinephrine, acetylcholine, GABA, and histamine.[150,151] Research suggests that dietary choices and nutrients significantly impact the balance and production of neurotransmitters in the brain.[152] Neurotransmitters are chemical messengers that transmit signals between nerve cells and play a crucial role in regulating cognitive function, behavior, and mood.

Nutrients play an essential role as co-factors in the production of neurotransmitters. Many neurotransmitters are derived from dietary amino acids, such as tryptophan, tyrosine, and phenylalanine. These amino acids serve as precursors for the synthesis of neurotransmitters, including dopamine, serotonin, and norepinephrine. For example, the cofactors vitamin B6 and iron are required to convert tryptophan to serotonin.[153] Vitamin C, folate, and iron are needed to synthesize dopamine and norepinephrine.[154] Other dietary co-factors, such as magnesium, zinc, and vitamin D, are also important in the production of neurotransmitters. Magnesium plays a role in the regulation and synthesis of acetylcholine, which plays an important role in learning and memory, and other neurotransmitter systems.[155,156] Zinc is necessary to modulate GABA, which helps regulate mood and anxiety.[157] Vitamin D is involved in synthesizing brain-derived neurotrophic factor, which is a protein that supports the survival and growth of neurons.[158] Therefore, balanced diets incorporating nutrient-dense, plant-based foods can support neurotransmitter production by providing nutrients necessary for their synthesis and protection against inflammation and oxidative stress. Healthy dietary interventions in patients with mental health conditions may help to reduce the risk or severity of mental illnesses, improve mood, and enhance cognitive function.

19.13 MATERNAL–FETAL NUTRITIONAL NEUROSCIENCE: THE FUTURE

Nutrition, mental health status, and environment during pregnancy may have both immediate and long-lasting impacts on offspring health outcomes. A pregnant person's diet can lead to epigenetic changes in the developing fetus, altering gene expression and increasing risk of mental health disorders in offspring. Epigenetic changes induced by events, including quality and quantity of nutrients, during embryonic, fetal, or neonatal development may alter mechanisms underlying growth, metabolism, temperament/personality, intelligence, and susceptibility to chronic disease in offspring that may manifest in childhood and often persist into adulthood.[159–161] Global epidemiological data have revealed that one-third of those afflicted by mental health disorders experience onset of their first mental health disorder before the age of 14, almost half by the age of 18, and over half before the age of 25.[162] Therefore, clinical applications of nutritional interventions via lifestyle psychiatry may be especially crucial in pregnant populations and offspring throughout key developmental periods. The pre-conception, pregnancy, perinatal, and early postnatal time periods are key developmental phases during which rapid and critical maturation processes occur in neural, endocrine, immune, and metabolic systems of offspring.[163–171] These time windows of development are extremely sensitive to internal and external stimuli and pivotal predictors of neurocognitive development, as well as BGM axis and immune system function, of offspring across the lifespan. The microbiome of offspring is influenced by maternal diet during pregnancy.[172] A period of development with irreversible health implications occurs as early as the first few months of life when bacterial signals are required for the normal development of neurobehavioral systems. Some studies have demonstrated that the standardized coefficients for the relationship between dietary exposure in pregnant people and mental health outcomes for offspring are similar in magnitude to those for depression, which is a well-established risk factor for poor mental health disorders in children.[160,173]

19.14 HUMAN STUDIES SURROUNDING NUTRITION

The most affordable and cost-effective dietary patterns are plant-predominant in nature.[174] Studies have shown that prescribing healthful foods and diets to patient populations, including those at high risk for poor health outcomes (e.g., individuals with lower socioeconomic status, individuals with disabilities, the elderly), can be a highly cost-effective and cost-saving method of providing healthcare that also results in improved health outcomes.[175] Of note, research findings that support the implementation of nutrition programs within public and private healthcare systems are consistent across patient population subgroups, such as those related to race, ethnicity, age, education, socioeconomic status, and status of participation in the Supplemental Nutrition Assistance Program (SNAP).[5]

Research evaluating the link between healthy dietary patterns and disease outcomes has largely focused on specific dietary components (e.g., vitamins, minerals, phytonutrients), dietary indices (e.g., inflammatory, glycemic), and healthy eating frameworks such as the Mediterranean diet or the Dietary Approaches to Stop Hypertension (DASH). Recent literature has shown that adherence to the Mediterranean-DASH Intervention for Neurodegenerative Delay (MIND) diet, Mediterranean diet, and DASH diet is associated with decreased risk of psychiatric and neurodegenerative conditions, increased cognitive function, and protection against cognitive decline.[176–179] The Mediterranean, DASH, and MIND dietary patterns include the following: emphasize whole, nutrient-dense foods; limit unhealthy, processed foods and refined sugars; promote plant-based sources of healthy fats; and have been shown to exert a positive impact on mental health. The MIND diet may improve mental health and brain health via anti-inflammatory and antioxidant mechanisms, as well as contain fewer unhealthy foodstuffs, such as processed foods, red meat, and refined sugars, than typical Western eating patterns. Greater adherence to the MIND diet has been correlated with increased mental health and brain health benefits.[180] It has also been noted that those who follow the MIND diet have lower stress levels due to dietary neuroprotective factors.[181] Emerging data suggest that the MIND diet can reverse the harmful implications of obesity on cognition and brain structure.[182]

Plant-predominant eating patterns that incorporate minimally processed foods and include vegetables, fresh fruits, legumes, and whole grains and lower intakes of saturated fats, trans-fats, sodium, refined sugar, and animal proteins are linked to and predictive of better mental health and physical health outcomes.[9] Literature indicates that whole food eating patterns are protective against mental health symptoms and increase quality of life, while processed food intake is a risk factor for poor mental health and mental illnesses and lower quality of life.[183,184] Increased consumption of whole foods is associated with attenuated mental health symptoms and decreased risk of mental illness. In conclusion, intervention programs aiming to improve physical health can also significantly improve mental health, furthering previous evidence regarding the bidirectional entanglement of mental health, physical health, and nutrition.[185]

REFERENCES

1. GBD 2019 Risk Factors Collaborators. Global burden of 87 risk factors in 204 countries and territories, 1990–2019: A systematic analysis for the global burden of disease study 2019. *Lancet.* 2020;396(10258):1223–1249. doi:10.1016/S0140-6736(20)30752-2

2. WHO. Healthy diet. Accessed April 24, 2023. https://www.who.int/news-room/fact-sheets/detail/healthy-diet

3. Murphy MM, Barraj LM, Spungen JH, Herman DR, Randolph RK. Global assessment of select phytonutrient intakes by level of fruit and vegetable consumption. *Br J Nutr.* 2014;112(6):1004–1018. doi:10.1017/S0007114514001937

4. CDC. Diabetes and Mental Health. Centers for Disease Control and Prevention. Accessed April 19, 2023. https://www.cdc.gov/diabetes/managing/mental-health.html

5. Lee Y, Mozaffarian D, Sy S, et al. Cost-effectiveness of financial incentives for improving diet and health through medicare and medicaid: A microsimulation study. *PLoS Med.* 2019;16(3):e1002761. doi:10.1371/journal.pmed.1002761

6. Physical Health and Mental Health. Accessed April 24, 2023. https://www.mental-health.org.uk/explore-mental-health/a-z-topics/physical-health-and-mental-health

7. Merlo G, Vela A. Mental health in lifestyle medicine: A call to action. *Am J Lifestyle Med.* 2022;16(1):7–20. doi:10.1177/15598276211013313

8. Bobo WV, Grossardt BR, Virani S, St Sauver JL, Boyd CM, Rocca WA. Association of depression and anxiety with the accumulation of chronic conditions. *JAMA Netw Open.* 2022;5(5):e229817. doi:10.1001/jamanetworkopen.2022.9817

9. Jacka FN, O'Neil A, Opie R, et al. A randomised controlled trial of dietary improvement for adults with major depression (the "SMILES" trial). *BMC Med.* 2017;15(1):23. doi:10.1186/s12916-017-0791-y

10. Gall SL, Sanderson K, Smith KJ, Patton G, Dwyer T, Venn A. Bi-directional associations between healthy lifestyles and mood disorders in young adults: The childhood determinants of adult health study. *Psychol Med.* 2016;46(12):2535–2548. doi:10.1017/S0033291716000738

11. Owen L, Corfe B. The role of diet and nutrition on mental health and wellbeing. *Proc Nutr Soc.* 2017;76(4):425–426. doi:10.1017/S0029665117001057

12. WHO. World Mental Health Report. Accessed April 19, 2023. https://www.who.int/teams/mental-health-and-substance-use/world-mental-health-report

13. Burrows T, Teasdale S, Rocks T, et al. Effectiveness of dietary interventions in mental health treatment: A rapid review of reviews. *Nutr Diet.* 2022;79(3):279–290. doi:10.1111/1747-0080.12754

14. Çelik Ince S, Partlak Günüşen N. The views and habits of the individuals with mental illness about physical activity and nutrition. *Perspect Psychiatr Care.* 2018;54(4):586–595. doi:10.1111/ppc.12289

15. Carson N, Blake C, Saunders R, O'Brien J. Influences on the food choice behaviors of adults with severe mental illness. *Occup Ther Ment Health.* 2013;29:361–384. doi:10.1080/0164212X.2013.848396

16. Barre LK, Ferron JC, Davis KE, Whitley R. Healthy eating in persons with serious mental illnesses: Understanding and barriers. *Psychiatr Rehabil J.* 2011;34(4):304–310. doi:10.2975/34.4.2011.304.310

17. National Institute of Mental Health (NIMH). Mental Illness. Accessed April 19, 2023. https://www.nimh.nih.gov/health/statistics/mental-illness

18. Mental Health America. The State of Mental Health in America. Accessed April 19, 2023. https://mhanational.org/issues/state-mental-health-america

19. Shortage Areas. Accessed April 19, 2023. https://data.hrsa.gov/topics/health-workforce/shortage-areas

20. Teasdale SB, Burrows TL, Hayes T, et al. Dietary intake, food addiction and nutrition knowledge in young people with mental illness. *Nutr Diet.* 2020;77(3):315–322. doi:10.1111/1747-0080.12550

21. Teasdale SB, Samaras K, Wade T, Jarman R, Ward PB. A review of the nutritional challenges experienced by people living with severe mental illness: A role for dietitians in addressing physical health gaps. *J Hum Nutr Diet.* 2017;30(5):545–553. doi:10.1111/jhn.12473

22. Elfhag K, Morey LC. Personality traits and eating behavior in the obese: Poor self-control in emotional and external eating but personality assets in restrained eating. *Eat Behav.* 2008;9(3):285–293. doi:10.1016/j.eatbeh.2007.10.003

23. Abayomi J, Hackett A. Assessment of malnutrition in mental health clients: Nurses' judgement vs. a nutrition risk tool. *J Adv Nurs.* 2004;45(4):430–437. doi:10.1046/j.1365-2648.2003.02926.x

24. Adan RAH, van der Beek EM, Buitelaar JK, et al. Nutritional psychiatry: Towards improving mental health by what you eat. *Eur Neuropsychopharmacol.* 2019;29(12):1321–1332. doi:10.1016/j.euroneuro.2019.10.011

25. Nathan PE, Gorman JM, eds. *A Guide to Treatments That Work, 4th ed.* Oxford University Press; 2015.

26. Leichsenring F, Abbass A, Hilsenroth MJ, et al. Biases in research: Risk factors for non-replicability in psychotherapy and pharmacotherapy research. *Psychol Med.* 2017;47(6):1000–1011. doi:10.1017/S003329171600324X

27. Patel JC, Carr KD, Rice ME. Actions and consequences of insulin in the striatum. *Biomolecules.* 2023;13(3):518. doi:10.3390/biom13030518

28. Jorm AF, Patten SB, Brugha TS, Mojtabai R. Has increased provision of treatment reduced the prevalence of common mental disorders? Review of the evidence from four countries. *World Psychiatry.* 2017;16(1):90–99. doi:10.1002/wps.20388

29. Leucht S, Hierl S, Kissling W, Dold M, Davis JM. Putting the efficacy of psychiatric and general medicine medication into perspective: Review of meta-analyses. *Br J Psychiatry.* 2012;200(2):97–106. doi:10.1192/bjp.bp.111.096594

30. Semahegn A, Torpey K, Manu A, Assefa N, Tesfaye G, Ankomah A. Psychotropic medication non-adherence and associated factors among adult patients with major psychiatric disorders: A protocol for a systematic review. *Syst Rev.* 2018;7(1):10. doi:10.1186/s13643-018-0676-y

31. Swift JK, Greenberg RP, Tompkins KA, Parkin SR. Treatment refusal and premature termination in psychotherapy, pharmacotherapy, and their combination: A meta-analysis of head-to-head comparisons. *Psychotherapy.* 2017;54(1):47–57. doi:10.1037/pst0000104

32. Gomes-da-Costa S, Marx W, Corponi F, et al. Lithium therapy and weight change in people with bipolar disorder: A systematic review and meta-analysis. *Neurosci Biobehav Rev.* 2022;134:104266. doi:10.1016/j.neubiorev.2021.07.011

33. Carvalho AF, Sharma MS, Brunoni AR, Vieta E, Fava GA. The safety, tolerability and risks associated with the use of newer generation antidepressant drugs: A critical review of the literature. *Psychother Psychosom.* 2016;85(5):270–288. doi:10.1159/000447034

34. Leucht S, Cipriani A, Spineli L, et al. Comparative efficacy and tolerability of 15 antipsychotic drugs in schizophrenia: A multiple-treatments meta-analysis. *Lancet.* 2013;382(9896):951–962. doi:10.1016/S0140-6736(13)60733-3

35. Panizzutti B, Bortolasci CC, Spolding B, et al. Biological mechanism(s) underpinning the association between antipsychotic drugs and weight gain. *J Clin Med.* 2021; 10(18):4095. doi:10.3390/jcm10184095

36. Bourin M, Briley M. Sedation, an unpleasant, undesirable and potentially dangerous side-effect of many psychotropic drugs. *Hum Psychopharmacol Clin Exp.* 2004;19: 135–139. doi:10.1002/hup.561

37. Homberg JR, Schubert D, Gaspar P. New perspectives on the neurodevelopmental effects of SSRIs. *Trends Pharmacol Sci.* 2010;31(2):60–65. doi:10.1016/j.tips.2009.11.003

38. Berger M, Gray JA, Roth BL. The expanded biology of serotonin. *Annu Rev Med.* 2009;60:355–366. doi:10.1146/annurev.med.60.042307.110802

39. Sanacora G, Zarate CA, Krystal JH, Manji HK. Targeting the glutamatergic system to develop novel, improved therapeutics for mood disorders. *Nat Rev Drug Discov.* 2008;7(5):426–437. doi:10.1038/nrd2462

40. Lapidus KA, Soleimani L, Murrough JW. Novel glutamatergic drugs for the treatment of mood disorders. *Neuropsychiatr Dis Treat.* 2013;9:1101–1112. doi:10.2147/NDT. S36689

41. Almutabagani LF, Almanqour RA, Alsabhan JF, et al. Inflammation and treatment-resistant depression from clinical to animal study: A possible link? *Neurol Int.* 2023; 15(1):100–120. doi:10.3390/neurolint15010009

42. Kiecolt-Glaser JK, Derry HM, Fagundes CP. Inflammation: Depression fans the flames and feasts on the heat. *Am J Psychiatry.* 2015;172(11):1075–1091. doi:10.1176/appi.ajp. 2015.15020152

43. Arteaga-Henríquez G, Simon MS, Burger B, et al. Low-grade inflammation as a predictor of antidepressant and anti-inflammatory therapy response in MDD patients: A systematic review of the literature in combination with an analysis of experimental data collected in the EU-MOODINFLAME consortium. *Front Psychiatry.* 2019;10:458. doi:10.3389/fpsyt.2019.00458

44. Carvalho LA, Torre JP, Papadopoulos AS, et al. Lack of clinical therapeutic benefit of antidepressants is associated overall activation of the inflammatory system. *J Affect Disord.* 2013;148(1):136–140. doi:10.1016/j.jad.2012.10.036

45. Kurowska A, Ziemichód W, Herbet M, Piątkowska-Chmiel I. The role of diet as a modulator of the inflammatory process in the neurological diseases. *Nutrients.* 2023; 15(6):1436. doi:10.3390/nu15061436

46. Firth J, Siddiqi N, Koyanagi A, et al. The lancet psychiatry commission: A blueprint for protecting physical health in people with mental illness. *Lancet Psychiatry.* 2019;6(8):675–712. doi:10.1016/S2215-0366(19)30132-4

47. Penninx BWJH, Lange SMM. Metabolic syndrome in psychiatric patients: Overview, mechanisms, and implications. *Dialogues Clin Neurosci.* 2018;20(1):63–73. doi:10.31887/ DCNS.2018.20.1/bpenninx

48. Mather AA, Cox BJ, Enns MW, Sareen J. Associations of obesity with psychiatric disorders and suicidal behaviors in a nationally representative sample. *J Psychosom Res.* 2009;66(4):277–285. doi:10.1016/j.jpsychores.2008.09.008

49. Simon GE, Von Korff M, Saunders K, et al. Association between obesity and psychiatric disorders in the US adult population. *Arch Gen Psychiatry.* 2006;63(7):824–830. doi:10.1001/archpsyc.63.7.824

50. Backholer K, Wong E, Freak-Poli R, Walls HL, Peeters A. Increasing body weight and risk of limitations in activities of daily living: A systematic review and meta-analysis. *Obes Rev.* 2012;13(5):456–468. doi:10.1111/j.1467-789X.2011.00970.x

51. Jia H, Lubetkin EI. The impact of obesity on health-related quality-of-life in the general adult US population. *J Public Health.* 2005;27(2):156–164. doi:10.1093/pubmed/fdi025

52. Vancampfort D, Stubbs B, Mitchell AJ, et al. Risk of metabolic syndrome and its components in people with schizophrenia and related psychotic disorders, bipolar

disorder and major depressive disorder: A systematic review and meta-analysis. *World Psychiatry.* 2015;14(3):339–347. doi:10.1002/wps.20252

53. Walker ER, McGee RE, Druss BG. Mortality in mental disorders and global disease burden implications: A systematic review and meta-analysis. *JAMA Psychiatry.* 2015;72(4):334–341. doi:10.1001/jamapsychiatry.2014.2502

54. Curtis J, Watkins A, Rosenbaum S, et al. Evaluating an individualized lifestyle and life skills intervention to prevent antipsychotic-induced weight gain in first-episode psychosis. *Early Interv Psychiatry.* 2016;10(3):267–276. doi:10.1111/eip.12230

55. Evans S, Newton R, Higgins S. Nutritional intervention to prevent weight gain in patients commenced on olanzapine: A randomized controlled trial. *Aust N Z J Psychiatry.* 2005;39(6):479–486. doi:10.1080/j.1440-1614.2005.01607.x

56. Druss BG, Walker ER. Mental disorders and medical comorbidity. *Synth Proj Res Synth Rep.* 2011;(21):1–26. PMID: 21675009.

57. Druss BG, Rosenheck RA, Desai MM, Perlin JB. Quality of preventive medical care for patients with mental disorders. *Med Care.* 2002;40(2):129–136. doi:10.1097/00005650-200202000-00007

58. Kleinridders A, Cai W, Cappellucci L, et al. Insulin resistance in brain alters dopamine turnover and causes behavioral disorders. *Proc Natl Acad Sci USA.* 2015;112(11): 3463–3468. doi:10.1073/pnas.1500877112

59. Milstein JL, Ferris HA. The brain as an insulin-sensitive metabolic organ. *Mol Metab.* 2021;52:101234. doi:10.1016/j.molmet.2021.101234

60. Spinelli M, Fusco S, Grassi C. Brain insulin resistance impairs hippocampal plasticity. *Vitam Horm.* 2020;114:281–306. doi:10.1016/bs.vh.2020.04.005

61. Spinelli M, Fusco S, Grassi C. Brain insulin resistance and hippocampal plasticity: Mechanisms and biomarkers of cognitive decline. *Front Neurosci.* 2019;13:788. doi:10.3389/fnins.2019.00788

62. Kleinridders A, Ferris HA, Cai W, Kahn CR. Insulin action in brain regulates systemic metabolism and brain function. *Diabetes.* 2014;63(7):2232–2243. doi:10.2337/db14-0568

63. Cetinkalp S, Simsir IY, Ertek S. Insulin resistance in brain and possible therapeutic approaches. *Curr Vasc Pharmacol.* 2014;12(4):553–564. doi:10.2174/1570161112999140206130426

64. Rasgon NL, McEwen BS. Insulin resistance—a missing link no more. *Mol Psychiatry.* 2016;21(12):1648–1652. doi:10.1038/mp.2016.162

65. Singh MK, Leslie SM, Packer MM, et al. Brain and behavioral correlates of insulin resistance in youth with depression and obesity. *Horm Behav.* 2019;108:73–83. doi:10.1016/j.yhbeh.2018.03.009

66. Watson KT, Simard JF, Henderson VW, et al. Association of insulin resistance with depression severity and remission status: Defining a metabolic endophenotype of depression. *JAMA Psychiatry.* 2021;78(4):439–441. doi:10.1001/jamapsychiatry.2020.3669

67. Lyra E Silva N de M, Lam MP, Soares CN, Munoz DP, Milev R, De Felice FG. Insulin resistance as a shared pathogenic mechanism between depression and type 2 diabetes. *Front Psychiatry.* 2019;10:57. doi:10.3389/fpsyt.2019.00057

68. Golden SH. A review of the evidence for a neuroendocrine link between stress, depression and diabetes mellitus. *Curr Diabetes Rev.* 2007;3(4):252–259. doi:10.2174/157339907782330021

69. Muscogiuri G, Barrea L, Caprio M, et al. Nutritional guidelines for the management of insulin resistance. *Crit Rev Food Sci Nutr.* 2022;62(25):6947–6960. doi:10.1080/10408398.2021.1908223

70. Satija A, Bhupathiraju SN, Rimm EB, et al. Plant-based dietary patterns and incidence of type 2 diabetes in US men and women: Results from three prospective cohort studies. *PLoS Med.* 2016;13(6):e1002039. doi:10.1371/journal.pmed.1002039

71. McGrath L, Fernandez ML. Plant-based diets and metabolic syndrome: Evaluating the influence of diet quality. *J Agric Food Res.* 2022;9:100322. doi:10.1016/j.jafr.2022.100322

72. Tanaka M, Tóth F, Polyák H, Szabó Á, Mándi Y, Vécsei L. Immune influencers in action: Metabolites and enzymes of the tryptophan-kynurenine metabolic pathway. *Biomedicines.* 2021;9(7):734. doi:10.3390/biomedicines9070734

73. Vécsei L, Szalárdy L, Fülöp F, Toldi J. Kynurenines in the CNS: Recent advances and new questions. *Nat Rev Drug Discov.* 2013;12(1):64–82. doi:10.1038/nrd3793

74. Colle R, Masson P, Verstuyft C, et al. Peripheral tryptophan, serotonin, kynurenine, and their metabolites in major depression: A case-control study. *Psychiatry Clin Neurosci.* 2020;74(2):112–117. doi:10.1111/pcn.12944

75. Oxenkrug G. Serotonin-kynurenine hypothesis of depression: Historical overview and recent developments. *Curr Drug Targets.* 2013;14(5):514–521. doi:10.2174/1389450111314050002

76. Miura H, Ozaki N, Sawada M, Isobe K, Ohta T, Nagatsu T. A link between stress and depression: Shifts in the balance between the kynurenine and serotonin pathways of tryptophan metabolism and the etiology and pathophysiology of depression. *Stress.* 2008;11(3):198–209. doi:10.1080/10253890701754068

77. Roth W, Zadeh K, Vekariya R, Ge Y, Mohamadzadeh M. Tryptophan metabolism and gut-brain homeostasis. *Int J Mol Sci.* 2021;22(6):2973. doi:10.3390/ijms22062973

78. Gao K, Mu CL, Farzi A, Zhu WY. Tryptophan metabolism: A link between the gut microbiota and brain. *Adv Nutr.* 2020;11(3):709–723. doi:10.1093/advances/nmz127

79. Kaur H, Bose C, Mande SS. Tryptophan metabolism by gut microbiome and gut-brain-axis: An *in silico* analysis. *Front Neurosci.* 2019;13. doi:10.3389/fnins.2019.01365

80. Agus A, Planchais J, Sokol H. Gut microbiota regulation of tryptophan metabolism in health and disease. *Cell Host Microbe.* 2018;23(6):716–724. doi:10.1016/j.chom.2018.05.003

81. Kałużna-Czaplińska J, Gątarek P, Chirumbolo S, Chartrand MS, Bjørklund G. How important is tryptophan in human health? *Crit Rev Food Sci Nutr.* 2019;59(1):72–88. doi:10.1080/10408398.2017.1357534

82. Henningsen P, Zimmermann T, Sattel H. Medically unexplained physical symptoms, anxiety, and depression: A meta-analytic review. *Psychosom Med.* 2003;65(4):528–533. doi:10.1097/01.psy.0000075977.90337.e7

83. Shabbir F, Patel A, Mattison C, et al. Effect of diet on serotonergic neurotransmission in depression. *Neurochem Int.* 2013;62(3):324–329. doi:10.1016/j.neuint.2012.12.014

84. Chojnacki C, Gąsiorowska A, Popławski T, et al. Beneficial effect of increased tryptophan intake on its metabolism and mental state of the elderly. *Nutrients.* 2023;15(4):847. doi:10.3390/nu15040847

85. Reuter M, Zamoscik V, Plieger T, et al. Tryptophan-rich diet is negatively associated with depression and positively linked to social cognition. *Nutr Res.* 2021;85:14–20. doi:10.1016/j.nutres.2020.10.005

86. Suga H, Asakura K, Kobayashi S, Nojima M, Sasaki S, Three-Generation Study of Women on Diets and Health Study Group. Association between habitual tryptophan intake and depressive symptoms in young and middle-aged women. *J Affect Disord.* 2018;231:44–50. doi:10.1016/j.jad.2018.01.029

87. Lieberman HR, Agarwal S, Fulgoni VL. Tryptophan intake in the US adult population is not related to liver or kidney function but is associated with depression and sleep outcomes. *J Nutr.* 2016;146(12):2609S–2615S. doi:10.3945/jn.115.226969

88. Lindseth G, Helland B, Caspers J. The effects of dietary tryptophan on affective disorders. *Arch Psychiatr Nurs.* 2015;29(2):102–107. doi:10.1016/j.apnu.2014.11.008

89. Bosi A, Banfi D, Bistoletti M, Giaroni C, Baj A. Tryptophan metabolites along the microbiota-gut-brain axis: An interkingdom communication system influencing the gut in health and disease. *Int J Tryptophan Res IJTR.* 2020;13:1–25. doi:10.1177/1178646920928984

90. Berding K, Vlckova K, Marx W, et al. Diet and the microbiota-gut-brain axis: Sowing the seeds of good mental health. *Adv Nutr.* 2021;12(4):1239–1285. doi:10.1093/advances/nmaa181

91. Badal VD, Vaccariello ED, Murray ER, et al. The gut microbiome, aging, and longevity: A systematic review. *Nutrients.* 2020;12(12):3759. doi:10.3390/nu12123759

92. Appleton J. The gut-brain axis: Influence of microbiota on mood and mental health. *Integr Med.* 2018;17(4):28–32.

93. Osadchiy V, Martin CR, Mayer EA. Gut microbiome and modulation of CNS function. *Compr Physiol.* 2019;10(1):57–72. doi:10.1002/cphy.c180031

94. Farzi A, Fröhlich EE, Holzer P. Gut Microbiota and the neuroendocrine system. *Neurotherapeutics.* 2018;15(1):5–22. doi:10.1007/s13311-017-0600-5

95. Selma-Royo M, Calatayud Arroyo M, García-Mantrana I, et al. Perinatal environment shapes microbiota colonization and infant growth: Impact on host response and intestinal function. *Microbiome.* 2020;8(1):167. doi:10.1186/s40168-020-00940-8

96. Eltokhi A, Sommer IE. A reciprocal link between gut microbiota, inflammation and depression: A place for probiotics? *Front Neurosci.* 2022;16:852506. doi:10.3389/fnins.2022.852506

97. Sandhu KV, Sherwin E, Schellekens H, Stanton C, Dinan TG, Cryan JF. Feeding the microbiota-gut-brain axis: Diet, microbiome, and neuropsychiatry. *Transl Res.* 2017;179:223–244. doi:10.1016/j.trsl.2016.10.002

98. Su Q, Liu Q. Factors affecting gut microbiome in daily diet. *Front Nutr.* 2021;8. doi:10.3389/fnut.2021.644138

99. Hrncir T. Gut Microbiota dysbiosis: Triggers, consequences, diagnostic and therapeutic options. *Microorganisms.* 2022;10(3):578. doi:10.3390/microorganisms10030578

100. Dash S, Syed YA, Khan MR. Understanding the role of the gut microbiome in brain development and its association with neurodevelopmental psychiatric disorders. *Front Cell Dev Biol.* 2022;10:880544. doi:10.3389/fcell.2022.880544

101. Safadi JM, Quinton AMG, Lennox BR, Burnet PWJ, Minichino A. Gut dysbiosis in severe mental illness and chronic fatigue: A novel trans-diagnostic construct? A systematic review and meta-analysis. *Mol Psychiatry.* 2022;27(1):141–153. doi:10.1038/s41380-021-01032-1

102. Bull MJ, Plummer NT. Part 1: The human gut microbiome in health and disease. *Integr Med.* 2014;13(6):17–22.

103. Sheng JA, Bales NJ, Myers SA, et al. The hypothalamic-pituitary-adrenal axis: Development, programming actions of hormones, and maternal-fetal interactions. *Front Behav Neurosci.* 2020;14:601939. doi:10.3389/fnbeh.2020.601939

104. Makris AP, Karianaki M, Tsamis KI, Paschou SA. The role of the gut-brain axis in depression: Endocrine, neural, and immune pathways. *Hormones.* 2021;20(1):1–12. doi:10.1007/s42000-020-00236-4

105. Sudo N, Chida Y, Aiba Y, et al. Postnatal microbial colonization programs the hypothalamic-pituitary-adrenal system for stress response in mice. *J Physiol.* 2004;558(Pt 1):263–275. doi:10.1113/jphysiol.2004.063388

106. Zou XH, Sun LH, Yang W, Li BJ, Cui RJ. Potential role of insulin on the pathogenesis of depression. *Cell Prolif.* 2020;53(5):e12806. doi:10.1111/cpr.12806

107. Chong ACN, Vogt MC, Hill AS, Brüning JC, Zeltser LM. Central insulin signaling modulates hypothalamus-pituitary-adrenal axis responsiveness. *Mol Metab.* 2015;4(2):83–92. doi:10.1016/j.molmet.2014.12.001

108. Haroon E, Raison CL, Miller AH. Psychoneuroimmunology meets neuropsychopharmacology: Translational implications of the impact of inflammation on behavior. *Neuropsychopharmacology.* 2012;37(1):137–162. doi:10.1038/npp.2011.205

109. Kastorini CM, Milionis HJ, Esposito K, Giugliano D, Goudevenos JA, Panagiotakos DB. The effect of mediterranean diet on metabolic syndrome and its components: A meta-analysis of 50 studies and 534,906 individuals. *J Am Coll Cardiol.* 2011;57(11):1299–1313. doi:10.1016/j.jacc.2010.09.073

110. Hlebowicz J, Persson M, Gullberg B, et al. Food patterns, inflammation markers and incidence of cardiovascular disease: The Malmö diet and cancer study. *J Intern Med.* 2011;270(4):365–376. doi:10.1111/j.1365-2796.2011.02382.x

111. Meyer J, Döring A, Herder C, Roden M, Koenig W, Thorand B. Dietary patterns, subclinical inflammation, incident coronary heart disease and mortality in middle-aged men from the MONICA/KORA Augsburg cohort study. *Eur J Clin Nutr.* 2011; 65(7):800–807. doi:10.1038/ejcn.2011.37

112. Giugliano D, Ceriello A, Esposito K. The effects of diet on inflammation: Emphasis on the metabolic syndrome. *J Am Coll Cardiol.* 2006;48(4):677–685. doi:10.1016/j. jacc.2006.03.052

113. Esposito K, Marfella R, Ciotola M, et al. Effect of a mediterranean-style diet on endothelial dysfunction and markers of vascular inflammation in the metabolic syndrome: A randomized trial. *JAMA.* 2004;292(12):1440–1446. doi:10.1001/jama.292.12.1440

114. Samara A, Murphy T, Strain J, et al. Neuroinflammation and white matter alterations in obesity assessed by diffusion basis spectrum imaging. *Front Hum Neurosci.* 2020;13:464. doi:10.3389/fnhum.2019.00464

115. Muñoz A, Costa M. Nutritionally mediated oxidative stress and inflammation. *Oxid Med Cell Longev.* 2013;2013:610950. doi:10.1155/2013/610950

116. Salim S. Oxidative stress and psychological disorders. *Curr Neuropharmacol.* 2014;12(2):140–147. doi:10.2174/1570159X11666131120230309

117. Halliwell B. Oxidative stress, nutrition and health. Experimental strategies for optimization of nutritional antioxidant intake in humans. *Free Radic Res.* 1996;25(1):57–74. doi:10.3109/10715769609145656

118. Sergi D, Luscombe-Marsh N, Naumovski N, Abeywardena M, O'Callaghan N. Palmitic acid, but not lauric acid, induces metabolic inflammation, mitochondrial fragmentation, and a drop in mitochondrial membrane potential in human primary myotubes. *Front Nutr.* 2021;8. doi:10.3389/fnut.2021.663838

119. Yuan JP, Ho TC, Coury SM, Chahal R, Colich NL, Gotlib IH. Early life stress, systemic inflammation, and neural correlates of implicit emotion regulation in adolescents. *Brain Behav Immun.* 2022;105:169–179. doi:10.1016/j.bbi.2022.07.007

120. Aleksandrova K, Koelman L, Rodrigues CE. Dietary patterns and biomarkers of oxidative stress and inflammation: A systematic review of observational and intervention studies. *Redox Biol.* 2021;42:101869. doi:10.1016/j.redox.2021.101869

121. Ortega MA, Fraile-Martínez Ó, García-Montero C, et al. Biological role of nutrients, food and dietary patterns in the prevention and clinical management of major depressive disorder. *Nutrients.* 2022;14(15):3099. doi:10.3390/nu14153099

122. Stevens AJ, Rucklidge JJ, Kennedy MA. Epigenetics, nutrition and mental health. Is there a relationship? *Nutr Neurosci.* 2018;21(9):602–613. doi:10.1080/1028415X.2017. 1331524

123. Nestler EJ, Peña CJ, Kundakovic M, Mitchell A, Akbarian S. Epigenetic basis of mental illness. *Neuroscientist.* 2016;22(5):447–463. doi:10.1177/1073858415608147

124. Chen J, Xu X. Diet, epigenetic, and cancer prevention. *Adv Genet.* 2010;71:237–255. doi:10.1016/B978-0-12-380864-6.00008-0

125. Tiffon C. The impact of nutrition and environmental epigenetics on human health and disease. *Int J Mol Sci.* 2018;19(11):3425. doi:10.3390/ijms19113425

126. Dauncey MJ. New insights into nutrition and cognitive neuroscience. *Proc Nutr Soc.* 2009;68(4):408–415. doi:10.1017/S0029665109990188

127. Dauncey MJ. Recent advances in nutrition, genes and brain health. *Proc Nutr Soc.* 2012;71(4):581–591. doi:10.1017/S0029665112000237

128. Lane MM, Gamage E, Travica N, et al. Ultra-processed food consumption and mental health: A systematic review and meta-analysis of observational studies. *Nutrients.* 2022;14(13):2568. doi:10.3390/nu14132568

129. Monteiro CA, Cannon G, Levy RB, et al. Ultra-processed foods: What they are and how to identify them. *Public Health Nutr.* 2019;22(5):936–941. doi:10.1017/S1368980018003762
130. Juul F, Parekh N, Martinez-Steele E, Monteiro CA, Chang VW. Ultra-processed food consumption among US adults from 2001 to 2018. *Am J Clin Nutr.* 2022;115(1):211–221. doi:10.1093/ajcn/nqab305
131. Li H, Li S, Yang H, et al. Association of ultraprocessed food consumption with risk of dementia: A prospective cohort. *Neurology.* 2022. doi:10.1212/WNL.0000000000200871
132. Coletro HN, Mendonça R de D, Meireles AL, Machado-Coelho GLL, de Menezes MC. Ultra-processed and fresh food consumption and symptoms of anxiety and depression during the COVID-19 pandemic: COVID inconfidentes. *Clin Nutr ESPEN.* 2022;47:206–214. doi:10.1016/j.clnesp.2021.12.013
133. Godos J, Bonaccio M, Al-Qahtani WH, et al. Ultra-processed food consumption and depressive symptoms in a mediterranean cohort. *Nutrients.* 2023;15(3):504. doi:10.3390/nu15030504
134. Hecht EM, Rabil A, Martinez Steele E, et al. Cross-sectional examination of ultra-processed food consumption and adverse mental health symptoms. *Public Health Nutr.* 2022;25(11):3225–3234. doi:10.1017/S1368980022001586
135. Martínez Leo EE, Segura Campos MR. Effect of ultra-processed diet on gut microbiota and thus its role in neurodegenerative diseases. *Nutrients.* 2020;71:110609. doi:10.1016/j.nut.2019.110609
136. Shi Z. Gut Microbiota: An important link between western diet and chronic diseases. *Nutrients.* 2019;11(10):2287. doi:10.3390/nu11102287
137. Teleanu RI, Niculescu AG, Roza E, Vladâcenco O, Grumezescu AM, Teleanu DM. Neurotransmitters-key factors in neurological and neurodegenerative disorders of the central nervous system. *Int J Mol Sci.* 2022;23(11):5954. doi:10.3390/ijms23115954
138. Verma H, Phian S, Lakra P, et al. Human gut microbiota and mental health: Advancements and challenges in microbe-based therapeutic interventions. *Indian J Microbiol.* 2020;60(4):405–419. doi:10.1007/s12088-020-00898-z
139. Valles-Colomer M, Falony G, Darzi Y, et al. The neuroactive potential of the human gut microbiota in quality of life and depression. *Nat Microbiol.* 2019;4(4):623–632. doi:10.1038/s41564-018-0337-x
140. Jiang H, Ling Z, Zhang Y, et al. Altered fecal microbiota composition in patients with major depressive disorder. *Brain Behav Immun.* 2015;48:186–194. doi:10.1016/j.bbi.2015.03.016
141. Foster JA, McVey Neufeld KA. Gut-brain axis: How the microbiome influences anxiety and depression. *Trends Neurosci.* 2013;36(5):305–312. doi:10.1016/j.tins.2013.01.005
142. Liu T, Huang Z. Evidence-based analysis of neurotransmitter modulation by gut microbiota: 8th international conference on health information science, HIS 2019. Wang H, Siuly S, Zhang Y, Zhou R, Martin-Sanchez F, Huang Z, eds. *Health Information Science.* Springer; 2019:238–249. doi:10.1007/978-3-030-32962-4_22
143. Caspani G, Swann J. Small talk: Microbial metabolites involved in the signaling from microbiota to brain. *Curr Opin Pharmacol.* 2019;48:99–106. doi:10.1016/j.coph.2019.08.001
144. Yang NJ, Chiu IM. Bacterial signaling to the nervous system via toxins and metabolites. *J Mol Biol.* 2017;429(5):587–605. doi:10.1016/j.jmb.2016.12.023
145. Chen Y, Xu J, Chen Y. Regulation of neurotransmitters by the gut Microbiota and effects on cognition in neurological disorders. *Nutrients.* 2021;13(6):2099. doi:10.3390/nu13062099
146. Terry N, Margolis KG. Serotonergic mechanisms regulating the GI tract: Experimental evidence and therapeutic relevance. *Handb Exp Pharmacol.* 2017;239:319–342. doi:10.1007/164_2016_103

147. Yano JM, Yu K, Donaldson GP, et al. Indigenous bacteria from the gut microbiota regulate host serotonin biosynthesis. *Cell.* 2015;161(2):264–276. doi:10.1016/j.cell. 2015.02.047

148. Xue R, Zhang H, Pan J, et al. Peripheral dopamine controlled by gut microbes inhibits invariant natural killer T cell-mediated hepatitis. *Front Immunol.* 2018;9:2398. doi:10.3389/fimmu.2018.02398

149. Eisenhofer G, Aneman A, Friberg P, et al. Substantial production of dopamine in the human gastrointestinal tract. *J Clin Endocrinol Metab.* 1997;82(11):3864–3871. doi:10.1210/jcem.82.11.4339

150. Strandwitz P, Kim KH, Terekhova D, et al. GABA-modulating bacteria of the human gut microbiota. *Nat Microbiol.* 2019;4(3):396–403. doi:10.1038/s41564-018-0307-3

151. Oleskin AV, El'-Registan GI, Shenderov BA. Role of neuromediators in the functioning of the human microbiota: "Business talks" among microorganisms and the microbiota-host dialogue. *Microbiology.* 2016;85(1):1–22. doi:10.1134/S0026261716010082

152. Duff J. Chapter fourteen-nutrition for ADHD and autism. In: Cantor DS, Evans JR, eds. *Clinical Neurotherapy.* Academic Press; 2014:357–381. doi:10.1016/B978-0-12-396988-0.00014-3

153. Mikawa Y, Mizobuchi S, Egi M, Morita K. Low serum concentrations of vitamin B6 and iron are related to panic attack and hyperventilation attack. *Acta Med Okayama.* 2013;67(2):99–104. doi:10.18926/AMO/49668

154. Harrison FE, May JM. Vitamin c function in the brain: Vital role of the ascorbate transporter SVCT2. *Free Radic Biol Med.* 2009;46(6):719–730. doi:10.1016/j. freeradbiomed.2008.12.018

155. Vink R, Nechifor M, eds. *Magnesium in the Central Nervous System.* University of Adelaide Press; 2011. Accessed April 19, 2023. http://www.ncbi.nlm.nih.gov/books/NBK507264/

156. Modak AT, Montanez J, Stavinoha WB. Magnesium deficiency: Brain acetylcholine and motor activity. *Neurobehav Toxicol.* 1979;1(3):187–191.

157. Takeda A, Minami A, Seki Y, Oku N. Differential effects of zinc on glutamatergic and GABAergic neurotransmitter systems in the hippocampus. *J Neurosci Res.* 2004;75(2):225–229. doi:10.1002/jnr.10846

158. Khairy EY, Attia MM. Protective effects of vitamin D on neurophysiologic alterations in brain aging: Role of brain-derived neurotrophic factor (BDNF). *Nutr Neurosci.* 2021;24(8):650–659. doi:10.1080/1028415X.2019.1665854

159. Koletzko B, Brands B, Grote V, et al. Long-term health impact of early nutrition: The power of programming. *Ann Nutr Metab.* 2017;70(3):161–169. doi:10.1159/000477781

160. Jacka FN, Ystrom E, Brantsaeter AL, et al. Maternal and early postnatal nutrition and mental health of offspring by age 5 years: A prospective cohort study. *J Am Acad Child Adolesc Psychiatry.* 2013;52(10):1038–1047. doi:10.1016/j.jaac.2013.07.002

161. Capra L, Tezza G, Mazzei F, Boner AL. The origins of health and disease: The influence of maternal diseases and lifestyle during gestation. *Ital J Pediatr.* 2013;39(1):7. doi:10.1186/1824-7288-39-7

162. Solmi M, Radua J, Olivola M, et al. Age at onset of mental disorders worldwide: Large-scale meta-analysis of 192 epidemiological studies. *Mol Psychiatry.* 2022;27(1):281–295. doi:10.1038/s41380-021-01161-7

163. Cowan CSM, Dinan TG, Cryan JF. Annual research review: Critical windows-the microbiota-gut-brain axis in neurocognitive development. *J Child Psychol Psychiatry.* 2020;61(3):353–371. doi:10.1111/jcpp.13156

164. Robertson RC, Manges AR, Finlay BB, Prendergast AJ. The human microbiome and child growth-first 1000 days and beyond. *Trends Microbiol.* 2019;27(2):131–147. doi:10.1016/j.tim.2018.09.008

165. Codagnone MG, Spichak S, O'Mahony SM, et al. Programming bugs: Microbiota and the developmental origins of brain health and disease. *Biol Psychiatry.* 2019;85(2): 150–163. doi:10.1016/j.biopsych.2018.06.014
166. Ismail FY, Fatemi A, Johnston MV. Cerebral plasticity: Windows of opportunity in the developing brain. *Eur J Paediatr Neurol.* 2017;21(1):23–48. doi:10.1016/j.ejpn. 2016.07.007
167. Macpherson AJ, de Agüero MG, Ganal-Vonarburg SC. How nutrition and the maternal microbiota shape the neonatal immune system. *Nat Rev Immunol.* 2017;17(8):508–517. doi:10.1038/nri.2017.58
168. Burggren WW, Mueller CA. Developmental critical windows and sensitive periods as three-dimensional constructs in time and space. *Physiol Biochem Zool PBZ.* 2015;88(2):91–102. doi:10.1086/679906
169. Goyal MS, Venkatesh S, Milbrandt J, Gordon JI, Raichle ME. Feeding the brain and nurturing the mind: Linking nutrition and the gut microbiota to brain development. *Proc Natl Acad Sci USA.* 2015;112(46):14105–14112. doi:10.1073/pnas.1511465112
170. Abrahamsson TR, Wu RY, Jenmalm MC. Gut microbiota and allergy: The importance of the pregnancy period. *Pediatr Res.* 2015;77(1–2):214–219. doi:10.1038/pr.2014.165
171. Marques AH, O'Connor TG, Roth C, Susser E, Bjørke-Monsen AL. The influence of maternal prenatal and early childhood nutrition and maternal prenatal stress on offspring immune system development and neurodevelopmental disorders. *Front Neurosci.* 2013;7. doi:10.3389/fnins.2013.00120
172. Chu DM, Antony KM, Ma J, et al. The early infant gut microbiome varies in association with a maternal high-fat diet. *Genome Med.* 2016;8(1):77. doi:10.1186/s13073-016-0330-z
173. Steenweg-de Graaff J, Tiemeier H, Steegers-Theunissen RPM, et al. Maternal dietary patterns during pregnancy and child internalising and externalising problems. The generation R study. *Clin Nutr Edinb Scotl.* 2014;33(1):115–121. doi:10.1016/j.clnu.2013. 03.002
174. Springmann M, Clark MA, Rayner M, Scarborough P, Webb P. The global and regional costs of healthy and sustainable dietary patterns: A modelling study. *Lancet Planet Health.* 2021;5(11):e797–e807. doi:10.1016/S2542-5196(21)00251-5
175. Downer S, Berkowitz SA, Harlan TS, Olstad DL, Mozaffarian D. Food is medicine: Actions to integrate food and nutrition into healthcare. *BMJ.* 2020;369:m2482. doi:10.1136/bmj.m2482
176. Gu Y, Brickman AM, Stern Y, et al. Mediterranean diet and brain structure in a multiethnic elderly cohort. *Neurology.* 2015;85(20):1744–1751. doi:10.1212/WNL. 0000000000002121
177. Valls-Pedret C, Sala-Vila A, Serra-Mir M, et al. Mediterranean diet and age-related cognitive decline: A randomized clinical trial. *JAMA Intern Med.* 2015;175(7): 1094–1103. doi:10.1001/jamainternmed.2015.1668
178. Martínez-Lapiscina EH, Clavero P, Toledo E, et al. Mediterranean diet improves cognition: The PREDIMED-NAVARRA randomised trial. *J Neurol Neurosurg Psychiatry.* 2013;84(12):1318–1325. doi:10.1136/jnnp-2012-304792
179. Psaltopoulou T, Sergentanis TN, Panagiotakos DB, Sergentanis IN, Kosti R, Scarmeas N. Mediterranean diet, stroke, cognitive impairment, and depression: A meta-analysis. *Ann Neurol.* 2013;74(4):580–591. doi:10.1002/ana.23944
180. Morris MC, Tangney CC, Wang Y, et al. MIND diet slows cognitive decline with aging. *Alzheimers Dement J Alzheimers Assoc.* 2015;11(9):1015–1022. doi:10.1016/j. jalz.2015.04.011
181. Koch M, Jensen MK. Limitations of the review and meta-analysis of fish and PUFA intake and mild-to-severe cognitive impairment risks: A dose-response meta-analysis of 21 cohort studies. *Am J Clin Nutr.* 2016;104(2):537. doi:10.3945/ajcn.116.133397

182. Arjmand G, Abbas-Zadeh M, Eftekhari MH. Effect of MIND diet intervention on cognitive performance and brain structure in healthy obese women: A randomized controlled trial. *Sci Rep*. 2022;12(1):2871. doi:10.1038/s41598-021-04258-9

183. Bayes J, Schloss J, Sibbritt D. The effect of a mediterranean diet on the symptoms of depression in young males (the "AMMEND: A mediterranean diet in MEN with depression" study): A randomized controlled trial. *Am J Clin Nutr*. 2022;116(2): 572–580. doi:10.1093/ajcn/nqac106

184. Akbaraly TN, Brunner EJ, Ferrie JE, Marmot MG, Kivimaki M, Singh-Manoux A. Dietary pattern and depressive symptoms in middle age. *Br J Psychiatry J Ment Sci*. 2009;195(5):408–413. doi:10.1192/bjp.bp.108.058925

185. Nanri A, Kimura Y, Matsushita Y, et al. Dietary patterns and depressive symptoms among Japanese men and women. *Eur J Clin Nutr*. 2010;64(8):832–839. doi:10.1038/ejcn.2010.86

20 Stress, Diet, and Metabolic Processes

Dorothy T. Chiu, PhD and
A. Janet Tomiyama, PhD

KEY POINTS

- The impact of stress on metabolic health is partially mediated by eating and dietary behaviors. Through the intricately woven system of psychological, behavioral, and physiological processes that compose the body's stress response, stress exerts strong biopsychosocial influences on diet. To a slightly lesser extent, diet and eating behaviors likewise impact stress.
- Both stress and diet are individual determinants of metabolic health. However, with the connections between them, dietary behaviors can augment or exacerbate stress effects on disease and other metabolic and physiological consequences, and vice versa.
- Interventions aiming to improve stress and diet may be effective in mitigating their respective and cumulative impacts on metabolic health.

20.1 INTRODUCTION

Globally, unhealthy diets pose a greater risk to morbidity and mortality than unsafe sex, alcohol, drug, and tobacco combined.[1] However, while there are many determinants of poor diets and eating behaviors, an arguably overlooked risk factor is stress—a factor that exerts its own influence on metabolism and health. Clearly, stress is an inevitable part of life. In the US, for example, Americans report having average past month levels of stress higher than what they perceive to be healthy.[2] Worldwide, negative experiences like stress and worry have gradually risen over the years.[3] Despite normal variation in specific sources and magnitudes of stress across sociodemographic groups and over time, the toll stress can potentially take on people's health is universal. This chapter will focus on the intersection of stress, diet, and metabolic processes, wherein the intricate and complex interplay of a multitude of systems—particularly the psychological, behavioral (i.e., diet/eating), and physiological—come together to exemplify the utility of the biopsychosocial model and bolster the need for applying such holistic frameworks to health. Figure 20.1 illustrates the overarching relations reviewed in this chapter.

For this chapter, we use Baum's[4] definition of stress as "a negative emotional experience accompanied by predictable biochemical, physiological, cognitive, and behavioral changes that are directed either toward altering the stressful event or accommodating to its effects" (p. 653). One important point is that "stress" comprises

DOI: 10.1201/b22810-23

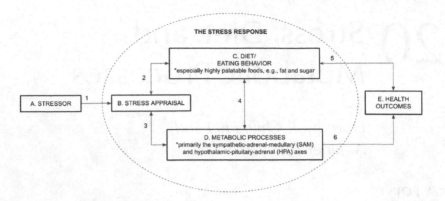

FIGURE 20.1 Conceptual framework relating stress, diet, and metabolic processes. Boxes A-E and Pathways 1–6 will be described within the text. Also, note the conceptualization of the stress response (dotted circle) to be composed of Boxes B–D.

two main parts: a *stressor* or stimulus (Box A) that triggers (Path 1) an accompanying stress *response* (dotted circle), which comprises one's perceived or subjective appraisal (Box B) of the exposure as well as its correspondent behavioral (Box C) and physiological (Box D) reactions.[5,6] As such, the variability in individual stress responses and their influence on health (Box E) is explicably wide, contextually dependent, and critically deterministic. A multitude of factors weigh in, including person-level characteristics such as genetics, developmental processes, personal histories of stressor exposure, and current stress loads; macrolevel influences such as one's socio-economic standing and cultural environment; and the existence of social, psychological, and behavioral protections.[5–7]

Stress may be acute, event-based, daily, or chronic.[5] More frequent and/or severe bouts of stressor exposures, however, will affect a more long-lasting stress response through repeated and/or intense activation of stress response pathways. Additionally, stressors that are difficult to control and pose a distinct threat to one's physical or social evaluation or integrity of being (i.e., one's perceived value, self-esteem, status) have been observed to figure especially prominently in metabolic processes via more pronounced cortisol and related hormone changes and perturbations.[5,8,9] Examples of threats of these type include weight stigma and racial discrimination.[5,8] Given this chapter's focus on diet and metabolic processes, which together can foster the development of chronic conditions and/or disease over the long term, more chronic and severe-type stress experiences are most relevant. Indeed, seminal research on stress and diet established differential effects between chronic and acute stress: while acute stress decreases appetite, chronic stress is more likely to drive the processes described herein.[10]

20.2 THE PHYSIOLOGICAL STRESS RESPONSE IN THE CONTEXT OF DIET

Overall, the stress response is an evolutionarily conserved phenomenon.[8] Stemming from genetic polymorphisms likely naturally selected during trying environments,[11] cellular level reactions to stress spur adaptive changes in body cells and tissues intended to protect an organism and promote its survival.[6] Ultimately, these adaptations can serve to dampen psychological and physiological stress reactions and reduce stress-related behaviors.[8]

Two principal pathways mediate the physiologic stress response after exposure to a stressor: the autonomic nervous system's sympathetic-adrenal-medullary (SAM) axis and the HPA axis. The primary goal of these axes is to conserve energy expenditure and increase the availability of fuel substrates for action.[7,12,13] In the SAM axis, stress exposure stimulates the adrenal glands to release the catecholamines epinephrine and norepinephrine, eliciting a "fight-or-flight" physiological state. Heart rate, myocardial contraction intensity and cardiac output, arterial blood pressure, blood coagulation, and plasma glucose levels are all increased.[7,12]

At the same time, a cascade is initiated in the HPA axis that stimulates the adrenal glands to release glucocorticoids (e.g., cortisol) into the blood, which then increases body metabolism, blood pressure, and retention of sodium and water.[7,8,12] On its own, cortisol mobilizes amino acids from muscle and free fatty acids (FFAs) from adipocytes and increases hepatic gluconeogenesis.[13] It also inhibits pancreatic beta-cells from secreting insulin. However, in excess levels due to stress, cortisol will work to enhance insulin secretion. Excess cortisol levels in combination with insulin will then upregulate lipoprotein lipase, an enzyme that liberates FFAs from lipoprotein triglycerides. Insulin will also assist in the transport of glucose and activate necessary enzymes that will ultimately facilitate triglyceride accumulation in adipocytes.[12,14] Such adipocytes are primarily situated in the visceral area as visceral adipose tissue has a high density of glucocorticoid receptors. As cortisol functions to regulate the differentiation, function, and distribution of adipose tissue, body fat is shuttled to areas of high glucocorticoid activity. The high cellular density of visceral tissue also contributes to its high metabolic activity and adipocyte turnover. The presence of more cells commands greater blood flow and innervation to the area,[14] for example, by catecholamines that assume lipolytic capacity in the presence of cortisol post-HPA axis activation.[14,15]

This activity has key implications for metabolic health. As catecholamines are attracted to visceral fat cells, the stage is set for insulin resistance. Catecholamines cause visceral adipose cells to release FFAs, resulting in high FFA concentrations in the portal vein. This leads to increased glucose production and decreased insulin clearance in the liver. FFAs, in conjunction with cortisol, also work to stimulate very-low-density lipoprotein (VLDL) secretion and promote hepatic triglyceride synthesis, as well as inhibit insulin secretion and increase insulin insensitivity in tissues. One of insulin's primary functions is the regulation of triglyceride and VLDL synthesis. Thus, when stress acts to reduce insulin activity, regulation of triglycerides and VLDL production become inhibited. Moreover, insulin resistance and cortisol transpire to hinder LDL clearance from the blood by suppressing hepatic LDL receptors and LDL breakdown.[14,15]

Repeated and/or intense activation of stress-related pathways can lead to lasting changes to the stress response, facilitated by stress-induced alterations to synaptic plasticity and gene expression.[16] Metabolic regulatory systems are particularly vulnerable as they are often the target of stress mediators such as cortisol.[17] Ultimately, these changes heighten the excitability and tone of the HPA and SAM axes, enabling their ability to continually rise to the demands of new subsequent stressors the body meets.[17] However, it also fosters a metabolically dysfunctional state of allostatic load, or the overactivation of stress systems that leads to wear and tear on the body.[9,18]

Insulin resistance and compensatory hyperinsulinemia, abdominal adiposity, athero-genic dyslipidemia, and hypertension are collectively recognized as metabolic syn-drome, a condition attributed to "stress of diverse origins"[7] (p. 717) and a potent risk factor for chronic conditions including diabetes, cardiovascular disease, and kidney disease, as well as premature mortality.[7,12,14,15]

Finally, a host of additional hormones, neuropeptides, and related systems have likewise been implicated in these stress-related processes and their metabolically dys-functional aftermath. These will be further discussed in the context of stress eating.

20.3   STRESS EATING

A common behavioral response or coping behavior to stress is eating. More specifi-cally, **stress eating** (also *stress-induced eating, comfort eating,* or *emotional eat-ing*) is defined as eating in response to negative affect or stimuli.[19] The prevalence of stress eating is sizeable, hovering around 15–46% in the general population or 47–71% in clinical samples with obesity or eating disorders.[19,20]

Cortisol, the primary actor of the HPA stress response, promotes eating both directly[21] and indirectly. For example, cortisol (1) reduces sensitivity to leptin, an appetite-reducing hormone in the brain, (2) stimulates the expression of neuropep-tide Y (NPY), an appetite-increasing hormone, and (3) potentiates reward processing pathways (e.g., dopamine release)[22] by sensitizing neural reward centers to foods that are highly palatable (e.g., sweet, fatty).[8] Sweet and fatty food consumption, driven by cortisol and insulin, stimulate pleasure centers of the nucleus accumbens while reducing discomfort arising from stimulation of its stress-sensitive centers.[23] Thus, consuming such "comfort" foods expedites psychological relief and reduces feelings of stress, incentivizing such behavior to become a habit.[8] Interestingly, sugar itself may have inhibitory effects on HPA reactivity as well via heightened opioidergic activity that inhibits HPA axis activity.[24]

Preferred foods during stress are often calorically-dense and highly-palatable (sweet and fatty or salty and fatty);[25] "comfort" foods replete with energy, sugar, and fat are especially coveted.[19,26] Accordingly, there is just cause for public health concern. Stress eating and comfort foods have been epidemiologically linked to abdominal obesity and poor metabolic health reflected through elevated glucose, insulin, insulin resistance, and glycosylated hemoglobin, as well as higher risks for prediabetes, diabetes, cardiovascular disease, and mortality.[19,26,27]

Metabolic dysfunction is further assisted by leptin, NPY, and the gut microbiota (microbiome). In excess, cortisol may interfere with leptin signaling and facilitate stress-related overeating.[22,28] Second, NPY can facilitate the development of abdom-inal obesity and metabolic syndrome-like symptoms under conditions of stress and consumption of high fat and high sugar foods.[29] NPY may additionally modulate reward processing pathways (e.g., dopaminergic and serotoninergic networks) to promote hedonic eating of palatable foods.[30] Lastly, microbiome constituency can impact stress and eating and be affected by these factors – e.g., via physiological stress responsivity and HPA axis activity and by appetite and sweet/fatty food prefer-ences, respectively.[8]

Beyond metabolism, other impacts of stress on diet and health have been estab-lished.[31] A recent meta-analysis found stress was associated with increased overall intake and intakes of unhealthy foods with decreased intake of healthy foods.[32] While another review and meta-analysis found associations between stress and overall diet quality to be mixed,[33] attributes of diets associated with stress include higher consumption of saturated fats, added sugars, sweets, snacks, fast foods, red/processed meat, and/or ultra-processed foods[33-36] simultaneous to lower intakes of fruits, vegetables, fish, unsaturated fats, fiber, and an assortment of micronutrients.[33,35,36]

Finally, increasing evidence demonstrates the powerful impact of diet on stress and mental health.[37] Healthier dietary patterns have also been associated with more diverse and beneficial microbiomes[38] as well as lower odds for allostatic load.[39] Indeed, one intervention found improvements in perceived stress and allostatic loads with higher vegetable consumption and less sodium.[40]

20.4   IMPLICATIONS FOR INTERVENTION AND FUTURE WORK

Lifestyle interventions to improve metabolic health and other health outcomes may focus on Boxes A, B, and/or C (Figure 20.1). Possible strategies include those to improve stress management—such as mindfulness[41] or physical activity[42]—as well as those to improve diet—such as disseminating strategies to consume less fat, sugar, and/or convenience foods when stressed or finding alternatively acceptable comfort foods. Our group found that comfort foods may not need to be unhealthy as after a laboratory stressor, fruits and vegetables provided equal stress relief to unhealthy comfort foods.[43]

Additionally, the role of moderators is a noted investigative need. Gender, body weight status, age, eating styles (i.e., dietary restraint, emotional and external eating), dispositional factors, and individual differences (e.g., cortisol reactivity) may all be important to account for, but research is lacking in these areas.[32]

20.5   SUMMARY

Stress and diet are powerful individual determinants of metabolic health. However, because of the multitude of pathways between them, dietary behaviors can augment or exacerbate stress effects on disease and other metabolic and physiological consequences, and vice versa. Interventions aiming to improve stress and diet health may effectively mitigate their respective and cumulative impacts on metabolic health and disease outcomes.

REFERENCES

1. Willett W, Rockström J, Loken B, et al. Food in The Anthropocene: The EAT–lancet commission on healthy diets from sustainable food systems. *Lancet.* 2019;393(10170): 447–492. doi:10.1016/S0140-6736(18)31788-4
2. American Psychological Association. Stress level trends. https://www.apa.org/news/press/releases/stress/interactive-graphics.
3. *Gallup Global Emotions 2021.* 2021. https://www.gallup.com/file/analytics/349280/Gallup_Global_Emotions_2021_Report.pdf.
4. Baum A. Stress, intrusive imagery, and chronic distress. *Heal Psychol.* 1990;9(6): 653–675. doi:10.1037//0278-6133.9.6.653

5. Epel ES, Crosswell AD, Mayer SE, et al. More than a feeling: A unified view of stress measurement for population science. *Front Neuroendocrinol.* 2018;49:146–169. doi:10.1016/j.yfrne.2018.03.001

6. McEwen BS. Stress, definitions and concepts of. *Encyclopedia of Stress.* 2nd edition. Elsevier Inc.; 2007:653.

7. Keltikangas-Järvinen L. Metabolic syndrome. *Encyclopedia of Stress.* 2nd edition. Elsevier Inc.; 2007:717–721.

8. Tomiyama AJ. Stress and obesity. *Annu Rev Psychol.* 2019;70:703–718.

9. Dickerson SS, Kemeny ME. Acute stressors and cortisol responses: A theoretical integration and synthesis of laboratory research. *Psychol Bull.* 2004;130(3):355–391. doi:10.1037/0033-2909.130.3.355

10. Torres SJ, Nowson CA. Relationship between stress, eating behavior, and obesity. *Nutrition.* 2007;23(11–12):887–894. doi:10.1016/j.nut.2007.08.008

11. Ellis BJ, Jackson JJ, Boyce WT. The stress response systems: Universality and adaptive individual differences. *Dev Rev.* 2006;26(2):175–212. doi:10.1016/j.dr.2006.02.004

12. Rosmond R. Metabolic syndrome and stress. *Encyclopedia of Stress.* 2nd edition. Elsevier Inc.; 2007:721–723.

13. Dallman MF, Bhatnagar S, Viau V. Hypothalamic-pituitary-adrenal axis. *Encyclopedia of Stress.* 2nd edition. Elsevier Inc.; 2007:421–428.

14. Rosmond R. Waist-hip ratio. *Encyclopedia of Stress.* 2nd edition. Elsevier Inc.; 2007: 853–855.

15. Stoney CM. Cholesterol and lipoproteins. In: *Encyclopedia of Stress.* Second. Elsevier Inc.; 2007:478–483. doi:10.1016/B978-012373947-6.00080-5

16. Ulrich-Lai YM, Herman JP. Neural regulation of endocrine and autonomic stress responses. *Nat Rev Neurosci.* 2009;10:397–409. doi:10.1038/nrn2647

17. Ulrich-Lai YM, Ryan KK. Neuroendocrine circuits governing energy balance and stress regulation: Functional overlap and therapeutic implications. *Cell Metab.* 2014; 19(6):910–925. doi:10.1016/j.cmet.2014.01.020

18. McEwen BS, Wingfield JC. Allostasis and allostatic load. *Encyclopedia of Stress.* 2nd edition. Elsevier Inc.; 2007:135–141.

19. Gibson EL. The psychobiology of comfort eating: Implications for neuropharmacological interventions. *Behav Pharmacol.* 2012;23(5–6):442–460. doi:10.1097/FBP. 0b013e328357bd4e

20. Cummings JR, Mason AE, Puterman E, Tomiyama AJ. Comfort eating and all-cause mortality in the U.S. Health and retirement study. *Int J Behav Med.* 2018;25(4): 473–478. doi:10.1007/s12529-017-9706-8

21. Tataranni PA, Larson DE, Snitker S, Young JB, Flatt JP, Ravussin E. Effects of glucocorticoids on energy metabolism and food intake in humans. *Am J Physiol.* 1996; 271(2 Pt. 1):E317–E325. doi:10.1152/ajpendo.1996.271.2.E317

22. Wardle J, Gibson EL. Diet and stress, non-psychiatric. *Encyclopedia of Stress.* 2nd edition. Elsevier Inc.; 2007:797–805.

23. Dallman MF, Pecoraro NC, Fleur SE. Chronic stress and comfort foods: Self-medication and abdominal obesity. *Brain Behav Immun.* 2005;19:275–280. doi:10.1016/j.bbi.2004. 11.004

24. Tryon MS, Stanhope KL, Epel ES, et al. Excessive sugar consumption may be a difficult habit to break: A view from the brain and body. *J Clin Endocrinol Metab.* 2015;100(6):2239–2247. doi:10.1210/jc.2014-4353

25. March V, Fernstrom MH. Diet and stress, psychiatric. In: *Encyclopedia of Stress.* 2nd edition. Elsevier Inc.; 2007:806–811. doi:10.1016/B978-012373947-6.00473-6

26. Dallman MF, Pecoraro N, Akana SF, et al. Chronic stress and obesity: A new view of "comfort food." *Proc Natl Acad Sci USA.* 2003;100(20):11696–11701. doi:10.1073/ pnas.1934666100

27. Tsenkova V, Boylan JM, Ryff C. Stress eating and health: Findings from MIDUS, a national study of U.S. Adults. *Appetite*. 2013;69:151–155. doi:10.1016/j.appet.2013.05.020.

28. Rosmond R. Obesity, stress and. *Encyclopedia of Stress*. 2nd edition. Elsevier Inc.; 2007:1–3.

29. Kuo LE, Czarnecka M, Kitlinska JB, Tilan JU, Kvetnansk R, Zukowska Z. Chronic stress, combined with a high-fat/high-sugar diet, shifts sympathetic signaling toward neuropeptide Y and leads to obesity and the metabolic syndrome Lydia. *Ann N Y Acad Sci*. 2008;1148:232–237. doi:10.1196/annals.1410.035

30. Rezitis J, Herzog H, Ip CK. Neuropeptide Y interaction with dopaminergic and sero-tonergic pathways: Interlinked neurocircuits modulating hedonic eating behaviours. *Prog Neuro-Psychopharmacology Biol Psychiatry*. 2022;113:110449. doi:10.1016/j.pnpbp.2021.110449

31. Epel E, Jimenez S, Brownell K, Stroud L, Stoney C, Niaura R. Are stress eaters at risk for the metabolic syndrome? *Ann N Y Acad Sci*. 2004;1032:208–210. doi:10.1196/annals.1314.022

32. Hill D, Conner M, Clancy F, et al. Stress and eating behaviours in healthy adults: A systematic review and meta-analysis. *Health Psychol Rev*. 2021;0(0):1–25. doi:10.1080/17437199.2021.1923406

33. Khaled K, Tsofliou F, Hundley V, Helmreich R, Almilaji O. Perceived stress and diet quality in women of reproductive age: A systematic review and meta-analysis. *Nutr J*. 2020;19(1):1–15. doi:10.1186/s12937-020-00609-w

34. Lopes Cortes M, Andrade Louzado J, Galvão Oliveira M, et al. Unhealthy food and psychological stress: The association between ultra-processed food consumption and perceived stress in working-class young adults. *Int J Environ Res Public Health*. 2021;18:3863. doi:10.3390/ijerph18083863

35. Khaled K, Hundley V, Tsofliou F. Poor dietary quality and patterns are associated with higher perceived stress among women of reproductive age in the UK. *Nutrients*. 2021;13:2588. doi:10.3390/nu13082588

36. Lopez-Cepero A, O'Neill J, Tamez M, et al. Associations between perceived stress and dietary intake in adults in Puerto Rico. *J Acad Nutr Diet*. 2021;121(4):762–769.

37. Marx W, Moseley G, Berk M, Jacka F. Nutritional psychiatry: The present state of the evidence. *Proc Nutr Soc*. 2017;76(4):427–436. doi:10.1017/S0029665117002026

38. Garcia-Vega AS, Corrales-Agudelo V, Reyes A, Escobar JS. Diet quality, food groups and nutrients associated with the gut microbiota in a nonwestern population. *Nutrients*. 2020;12:2938.

39. Zhou MS, Hasson RE, Baylin A, Leung CW. Associations between diet quality and allostatic load in U.S. Adults: Findings from the national health and nutrition examina-tion survey, 2015-2018. *J Acad Nutr Diet*. 2022;122:2207–2217.

40. Soltani H, Keim NL, Laugero KD. Diet quality for sodium and vegetables mediate effects of whole food diets on 8-week changes in stress load. *Nutrients*. 2018;10(11). doi:10.3390/nu10111606

41. Epel E, Laraia B, Coleman-Phox K, et al. Effects of a mindfulness-based intervention on distress, weight gain, and glucose control for pregnant low-income women: A quasi-experimental trial using the ORBIT model. *Int J Behav Med*. 2019;26(5):461–473. doi:10.1007/s12529-019-09779-2

42. Schultchen D, Reichenberger J, Mittl T, et al. Bidirectional relationship of stress and affect with physical activity and healthy eating. *Br J Health Psychol*. 2019;24(2):315–333. doi:10.1111/bjhp.12355

43. Finch LE, Cummings JR, Tomiyama AJ. Cookie or clementine? Psychophysiological stress reactivity and recovery after eating healthy and unhealthy comfort foods. *Psy-choneuroendocrinology*. 2019;107:26–36. doi:10.1016/j.psyneuen.2019.04.022

21 Social Connections in Health and Well-Being

Bert N. Uchino, PhD, Joshua Landvatter, MA and Tracey Tacana, BS

KEY POINTS

- Social connections appear as important to health as standard biomedical risk factors.
- Existing research finds that difficulties with social relationships can directly or indirectly impede medical care.
- Healthcare professionals will play a crucial role in helping advance social connections as a medical priority.

21.1 INTRODUCTION AND OVERVIEW

A patient comes into your office presenting with chest pains. An assessment of their blood pressure reveals that they are hypertensive. The patient starts complaining about a bad marriage and that others treat them poorly. How would you respond? Such medical communications related to psychosocial issues are not uncommon.[1] Do you think this additional information on the quality of their social connections matters for their current condition? The main goal of this chapter is to provide health professionals with general information that will help inform the answers to these questions. What we hope to do is to provide evidence that such issues are of great importance to the goal of understanding part of the etiology of your patient's physical health problems and have significant prognostic value for its clinical course.

21.2 WHAT DO WE MEAN BY SOCIAL CONNECTIONS?

Social connections can be defined at both broad and more specific levels. At a broad level, there is a distinction between positive and negative aspects of social relationships.[2] The more specific positive aspects include social integration, perceived support, and received support. Social integration examines the extent of social connections (e.g., number of friends, amount of contact); perceived support is the perception that support would be available if needed; and received support is the actual support received.[3] The more specific negative aspects include social negativity and loneliness.[2] Social negativity refers to adverse social behaviors by others (e.g., criticism, undermining), whereas loneliness is the perception that one lacks close connections.[2] These broad and specific distinctions are important as not all of these measures are related to health outcomes equally or via similar processes as will be

DOI: 10.1201/b22810-24

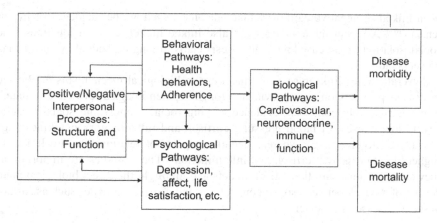

FIGURE 21.1   General mechanistic model linking social connections to health.

discussed below.[4] For instance, receiving support from others is not always helpful if it is not communicated in a caring manner.[5]

A general model linking relationships to health is depicted in Figure 21.1. As shown in the first box, social networks provide the interpersonal context (e.g., family, friends) for positive and negative interactions and perceptions. These social processes have bidirectional links with behavioral and psychological pathways, which, in turn, have documented links to health-relevant autonomic, neuroendocrine, and immune system functioning. Alterations in these biological pathways are predicted to influence disease development (i.e., morbidity) and/or course (i.e., mortality). It is also clear that coping with a chronic disease may influence relationship processes and psychological processes for better or worse (e.g., relationship growth, stress of caregiving) and is depicted as feedback loops in the model.

21.3   WHAT IS THE EVIDENCE LINKING SOCIAL CONNECTIONS TO HEALTH?

It is clear that close relationships are related to significant mental health outcomes such as depression.[6] However, less known is the equally strong and rapidly increasing evidence base linking social connections to physical health outcomes such as cardiovascular disease, cancer, and longevity.[2] At this point in time, there is ample epidemiological evidence linking social connections to health. A meta-analysis was consistent with early data indicating that positive aspects of relationships (i.e., perceived social support) were associated with a lower risk for mortality.[7] Indeed, effect sizes from the meta-analysis appeared as large as, if not larger than, standard risk factors such as exercise and obesity. Moreover, the links between social relationships and mortality were found across a number of diseases,[7] especially cardiovascular disease.[8] There is also meta-analytic evidence linking social support and social integration to lower cancer mortality.[9] Although less epidemiological evidence is available currently, negative aspects of relationships, such as criticism and conflict, have been linked to negative cardiovascular outcomes, such as the incidence of hypertension.[10,11] A recent meta-analysis has also linked higher levels of loneliness and social isolation to increased mortality – especially among individuals younger than 65 years old.[12]

Several studies linking social connections to biological mechanisms implicated in disease provide converging evidence for the epidemiological evidence to date.[13] There is relatively consistent evidence linking social support and social integration to lower levels of blood pressure, cortisol, and inflammatory cytokines (e.g., C-reactive protein, IL-6), whereas negative aspects of relationships are linked to higher blood pressure, cortisol, and inflammation[13] These studies are important as they are consistent with theoretical models and highlight the direct biological plausibility of the link between social connections and disease outcomes such as cardiovascular disease and cancer.

21.4   CAN INTERVENTIONS IMPROVE RELATIONSHIPS AND IMPACT HEALTH?

One of the most pressing issues in this literature is whether we can leverage the epidemiological evidence to date to design effective interventions. Randomized clinical trials (RCTs) are critically important given that the epidemiological literature relies on cross-sectional/observational studies which raise questions about confounding and causality. On the other hand, designing an effective relationship intervention to impact health is a tall task considering the complexity of relationships ranging from their simple presence, past history, how they are perceived, and what they actually do to promote the health of others. Relationship interventions are further complicated when considering that one is trying to modify health outcomes that are multiply-determined and can have a long-term course. For instance, the development of chronic conditions like heart disease is years in the making, and at advanced stages might be more difficult to alter given their clinical status.[4] Taking into account these complexities at both the social and biomedical levels is key in adhering to an important support doctrine to "do no harm." If researchers are not careful, individuals in support interventions may get ineffective information, feel frustrated with their relationships, feel let down by the support provider, or incur costs due to suboptimal support.

Two recent reviews paint a promising picture of interventions targeting social connections aimed at impacting health.[13,14] The National Academies of Science, Engineering, and Medicine formed an expert interdisciplinary panel. The panel found that interventions to reduce loneliness and isolation have produced some successes. Still, most work in the area has suffered from (1) limited sample size, (2) short follow-up periods, (3) lack of randomized controlled trials, and (4) lack of theory.[13] However, some findings appear more robust and include evidence from a meta-analysis indicating that cognitive-behavioral approaches that focused on maladaptive thoughts were more effective in reducing loneliness compared to social skills training.[15] More recent approaches include mindfulness-based interventions that appear to have positive influences on both relationships and biological function.[16] Finally, one limitation of existing interventions is that they tend to focus on the individual. There is increasing evidence that interventions that actively include family members (e.g., spouses, parents) may be superior as they consider the social context of health maintenance in which close others play an active role.[17]

A second recent review was a meta-analysis to test if psychosocial support interventions impacted survival in healthcare settings.[14] The review included 106 RCTs comprising over 40,000 inpatient/outpatient participants. Of the health conditions, 42% had cardiovascular disease, 36% had cancer, and 22% had other conditions. Across all RCTs, there was a statistically significant 20% increased likelihood of survival (discrete time period), and 29% increased survival over time for participants provided with psychosocial support compared to standard medical care.[14] These results were more robust when RCTs focused on health behavior change and patients with less severe disease. There was evidence of bias in only one of three subgroup analyses.[14] However, given the nature of such interventions, the authors noted the difficulties in blinding study personnel to the intervention conditions. The authors concluded that the current status of the literature suggests that psychosocial support RCTs have comparable effects on survival to most rehabilitation programs (e.g., exercise, alcohol interventions). The evidence linking interventions that focus on social connections is thus promising and refinements based on theory and new technology will be important to maximize positive outcomes. These refinements include the need to consider indirect intervention approaches such as participation in activity groups (e.g., exercise) that can benefit relationship processes[18] and the use of interventions delivered online (e.g., apps) which are important for individuals who have mobility limitations or social anxiety.

An alternative way of thinking about interpersonal interventions is as a form of primary prevention.[19] Most interventions focus on individuals who already have health problems. These are often referred to as secondary prevention efforts, which stand in contrast to primary prevention efforts that focus on preventing problems in healthy individuals. In a compelling analysis, Kaplan[19] argued for the promise of primary prevention efforts, especially in light of the more limited public health benefits that seem to arise from secondary prevention. Repetti et al.[20] have argued that early familial interventions are an important starting point and may pay large dividends in the long term. A focus on primary prevention thus raises the interesting possibility that support interventions aimed at improving relationship functioning may be useful if applied early on with children and adolescents to place them on healthier trajectories. In one example, Miller et al.[21] found that training parents in nurturance, monitoring, and communication skills was associated with lower levels of inflammation in the adolescent 8 years later.

21.5   WHAT ARE THE PRACTICE AND POLICY IMPLICATIONS OF WORK ON RELATIONSHIPS AND HEALTH?

Given the epidemiological evidence to date, an important practice issue that has been highlighted is if healthcare professionals should screen to identify people who are low in support or socially isolated in order to facilitate treatment outcomes.[22] Critics of such an approach would argue that we do not know enough regarding what screening measures to use, what would be an appropriate cut-off score, and perhaps more importantly what exactly we can do to help them.[23] Proponents, on the other hand, argue that there are scales based on the available epidemiological evidence that could be developed for such purposes and promising treatment protocols.[22,24] Work in this area is rapidly expanding, and several brief instruments are now available to screen for the social determinants of health.[25,26] Even if we might have difficulty treating low support, it can still be assessed for prognostic or predictive purposes along with other factors like age, sex, and family history.[27] In fact, regardless of its treatment, such information might be used to inform individualized treatment protocols such as more intensive monitoring or follow-ups.

The work linking social connections to health also has important policy implications. Public policies can be aimed at increasing funding for understanding the more specific nature of such links or at fostering better interpersonal functioning.[28] As an example, the Deficit Reduction Act of 2005 devoted significant funds to the Healthy Marriage Initiative (HMI) to help build stronger, stable marriages.[29] The HMI focused on research and demonstration projects regarding relationship education and skill-building (e.g., listening, problem-solving), which have produced small effect sizes on relationship quality and communication patterns with considerable variability, highlighting the complexity of such interventions.[29] Most recently, the importance of social relationships was acknowledged explicitly in Healthy People 2020, a nationwide health promotion plan that seeks to create social and physical environments that promote good health for everyone. It has explicit goals for increasing social connections (e.g., increasing the proportion of adolescents with a support figure in their lives) that can guide program development, funding, and assessment. From a policy standpoint, it would also be important to evaluate existing or future policies regarding their impact on social connections (e.g., open spaces, end-of-life issues).

21.6 WHAT ARE THE CRITICAL FUTURE QUESTIONS IN NEED OF ANSWERS IF WE ARE TO FULLY CAPITALIZE ON THE RESEARCH LINKING RELATIONSHIPS TO HEALTH?

Although there is ample evidence to act on the research linking social connections to health, several important questions will require future work. First is the need for more theoretical development on social connections. What are the critical social constructs that impact health and longevity? Most work in the area focuses on distinct measures of relationships (e.g., social support, loneliness), but few studies compare constructs that might differ in their mechanisms and implications for intervention development. One area with some history in addressing such issues is the work on a social negativity bias.[30] It has been proposed that negative aspects of relationships (e.g., conflict) might have stronger links to health than positive aspects (e.g., support). There is some evidence to this point as studies that directly contrasted both positive and negative relationship measures show that links appear stronger for negative relationship processes.[10] More work that directly compares different measures of social connections will help with theory and intervention development.

A second important issue is the need to test and refine interventions. There are certain animal models of social connection that highlight its causal impact on health.[31] Such causal studies are challenging to do with humans, but short-term laboratory studies find that receiving comforting social support from others decreases cardio-vascular reactions to stress.[32] As noted above, RCTs provide an opportunity to not only capitalize on this literature but also strengthen causal inferences. RCTs that are replicable and generalizable are the gold standard for evidence-based practice and should be a priority for future work.

Finally, understanding antecedent processes that give rise to health-relevant social connections will be important. By antecedent processes, we mean the factors that contribute to developing strong or poor social connections. Highlighting the role of epigenetic processes on social connections and health is important work.[33] There is also emerging evidence that adult support and conflict processes have their origins in the early family environment which influences later health[34] More proximal ante-cedent processes facilitating smooth interpersonal functioning are also important to understand (e.g., sexual behavior).[35] The lack of a clear understanding of these antecedent factors will limit primary prevention efforts that are likely to be highly cost-effective.

21.7   CONCLUSIONS

Social connections are a reliable and often robust predictor of physical health and longevity. Decades of research across disciplines have found that positive and nega-tive aspects of relationships (e.g., support, conflict) are related to the major causes of morbidity and mortality in the world including cancer, cardiovascular disease, and infectious illnesses. Mounting research suggests that social connections directly influence biology, which may mediate links to both acute and chronic disease devel-opment and its clinical course. More work is needed on intervention development to complete this research circle but promising examples exist.[2]

Let's return to our hypothetical example where a patient starts disclosing a bad relationship with their spouse and other interpersonal problems. How would you now respond to such information? First, we hope that you can convey that such relationship issues are tied to both the development and clinical course of health conditions – perhaps the very health condition with which the patient has been diagnosed. Second, you could consider screening for relationship issues as such instruments are now available. Third, in collaboration with clinical/counseling psy-chologists and social or community workers, treatment referrals might benefit the patient's relationships and their physical health condition. We believe that medical professionals will play a critical role in advancing and applying this robust literature. The extent of these collaborations will ultimately enable biomedical and behavioral professionals to assist individuals in living happier and healthier lives.

REFERENCES

1. Roter DL, Stewart M, Putnam SM, Lipkin MJ, Stiles W, Inui TS. Communication pat-terns of primary care physicians. *J Am Med Assoc.* 1997;277(4):350–356. doi:10.1001/jama.1997.03540280088045
2. Holt-Lunstad J. Why social relationships are important for physical health: A systems approach to understanding and modifying risk and protection. *Annu Rev Psychol.* 2018;69(1):437–458. doi:10.1146/annurev-psych-122216-011902

3. Uchino BN. *Social Support and Physical Health: Understanding the Health Consequences of Relationships.* Yale University Press; 2004. doi:10.1093/aje/kwi036

4. Uchino BN. Understanding the links between social support and physical health: A life-span perspective with emphasis on the separability of perceived and received support. *Perspect Psychol Sci.* 2009;4(3):236–255. doi:10.1111/j.1745-6924.2009.01122.x

5. Selcuk E, Ong AD. Perceived partner responsiveness moderates the association between received emotional support and all-cause mortality. *Heal Psychol.* 2013;32(2):231–235. doi:10.1037/a0028276

6. Gariépy G, Honkaniemi H, Quesnel-Vallée A. Social support and protection from depression: Systematic review of current findings in western countries. *Br J Psychiatry.* 2016;209(4):284–293. doi:10.1192/bjp.bp.115.169094

7. Holt-Lunstad J, Smith TB, Layton JB. Social relationships and mortality risk: A meta-analytic review. *PLoS Med.* 2010;7(7). doi:10.1371/journal.pmed.1000316

8. Barth J, Schneider S, von Känel R. Lack of social support in the etiology and the prognosis of coronary heart disease: A systematic review and meta-analysis. *Psychosom Med.* 2010;72(3):229–238. doi:10.1097/PSY.0b013e3181d01611

9. Pinquart M, Duberstein PR. Associations of social networks with cancer mortality: A meta-analysis. *Crit Rev Oncol Hematol.* 2010;75(2):122–137. doi:10.1016/j.critrevonc.2009.06.003

10. De Vogli R, Chandola T, Marmot MG. Negative aspects of close relationships and heart disease. *Arch Intern Med.* 2007;167(18):1951–1957. doi:10.1001/archinte.167.18.1951

11. Sneed RS, Cohen S. Negative social interactions and incident hypertension among older adults. *Heal Psychol.* 2014;33(6):554–565. doi:10.1037/hea0000057

12. Holt-Lunstad J, Smith TB, Baker M, Harris T, Stephenson D. Loneliness and social isolation as risk factors for mortality: A meta-analytic review. *Perspect Psychol Sci.* 2015;10(2):227–237. doi:10.1177/1745691614568352

13. National Academies of Sciences, Engineering, and Medicine. *Social Isolation and Loneliness in Older Adults: Opportunities for the Health Care System.* Washington, DC: The National Academies Press; 2020. doi:10.17226/25663

14. Smith TB, Workman C, Andrews C, et al. Effects of psychosocial support interventions on survival in inpatient and outpatient healthcare settings: A meta-analysis of 106 randomized controlled trials. *PLoS Med.* 2021;18(5):1–25. doi:10.1371/journal.pmed.1003595

15. Masi CM, Chen H-Y, Hawkley LC, Cacioppo JT. A meta-analysis of interventions to reduce loneliness. *Personal Soc Psychol Rev.* 2011;15(3):219–266. doi:10.1177/1088868310377394

16. Lindsay EK, Young S, Smyth JM, Brown KW, Creswell JD. Acceptance lowers stress reactivity: Dismantling mindfulness training in a randomized controlled trial. *Psychoneuroendocrinology.* 2018;87:63–73. doi:10.1016/j.psyneuen.2017.09.015

17. Martire LM, Helgeson VS. Close relationships and the management of chronic illness: Associations and interventions. *Am Psychol.* 2017;72(6):601–612. doi:10.1037/amp0000066

18. Rook KS. Facilitating friendship formation in late life: Puzzles and challenges. *Am J Community Psychol.* 1991;19(1):103–110. doi:10.1007/BF00942258

19. Kaplan RM. Two pathways to prevention. *Am Psychol.* 2000;55:382–396.

20. Repetti RL, Robles TF, Reynolds B. Allostatic processes in the family. *Dev Psychopathol.* 2011;23(3):921–938. doi:10.1017/S095457941100040X

21. Miller GE, Brody GH, Yu T, Chen E. A family-oriented psychosocial intervention reduces inflammation in low-SES African American youth. *Proc Natl Acad Sci.* 2014; 111(31):11287–11292. doi:10.1073/pnas.1406578111

22. Lett HS, Blumenthal JA, Babyak MA, et al. Social support and prognosis in patients at increased psychosocial risk recovering from myocardial infarction. *Heal Psychol.* 2007;26(4):418–427. doi:10.1037/0278-6133.26.4.418

23. Bucholz EM, Krumholz HM. Loneliness and living alone. *Arch Intern Med.* 2012; 172(14):1084–1085. doi:10.1001/archinternmed.2012.2649

24. Butler AC, Chapman JE, Forman EM, Beck AT. The empirical status of cognitive-behavioral therapy: A review of meta-analyses. *Clin Psychol Rev.* 2006;26(1):17–31. doi:10.1016/j.cpr.2005.07.003

25. Andermann A. Screening for social determinants of health in clinical care: Moving from the margins to the mainstream. *Public Health Rev.* 2018;39(1):1–17. doi:10.1186/s40985-018-0094-7

26. O'Gurek DT, Henke C. A practical approach to screening for social determinants of health. *Fam Pract Manag.* 2018;25(3):7–11.

27. Lett HS, Blumenthal JA, BabLett HS, et al. Perceived social support predicts outcomes following myocardial infarction: A call for screening - in response. *Heal Psychol.* 2008;27(1):1–3.

28. Umberson D, Montez JKJ. Social relationships and health: A flashpoint for health policy. *J Health Soc Behav.* 2010;51(Suppl):S54–S66. doi:10.1177/0022146510383501

29. Bradbury TN, Bodenmann G. Interventions for couples. *Annu Rev Clin Psychol.* 2020;16:99–123. doi:10.1146/annurev-clinpsy-071519-020546

30. Taylor SE. Asymmetrical effects of positive and negative events: The mobilization-minimization hypothesis. *Psychol Bull.* 1991;110(1):67–85. doi:10.1037/0033-2909.110.1.67

31. Snyder-Mackler N, Burger JR, Gaydosh L, et al. Social determinants of health and survival in humans and other animals. *Science (80-).* 2020;368(6493). doi:10.1126/science.aax9553

32. Teoh AN, Hilmert C. Social support as a comfort or an encouragement: A systematic review on the contrasting effects of social support on cardiovascular reactivity. *Br J Health Psychol.* 2018;23(4):1040–1065. doi:10.1111/bjhp.12337

33. Spithoven AWM, Cacioppo S, Goossens L, Cacioppo JT. Genetic contributions to loneliness and their relevance to the evolutionary theory of loneliness. *Perspect Psychol Sci.* 2019;14(3):376–396. doi:10.1177/1745691618812684

34. Chen E, Brody GH, Miller GE. Childhood close family relationships and health. *Am Psychol.* 2017;72(6):555–566. doi:10.1037/amp0000067

35. Diamond LM, Huebner DM. Is good sex good for you? Rethinking sexuality and health. *Soc Personal Psychol Compass.* 2011;6(1):54–69. doi:10.1111/j.1751-9004.2011.00408.x

22 Substance Use Approaches

Autena Torbati, PhD and
Marcel A. de Dios, MS, PhD

KEY POINTS

- Substance use is a significant public health concern.
- The impact of substance use is far-reaching and can have effects on a variety of areas of a person's life, including, but not limited to, physical health, mental well-being, social connections, sleep, and more.
- Interventions aimed at reducing substance use must be integrative and consider the interrelationships that exist between substance use and other lifestyle domains.

22.1 INTRODUCTION

Substance use is a significant public health concern. According to a 2021 survey by the Substance Abuse and Mental Health Services Administration (SAMHSA), approximately 16.5% of people aged 12 years and older in the United States (US) reported having a substance use disorder (SUD) in the past year.[1] Of these 46.3 million people with an SUD, 29.5 million struggled with alcohol use disorder specifically.[1] Moreover, research has identified overconsumption of alcohol as a leading cause of preventable death among individuals living in the US,[2] with the Centers for Disease Control (CDC) estimating an average of 95,158 alcohol-attributable deaths occurring per year between 2011-2015.[3] Moreover, consequences associated with excessive alcohol use come at a significant economic cost to the US. For example, in 2010, costs related to criminal justice, healthcare, and workplace productivity losses stemming from excessive alcohol use totaled $249 billion.[4] In addition to alcohol, tobacco use is another notable public health concern. According to SAMHSA,[1] of people aged 12 years or older in the US, 19.5% (or 54.7 million) report having used tobacco in the past month, with cigarette smokers comprising 43.6 of those 54.7 million. Importantly, cigarette smoking continues to be the leading cause of preventable death and disease in the US.[5] In fact, over 480,000 US adults die annually from consequences related to cigarettes, and 16 million have a smoking-related illness.[6]

22.2 SCOPE OF THE PROBLEM

Alcohol and tobacco use have numerous deleterious effects on one's physical and mental health. Alcohol use is associated with several diseases, including liver

 DOI: 10.1201/b22810-25

cirrhosis, cardiovascular diseases, and some cancers.[7] In addition to health risks at the individual level, alcohol use can lead to violence, road traffic crashes,[7] and increased contraction and transmission of communicable diseases such as HIV[8] and tuberculosis.[9] Smoking is also associated with increased risk for tuberculosis,[10] as well as several other illnesses including, but not limited to, heart disease, cancer, lung diseases, and immune system complications.[11] Alcohol and tobacco also have harmful consequences for other areas of one's life. For example, alcohol use has been shown to be associated with marital dissatisfaction, higher levels of marital violence,[12] and poorer cognitive functioning.[13] Early tobacco use has also been associated with negative outcomes later in life, including low academic achievement, delinquent behaviors such as stealing, use of violence, early pregnancy, and poly-substance problems.[14] Unsurprisingly, given the vast impact alcohol and tobacco use can have on health and functioning, they each are also associated with significant healthcare costs. In 2012, the global economic cost of smoking was over $1.4 trillion, with treatment for smoking-related illnesses comprising $422 billion.[15] According to the 2020 Surgeon General's Report, in the US, smoking-related illnesses cost over $300 billion per year.[16] Considering these associations, both alcohol and tobacco use represent a substantial global health problem.

22.3 PHYSICAL AND MENTAL HEALTH OVERLAP

The many negative consequences of using alcohol, tobacco, and other substances cut across various domains of one's life, including physical, mental, and social well-being, it is important to assess and treat substance use in the context of integrated health care. A more recent framework proposed for the delivery of integrated healthcare is *Lifestyle Medicine*.[17,18] *Lifestyle Medicine* (LM) attempts to prevent, treat, or reverse lifestyle-related disease by implementing behavioral modifications across six pillars of life: nutrition, physical activity, stress management, restorative sleep, social connection, and the avoidance of risky substance use.[17] Decades of research have supported the association between the aforementioned pillars and various physical health outcomes. For example, a study examining the relationship between diet and COVID-19 outcomes among a sample of nearly 3000 healthcare workers across six countries found that participants who adhered to a plant-based or pescatarian diet and consumed more vegetables, legumes, and nuts had lower odds of contracting moderate-to-severe COVID-19 than those who adhered to a high protein, low carbohydrate diet.[19]

The interrelationships between substance use and other LM pillars are particularly complex, and a nuanced emphasis on substance use can play a pivotal role in negatively impacting one's ability to improve or maintain optimal functioning in the other LM pillars. For example, excessive alcohol use can damage organs, which over time may lead to nutritional deficiencies among individuals who drink heavily.[20,21] Research has also found a negative relationship between cigarette use and physical activity in young adults.[22] Both alcohol and tobacco use are particularly intertwined with the experience of stress over time. While alcohol and tobacco may diminish the experience of stress in the short-term, both have been linked to higher levels of long-term stress.[23,24] Excessive drinking, for example, can cause an individual to release higher amounts of cortisol, which can lead an individual to experience higher anxiety when confronted with stressful situations compared to less excessive drinkers.[23] Cigarette smoking has also been shown to generate or exacerbate negative emotional states and promote negative coping strategies, leading to increased experience of stress over time.[25,26] Sleep is also known to be negatively impacted by alcohol use. Similar to stress, many individuals turn to alcohol to aid sleep, but over time, alcohol use leads to disrupted and fragmented sleep.[27] Substances, particularly alcohol use, can also negatively impact social relationships. In fact, roughly 20% of adults in the US report experiencing harm due to another's alcohol use each year.[28]

While substance use can clearly have a negative impact on functioning across the pillars targeted by LM, many individuals may use substances as a way to improve their functioning with respect to the other pillars of the LM model. For example, nicotine has been shown to reduce appetite, which has led many to turn to smoking for the management of body weight.[29] While tobacco use has been inversely related to physical activity, several research studies have found a positive association between moderate drinking and physical activity levels.[30,31] Both tobacco and alcohol are also commonly used as forms of stress management. Perceived stress has been linked to the onset and maintenance of smoking in several research studies.[32,33] Additionally, coping with stress has been identified as a major reason individuals drink alcohol.[34] Similarly, many individuals turn to alcohol to induce sleep, as alcohol can initially have a sedating effect.[27] Moreover, vivid dreams and insomnia can often occur in chronic drinkers who are practicing abstinence, which can lead to relapse.[27] Finally, both tobacco and alcohol use play an important role in the social connections of many individuals. For example, young adults identify alcohol as a means for developing and maintaining social connectedness.[35]

22.4   INTERVENTIONS

Given the complex, interrelated nature of substance use and the LM pillars, it is important for interventions aimed at reducing substance use to integrate the other lifestyle pillars simultaneously. Such interventions have been developed and used with some success. For example, noting that stress is often a precipitating factor for tobacco use, and can maintain tobacco use, interventions that incorporate stress management skills both prior to quitting and during quit attempts have been shown to be particularly effective in reducing tobacco use.[36,37] In addition, researchers have found that supplementing an existing alcohol intervention with relaxation training and psychoeducation regarding stress management resulted in lasting reductions in alcohol use among college students.[38] Sleep difficulties have often been shown to lead to relapse in individuals with alcohol use disorders.[39] Thus, clinical studies have attempted to address sleep quality as a means for reducing alcohol use. Research has thus far found support for pharmacological treatment in improving sleep and reducing risk of alcohol relapse in individuals with alcohol use disorders,[40,41] and research continues to be done on psychological interventions, such as cognitive behavioral therapy for insomnia, that may aid existing alcohol use disorder treatments.[42] Clinical studies have also sought to develop and test interventions that target alcohol reduction through increasing physical activity. One such study found that women who engaged in physical activity to cope with negative mood and alcohol cravings were better able to maintain abstinence from alcohol.[43] Similarly, research has shown that an increase in physical activity is associated with a greater likelihood of sustained abstinence from smoking. [44] Leveraging social relationships in an effort to reduce alcohol use is another method by which LM pillars may be integrated with substance use reduction strategies. Specifically, Behavioral Couples Therapy, which acknowledges that relationships and substance use are intertwined, has been effective in both improving relationship functioning and reducing alcohol use.[45] Research has also supported the efficacy of the "CATCH My Breath" intervention, a prevention program that centers on social competence, social influences, and refusal skills to reduce e-cigarette use among middle school students.[46] Research on programs that incorporate nutrition-related content with substance use cessation interventions is more limited. However, some research has outlined a link between smoking cessation and a greater readiness to increase fruit and vegetable intake,[47] while another study found that participants involved in an intervention for reducing smoking were more likely to also reduce binge drinking, increase exercise, and increase the number of days they ate healthy breakfasts.[48] These studies suggest that interventions that target multiple areas of healthy lifestyle may be effective.

22.5 SUMMARY

Decades of research have documented the negative effects of substance use on health and well-being. Nevertheless, the associations between substance use (alcohol and tobacco in particular) and other domains of LM are complex. Health care practitioners seeking to implement approaches that account for lifestyle and behavioral factors must carefully consider some of the less apparent ways that individuals use substances in an effort towards more optimal functioning. Healthcare systems and approaches that are designed with the aim of concurrent integration have the greatest potential for positively impacting health and wellness.

REFERENCES

1. Substance Abuse and Mental Health Services Administration. Key substance use and mental health indicators in the United States: Results from the 2021 National Survey on Drug Use and Health (HHS Publication No. PEP22-07-01-005, NSDUH Series H-57). Center for Behavioral Health Statistics and Quality, Substance Abuse and Mental Health Services Administration; 2022. https://www.samhsa.gov/data/report/2021-nsduh-annual-national-report
2. Mokdad AH, Ballestros K, Echko M, et al. US Burden of Disease Collaborators. The state of U.S. health, 1990–2016: Burden of diseases, injuries, and risk factors among U.S. states. *JAMA* 2018;319:1444–1472. 10.1001/jama.2018.0158
3. Esser MB, Sherk A, Liu Y, et al. Deaths and years of potential life lost from excessive alcohol use – United States, 2011–2015 [published correction appears in MMWR Morb Mortal Wkly Rep. 2020 Oct 02;69(39):1427]. *MMWR Morb Mortal Wkly Rep.* 2020;69(30):981–987. doi:10.15585/mmwr.mm6930a1

4. Sacks JJ, Gonzales KR, Bouchery EE, Tomedi LE, Brewer RD. 2010 national and state costs of excessive alcohol consumption. *Am J Prev Med*. 2015;49:e73–e79. doi:10.1016/j. amepre.2015.05.031

5. Cornelius ME, Wang TW, Jamal A, Loretan CG, Neff LJ. Tobacco product use among adults - United States, 2019. *MMWR Morb Mortal Wkly Rep*. 2020;69(46):1736–1742. doi:10.15585/mmwr.mm6946a4

6. Selby P, Zawertailo L. Tobacco addiction. *N Engl J Med*. 2022;387(4):345–354. doi:10. 1056/NEJMcp2032393

7. World Health Organization. Alcohol. https://www.who.int/news-room/fact-sheets/ detail/alcohol#:~:text=Worldwide%2C%203%20million%20deaths%20every,adjusted %20life%20years%20(DALYs). Accessed January 29, 2023.

8. Williams EC, Hahn JA, Saitz R, et al. Alcohol use and human immunodeficiency virus (HIV) infection: Current knowledge, implications, and future directions. *Alcohol Clin Exp Res*. 2016;40(10):2056–2072. doi:10.1111/acer.13204

9. Lönnroth K, Williams BG, Stadlin S, Jaramillo E, Dye C. Alcohol use as a risk factor for tuberculosis - a systematic review. *BMC Public Health*. 2008;8:289. doi:10.1186/ 1471-2458-8-289

10. Silva DR, Muñoz-Torrico M, Duarte R, et al. Risk factors for tuberculosis: Diabetes, smoking, alcohol use, and the use of other drugs. *J Bras Pneumol*. 2018;44(2):145–152. doi:10.1590/s1806-37562017000000443

11. Centers for Disease Control and Prevention. Health effects of cigarette smoking; 2021. https://www.cdc.gov/tobacco/data_statistics/fact_sheets/health_effects/effects_cig_ smoking/.

12. Marshal MP. For better or for worse? The effects of alcohol use on marital functioning. *Clin Psychol Rev*. 2003;23(7):959–997. doi:10.1016/j.cpr.2003.09.002

13. Lees B, Meredith LR, Kirkland AE, Bryant BE, Squeglia LM. Effect of alcohol use on the adolescent brain and behavior. *Pharmacol Biochem Behav*. 2020;192:172906. doi:10.1016/j.pbb.2020.172906

14. Ellickson PL, Tucker JS, Klein DJ. High-risk behaviors associated with early smoking: Results from a 5-year follow-up. *J Adolesc Health*. 2001;28(6):465–473. doi:10.1016/ s1054-139x(00)00202-0

15. Chaloupka FJ, Powell LM, Warner KE. The use of excise taxes to reduce tobacco, alcohol, and sugary beverage consumption. *Annu Rev Public Health*. 2019;40:187–201. doi:10.1146/annurev-publhealth-040218-043816

16. Centers for Disease Control and Prevention. Data and statistics; 2022. https://www.cdc. gov/tobacco/data_statistics/index.htm.

17. American College of Lifestyle Medicine. Home; 2023. https://lifestylemedicine.org/.

18. Katz DL, Karlsen MC, Chung M, et al. Hierarchies of evidence applied to lifestyle medicine (HEALM): Introduction of a strength-of-evidence approach based on a meth-odological systematic review. *BMC Med Res Methodol*. 2019;19(1):178. doi:10.1186/ s12874-019-0811-z

19. Kim H, Rebholz CM, Hegde S, et al. Plant-based diets, pescatarian diets and COVID-19 severity: A population-based case-control study in six countries. *BMJ Nutr Prev Health*. 2021;4(1):257–266. doi:10.1136/bmjnph-2021-000272

20. Bode C, Bode JC. Alcohol's role in gastrointestinal tract disorders. *Alcohol Health Res World*. 1997;21(1):76–83.

21. Mann J, Truswell AS. *Essentials of Human Nutrition*. Oxford University Press; 2017.

22. VanKim NA, Laska MN, Ehlinger E, Lust K, Story M. Understanding young adult physical activity, alcohol and tobacco use in community colleges and 4-year post-secondary institutions: A cross-sectional analysis of epidemiological surveillance data. *BMC Public Health*. 2010;10:208. doi:10.1186/1471-2458-10-208

23. National Institutes of Health. Alcohol alert number 85. https://pubs.niaaa.nih.gov/publications/AA85/AA85.pdf. Accessed January 28, 2023.
24. Lawless MH, Harrison KA, Grandits GA, Eberly LE, Allen SS. Perceived stress and smoking-related behaviors and symptomatology in male and female smokers. *Addict Behav.* 2015;51:80–83. doi:10.1016/j.addbeh.2015.07.011
25. Hajek P, Taylor T, McRobbie H. The effect of stopping smoking on perceived stress levels. *Addiction.* 2010;105(8):1466–1471. doi:10.1111/j.1360-0443.2010.02979.x
26. Stein RJ, Pyle SA, Haddock CK, Poston WS, Bray R, Williams J. Reported stress and its relationship to tobacco use among U.S. military personnel. *Mil Med.* 2008;173(3):271–277. doi:10.7205/milmed.173.3.271
27. Colrain IM, Nicholas CL, Baker FC. Alcohol and the sleeping brain. *Handb Clin Neurol.* 2014;125:415–431. doi:10.1016/B978-0-444-62619-6.00024-0
28. White AM. Gender differences in the epidemiology of alcohol use and related harms in the United States. *Alcohol Res.* 2020;40(2). doi:10.35946/arcr.v40.2.01
29. Chiolero A, Faeh D, Paccaud F, Cornuz J. Consequences of smoking for body weight, body fat distribution, and insulin resistance. *Am J Clin Nutr.* 2008;87(4):801–809. doi:10.1093/ajcn/87.4.801
30. French MT, Popovici I, Maclean JC. Do alcohol consumers exercise more? Findings from a national survey. *Am J Health Promot.* 2009;24(1):2–10. doi:10.4278/ajhp.0801104
31. Lisha NE, Martens M, Leventhal AM. Age and gender as moderators of the relationship between physical activity and alcohol use. *Addict Behav.* 2011;36(9):933–936. doi:10.1016/j.addbeh.2011.04.003
32. Bryant J, Bonevski B, Paul C, O'Brien J, Oakes W. Developing cessation interventions for the social and community service setting: A qualitative study of barriers to quitting among disadvantaged Australian smokers. *BMC Public Health.* 2011;11:493. doi:10.1186/1471-2458-11-493
33. Slopen N, Kontos EZ, Ryff CD, Ayanian JZ, Albert MA, Williams DR. Psychosocial stress and cigarette smoking persistence, cessation, and relapse over 9–10 years: A prospective study of middle-aged adults in the United States. *Cancer Causes Control.* 2013;24(10):1849–1863. doi:10.1007/s10552-013-0262-5
34. Condit M, Kitaji K, Drabble L, Trocki K. Sexual minority women and alcohol: Intersections between drinking, relational contexts, stress and coping. *J Gay Lesbian Soc Serv.* 2011;23(3):351–375. doi:10.1080/10538720.2011.588930
35. Brown R, Murphy S. Alcohol and social connectedness for new residential university students: Implications for alcohol harm reduction. *J Furth High Educ.* 2018;44(2):216–230. doi:10.1080/0309877X.2018.1527024
36. Farris SG, Aston ER, Leyro TM, Brown LA, Zvolensky MJ. Distress intolerance and smoking topography in the context of a biological challenge. *Nicotine Tob Res.* 2019;21(5):568–575. doi:10.1093/ntr/nty167
37. Volz AR, Dennis PA, Dennis MF, Calhoun PS, Wilson SM, Beckham JC. The role of daily hassles and distress tolerance in predicting cigarette craving during a quit attempt. *Nicotine Tob Res.* 2014;16(6):872–875. doi:10.1093/ntr/ntt286
38. Murphy JG, Dennhardt AA, Martens MP, Borsari B, Witkiewitz K, Meshesha LZ. A randomized clinical trial evaluating the efficacy of a brief alcohol intervention supplemented with a substance-free activity session or relaxation training. *J Consult Clin Psychol.* 2019;87(7):657–669. doi:10.1037/ccp0000412
39. Brower KJ, Aldrich MS, Robinson EA, Zucker RA, Greden JF. Insomnia, self-medication, and relapse to alcoholism. *Am J Psychiatry.* 2001;158(3):399–404. doi:10.1176/appi.ajp.158.3.399
40. Brower KJ, Myra Kim H, Strobbe S, Karam-Hage MA, Consens F, Zucker RA. A randomized double-blind pilot trial of gabapentin versus placebo to treat alcohol

dependence and comorbid insomnia. *Alcohol Clin Exp Res.* 2008;32(8):1429–1438. doi:10.1111/j.1530-0277.2008.00706.x

41. Anton RF, O'Malley SS, Ciraulo DA, et al. Combined pharmacotherapies and behavioral interventions for alcohol dependence: The COMBINE study: A randomized controlled trial. *JAMA.* 2006;295(17):2003–2017. doi:10.1001/jama.295.17.2003

42. Miller MB, Metrik J, McGeary JE, et al. Protocol for the Project SAVE randomised controlled trial examining CBT for insomnia among veterans in treatment for alcohol use disorder. *BMJ Open.* 2021;11(6):e045667. doi:10.1136/bmjopen-2020-045667

43. Abrantes AM, Blevins CE, Battle CL, Read JP, Gordon AL, Stein MD. Developing a Fitbit-supported lifestyle physical activity intervention for depressed alcohol dependent women. *J Subst Abuse Treat.* 2017;80:88–97. doi:10.1016/j.jsat.2017.07.006

44. Prochaska JJ, Hall SM, Humfleet G, et al. Physical activity as A strategy for maintaining tobacco abstinence: A randomized trial. *Prev Med.* 2008;47(2):215–220. doi:10.1016/j.ypmed.2008.05.006

45. Powers MB, Vedel E, Emmelkamp PM. Behavioral couples therapy (BCT) for alcohol and drug use disorders: A meta-analysis. *Clin Psychol Rev.* 2008;28(6):952–962. doi:10.1016/j.cpr.2008.02.002

46. Kelder SH, Mantey DS, Van Dusen D, Case K, Haas A, Springer AE. A middle school program to prevent e-cigarette use: A pilot study of "CATCH My Breath". *Public Health Rep.* 2020;135(2):220–229. doi:10.1177/0033354919900887

47. Vogel EA, Ramo DE. Smoking cessation, metabolic risk behaviors, and stress management over time in a sample of young adult smokers. *Transl Behav Med.* 2021;11(1): 189–197. doi:10.1093/tbm/ibz139

48. An LC, Demers MR, Kirch MA, et al. A randomized trial of an avatar-hosted multiple behavior change intervention for young adult smokers. *J Natl Cancer Inst Monogr.* 2013;2013(47):209–215. doi:10.1093/jncimonographs/lgt021

23 Brain Health

Daniel Argueta, BA and
Gia Merlo, MD, MBA, MEd

KEY POINTS

- Neuroinflammation is a fundamental mediator connecting deficiencies in connectivity and the brain gut microbiota system to brain health.
- Disorders like Alzheimer's disease, Parkinson's disease, and autism spectrum disorder are all deeply affected by neuroinflammation, connectivity, and the brain gut microbiota system.
- Brain health should be considered a priority in treatment and promotion of well-being in psychiatric practice.

23.1 INTRODUCTION

The brain is arguably the most complex and important organ in the human body. All functions of the body, including movement, sensation, perception, thought, and emotion, are controlled and coordinated by the brain. Brain health is an essential component to overall health and well-being. Therefore, maintaining brain health through healthy lifestyle choices may be considered a priority in medicine and public health.[1] Each of the aforementioned chapters in this section discusses one of the 6 pillars of lifestyle medicine, all of which partly contribute to brain health across the lifespan.

The role of the brain in medicine spans neurological, cognitive, and mental disorders. Nearly 300 million people globally experience neurological disorder to some degree,[2] but the brain has far-reaching effects and implications on health. Importantly, the concept of brain health is typically restricted to emotional, cognitive, and neural diagnoses. In other words, brain health is typically characterized by emotion regulation (e.g., Major Depressive Disorder, MDD), cognitive ability (e.g., Alzheimer's Disease, AD), or neural dysfunction (e.g., Multiple Sclerosis). We have made strides in combating such diseases, but health in general is an ongoing, lifestyle-centered process. We should therefore consider brain health to be a concept extending beyond deficiency or diagnosis. Brain health is specifically defined as the promotion of optimal brain development, cognitive health, connection to people and purpose, and well-being across the life course.[3] The interplay between well-being, wellness, mental health, and brain health is depicted in Figure 23.1.[4]

The characteristics of psychiatric conditions and their implications for lifestyle psychiatry should not be understated; without research, diagnosis, and treatment relating to the brain, the present topic would not be included in this volume. However, brain development and well-being across a lifetime require more than treatment or diagnosis; rather, they involve lifestyle factors that offer continual maintenance and improvement of the mind and body. These factors include mechanisms of social

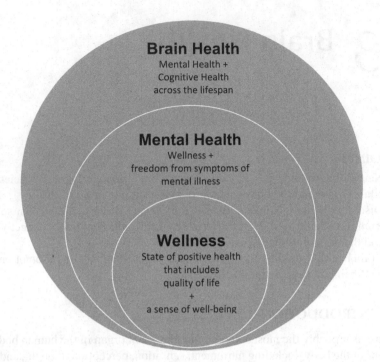

FIGURE 23.1   Relationship of wellness, mental health, and brain health.

connection, resilience, meaning and purpose in life, happiness, compassion, and spirituality. They also include mechanisms along the brain gut microbiota (BGM) system that have important implications for ongoing brain development and well-being.

This chapter will discuss inflammation as the mediator between factors and mechanisms that affect brain health. Inflammatory processes help to protect the body and promote healing and homeostasis in the setting of infection, injury, or tissue damage. However, chronic or prolonged inflammation can negatively impact brain health. Chronic inflammation in the brain, spine, and/or other nervous tissue (neuroinflammation) has been linked to a variety of brain-related issues. We will also describe the ways in which neuroinflammation contributes to Alzheimer's disease (AD), Parkinson's disease (PD), and autism spectrum disorder (ASD).

23.2   NEUROINFLAMMATION

Chapter 11 discusses the inflammatory response, described here in brief. Inflammation has evolved as an immune defense mechanism that prepares the body for injury. In the modern world, poor diet, lack of physical activity, toxins, and other frequent stressors activate this response maladaptively, overwhelming the immune system. The acute sympathetic nervous system response is characterized by the release of catecholamines that increase heart rate and blood pressure to prepare the body for stress.[5] Corticotropin-releasing hormone (CRH) is secreted from the hypothalamus, which activates adrenocorticotropic hormone (ACTH) release from the anterior pituitary gland. Cortisol, a glucocorticoid, is then released after ACTH binds to receptors in the adrenal cortex.[6] Glucocorticoids suppress the initial inflammatory response, reducing the expression of proinflammatory cytokines that signal and recruit monocytes to damaged or infected areas for tissue repair. However, chronic stress sometimes leads to glucocorticoid resistance, allowing for increased proinflammatory cytokine expression and circulation.[7-10] Chronic stress thereby contributes to low-grade inflammation.[8,10]

The peripheral immune response impacts and influences inflammation in the central nervous system. Neuroinflammation is characterized by the recruitment of immune cells to areas of the brain affected by inflammation. A balance between pro- and anti-inflammatory signaling is maintained by cytokines to reach homeostasis following stress. Cytokines also mediate monocyte function in the central nervous system (CNS) driven by microglia.[11] Increased pro-inflammatory cytokine production is associated with tissue damage[12] through decreased levels of brain-derived neurotrophic factor (BDNF).[13] A negative disruption of neural connectivity may occur due to disinhibited phagocytosis of neurons and glia in the CNS induced by inflammatory healing mechanisms.[12] Furthermore, areas in the brain involved in mood processes generally display a heightened immune response compared to other regions of the brain.[14] promoting negative alterations in neural connectivity due to disinhibited phagocytosis of neurons and glia in the CNS.[11] The specific roles of the hippocampus and prefrontal cortex have sensitive responses to pro-inflammatory signals,[10,11] suggesting glucocorticoid resistance to anti-inflammatory signaling can negatively affect hippocampal neurogenesis and executive brain function.

Chronic neuroinflammation is implicated in negative brain health outcomes, including inhibited neurodevelopment and neurogenesis, accelerated aging, and psychiatric disorders.[15-18] Neuroimmunological factors significantly impact brain health by influencing a diverse range of neural mechanisms in various psychiatric/ neurological disorders. A variety of symptoms associated with ASD have been attributed to immune dysfunction, including increased social withdrawal, disordered eating, and disordered sleeping.[19,20] ASD is characterized by deficits in social development, interaction, and repetitive interests or behaviors. A growing body of evidence suggests that neuroinflammation may be implicated in the pathogenesis, severity, and clinical presentation of ASD.[19] Patients with ASD have been found to have increased levels of CNS and circulating pro-inflammatory cytokines including tumor-necrosis factor-alpha (TNF-a) and interleukin-6 (IL-6).[20-26] Current research indicates that the pro-inflammatory phenotypes of microglia and astrocytes also contribute to ASD in similar ways to PD. Patients with ASD exhibit increased astrocyte and microglial markers compared to those of neurotypical controls.[21] Further evidence indicates microglia may be more densely located in the dorsolateral prefrontal cortices of patients with ASD. Therefore, neuroinflammation may significantly affect the cognitive, affective, or sensory differences between those with ASD and their neurotypical counterparts.[27]

Age-related increases in neuroinflammation are linked to decreased adult hippocampal neurogenesis (AHN), long-term potentiation, and maladaptive dendritic remodeling.[28] Current data suggest that aged microglia amplify cytokine production and activation during the aging process can lead to anorexia, social withdrawal, depressive behavior, and cognitive impairment, the most severe of which includes AD.[28,29] AD is a condition characterized by neurodegeneration and neurocognitive decline resulting from accumulations of amyloid-beta (Aβ) plaques and tau tangles.[30] Chronic microglial functional impairment related to neuroinflammation contributes to the pathogenesis of AD.[31] Although microglia can combat Aβ plaques, long-term exposure to plaque accumulation can result in increased levels of pro-inflammatory cytokines in the brain that alter the phago-cytic properties of microglia.[29] The pathogenesis of PD is also heavily mediated by neuroinflammation. PD is characterized by the death of dopaminergic neu-rons mediated by glial dysregulation.[32] Cell death leads to low dopamine levels resulting in motor dysfunction, cognitive impairment (including dementia), and psychiatric disorders.[32] Both cells have pro- and anti-inflammatory phenotypes, the balance of which is crucial to healthy cell and tissue maintenance in the brain. Apoptosis of such dopaminergic cells is induced by astrocytes and promoted by microglia, likely due to overexpression of pro-inflammatory phenotypes from both cells.[13]

23.3 CONNECTIVITY

Connections with people and purpose are important protective factors for mental and physical health. The concept of connectivity related to brain health is defined by 6 factors: social connectivity, resilience, meaning in life, happiness, compassion, and spirituality. The following section introduces these concepts and uses neuroinflam-mation to illustrate their impact on brain health.

23.3.1 SOCIAL CONNECTIVITY

As discussed in Chapter 21, social connection and integration are important for a variety of mental and physical health outcomes. A variety of mental and cognitive disorders are associated with deficits in social connectivity. Indeed, negative social experiences can trigger inflammation. This section introduces the ways in which brain health interacts with inflammation in the periphery and CNS, as well as the ways in which inflammation leads to deficiencies in social connection and interac-tion in ASD.

Human and non-human animal studies provide evidence that social defeat and related stress can promote heightened neuroinflammatory signaling in the brain and periphery.[33,34] Neuroinflammatory responses to social stress can lead to cog-nitive impairment.[35] Social processes and inflammation interact bidirectionally. Therefore, neuroinflammation can influence downstream social processes and functions. Increased social pain,[36] increased sensitivity to social information,[37] and increased desire and searching for social integration may induce neuroinflamma-tion that has the potential to engender negative depressive effects.[38] Current animal models provide evidence of the role of social desire, interaction, and response in brain health and function. There is little literature examining the effect of neuroin-flammation on social activity in neurotypical humans. However, emerging evidence indicates that endotoxins and inflammatory signaling can enhance feelings of social disconnection,[39] avoidance of stranger interactions,[40] and sensitivity to social reward and punishment.[41,42] Moreover, new research indicates that social connectivity plays a protective factor against suicidal ideation for adults with ASD.[43,44]

Recent data suggest that social cognitive deficits in people with ASD may be explained by neuroinflammation.[45] Rodent models demonstrated that mice with increased proinflammatory cytokines in the cerebellum displayed reduced social interaction and impaired play behaviors.[46] Social cognitive deficits in humans may also result from decreased reward and pleasure in social interaction.[47] Inflammation can lead to decreased communication in people with ASD and increased overall symptom severity.[48–50] Neuroimmune abnormality could also adversely affect dopamine reward processing that can contribute to ASD symptoms.[51] The link between ASD and neuroinflammation is complex and under investigation. However, research on impaired social function in patients with ASD reveals important mechanisms by which brain health and neuroinflammation interact in the etiology and maintenance of the disorder.[52] Targeting neuroinflammation may be a potential avenue for creating novel treatments for those with ASD.

23.3.2 RESILIENCE

Psychological and health resilience can positively impact brain health.[53,54] Current literature on stress and its impact on brain health is grounded in concepts related to resilience. This section aims to identify how stress can be combated, who is resilient, and the factors that contribute to resilience. Many definitions are used to describe resilience in many fields. To best illustrate brain health, we will discuss stress resilience specifically as the capability of achieving positive or neutral outcomes during adversity. In other words, those demonstrating resilience show little to no stress response when presented with stressful stimuli. In fact, resilient people may be affected positively by stress.[55] Health care professionals may be able to improve brain health, mental health, and physical health outcomes in patients by understanding the mechanisms behind resilience.

The brain coordinates physiological and behavioral responses to stressful stimuli, making brain health key towards the promotion of stress resilience. Normally, chronic stressors negatively influence this response by inducing a chronic, low-grade inflammation. As mentioned previously, this response is maladaptive and negatively impacts the health of the brain. However, considerable variability in stress response exists, and emerging evidence examines the mechanisms that allow some individuals to respond adaptively to stress. In rodent models, resilient individuals display decreased neuroinflammatory responses such as decreased corticotropin-releasing factor (CRF), cytokines, and monocytes in the brain in response to induced stress.[56,57] Resilience to neuroinflammation may be influenced by epigenetic factors that reduce the neuroinflammatory cytokine response, promoting resilience to depression-like behaviors. Specifically, Dihydrocaffeic acid (DHCA) and malvidin-3'-O glucoside (mal-gluc) are involved in expression inhibition of IL-6 production and synaptic plasticity sequences, respectively.[57] Resilience may also be mediated by adult hippocampal neurogenesis (AHN). While research surrounding AHN is under active investigation, some evidence suggests that increased AHN contributes to greater cognitive and emotional processing, thereby allowing for effective stress coping.[58] Neuroinflammation normally inhibits AHN such that a balance between pro- and anti-inflammatory responses could be important for stress resilience to promote AHN.[58]

Resilience in AD and PD helps illustrate the link between inflammation and neurocognitive decline. Patients with PD with greater psychological resilience displayed less disability, attenuated depressive symptoms, and greater of quality of life compared to those with less psychological resilience.[59] Other factors, like social connection, may be important for resilience directly related to disease in AD.[60] Social connectivity can buffer the compounding effects of a dysregulated stress response on the neurocognitive deficits associated with AD.[60]

Existing literature indicates that individuals can improve their resilience and ability to cope with stress and adversity by promoting brain health through positive social connectivity.[61,62] However, further research is needed to better understand the specific protective factors of psychological and inflammatory resilience in PD and AD to combat neurodegenerative disease.

23.3.3 COMPASSION, HAPPINESS, MEANING IN LIFE, AND SPIRITUALITY

Researchers are beginning to investigate compassion, happiness, meaning in life, and spirituality as factors influencing inflammation. However, emerging evidence indicates that lifestyle fulfillment and incorporation of each of the 4 topics can be protective for brain health. Increased self-compassion is associated with lower levels of IL-6 and better mental health.[63,64] Practicing compassion through kindness meditation may have protective age-related longevity effects.[65] Compassion training may help reduce amounts of circulating CRP for individuals who report early life adversity.[66] This effect was also uniquely observed in populations with a high-stress vulnerability, suggesting that compassion training may be uniquely effective for high-risk individuals.[67] Joy, contentment, and pride have also been shown to decrease inflammation, indicating that a happy disposition may be important in protecting the body from immunological stress.[68,69] Additionally, happiness measured by positive affect may help buffer the effect of stress on CRP levels.[70] Having both a meaning or purpose in life and a spiritual connection may be protective against the inflammatory effects of aging and stress.[71–73]

Each of the 6 factors influencing connectivity (social connectivity, resilience, compassion, happiness, meaning in life, and spirituality) needs more investigation on their neural and immunological effects. The incorporation of therapeutic modalities addressing the roles of each of these factors and quality of life may be fundamental to promoting brain health and well-being across the lifespan.

23.4 BGM SYSTEM

The brain gut microbiota (BGM) system influences brain health in ways that should be considered fundamental. Gut microbiota (GM) consist of the organisms that inhabit the gastrointestinal tract.[74] The GM produce vital chemical precursors to many neurotransmitters, immune cells, and hormones that are fundamental to the survival of host organisms.[75-77] This system is directly innervated and modulated by the vagus nerve, which serves as the main line of communication between the CNS and GM.[78,79] The BGM system also relies heavily on the enteric nervous system (ENS), the part of the peripheral nervous system that directly coordinates the functions of secretion, motility, and mucosal and immunologic maintenance.[80] A variety of factors can disrupt this system, including neuroinflammation, mental disorders, and psychological or immunological stress.[81-86]

The vagus nerve is fundamental to the communication between the GM and the brain. Bidirectional communication between the brain and gut relies on a system composed of 80% afferent and 20% efferent neurons.[79,80,87,88] An epithelial layer and proximal mucosal layer create the barrier between the vagus nerve afferent receptors in the GM. The afferent receptors end in the epithelium of the intestine and enteroendocrine cells reside in the mucosal layer.[89] Little to no bacteria reside in the epithelium under normal conditions. Still, GM products are detected by enteroendocrine cells (EECs), which release serotonin as a form of direct communication between bacteria and vagal receptors.[90] Vagal receptors throughout the gastrointestinal tract detect microbial metabolites and inflammatory signaling through EECs, thereby allowing for changes or disruption in the balance of organisms within the gut to be communicated with the CNS. Such balance disruption within the gut is known as dysbiosis and is involved in many of the adverse health outcomes described in this section.[80]

Efferent fibers of the vagus nerve can affect intestinal permeability and gut microbiota composition via communication from the CNS to the gut. Efferent vagal innervations within the gut reduce inflammation. Afferent fibers of the vagus nerve signal inflammation to the CNS during the stress response. Efferent fibers of the vagus nerve then release acetylcholine to activate the cholinergic anti-inflammatory pathway which inhibits cytokine production.[79] Enteric glial cells regulate the permeability of the gastrointestinal epithelium through a variety of mechanisms.[91,92] Chronic stress and inflammation suppress the parasympathetic response of the vagus nerve and can lead to increased intestinal permeability and dysbiosis.[79] Research currently examines the role of vagus nerve stimulation as a therapeutic approach and distinct parasympathetic responder to the effects of stress on the gut.[93] Researchers have shown that vagus nerve stimulation can prime the body for injury by maintaining low epithelial permeability,[94] and prevent common symptoms of gut dysbiosis, including body weight loss and increased defecation.[78] Studies have also demonstrated that vagus nerve stimulation can decrease pain in response to colorectal distension, a classic marker of irritable bowel syndrome in humans.[78] Limited research currently investigates the downstream effects of CNS vagus nerve stimulation on the gut microbiota. However, ongoing investigation of this relationship may provide further insight into how the gut microbiota can affect brain health.

The bidirectional relationship between inflammation and the BGM system is complex and still not fully understood. However, psychoneuroimmunology research reveals that disruptions to homeostasis or communication in the BGM pathway can significantly affect gut and brain health. Gut dysbiosis promotes and is promoted by elevated stress and the peripheral immune response.[77] Inflammation can alter the integrity of the intestinal barrier via the vagus nerve.[79] Factors including poor diet and stress that alter the composition of the GM enhance the epithelial immune response through increased recognition of pathogenic bacteria.[83,92] The blood-brain barrier (BBB) can be altered by increased inflammation in the periphery through reduced tight junction protein expression along the BGM system.[95,96] Gut permeability allows endotoxins secreted by bacteria, like lipopolysaccharide (LPS), to enter the bloodstream. Such endotoxins can then reach the brain after penetrating the BBB and influence the CNS inflammatory response.[97] LPS promotes the phagocytic and pro-inflammatory phenotypes of microglia in the brain, inducing cell death and brain dysfunction.[98]

The GM influence neurotransmitter precursors and inflammatory mediators that contribute to the pathology and development of AD, PD, and ASD. Enhanced permeability of the epithelium and BBB in patients with AD increases the risk of bacterial endotoxins reaching the brain.[99] LPS levels are much higher in patients with AD compared to healthy controls. Cerebrospinal fluid (CSF) concentrations of LPS specifically can increase neuroinflammation and Aβ accumulation.[100,101] Microbiota influences on microglia can also promote the progression of AD by exacerbating neuroinflammatory mechanisms. Indeed, the upregulation of proinflammatory cytokines is associated with increased levels of pathogenic species of bacteria and decreased levels of beneficial species of bacteria, which can contribute to chronic inflammation in the CNS.[76,82,102] Excessive inflammatory signaling can therefore cause microglia to cease phagocytic activity, thereby allowing for the progression of Aβ accumulation and subsequent dementia.[103]

Patients with PD are also more likely to present with dysbiosis. Less research has been done that examines the mechanisms between dysbiosis and dopaminergic cell death in patients or models of PD. Motor symptoms worsen with an accelerated decrease in the variability of intestinal microbiota,[104,105] and dysbiosis can lead to LPS accumulation.[106] The gut produces α-synuclein, a major component of Lewy bodies that characterize PD. Under dysbiosis, this protein can promote the development of Lewy bodies in the CNS.[107] The GM of patients with PD often resemble that of patients with irritable bowel syndrome, resulting in leaky gut syndrome and neuroinflammation.[108]

ASD is often associated with gastrointestinal issues and dysfunction. Research has demonstrated a link between severity of emotional, behavioral, and GI symptoms in patients with ASD.[109] Indeed, over half of the GI symptoms experienced by people with ASD are associated with dysbiosis. Patients with ASD often present with high levels of pathogenic bacteria and low levels of beneficial bacteria in the gut compared to neurotypical controls.[19,109] Dysbiosis, increased intestinal permeability, promotion of systemic inflammation, and decreased lactic acid production commonly present in patients with ASD.[74,109,110] Each of the mechanisms associated with dysbiosis and GI symptoms in patients with ASD promotes neuroinflammation, indicating the role of the BGM system in the expression, pathogenesis, and clinical presentation of ASD.

A variety of research establishes effective probiotic intervention in AD, PD, and ASD. Probiotic treatment through bacterial administration may improve memory and cognitive decline in AD.[108,111,112] The protective effects of probiotic administration on dopaminergic neuron loss have been demonstrated in rodent models.[113] Fecal matter transplant from a healthy donor to a child with ASD has been shown to alleviate characteristic behavioral symptoms.[114] Mechanistic research regarding the role of the gut brain system in AD, PD, and ASD is needed due to current lack of human studies in this space.

23.5 CONCLUSION

Overall well-being and brain health across the lifespan are dependent on mechanisms and communication within the BGM system that link lifestyle factors to psychiatric outcomes. Future assessments and interventions must rely on and consider how this relationship indicates organ functioning and well-being. Psychiatry cannot overlook lifestyle factors or brain health. Healthcare historically neglected and misunderstood brain health as a key process for improving overall health and well-being in patients. Neuroinflammation underlies many mental and brain health diseases, including neurodegenerative disorders. The emergence of this mechanism holds promise for advancing the diagnosis and treatment of brain health conditions. Lifestyle interventions can offer solutions that promote health across the lifespan by addressing the mind, brain, and body alike.

REFERENCES

1. Optimizing brain health across the life course: WHO position paper. https://www.who.int/publications-detail-redirect/9789240054561. Accessed April 24, 2023.
2. GBD 2016 Neurology Collaborators. Global, regional, and national burden of neurological disorders, 1990–2016: A systematic analysis for the Global Burden of Disease Study 2016. *Lancet Neurol.* 2019;18(5):459–480. doi:10.1016/S1474-4422(18)30499-X
3. Chapman SB, Fratantoni JM, Robertson IH, et al. A novel BrainHealth index prototype improved by telehealth-delivered training during COVID-19. *Front Public Health.* 2021;9:641754. doi:10.3389/fpubh.2021.641754
4. Merlo G, Sugden SG, Abascal L. Lifestyle psychiatry: An overview. In: *Lifestyle Medicine.* 4th ed. Boca Ratan, Florida: CRC Press/Taylor&Francis; 2023 (forthcoming).
5. Johnson JD, Campisi J, Sharkey CM, et al. Catecholamines mediate stress-induced increases in peripheral and central inflammatory cytokines. *Neuroscience.* 2005;135(4): 1295–1307. doi:10.1016/j.neuroscience.2005.06.090
6. Juruena MF, Eror F, Cleare AJ, Young AH. The role of early life stress in HPA axis and anxiety. In: Kim YK, ed. Advances in experimental medicine and biology. *Anxiety Disorders: Rethinking and Understanding Recent Discoveries.* Springer; 2020:141–153. doi:10.1007/978-981-32-9705-0_9
7. Barnes PJ, Adcock IM. Glucocorticoid resistance in inflammatory diseases. *The Lancet.* 2009;373(9678):1905–1917. doi:10.1016/S0140-6736(09)60326-3
8. Walsh CP, Bovbjerg DH, Marsland AL. Glucocorticoid resistance and β2-adrenergic receptor signaling pathways promote peripheral pro-inflammatory conditions associated with chronic psychological stress: A systematic review across species. *Neurosci Biobehav Rev.* 2021;128:117–135. doi:10.1016/j.neubiorev.2021.06.013
9. Furtado M, Katzman MA. Examining the role of neuroinflammation in major depression. *Psychiatry Res.* 2015;229(1):27–36. doi:10.1016/j.psychres.2015.06.009
10. Liu YZ, Wang YX, Jiang CL. Inflammation: The common pathway of stress-related diseases. *Front Hum Neurosci.* 2017;11:316. doi:10.3389/fnhum.2017.00316
11. DiSabato D, Quan N, Godbout JP. Neuroinflammation: The devil is in the details. *J Neurochem.* 2016;139(Suppl 2):136–153. doi:10.1111/jnc.13607

12. Berger A. Th1 and Th2 responses: What are they? *BMJ*. 2000;321(7258):424. doi:10.1136/bmj.321.7258.424

13. Rasheed M, Liang J, Wang C, Deng Y, Chen Z. Epigenetic regulation of neuroinflammation in Parkinson's disease. *Int J Mol Sci*. 2021;22(9):4956. doi:10.3390/ijms22094956

14. Kiecolt-Glaser JK, Derry HM, Fagundes CP. Inflammation: Depression fans the flames and feasts on the heat. *Am J Psychiatry*. 2015;172(11):1075–1091. doi:10.1176/appi.ajp.2015.15020152

15. Fan LW, Pang Y. Dysregulation of neurogenesis by neuroinflammation: Key differences in neurodevelopmental and neurological disorders. *Neural Regen Res*. 2017;12(3):366–371. doi:10.4103/1673-5374.202926

16. Kim YK, Na KS, Myint AM, Leonard BE. The role of pro-inflammatory cytokines in neuroinflammation, neurogenesis and the neuroendocrine system in major depression. *Prog Neuropsychopharmacol Biol Psychiatry*. 2016;64:277–284. doi:10.1016/j.pnpbp.2015.06.008

17. Millington C, Sonego S, Karunaweera N, et al. Chronic neuroinflammation in Alzheimer's disease: New perspectives on animal models and promising candidate drugs. *BioMed Res Int*. 2014;2014:e309129. doi:10.1155/2014/309129

18. Jauhari A, Baranov SV, Suofu Y, et al. Melatonin inhibits cytosolic mitochondrial DNA–induced neuroinflammatory signaling in accelerated aging and neurodegeneration. *J Clin Invest*. 2020;130(6):3124–3136. doi:10.1172/JCI135026

19. Matta SM, Hill-Yardin EL, Crack PJ. The influence of neuroinflammation in autism spectrum disorder. *Brain Behav Immun*. 2019;79:75–90. doi:10.1016/j.bbi.2019.04.037

20. Al-Ayadhi LY. Pro-inflammatory cytokines in autistic children in central Saudi Arabia. *Neurosci J*. 2005;10(2):155–158.

21. Vargas DL, Nascimbene C, Krishnan C, Zimmerman AW, Pardo CA. Neuroglial activation and neuroinflammation in the brain of patients with autism. *Ann Neurol*. 2005;57(1):67–81. doi:10.1002/ana.20315

22. Wei H, Zou H, Sheikh AM, et al. IL-6 is increased in the cerebellum of autistic brain and alters neural cell adhesion, migration and synaptic formation. *J Neuroinflammation*. 2011;8(1):52. doi:10.1186/1742-2094-8-52

23. Basheer S, Venkataswamy MM, Christopher R, et al. Immune aberrations in children with autism spectrum disorder: A case-control study from a tertiary care neuropsychiatric Hospital in India. *Psychoneuroendocrinology*. 2018;94:162–167. doi:10.1016/j.psyneuen.2018.05.002

24. Ashwood P, Krakowiak P, Hertz-Picciotto I, Hansen R, Pessah IN, Van de Water J. Altered T cell responses in children with autism. *Brain Behav Immun*. 2011;25(5):840–849. doi:10.1016/j.bbi.2010.09.002

25. Chez MG, Dowling T, Patel PB, Khanna P, Kominsky M. Elevation of tumor necrosis factor-alpha in cerebrospinal fluid of autistic children. *Pediatr Neurol*. 2007;36(6):361–365. doi:10.1016/j.pediatrneurol.2007.01.012

26. Ghaffari MA, Mousavinejad E, Riahi F, Mousavinejad M, Afsharmanesh MR. Increased serum levels of tumor necrosis factor-alpha, resistin, and visfatin in the children with autism spectrum disorders: A case-control study. *Neurol Res Int*. 2016;2016:e9060751. doi:10.1155/2016/9060751

27. Morgan JT, Chana G, Abramson I, Semendeferi K, Courchesne E, Everall IP. Abnormal microglial–neuronal spatial organization in the dorsolateral prefrontal cortex in autism. *Brain Res*. 2012;1456:72–81. doi:10.1016/j.brainres.2012.03.036

28. Norden DM, Godbout JP. Microglia of the aged brain: Primed to be activated and resistant to regulation. *Neuropathol Appl Neurobiol*. 2013;39(1):19–34. doi:10.1111/j.1365-2990.2012.01306.x

29. Heneka MT, Carson MJ, Khoury JE, et al. Neuroinflammation in Alzheimer's disease. *Lancet Neurol*. 2015;14(4):388–405. doi:10.1016/S1474-4422(15)70016-5

30. Scheltens P, Blennow K, Breteler MMB, et al. Alzheimer's disease. *The Lancet.* 2016 ;388(10043):505–517. doi:10.1016/S0140-6736(15)01124-1

31. Lyman M, Lloyd DG, Ji X, Vizcaychipi MP, Ma D. Neuroinflammation: The role and consequences. *Neurosci Res.* 2014;79:1–12. doi:10.1016/j.neures.2013.10.004

32. Badanjak K, Fixemer S, Smajić S, Skupin A, Grünewald A. The contribution of microglia to neuroinflammation in Parkinson's disease. *Int J Mol Sci.* 2021;22(9):4676. doi:10.3390/ijms22094676

33. Lisboa SF, Niraula A, Resstel LB, Guimaraes FS, Godbout JP, Sheridan JF. Repeated social defeat-induced neuroinflammation, anxiety-like behavior and resistance to fear extinction were attenuated by the cannabinoid receptor agonist WIN55,212-2. *Neuropsychopharmacology.* 2018;43(9):1924–1933. doi:10.1038/s41386-018-0064-2

34. Bravo-Tobar ID, Fernández P, Sáez JC, Dagnino-Subiabre A. Long-term effects of stress resilience: Hippocampal neuroinflammation and behavioral approach in male rats. *J Neurosci Res.* 2021;99(10):2493–2510. doi:10.1002/jnr.24902

35. Pfau ML, Russo SJ. Neuroinflammation regulates cognitive impairment in socially defeated mice. *Trends Neurosci.* 2016;39(6):353–355. doi:10.1016/j.tins.2016.04.004

36. Eisenberger NI, Inagaki TK, Rameson LT, Mashal NM, Irwin MR. An fMRI study of cytokine-induced depressed mood and social pain: The role of sex differences. *NeuroImage.* 2009;47(3):881–890. doi:10.1016/j.neuroimage.2009.04.040

37. Muscatell KA, Moieni M, Inagaki TK, et al. Exposure to an inflammatory challenge enhances neural sensitivity to negative and positive social feedback. *Brain Behav Immun.* 2016;57:21–29. doi:10.1016/j.bbi.2016.03.022

38. Willette AA, Lubach GR, Coe CL. Environmental context differentially affects behavioral, leukocyte, cortisol, and interleukin-6 responses to low doses of endotoxin in the rhesus monkey. *Brain Behav Immun.* 2007;21(6):807–815. doi:10.1016/j.bbi.2007.01.007

39. Eisenberger NI, Inagaki TK, Mashal NM, Irwin MR. Inflammation and social experience: An inflammatory challenge induces feelings of social disconnection in addition to depressed mood. *Brain Behav Immun.* 2010;24(4):558–563. doi:10.1016/j.bbi.2009.12.009

40. Jolink TA, Fendinger NJ, Alvarez GM, Feldman MJ, Gaudier-Diaz MM, Muscatell KA. Inflammatory reactivity to the influenza vaccine is associated with changes in automatic social behavior. *Brain Behav Immun.* 2022;99:339–349. doi:10.1016/j.bbi.2021.10.019

41. Eisenberger NI, Moieni M, Inagaki TK, Muscatell KA, Irwin MR. In sickness and in health: The co-regulation of inflammation and social behavior. *Neuropsychopharmacology.* 2017;42(1):242–253. doi:10.1038/npp.2016.141

42. Bower JE, Kuhlman KR. Psychoneuroimmunology: An introduction to immune-to-brain communication and its implications for clinical psychology. *Annu Rev Clin Psychol.* 2023;19(1): 331–359. doi:10.1146/annurev-clinpsy-080621-045153

43. Hedley D, Uljarević M, Foley KR, Richdale A, Trollor J. Risk and protective factors underlying depression and suicidal ideation in autism spectrum disorder. *Depress Anxiety.* 2018;35(7):648–657. doi:10.1002/da.22759

44. Mournet AM, Wilkinson E, Bal VH, Kleiman EM. A systematic review of predictors of suicidal thoughts and behaviors among autistic adults: Making the case for the role of social connection as a protective factor. *Clin Psychol Rev.* 2023;99:102235. doi:10.1016/j.cpr.2022.102235

45. Nakagawa Y, Chiba K. Involvement of neuroinflammation during brain development in social cognitive deficits in autism spectrum disorder and schizophrenia. *J Pharmacol Exp Ther.* 2016;358(3):504–515.

46. McFarlane HG, Kusek GK, Yang M, Phoenix JL, Bolivar VJ, Crawley JN. Autism-like behavioral phenotypes in BTBR T+tf/J mice. *Genes Brain Behav.* 2008;7(2):152–163. doi:10.1111/j.1601-183X.2007.00330.x

47. Kohls G, Chevallier C, Troiani V, Schultz RT. Social 'wanting' dysfunction in autism: Neurobiological underpinnings and treatment implications. *J Neurodev Disord*. 2012; 4(1):10. doi:10.1186/1866-1955-4-10

48. Ashwood P, Krakowiak P, Hertz-Picciotto I, Hansen R, Pessah I, Van de Water J. Elevated plasma cytokines in autism spectrum disorders provide evidence of immune dysfunction and are associated with impaired behavioral outcome. *Brain Behav Immun*. 2011;25(1):40–45. doi:10.1016/j.bbi.2010.08.003

49. Piras IS, Haapanen L, Napolioni V, Sacco R, Van de Water J, Persico AM. Anti-brain antibodies are associated with more severe cognitive and behavioral profiles in Italian children with autism spectrum disorder. *Brain Behav Immun*. 2014;38:91–99. doi:10.1016/j.bbi.2013.12.020

50. El Gohary TM, El Aziz NA, Darweesh M, Sadaa ES. Plasma level of transforming growth factor β 1 in children with autism spectrum disorder. *Egypt J Ear Nose Throat Allied Sci*. 2015;16(1):69–73. doi:10.1016/j.ejenta.2014.12.002

51. Greene RK, Walsh E, Mosner MG, Dichter GS. A potential mechanistic role for neuroinflammation in reward processing impairments in autism spectrum disorder. *Biol Psychol*. 2019;142:1–12. doi:10.1016/j.biopsycho.2018.12.008

52. El-Ansary A, Al-Ayadhi L. Neuroinflammation in autism spectrum disorders. *J Neuroinflammation*. 2012;9(1):265. doi:10.1186/1742-2094-9-265

53. Kong F, Ma X, You X, Xiang Y. The resilient brain: Psychological resilience mediates the effect of amplitude of low-frequency fluctuations in orbitofrontal cortex on subjective well-being in young healthy adults. *Soc Cogn Affect Neurosci*. 2018;13(7):755–763. doi:10.1093/scan/nsy045

54. Majnarić LT, Bosnić Z, Guljaš S, et al. Low psychological resilience in older individuals: An association with increased inflammation, oxidative stress and the presence of chronic medical conditions. *Int J Mol Sci*. 2021;22(16):8970. doi:10.3390/ijms22168970

55. Tugade MM, Fredrickson BL. Resilient individuals use positive emotions to bounce back from negative emotional experiences. *J Pers Soc Psychol*. 2004;86(2):320–333. doi:10.1037/0022-3514.86.2.320

56. Gururajan A, van de Wouw M, Boehme M, et al. Resilience to chronic stress is associated with specific neurobiological, neuroendocrine and immune responses. *Brain Behav Immun*. 2019;80:583–594. doi:10.1016/j.bbi.2019.05.004

57. Wang J, Hodes GE, Zhang H, et al. Epigenetic modulation of inflammation and synaptic plasticity promotes resilience against stress in mice. *Nat Commun*. 2018;9:477. doi:10.1038/s41467-017-02794-5

58. Vasic V, Schmidt MHH. Resilience and vulnerability to pain and inflammation in the hippocampus. *Int J Mol Sci*. 2017;18(4):739. doi:10.3390/ijms18040739

59. Robottom BJ, Gruber-Baldini AL, Anderson KE, et al. What determines resilience in patients with Parkinson's disease? *Parkinsonism Relat Disord*. 2012;18(2):174–177. doi:10.1016/j.parkreldis.2011.09.021

60. Perry BL, McConnell WR, Coleman ME, Roth AR, Peng S, Apostolova LG. Why the cognitive "fountain of youth" may be upstream: Pathways to dementia risk and resilience through social connectedness. *Alzheimers Dement*. 2022;18(5):934–941. doi:10.1002/alz.12443

61. O'Neal CW, Richardson EW, Mancini JA. Community, context, and coping: How social connections influence coping and well-being for military members and their spouses. *Fam Process*. 2020;59(1):158–172. doi:10.1111/famp.12395

62. Moore KA, March E. Socially connected during COVID-19: Online social connections mediate the relationship between loneliness and positive coping strategies. *J Stress Trauma Anxiety Resil J-STAR*. 2022;1(1). doi:10.55319/js.v1i1.9

63. Breines JG, Thoma MV, Gianferante D, Hanlin L, Chen X, Rohleder N. Self-compassion as a predictor of interleukin-6 response to acute psychosocial stress. *Brain Behav Immun*. 2014;37:109–114. doi:10.1016/j.bbi.2013.11.006

64. Lee EE, Govind T, Ramsey M, et al. Compassion toward others and self-compassion predict mental and physical well-being: A 5-year longitudinal study of 1090 community-dwelling adults across the lifespan. *Transl Psychiatry*. 2021;11(1):1–9. doi:10.1038/s41398-021-01491-8

65. Hoge EA, Chen MM, Orr E, et al. Loving-kindness meditation practice associated with longer telomeres in women. *Brain Behav Immun*. 2013;32:159–163. doi:10.1016/j.bbi.2013.04.005

66. Pace TWW, Negi LT, Dodson-Lavelle B, et al. Engagement with cognitively-based compassion training is associated with reduced salivary C-reactive protein from before to after training in foster care program adolescents. *Psychoneuroendocrinology*. 2013;38(2):294–299. doi:10.1016/j.psyneuen.2012.05.019

67. Puhlmann LMC, Engert V, Apostolakou F, et al. Only vulnerable adults show change in chronic low-grade inflammation after contemplative mental training: Evidence from a randomized clinical trial. *Sci Rep*. 2019;9(1):19323. doi:10.1038/s41598-019-55250-3

68. Stellar JE, John-Henderson N, Anderson CL, Gordon AM, McNeil GD, Keltner D. Positive affect and markers of inflammation: Discrete positive emotions predict lower levels of inflammatory cytokines. *Emotion*. 2015;15(2):129–133. doi:10.1037/emo0000033

69. Panagi L, Poole L, Hackett RA, Steptoe A. Happiness and inflammatory responses to acute stress in people with type 2 diabetes. *Ann Behav Med Publ Soc Behav Med*. 2018;53(4):309–320. doi:10.1093/abm/kay039

70. Blevins CL, Sagui SJ, Bennett JM. Inflammation and positive affect: Examining the stress-buffering hypothesis with data from the national longitudinal study of adolescent to adult health. *Brain Behav Immun*. 2017;61:21–26. doi:10.1016/j.bbi.2016.07.149

71. Guimond AJ, Shiba K, Kim ES, Kubzansky LD. Sense of purpose in life and inflammation in healthy older adults: A longitudinal study. *Psychoneuroendocrinology*. 2022;141:105746. doi:10.1016/j.psyneuen.2022.105746

72. Ferraro KF, Kim S. Health benefits of religion among black and white older adults? Race, religiosity, and C-reactive protein. *Soc Sci Med*. 2014;120:92–99. doi:10.1016/j.socscimed.2014.08.030

73. Hybels CF, George LK, Blazer DG, Pieper CF, Cohen HJ, Koenig HG. Inflammation and coagulation as mediators in the relationships between religious attendance and functional limitations in older adults. *J Aging Health*. 2014;26(4):679–697. doi:10.1177/0898264314527479

74. Gomaa EZ. Human gut microbiota/microbiome in health and diseases: A review. *Antonie Van Leeuwenhoek*. 2020;113(12):2019–2040. doi:10.1007/s10482-020-01474-7

75. Strandwitz P. Neurotransmitter modulation by the gut microbiota. *Brain Res*. 2018; 1693:128–133. doi:10.1016/j.brainres.2018.03.015

76. Schirmer M, Smeekens SP, Vlamakis H, et al. Linking the human gut microbiome to inflammatory cytokine production capacity. *Cell*. 2016;167(4):1125–1136.e8. doi:10.1016/j.cell.2016.10.020

77. Dinan TG, Cryan JF. Regulation of the stress response by the gut microbiota: Implications for psychoneuroendocrinology. *Psychoneuroendocrinology*. 2012;37(9):1369–1378. doi:10.1016/j.psyneuen.2012.03.007

78. Bonaz B, Picq C, Sinniger V, Mayol JF, Clarençon D. Vagus nerve stimulation: From epilepsy to the cholinergic anti-inflammatory pathway. *Neurogastroenterol Motil*. 2013; 25(3):208–221. doi:10.1111/nmo.12076

79. Bonaz B, Bazin T, Pellissier S. The vagus nerve at the interface of the Microbiota-gut-brain axis. *Front Neurosci*. 2018;12. doi:10.3389/fnins.2018.00049

80. Cryan JF, O'Riordan KJ, Cowan CSM, et al. The Microbiota-gut-brain axis. *Physiol Rev.* 2019;99(4):1877–2013. doi:10.1152/physrev.00018.2018
81. Suda K, Matsuda K. How microbes affect depression: Underlying mechanisms via the Gut–Brain axis and the modulating role of probiotics. *Int J Mol Sci.* 2022;23(3):1172. doi:10.3390/ijms23031172
82. Bairamian D, Sha S, Rolhion N, et al. Microbiota in neuroinflammation and synaptic dysfunction: A focus on Alzheimer's disease. *Mol Neurodegener.* 2022;17(1):19. doi:10.1186/s13024-022-00522-2
83. Rea K, Dinan TG, Cryan JF. The microbiome: A key regulator of stress and neuroinflammation. *Neurobiol Stress.* 2016;4:23–33. doi:10.1016/j.ynstr.2016.03.001
84. Bear T, Dalziel J, Coad J, Roy N, Butts C, Gopal P. The microbiome-gut-brain axis and resilience to developing anxiety or depression under stress. *Microorganisms.* 2021;9(4):723. doi:10.3390/microorganisms9040723
85. Rao M, Gershon MD. The bowel and beyond: The enteric nervous system in neurological disorders. *Nat Rev Gastroenterol Hepatol.* 2016;13(9):517–528. doi:10.1038/nrgastro.2016.107
86. Carlessi AS, Borba LA, Zugno AI, Quevedo J, Réus GZ. Gut microbiota–brain axis in depression: The role of neuroinflammation. *Eur J Neurosci.* 2021;53(1):222–235. doi:10.1111/ejn.14631
87. Agostoni E, Chinnock JE, Daly MDB, Murray JG. Functional and histological studies of the vagus nerve and its branches to the heart, lungs and abdominal viscera in the cat. *J Physiol.* 1957;135(1):182–205. doi:10.1113/jphysiol.1957.sp005703
88. Prechtl JC, Powley TL. B-afferents: A fundamental division of the nervous system mediating homeostasis? *Behav Brain Sci.* 1990;13(2):289–300. doi:10.1017/S0140525X00078729
89. Osadchiy V, Martin CR, Mayer EA. Gut microbiome and modulation of CNS function. *Compr Physiol.* 2019;10(1):57–72. doi:10.1002/cphy.c180031
90. Latorre R, Sternini C, De Giorgio R, Greenwood-Van Meerveld B. Enteroendocrine cells: A review of their role in brain-gut communication. *Neurogastroenterol Motil Off J Eur Gastrointest Motil Soc.* 2016;28(5):620–630. doi:10.1111/nmo.12754
91. Gulbransen BD, Sharkey KA. Purinergic neuron-to-glia signaling in the enteric nervous system. *Gastroenterology.* 2009;136(4):1349–1358. doi:10.1053/j.gastro.2008.12.058
92. Petra AI, Panagiotidou S, Hatziagelaki E, Stewart JM, Conti P, Theoharides TC. Gut-Microbiota-brain axis and its effect on neuropsychiatric disorders with suspected immune dysregulation. *Clin Ther.* 2015;37(5):984–995. doi:10.1016/j.clinthera.2015.04.002
93. Austelle CW, O'Leary GH, Thompson S, et al. A comprehensive review of vagus nerve stimulation for depression. *Neuromodulation Technol Neural Interface.* 2022;25(3):309–315. doi:10.1111/ner.13528
94. Costantini TW, Bansal V, Krzyzaniak M, et al. Vagal nerve stimulation protects against burn-induced intestinal injury through activation of enteric glia cells. *Am J Physiol-Gastrointest Liver Physiol.* 2010;299(6):G1308–G1318. doi:10.1152/ajpgi.00156.2010
95. Martin CR, Osadchiy V, Kalani A, Mayer EA. The brain-gut-microbiome axis. *Cell Mol Gastroenterol Hepatol.* 2018;6(2):133–148. doi:10.1016/j.jcmgh.2018.04.003
96. Braniste V, Al-Asmakh M, Kowal C, et al. The gut microbiota influences blood-brain barrier permeability in mice. *Sci Transl Med.* 2014;6(263):263ra158. doi:10.1126/scitranslmed.3009759
97. Varanoske AN, McClung HL, Sepowitz JJ, et al. Stress and the gut-brain axis: Cognitive performance, mood state, and biomarkers of blood-brain barrier and intestinal permeability following severe physical and psychological stress. *Brain Behav Immun.* 2022;101:383–393. doi:10.1016/j.bbi.2022.02.002
98. Ye X, Zhu M, Che X, et al. Lipopolysaccharide induces neuroinflammation in microglia by activating the MTOR pathway and downregulating Vps34 to inhibit

autophagosome formation. *J Neuroinflammation*. 2020;17(1):1–17. doi:10.1186/s12974-019-1644-8

99. Li Z, Zhu H, Zhang L, Qin C. The intestinal microbiome and Alzheimer's disease: A review. *Anim Models Exp Med*. 2018;1(3):180–188. doi:10.1002/ame2.12033

100. Jaeger LB, Dohgu S, Sultana R, et al. Lipopolysaccharide alters the blood–brain barrier transport of amyloid β protein: A mechanism for inflammation in the progression of Alzheimer's disease. *Brain Behav Immun*. 2009;23(4):507–517. doi:10.1016/j.bbi.2009.01.017

101. Kim H, Kim S, Shin SJ, et al. Gram-negative bacteria and their lipopolysaccharides in Alzheimer's disease: Pathologic roles and therapeutic implications. *Transl Neurodegener*. 2021;10(1):49. doi:10.1186/s40035-021-00273-y

102. Sharma VK, Singh TG, Garg N, et al. Dysbiosis and Alzheimer's disease: A role for chronic stress? *Biomolecules*. 2021;11(5):678. doi:10.3390/biom11050678

103. Krabbe G, Halle A, Matyash V, et al. Functional impairment of microglia coincides with Beta-amyloid deposition in mice with Alzheimer-like pathology. *PLoS ONE*. 2013; 8(4):e60921. doi:10.1371/journal.pone.0060921

104. Heintz-Buschart A, Pandey U, Wicke T, et al. The nasal and gut microbiome in Parkinson's disease and idiopathic rapid eye movement sleep behavior disorder. *Mov Disord*. 2018;33(1):88–98. doi:10.1002/mds.27105

105. Minato T, Maeda T, Fujisawa Y, et al. Progression of Parkinson's disease is associated with gut dysbiosis: Two-year follow-up study. *PLoS ONE*. 2017;12(11):e0187307. doi:10.1371/journal.pone.0187307

106. Hasegawa S, Goto S, Tsuji H, et al. Intestinal dysbiosis and lowered serum lipopolysaccharide-binding protein in Parkinson's disease. *PLoS ONE*. 2015;10(11):e0142164. doi:10.1371/journal.pone.0142164

107. Breydo L, Wu JW, Uversky VN. α-synuclein misfolding and Parkinson's disease. *Biochim Biophys Acta BBA - Mol Basis Dis*. 2012;1822(2):261–285. doi:10.1016/j.bbadis.2011.10.002

108. Baizabal-Carvallo JF, Alonso-Juarez M. The link between gut dysbiosis and neuroinflammation in Parkinson's disease. *Neuroscience*. 2020;432:160–173. doi:10.1016/j.neuroscience.2020.02.030

109. Xu M, Xu X, Li J, Li F. Association between gut microbiota and autism spectrum disorder: A systematic review and meta-analysis. *Front Psychiatry*. 2019;10. doi:10.3389/fpsyt.2019.00473

110. Rhee SH, Pothoulakis C, Mayer EA. Principles and clinical implications of the brain–gut–enteric microbiota axis. *Nat Rev Gastroenterol Hepatol*. 2009;6(5). doi:10.1038/nrgastro.2009.35

111. Kesika P, Suganthy N, Sivamaruthi BS, Chaiyasut C. Role of gut-brain axis, gut microbial composition, and probiotic intervention in Alzheimer's disease. *Life Sci*. 2021;264: 118627. doi:10.1016/j.lfs.2020.118627

112. Akbari E, Asemi Z, Daneshvar Kakhaki R, et al. Effect of probiotic supplementation on cognitive function and metabolic status in Alzheimer's disease: A randomized, double-blind and controlled trial. *Front Aging Neurosci*. 2016;8. doi:10.3389/fnagi.2016.00256

113. Tan AH, Hor JW, Chong CW, Lim SY. Probiotics for Parkinson's disease: Current evidence and future directions. *JGH Open*. 2021;5(4):414–419. doi:10.1002/jgh3.12450

114. Hughes HK, Rose D, Ashwood P. The gut microbiota and dysbiosis in autism spectrum disorders. *Curr Neurol Neurosci Rep*. 2018;18(11):81. doi:10.1007/s11910-018-0887-6

Section IV

Physical and Mental
Health Conditions

24 Cardiovascular Disease

Christopher P. Fagundes, PhD and
Lydia Wu-Chung, MA

KEY POINTS

- A healthy lifestyle can prevent 80% of sudden cardiac death and 72% of premature deaths due to heart disease; psychological stress is associated with a 40-60% excess risk of CVD.
- Both acute and chronic psychological stress alter physiological and biochemical processes related to CVD-related morbidity and mortality.
- Emotions and social relationship processes affect physiological and biochemical processes associated with CVD via the stress-response system.

24.1 INTRODUCTION

Cardiovascular disease (CVD) is the leading cause of death in the United States and globally. A healthy lifestyle can prevent 80% of sudden cardiac death and 72% of premature deaths due to heart disease. Emotions and social relationships shape health behaviors and affect physiological and biochemical processes associated with CVD via the stress-response system. Psychological stress is associated with a 40-60% excess risk of CVD.[1] Both acute and chronic psychological stress alter physiological and biochemical processes related to CVD-related morbidity and mortality. Stress and other negative emotions also adversely impact health behaviors associated with CVD-related morbidity and mortality. This chapter describes the interconnected effects of emotions and close relationship processes on CVD through psychobiological mechanisms. Our primary objective is to articulate how emotions and social connections interact to alter physiological and biochemical processes contributing to CVD-related morbidity and mortality. We also briefly describe how stress impacts sleep, a critical pathway to CVD-related morbidity and mortality.

24.2 ACUTE PSYCHOLOGICAL STRESS & CARDIOVASCULAR EVENTS

Stress can promote risk for acute cardiovascular events, especially for those with preexisting conditions. Data collected during natural disasters or other traumatic circumstances have provided some of the best "real-world" evidence linking acute stress to acute coronary events.[2] For example, New Yorkers who underwent implanted cardioverter-defibrillator interrogation in the month preceding the attack on the World Trade Center in 2001 exhibited a two-fold increase in tachyarrhythmias compared to those who received an implantable cardioverter-defibrillator between

DOI: 10.1201/b22810-28

3 and 12 months after the attacks.[2] When the eastern Gulf of Corinth, Greece, was struck by three severe earthquakes within two weeks in 1981, CVD-related deaths doubled among those with existing heart disease.[3] In the two weeks following a significant earthquake in the Los Angeles area in 1994, the average number of cardiac deaths among those with preexisting heart disease increased by 41% compared with the two weeks before the earthquake.[4]

24.2.1 IMPLICATIONS FOR CLOSE RELATIONSHIPS

"The "widowhood effect" is perhaps the most well-known example of a major life stressor boosting the risk for acute coronary events.[5,6] In a matched cohort study using a UK primary care database, older adults who were widowed in the past month experienced myocardial infarction (MI) and stroke at twice the rate of non-bereaved controls. Within 24 hours of learning of the death of a significant person, the rate of acute MI onset was elevated 21.1 fold.[7] Those hospitalized with MI were 21 times more likely to have experienced the death of a significant person within the last 24 hours compared with those demographically similar but not hospitalized for MI.[7]

24.2.2 BIOLOGICAL MECHANISMS LINKING ACUTE STRESS
TO CARDIOVASCULAR EVENTS

When confronted with a stressor, the limbic and cortical regions of the brain involved in attention, memory, and emotion processing initiate the fight-or-flight response, characterized by autonomic nervous system (ANS) and hypothalamic-pituitary-adrenal (HPA) axis activity.[8] When the autonomic nervous system is activated as part of a coordinated physiological stress-response, parasympathetic activity decreases, and sympathetic activity increases.[9] The neuroendocrine system is also highly responsive to psychological stress. When the brain signals a stress response, corticotropin-releasing hormone is secreted, which initiates a cascade of processes associated with HPA activation.[9] Corticotrophin-releasing hormone activates the release of adrenocorticotropic hormone from the anterior pituitary gland. In turn, the adrenal cortex secretes cortisol, the glucocorticoid secreted in humans.[9]

The link between acute stress and an acute cardiovascular event is likely mediated through sympathetic influences.[10] Adenosine triphosphate and the catecholamine norepinephrine interact to promote coronary artery vasoconstriction and reversible ischemia. Takotsubo cardiomyopathy, a transient left ventricular wall dysfunction, is caused by extreme acute emotional stress.[11] Colloquially called "broken heart syndrome," Takotsubo cardiomyopathy is triggered by an acute surge in the stress-hormones, norepinephrine, and epinephrine. Preexisting cardiovascular disease is common among those who experience a coronary event in the wake of a significant acute stressor.[10]

24.3 CHRONIC STRESS AND CORONARY ATHEROSCLEROSIS

Atherosclerosis can start developing early in life, decades before clinical manifestations of the disease emerge. Psychological stress can have a cumulative impact on subsequent CVD-related morbidity mortality. Workplace stress can alter CVD-related outcomes. A meta-analysis of 5 high-quality studies found that among employees with preexisting cardiovascular conditions, workplace stress is associated with a 65% excess risk of a heart attack.[12] More broadly, those exposed to high levels of work stress have an excess risk of CVD-related morbidity and mortality that ranges from 10-40%.[13] Those exposed to high levels of heart attack patients studied in Stockholm as part of the Whitehall II study were at a 2.15-fold increased risk for new coronary heart disease if they were employed in jobs where they experienced a mismatch between effort and reward.[14]

24.3.1 IMPLICATIONS FOR CLOSE RELATIONSHIP

Relationships have a powerful impact on CVD-related morbidity and mortality. Indeed, both the presence and quality of close interpersonal relationships confer risk. The effect relational stress has on cardiovascular disease commences early in life.[15] Over twenty high-quality studies have linked childhood abuse and neglect to adult CVD-related morbidity and mortality.[16] As the central, close relationship for most adults, several studies have linked marital status and quality to CVD. More significant marital conflict increases the risk of both non-fatal and fatal myocardial infarctions and the rate of coronary atherosclerosis progression.[17] Hostility within close interpersonal relationships such as marriage appears to confer a unique risk. A meta-analysis that included 25 studies investigating CVD-related morbidity and mortality among initially healthy adults found those reporting high levels and anger and hostility more likely to have a subsequent coronary event than those with lower levels of anger and hostility. Furthermore, anger and hostility were associated with a poorer prognosis among those who had a CVD event.[18] In a study of over 97,000 women free of cardiovascular disease at study entry, those who reported being more optimistic had lower age-adjusted rates of cardiovascular disease and total mortality than those who reported less optimism. A similar effect exists for hostility; however, optimism and hostility were independently associated with these cardiovascular outcomes.[19]

In addition to its immediate acute effects on cardiovascular events, the link between CVD-related morbidity and mortality and widowhood persists.[20] The risk for CVD-related morbidity and mortality continues throughout the first two years of widowhood. One study showed a 30–90% increased risk of mortality in the first six months of widowhood.[5,6] Another study showed that widow(er)s had 61% greater odds of death in the first six months of widowhood. Even two years after the death of a spouse, widow(er)s have 18% greater odds of death.[21]

In a study of 30,447 individuals aged 60 to 90, widow(er)s had a 25% higher mortality risk in the first year post-loss.[22] Cardiovascular-related death was the most common cause of death. In a study of 373,189 older American couples, the effect of widowhood on mortality was higher for husbands than wives, but substantial for both males and females[5]; the study showed an association between widowhood and partners' mortality from vascular diseases for men and women. The effect was equivalent to or exceeded CVD's established risk factors for all four cardiovascular disease categories.[5]

24.3.2 BIOLOGICAL MECHANISMS UNDERLYING ATHEROSCLEROSIS

Chronic activation of the stress-response system mobilizes plasma lipids and promotes changes in blood platelet aggregation and inflammatory activity.[23] Inflammation serves as a primary route linking stress to atherosclerosis. Atherosclerosis is a condition where the artery wall develops lesions that narrow due to plaque that builds up in the artery walls, consisting of calcium, fat, cholesterol, and other circulating substances in the blood.[24] Under normal conditions, when inflammation is low, immune cells (i.e., lymphocytes) interact with the cells that layer the inside surface of blood vessels (i.e., endothelial cells).[25-28] However, when the stress response activates proinflammatory cytokine production, endothelial cells increase molecules that facilitate cells binding to the endothelium via upregulation of adhesion molecules.[24] Endothelial cells also selectively recruit immune cells (e.g., monocytes, macrophages, helper T cells) that release proinflammatory cytokines. When macrophages are activated in these conditions, they also store fat. Therefore, they are referred to as 'foamy macrophages.'[23] These foamy macrophages bind to the blood vessel wall and induce a local immune response, finally damaging the vessel wall. Proinflammatory cytokines simultaneously inhibit collagen production (i.e., connective tissue made up of protein), weakening the fibrous cap that forms over plaque buildup in the blood vessel wall.[24] When the fibrous plaque eventually breaks, a thrombus (i.e., blood clot) develops, the event responsible for most heart attacks.[29-33] Inflammatory biomarkers assessed in the blood are reliable predictors of cardiovascular events in males and females. C-reactive protein (CRP), an acute-phase protein produced primarily by the liver, serves as a relatively stable index of systemic inflammation.[34]

Sympathetic activation produces transient increases in proinflammatory cytokine production. Specifically, norepinephrine induces nuclear factor kB (NF-kB) transcription, an intracellular signaling molecule that controls proinflammatory cytokine gene expression.[23] Acetylcholine can inhibit proinflammatory cytokine production by partially inhibiting this response through the cholinergic anti-inflammatory pathway.[23] Functionally slower, the cortisol inhibits inflammation. Yet when cortisol is chronically elevated, glucocorticoid insensitivity can develop, which sometimes leads to glucocorticoid resistance.[35] This phenomenon indirectly leads to higher levels of systemic inflammation by producing an unregulated proinflammatory environment.[35] Recent work suggests that acute stress increases proinflammatory cytokine production which may also play an etiological role in Takotsubo cardiomyopathy. We recently demonstrated that grief primes the acute inflammatory stress response in recently widowed older adults, which may help explain the link between grief and Takotsubo cardiomyopathy.[36]

Chronic stress primes the inflammatory stress response.[35] Experimental laboratory stress reliably elevates the proinflammatory cytokine, IL-6. We have demonstrated that grief and depressive symptoms independently promote an exaggerated proinflammatory response to acute stress. Loneliness is also a potent predictor of an exaggerated proinflammatory response to acute stress. In addition, work from our lab and others has shown that chronic stress of widowhood promotes elevated proinflammatory cytokine activity.[37] This dovetail will work showing that early life stress, depression, adverse interpersonal events, relationship insecurity, dementia spousal caregiving, and being of low socioeconomic status (SES) is associated with an over-active proinflammatory state.[36,38]

24.3.3 ROLE OF THE PARASYMPATHETIC NERVOUS SYSTEM

Historically, most of the work linking stress to cardiovascular disease has focused on the impact of the sympathetic branch of the autonomic nervous system; however, the parasympathetic branch of the autonomic nervous system also plays a central role.[39] The mechanisms by which lower vagally mediated heart rate variability (HRV) boosts CVD risk, heart attack, and CVD-related mortality are multifactorial—higher vagally mediated HRV indexes suggest higher parasympathetic nervous system activity, which reflects a well-regulated autonomic nervous system. Parasympathetic activity promotes energy conversation and allows the body to be more dynamic and flexible when psychological stressors or other perturbations that impact poor health emerge. When under tonic inhibition by parasympathetic activity (reflected as higher vagally mediated HRV), people can adaptively react to stressors and recover, thus avoiding the negative repercussions of the physiological (e.g., high blood pressure).[39] Likewise, because the vagus innervates the heart's pacemaker, it can modulate rapid fluctuations in heart rate to restore normal function. Low parasympathetic activity (reflected as low vagally mediated HRV) is also related to hypertension, diabetes, and high high-density lipoprotein (HDL), even after accounting for age, body mass index (BMI), smoking, alcohol consumption, and unfavorable cholesterol (lipid) levels.[39] Lower HRV increases the risk for atherosclerosis, incident myocardial infarction, incident coronary heart disease (CHD), fatal coronary heart disease, and all-cause mortality.[39] For example, after a myocardial infarction (MI) (i.e., heart attack), having lower vagally mediated HRV was a significant independent predictor of mortality.[39] In an older adult sample within the Framingham Heart Study (736 men and women with an average age of 72), vagally mediated lower HRV was associated with higher all-cause mortality.[40] Although studies typically adjust for standard risk factors, lower HRV is prognostic for high blood pressure (hypertension), diabetes, high triglycerides, and elevated low-density lipoproteins (LDL).[40]

24.4 STRESS, SLEEP, AND CARDIOVASCULAR DISEASE

In addition to the impact of stress and close relationships on CVD through a dys-regulated stress-response system, health behaviors are influenced by stress and close interpersonal relationships. Stress's impact on health behaviors is significant; 80% of cardiovascular and coronary heart disease events can be attributed to the following health behaviors: poor-quality diet, excess calorie intake, physical inactivity, sleep, and smoking.[41] Detailing how each health behavior is associated with CVD-related morbidity and mortality is beyond the scope of this chapter. However, here is a brief outline of recent work describing sleep's impact on cardiovascular risk.

Given the importance of sleep to long-term health outcomes, researchers have been increasingly interested in characterizing the mechanisms linking sleep to increased risk of cardiovascular events. Sleep is vital for maintaining physiological homeostasis. Sleep generally supports cardiovascular relaxation (e.g., decreases in heart rate, blood pressure, and cardiac output; increases in parasympathetic activity) and preserves immune competence.[42,43] In contrast, sleep disturbances are linked with increased cardiovascular risk. Indeed, meta-analyses demonstrate that those reporting shorter (<= 5 hours) and longer sleep duration (>=9 hours) have an increased risk of hypertension and developing other cardiovascular events.[44–46] Poor sleep quality is also associated with less adaptive responses to infection and elevated levels of proinflammatory biomarkers.

Shorter sleep duration is associated with less adaptive patterns of stress reactivity and recovery, such as higher blood pressure reactivity to stress,[47] more significant increases in proinflammatory cytokines (IL-6, TNF-a) during marital conflict,[48] and prolonged elevations in blood pressure post-stressor.[49] The link between greater blood pressure reactivity to stress, prolonged heart rate recovery following stress, and poorer longitudinal cardiometabolic outcomes is consistently supported by several studies.[50] Exaggerated stress-induced increases in IL-6 have also previously been linked with indicators of poorer cardiometabolic health 12 years later.[51] Sleep may also be a protective factor against stress-induced changes in surrogate markers of atherosclerosis. In a sample of 99 middle-aged participants, increased stress reactivity predicted greater carotid artery intima-media thickness only in those showing lower slow-wave sleep, the sleep stage crucial for cardiovascular rest and recovery.[52] In sum, research suggests that poor sleep quality exaggerates the physiological stress response, which, in turn, can shape downstream health. In contrast, good quality sleep protects against the negative consequences of stress on cardiovascular physiology.

Psychosocial factors affect the relationship between sleep and health. Being more socially integrated protects against the adverse effects of sleep on physiology. Indeed, in a sample of middle-aged men[53] and individuals at risk for cardiovascular disease,[54] poorer subjective sleep quality was associated with increased levels of proinflammatory biomarkers only in those reporting low social support, not high social support. Sleep behaviors may also explain the benefits of social integration on health. Higher levels of social integration were associated with greater blood pressure dipping, which is more adaptive; this relationship was partially explained by greater sleep regularity among more socially-integrated individuals.[55]

24.5 CONCLUSION

Cardiovascular health is governed by biological, psychological, and social factors that interact to impact disease.[56] Psychological stress, especially if interpersonal, profoundly impacts autonomic, neuroendocrine, and immune processes associated with CVD-related morbidity and mortality.[57] These same psychosocial processes also influence health behaviors; indeed, poor health behaviors such as physical inactivity, high caloric intake, poor sleep, diet, smoking, and excess alcohol consumption are all risk factors for the development and progression of CVD.[58] By emphasizing positive social connections, stress management, and good health behaviors, lifestyle medicine can significantly reduce CVD-related morbidity and mortality.[58]

REFERENCES

1. Steptoe A. Stress, inflammation, and coronary heart disease. *Stress and Cardiovascular Disease.* Springer; 2012:111–128.
2. Steinberg JS, Arshad A, Kowalski M, et al. Increased incidence of life-threatening ventricular arrhythmias in implantable defibrillator patients after the World Trade Center attack. *J Am Coll Cardiol.* 2004;44(6):1261–1264. doi:10.1016/j.jacc.2004.06.032
3. Ambraseys NN, Jackson JA. Earthquake hazard and vulnerability in the northeastern Mediterranean: The Corinth earthquake sequence of February-March 1981. *Disasters.* 1981;5(4):355–368. doi:10.1111/j.1467-7717.1981.tb01108.x
4. Kloner RA, Leor J, Poole WK, Perritt R. Population-based analysis of the effect of the Northridge earthquake on cardiac death in Los Angeles County, California. *J Am Coll Cardiol.* 1997;30(5):1174–1180. doi:10.1016/s0735-1097(97)00281-7
5. Elwert F, Christakis NA. The effect of widowhood on mortality by the causes of death of both spouses. *Am J Public Health.* 2008;98(11):2092–2098. doi:10.2105/AJPH.2007.114348
6. Martikainen P, Valkonen T. Mortality after death of spouse in relation to duration of bereavement in Finland. *J Epidemiol Community Health.* 1996;50(3):264–268. doi:10.1136/jech.50.3.264
7. Mostofsky E, Maclure M, Sherwood JB, Tofler GH, Muller JE, Mittleman MA. Risk of acute myocardial infarction after the death of a significant person in one's life: The Determinants of Myocardial Infarction Onset Study. *Circulation.* 2012;125(3): 491–496. doi:10.1161/CIRCULATIONAHA.111.061770
8. Kraynak TE, Marsland AL, Gianaros PJ. Neural mechanisms linking emotion with cardiovascular disease. *Curr Cardiol Rep.* 2018;20(12):128. doi:10.1007/s11886-018-1071-y
9. Gianaros PJ, Wager TD. Brain-body pathways linking psychological stress and physical health. *Curr Dir Psychol Sci.* 2015;24(4):313–321. doi:10.1177/0963721415581476
10. Steptoe A, Kivimäki M. Stress and cardiovascular disease. *Nat Rev Cardiol.* 2012; 9(6):360–370. doi:10.1038/nrcardio.2012.45
11. Sealove BA, Tiyyagura S, Fuster V. Takotsubo cardiomyopathy. *J Gen Intern Med.* 2008;23(11):1904–1908. doi:10.1007/s11606-008-0744-4
12. Li J, Zhang M, Loerbroks A, Angerer P, Siegrist J. Work stress and the risk of recurrent coronary heart disease events: A systematic review and meta-analysis. *Int J Occup Med Environ Health.* 2015;28(1):8–19. doi:10.2478/s13382-014-0303-7
13. Kivimäki M, Kawachi I. Work stress as a risk factor for cardiovascular disease. *Curr Cardiol Rep.* 2015;17(9):630. doi:10.1007/s11886-015-0630-8
14. Bosma H, Peter R, Siegrist J, Marmot M. Two alternative job stress models and the risk of coronary heart disease. *Am J Public Health.* 1998;88(1):68–74.
15. Dong M, Giles WH, Felitti VJ, et al. Insights into causal pathways for ischemic heart disease: Adverse childhood experiences study. *Circulation.* 2004;110(13):1761–1766. doi:10.1161/01.CIR.0000143074.54995.7F
16. Basu A, McLaughlin KA, Misra S, Koenen KC. Childhood maltreatment and health impact: The examples of cardiovascular disease and type 2 diabetes mellitus in adults. *Clin Psychol Publ Div Clin Psychol Am Psychol Assoc.* 2017;24(2):125–139. doi:10.1111/cpsp.12191
17. De Vogli R, Chandola T, Marmot MG. Negative aspects of close relationships and heart disease. *Arch Intern Med.* 2007;167(18):1951–1957. doi:10.1001/archinte.167.18.1951
18. Chida Y, Steptoe A. The association of anger and hostility with future coronary heart disease: A meta-analytic review of prospective evidence. *J Am Coll Cardiol.* 2009;53(11):936–946. doi:10.1016/j.jacc.2008.11.044

19. Tindle HA, Chang YF, Kuller LH, et al. Optimism, cynical hostility, and incident coronary heart disease and mortality in the Women's health initiative. *Circulation.* 2009;120(8):656–662. doi:10.1161/CIRCULATIONAHA.108.827642

20. Fagundes CP, Wu EL. Matters of the heart: Grief, morbidity, and mortality. *Curr Dir Psychol Sci.* 2020;29(3):235–241. doi:10.1177/0963721420917698

21. Sullivan AR, Fenelon A. Patterns of widowhood mortality. *J Gerontol Ser B.* 2014; 69B(1):53–62. doi:10.1093/geronb/gbt079

22. Carey IM, Shah SM, DeWilde S, Harris T, Victor CR, Cook DG. Increased risk of acute cardiovascular events after partner bereavement: A matched cohort study. *JAMA Intern Med.* 2014;174(4):598–605.

23. Libby P. The changing landscape of atherosclerosis. *Nature.* 2021;592(7855):524–533. doi:10.1038/s41586-021-03392-8

24. Geovanini GR, Libby P. Atherosclerosis and inflammation: Overview and updates. *Clin Sci.* 2018;132(12):1243–1252. doi:10.1042/CS20180306

25. Dentino AN, Pieper CF, Rao KMK, et al. Association of interleukin-6 and other biologic variables with depression in older people living in the community. *J Am Geriatr Soc.* 1999;47(1):6–11. doi:10.1111/j.1532-5415.1999.tb01894.x

26. Lutgendorf SK, Garand L, Buckwalter KC, Reimer TT, Hong SY, Lubaroff DM. Life stress, mood disturbance, and elevated interleukin-6 in healthy older women. *J Gerontol Ser A.* 1999;54(9):M434–M439. doi:10.1093/gerona/54.9.M434

27. Maes M, Lin A-H, Delmeire L, et al. Elevated serum interleukin-6 (IL-6) and IL-6 receptor concentrations in posttraumatic stress disorder following accidental manmade traumatic events. *Biol Psychiatry.* 1999;45(7):833–839. doi:10.1016/S0006-3223(98)00131-0

28. Maes M, Song C, Lin A, et al. The effects of psychological stress on humans: Increased production of pro-inflammatory cytokines and Th1-like response in stress-induced anxiety. *Cytokine.* 1998;10(4):313–318. doi:10.1006/cyto.1997.0290

29. Ellenbogen MA, Schwartzman AE, Stewart J, Walker CD. Stress and selective attention: The interplay of mood, cortisol levels, and emotional information processing. *Psychophysiology.* 2002;39(6):723–732.

30. Libby P. Inflammation and cardiovascular disease mechanisms. *Am J Clin Nutr.* 2006; 83(2):456S–460S. doi:10.1093/ajcn/83.2.456S

31. Lai JY, Linden W. Gender, anger expression style, and opportunity for anger release determine cardiovascular reaction to and recovery from anger provocation. *Psychosom Med.* 1992;54(3):297–310. doi:10.1097/00006842-199205000-00006

32. Ridker PM, Rifai NMF, Stampfer MJ, Hennekens CH. Plasma concentration of interleukin-6 and the risk of future myocardial infarction among apparently healthy men. *Circulation.* 2000;101(15):1767–1772.

33. Roy MP, Kirschbaum C, Steptoe A. Psychological, cardiovascular, and metabolic correlates of individual differences in cortisol stress recovery in young men. *Psychoneuroendocrinology.* 2001;26(4):375–391. doi:10.1016/S0306-4530(00)00061-5

34. Ridker PM. A test in context: High-sensitivity C-reactive protein. *J Am Coll Cardiol.* 2016;67(6):712–723. doi:10.1016/j.jacc.2015.11.037

35. Miller GE, Cohen S, Ritchey AK. Chronic psychological stress and the regulation of pro-inflammatory cytokines: A glucocorticoid-resistance model. *Health Psychol.* 2002;21(6):531–541. doi:10.1037/0278-6133.21.6.531

36. Brown RL, LeRoy AS, Chen MA, et al. Grief symptoms promote inflammation during acute stress among bereaved spouses. *Psychol Sci.* 2022;33(6):859–873. doi:10.1177/09567976211059502

37. Jaremka LM, Fagundes CP, Peng J, et al. Loneliness promotes inflammation during acute stress. *Psychol Sci.* 2013;24(7):1089–1097. doi:10.1177/0956797612464059

38. Kiecolt-Glaser JK, Renna ME, Shrout MR, Madison AA. Stress reactivity: What pushes us higher, faster, and longer—and why it matters. *Curr Dir Psychol Sci*. 2020; 29(5):492–498. doi:10.1177/0963721420949521

39. Thayer JF, Yamamoto SS, Brosschot JF. The relationship of autonomic imbalance, heart rate variability and cardiovascular disease risk factors. *Int J Cardiol*. 2010;141(2): 122–131. doi:10.1016/j.ijcard.2009.09.543

40. Tsuji H, Larson MG, Venditti FJ, et al. Impact of reduced heart rate variability on risk for cardiac events. The framingham heart study. *Circulation*. 1996;94(11):2850–2855. doi:10.1161/01.cir.94.11.2850

41. Spring B, Ockene JK, Gidding SS, et al. Better population health through behavior change in adults. *Circulation*. 2013;128(19):2169–2176. doi:10.1161/01.cir.0000435173. 25936.e1

42. Irwin MR. Why sleep is important for health: A psychoneuroimmunology perspective. *Annu Rev Psychol*. 2015;66(1):143–172. doi:10.1146/annurev-psych-010213-115205

43. Leung RST, Douglas Bradley T. Sleep apnea and cardiovascular disease. *Am J Respir Crit Care Med*. 2001;164(12):2147–2165. doi:10.1164/ajrccm.164.12.2107045

44. Cappuccio FP, Cooper D, D'Elia L, Strazzullo P, Miller MA. Sleep duration predicts cardiovascular outcomes: A systematic review and meta-analysis of prospective studies. *Eur Heart J*. 2011;32(12):1484–1492. doi:10.1093/eurheartj/ehr007

45. Guo X, Zheng L, Wang J, et al. Epidemiological evidence for the link between sleep duration and high blood pressure: A systematic review and meta-analysis. *Sleep Med*. 2013;14(4):324–332. doi:10.1016/j.sleep.2012.12.001

46. Wang Q, Xi B, Liu M, Zhang Y, Fu M. Short sleep duration is associated with hypertension risk among adults: A systematic review and meta-analysis. *Hypertens Res*. 2012;35(10):1012–1018. doi:10.1038/hr.2012.91

47. Franzen PL, Gianaros PJ, Marsland AL, et al. Cardiovascular reactivity to acute psychological stress following sleep deprivation. *Psychosom Med*. 2011;73(8):679–682. doi:10.1097/PSY.0b013e31822ff440

48. Wilson SJ, Jaremka LM, Fagundes CP, et al. When couples' hearts beat together: Linkages in heart rate variability during conflict predict heightened inflammation throughout the day. *Brain Behav Immun*. 2017;66:e20–e21. doi:10.1016/j.bbi.2017.07.081

49. Mezick EJ, Matthews KA, Hall MH, Richard Jennings J, Kamarck TW. Sleep duration and cardiovascular responses to stress in undergraduate men. *Psychophysiology*. 2014;51(1):88–96. doi:10.1111/psyp.12144

50. Whittaker AC, Ginty A, Hughes BM, Steptoe A, Lovallo WR. Cardiovascular stress reactivity and health: Recent questions and future directions. *Psychosom Med*. 2021; 83(7):756–766. doi:10.1097/PSY.0000000000000973

51. Zannas AS, Gordon JL, Hinderliter AL, Girdler SS, Rubinow DR. IL-6 response to psychosocial stress predicts 12-month changes in cardiometabolic biomarkers in perimenopausal women. *J Clin Endocrinol Metab*. 2020;105(10):e3757–e3765. doi:10.1210/clinem/dgaa476

52. Brindle RC, Duggan KA, Cribbet MR, et al. Cardiovascular stress reactivity and carotid intima-media thickness: The buffering role of slow-wave sleep. *Psychosom Med*. 2018; 80(3):301–306. doi:10.1097/PSY.0000000000000560

53. Friedman EM. Sleep quality, social well-being, gender, and inflammation: An integrative analysis in a national sample. *Ann N Y Acad Sci*. 2011;1231(1):23–34. doi:10.1111/j.1749-6632.2011.06040.x

54. Tomfohr LM, Edwards KM, Madsen JW, Mills PJ. Social support moderates the relationship between sleep and inflammation in a population at high risk for developing cardiovascular disease. *Psychophysiology*. 2015;52(12):1689–1697. doi:10.1111/psyp.12549

55. Chin BN, Dickman KD, Koffer RE, Cohen S, Hall MH, Kamarck TW. Sleep and daily social experiences as potential mechanisms linking social integration to nocturnal blood pressure dipping. *Psychosom Med.* 2022;84(3):368. doi:10.1097/PSY. 0000000000001045

56. Adler RH. Engel's biopsychosocial model is still relevant today. *J Psychosom Res.* 2009;67(6):607–611. doi:10.1016/j.jpsychores.2009.08.008

57. Smith TW, Baron CE, Caska CM. On marriage and the heart: Models, methods, and mechanisms in the study of close relationships and cardiovascular disease. In: *Interpersonal Relationships and Health: Social and Clinical Psychological Mechanisms.* Oxford University Press; 2014:34–70. doi:10.1093/acprof:oso/9780199936632.003.0003

58. Bacon SL, Campbell TS, Lavoie KL. Rethinking how to expand the evidence base for health behavior change in cardiovascular disease prevention. *J Am Coll Cardiol.* 2020;75(20):2619–2622. doi:10.1016/j.jacc.2020.03.055

25 Cardiometabolic Disease

Martha A. Belury, PhD, RDN
and Annelise A. Madison, MA

KEY POINTS

- The metabolic syndrome, a cluster of conditions that increase risk for cardiometabolic disease (CMD), is both a cause and consequence of psychological distress.
- Many, but not all, studies show that long-chain n3 polyunsaturated fatty acids (LCn3PUFAs) impact dyslipidemia and chronic inflammation, two risk factors that contribute to CMD.
- In addition to affecting dyslipidemia and acute inflammation through oxylipin metabolites, LCn3PUFAs may attenuate the chronic inflammation that underlies some cases of depression.
- There is mixed evidence in randomized controlled trials for whether LCn3PUFAs decrease CMD risk and reduce distress or depression. Rigorous randomized controlled trials are needed before recommendations can be made to use LCn3PUFAs in the treatment of distress, depression, and CMD.

25.1 OVERVIEW

Cardiometabolic disease (CMD) is a group of co-morbid diseases that are the most prevalent non-communicable diseases in the United States.[1,2] These diseases include cardiovascular disease, diabetes mellitus, and chronic renal failure. One in three adults has CMD risk factors, such as elevated waist circumference, triglycerides, blood pressure, and fasting glucose, along with low high-density lipoprotein (HDL) cholesterol – all encompassed in the metabolic syndrome designation.[1-3] Major depressive disorder is also a leading cause of disability, and one in five US adults has had at least one major depressive episode.[4] There is a bi-directional relationship between CMD and clinical depression, and diet can influence both.

In fact, the nearly 60-fold variance in the annual prevalence of major depression across countries is very similar to the pattern for cardiovascular disease, which shows a strong comorbidity for depression.[5] Long-chain omega-3 polyunsaturated fatty acids (LCn3PUFAs), found in cold-water fish and from some algae, may modulate inflammation, metabolism, and at least for some at-risk individuals, it may affect mood. This review captures some potential mechanistic links from clinical research studies concerning LCn3PUFAs and mood and describes a theoretical mechanistic link for LCn3PUFAs as potential therapy for reducing the risk for CMD (Figure 25.1).

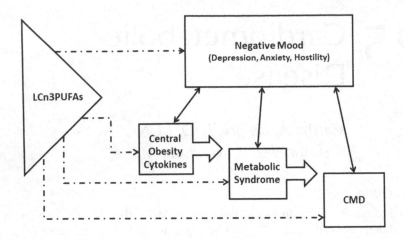

FIGURE 25.1 Schematic diagram showing proposed interplay between LCn3PUFAs, negative mood (also called negative affect or stress symptoms), central obesity, and cardiometabolic disease (CMD).

25.2 MECHANISMS CONNECTING DISTRESS TO CMD

Central obesity (waist circumference $\geq$ 88 cm for women or $\geq$ 102 cm for men) is a leading contributor to CMD. Central obesity, as a marker of excessive visceral adipose tissue, is a cornerstone of CMD risk.[6] Of note, visceral adipose tissue is to blame for approximately one-third of the circulating inflammatory marker interleukin-6 (IL-6), which stimulates the liver to produce the acute phase protein C-reactive protein (CRP).[7] CRP appears to be a stronger predictor of cardiovascular events than other more commonly monitored risk factors, like low-density lipoproteins (LDL) cholesterol, and in one study among women, those who had the highest quintile of CRP were 2.3 times more likely to have a subsequent cardiovascular event than those in the lowest quintile.[8] In addition to central obesity, multiple factors, including genetics, poor diet quality, excessive intake of calories, and inactivity are dominant risk factors for CMD.[9]

Psychological factors that increase distress (e.g., depression, anxiety, hostility) are now receiving recognition as other important contributors to central obesity and CMD development. Cross-sectional studies have linked abdominal obesity with depression,[10–12] and a large community-based prospective study replicated and extended these findings: Older depressed adults gained an average of 9 cm^2 of visceral fat over five years, while study participants who were not depressed lost 7 cm^2 of visceral fat.[13] Importantly, the association between depression and central adiposity was independent of overall obesity, which suggested that depressive symptoms were specifically associated with changes in visceral adipose tissue. Given the connection between distress and visceral fat accumulation, it makes sense that chronic stressors and stressful life events enhance the development of CMD.[14] In this regard, it is notable that chronic work stressors over 14 years showed a dose-response relationship with development of CMD.[15] In a different study, chronic interpersonal strain also heightened risk: Women who were dissatisfied with their marriages had greater odds of developing metabolic syndrome than their peers who were satisfied.[16] Therefore, distress-related psychological factors are a linchpin of the CMD-risk profile.

In an effort to understand whether distress changes metabolism, we conducted a trial evaluating whether depression and recent stress affect women's energy metabolism after a high-fat meal (60% calories from fat).[17] Women with greater numbers of stressors on the day prior to their clinical visit exhibited lower post-meal resting energy expenditure, fat oxidation, and higher insulin levels. If women had a history of major depressive disorder, they had higher post-meal cortisol and fat oxidation. If women reported stress the day before and a history of major depressive disorder, they exhibited an exaggerated and prolonged elevation of triglycerides after the meal.[17] In a separate study, we had married couples eat a high-fat meal and then, two hours later, try to resolve an ongoing, central disagreement during a 20-minute discussion.[18] Participants with a mood disorder and who exhibited more hostile behaviors (e.g., eye rolling) during the discussion exhibited reduced postprandial resting energy expenditure and higher peak triglycerides and insulin. Participants with a mood disorder also had a steeper rise of interleulin-6 and glucose. Higher levels of hostility were associated with elevated post-meal tumor necrosis factor-alpha (TNF-α).[18] The findings from our studies suggest that distress may alter aspects of postprandial metabolism that contribute to CMD risk.

As another mechanism, depression is associated with the dysregulation of the hypothalamic-pituitary-adrenal axis, including chronically elevated cortisol levels.[13] The sustained levels of cortisol increase adipocyte differentiation and lipid filling especially in visceral adipose tissues (e.g., those adipose tissues immediately adjacent to the internal organs). Cortisol also affects fat distribution, such that more is stored in the lower abdomen. Visceral fat has more glucocorticoid receptors than other tissue types, and therefore it is more responsive to cortisol's fat-enhancing effects.[13] Cross-sectionally, stress-induced cortisol responses are larger among women with central obesity than women without central obesity.[19] In further work, women who had larger stress-induced cortisol responses also ate more snack foods following a laboratory stressor than when they were not stressed, and post-stress mood worsening promoted more snack consumption.[20] A field study confirmed and extended these findings: High-cortisol responders who reported more daily stressors ate more snacks, a pattern not found among the low-cortisol responders.[21] Putting these studies together, stress and visceral adiposity promote hypercortisolemia as well as greater consumption of calorically-dense, high-fat foods, all of which further enhance adipocyte accumulation.[6,22]

Stress, anxiety, and low mood additively contribute to sustained increases of pro-inflammatory cytokines, especially IL-6.[5,23–25] Ex vivo studies, in which human immune cells are stimulated with antigens, have shown that both clinical depression and subthreshold depressive symptoms may sensitize the inflammatory response, particularly in men.[26] Also, those with mild depressive symptoms as well as clinical depression have higher inflammatory responses to psychological stressors.[27] Further compounding this issue, women with greater central adiposity produced larger inflammatory responses to a laboratory stress task than their leaner counterparts.[28] Therefore, the combination of depression and obesity, which is prevalent, may be especially problematic in terms of inflammatory responsivity to acute stress. Additionally, in the context of frequent stress exposure, inflammation levels may not fully return to baseline (i.e., recover), ultimately leading to elevated basal levels of inflammation. Indeed, the combination of greater inflammatory reactivity to stress and frequent social stress exposure in daily life predicted depressive symptom worsening over time.[29] Heightened basal inflammation itself also longitudinally predicts depressive symptom worsening, and vice versa – a vicious cycle.[30]

25.3 CHRONIC INFLAMMATION UNDERLYING CMD AND DEPRESSION: A POTENTIAL TREATMENT AND PREVENTION TARGET

Chronic inflammation may link stress with central obesity and depression. Recently, a meta-analysis identified a strong relationship among depression, stress, and central obesity.[13] Many pro-inflammatory cytokines [e.g., TNF-α, IL-6, C-reactive protein (CRP)] contribute to accumulation of visceral adipose tissue mass, in part, by diminishing insulin-mediated metabolism in key tissues such as adipose and muscle. Also, chronic inflammation may contribute to CMD by increasing oxidative stress and redox-sensitive transcription factors leading to transcription of TNF-α, IL-6, and other chemokine genes. In essence, chronic or repetitive stress may provoke sustained increases in basal inflammation, which is a shared etiological factor in CMD and some cases of depression. Therefore, strategies to reduce inflammation may do double duty by lowering risk for both clinical depression and CMD.

Possible anti-inflammatory treatments that have been proposed or tested range from inexpensive non-steroidal anti-inflammatory drugs (e.g., aspirin, acetaminophen, etc.) to expensive biologic injectables (e.g., pharmaceuticals that oppose the effects of proinflammatory cytokines). For instance, a seminal study showed that infliximab, a biologic anti-inflammatory treatment commonly used to treat Crohn's disease, effectively treated intractable cases of major depressive disorder among people who had high levels of inflammation at the start of the intervention.[31] Even so, such biologic anti-inflammatory treatments are expensive and carry risks.[32] As a less expensive option, low-dose aspirin has been a mainstay of cardiovascular disease (CVD) prevention in clinical care for decades. Yet, meta-analytic evidence suggests that, at least for the prevention of a first cardiovascular event, the harm of excessive bleeding may outweigh the benefits – even among those at high risk for CVD.[33] In short, pharmacological interventions to reduce inflammation to treat or prevent depression or CMD have downsides.

25.4 LCn3PUFAs MAY LOWER INFLAMMATION, DEPRESSION, AND CMD RISK

LCn3PUFAs [e.g., eicosapentaenoate (EPA, 20:5n3), docosapentaenoate (DPA, 22:5n3) and docosahexaenoate (DHA, 22:6n3) may be an inexpensive, low-risk mechanism to reduce inflammation.[34] LCn3PUFAs are readily esterified into phospholipids of cell membranes. If hydrolyzed from phospholipid membranes via phospholipase activity, LCn3PUFAs may be enzymatically metabolized to form oxylipins. Oxylipins have relatively short-lived effects on inflammation and work in a paracrine manner to affect cellular events in nearby tissues.[35,36] Several epidemiological studies have linked higher dietary intakes of LCn3PUFAs with lower serum proinflammatory cytokine levels.[37-40] Data from food frequency questionnaires showed that higher fish or other n-3 consumption was associated with lower IL-6[39] and lower TNF-α[37] which was corroborated in a recent meta-analysis. Although food frequency questionnaires are well validated and widely used, fatty acid exposure depends not only on intake, but also absorption and metabolism.[41] Therefore, LCn3PUFA in the blood may more reliably track with inflammation. The association of blood levels of LCn3PUFAs with cytokines has been shown in some,[34,42-44] but not all,[45] studies. Differences between studies can be due to a variety of differences in methods. Methods such as measuring cytokines isolated from plasma vs. isolated and stimulated ex vivo may introduce different conditions that need consideration.

Although prior research shows a promising anti-inflammatory effect of LCn3PUFA, which may in turn lower CMD risk, it is important to note that the most recent Cochrane review does not suggest that omega-3 supplementation is helpful in preventing CVD.[46] Therefore, omega-3 supplementation for the purpose of reducing CVD risk is not a staple of current medical care. This null finding may result from not enough high-quality, randomized, controlled trials, or it is also possible that omega-3 is helpful only for some people, and perhaps especially for those with elevated inflammatory markers.

Moving on to depression risk, there is an inverse relationship between LCn3PUFA consumption and prevalence of major depression.[47] Also, higher dietary intake of LCn3PUFAs was related to lower hostility.[48] These findings are echoed in studies that measure LCn3PUFA in the blood: People who have lower blood levels of LCn3PUFA tend to have higher depressive symptoms.[5,24,49-52] As one example, in older adults, we showed that lower levels of LCn3PUFAs in plasma predicted for increased levels of markers of inflammation in older people who have depression.[53] Also, in a seminal study in medical students, baseline levels of LCn3PUFAs moderated the proinflammatory response to examination stress.[54] Students who had lower serum LCn3PUFA levels (below the median at baseline, several weeks before exams) demonstrated greater increases in stimulated IL-6 and TNF-α production during exams than those with higher levels, while LCn3PUFA levels, measured at each of the three time points in the study, did not change significantly.

After this study, we conducted a randomized controlled double-blinded study on medical students who were supplemented with a placebo or 2.5 g/LCn3PUFA oil per day for 12 weeks.[55] Supplementation with LCn3PUFA oil for 12 weeks resulted in decreased lipopolysaccharide-induction of IL-6. In addition, anxiety, as measured using the Beck Anxiety Inventory, was reduced after 12 weeks of intervention with LCn3PUFA, but depressive symptoms were unchanged. We had similar results from a subsequent double-blinded randomized controlled trial in older adults testing two doses of LCn3PUFA oil (1.25 g/day and 2.50 g/day) supplementation.[55] Indeed, both doses reduced inflammation but had no effect on depressive symptoms, which were low at baseline and remained low at follow-up. Additionally, in this study, we demonstrated that both doses of omega-3 lowered oxidative stress by about 15% compared to the placebo group.[56] Using data from this trial, we also tested whether omega-3 supplementation could blunt the physiological toll of an acute speech stressor. Indeed, we reported that both doses of LCn3PUFA oil supplementation prevented the placebo-group's post-stress declines of the anti-aging enzyme telomerase and the anti-inflammatory cytokine IL10. In addition, adults in the 2.5 gram per day supplement group had lower salivary cortisol and plasma IL-6 throughout the duration of the stress test, compared to the placebo group. Overall, the LCn3PUFA oil groups had a stress response profile that was more resilient, which over time may promote healthy biological aging trajectories, especially among those who experience frequent stress. Overall, our omega-3 randomized controlled trials demonstrated that regardless of age, omega-3 can reduce chronic inflammation. In our younger population, we also showed that it could reduce anxiety, and in our older population, we showed that it can increase physiological resilience in the face of acute stress. The collective findings are notable because the cohorts were consuming a typical "Western" diet, and thus supplementation could be applicable to other populations consuming their personalized/typical diets. However, we also showed that regardless of age, omega-3 supplementation did not impact depressive symptoms.

Consistent with our null findings concerning depressive symptoms, the most recent Cochrane review did not find an effect of omega-3 on depression in adults, even though there are some positive reports.[50,57] The ambiguous reports raise the urgency for rigorous randomized controlled trials to test the effects in various types of mood and distressed populations. Indeed, inflammation is only elevated in approximately one-third of depression cases.[58] Omega-3 may have an anti-depressant effect among those who have, or are at risk for, the inflammatory subtype of depression. Indeed, future studies should investigate whether it boosts the efficacy of traditional antidepressant medications, especially among those with heightened levels of inflammation. Although the null Cochrane review findings for omega-3 and its effect on CVD and depression are disappointing, they point to the need for a more personalized approach that recognizes that the etiology of disorders and diseases varies, and some may benefit more than others from preventative strategies and treatments.

25.5   SUMMARY AND CONCLUSIONS

There are no recommendations of optimal levels of LCn3PUFAs for reducing the risk for depression and CMD. The American Heart Association recommends that all adults consume 1-2 servings of oily fish per week (averaging between 0.25 g/d - 0.50 g/d of LCn3PUFA) to achieve a level of EPA and DHA that may reduce risk for cardiovascular diseases.[59,60] Yet, we predict that adults are getting far less than this: Estimates from NHANES suggest that US adults are consuming less than 100 mg/day.[61] Adequately powered studies are needed to define whether LCn3PUFAs are effective for altering mood and CMD risk factors. In addition, further work is needed to identify whether, under what conditions, and for whom LCn3PUFAs complement pharmaceutical management of chronic inflammation, e.g., cytokines responses, with depression will reduce CMD risk. Overall, LCn3PUFA's anti-inflammatory effect is clear, and systemic inflammation is certainly an etiological factor in CMD and some cases of depression. Therefore, it is plausible that increasing LCn3PUFA in the diet, even via supplementation, may help to reduce CMD and depression risk for certain individuals, especially those with elevated stress levels or inflammation.

REFERENCES

1. Ford ES, Giles WH, Dietz WH. Prevalence of the metabolic syndrome among US adults: Findings from the third National Health and Nutrition Examination Survey. *JAMA*. 2002;287(3):356–359.
2. Ervin RB. Prevalence of metabolic syndrome among adults 20 years of age and over, by sex, age, race and ethnicity, and body mass index: United States, 2003–2006. *Natl Health Stat Report*. 2009;5(13):1–7.
3. Beydoun MA, Wang Y. Gender-ethnic disparity in BMI and waist circumference distribution shifts in US adults. *Obesity*. 2009;17(1):169–176.
4. National Institute of Mental Health NIoH. Major depression. https://www.nimh.nih.gov/health/statistics/major-depression#:~:text=The%20prevalence%20of%20major%20depressive%20episode%20was%20highest,episode%20was%20highest%20among%20individuals%20aged%2018-25%20%2813.1%25%29. Published 2022.
5. Maes M, Smith RS. Fatty acids, cytokines, and major depression. *Biol Psychiatry*. 1998;43(5):313–314.
6. Kyrou I, Chrousos GP, Tsigos C. Stress, visceral obesity, and metabolic complications. *Ann N Y Acad Sci*. 2006;1083:77–110.
7. Mohamed-Ali V, Goodrick S, Rawesh A, et al. Subcutaneous adipose tissue releases interleukin-6, but not tumor necrosis factor-alpha, in vivo. *J Clin Endocrinol Metab*. 1997;82(12):4196–4200.
8. Ridker PM. Clinical application of C-reactive protein for cardiovascular disease detection and prevention. *Circulation*. 2003;107(3):363–369.
9. Mustelin L, Silventoinen K, Pietilainen K, Rissanen A, Kaprio J. Physical activity reduces the influence of genetic effects on BMI and waist circumference: A study in young adult twins. *Int J Obes*. 2009;33(1):29–36.
10. Ahlberg AC, Ljung T, Rosmond R, et al. Depression and anxicty symptoms in relation to anthropometry and metabolism in men. *Psychiatry Res*. 2002;112(2):101–110.
11. Weber-Hamann B, Hentschel F, Kniest A, et al. Hypercortisolemic depression is associated with increased intra-abdominal fat. *Psychosom Med*. 2002;64(2):274–277.
12. Thakore JH, Richards PJ, Reznek RH, Martin A, Dinan TG. Increased intra-abdominal fat deposition in patients with major depressive illness as measured by computed tomography. *Biol Psychiatry*. 1997;41(11):1140–1142.
13. Vogelzangs N, Kritchevsky SB, Beekman AT, et al. Depressive symptoms and change in abdominal obesity in older persons. *Arch Gen Psychiatry*. 2008;65(12):1386–1393.
14. Raikkonen K, Matthews KA, Kuller LH. Depressive symptoms and stressful life events predict metabolic syndrome among middle-aged women: A comparison of World Health Organization, Adult Treatment Panel III, and International Diabetes Foundation definitions. *Diabetes Care*. 2007;30(4):872–877.
15. Chandola T, Brunner E, Marmot M. Chronic stress at work and the metabolic syndrome: Prospective study. *BMJ*. 2006;332(7540):521–525.
16. Troxel W, Matthews KA, Gallo LC, Kuller LH. Marital quality and occurrence of the metabolic syndrome in women. *Acrch Intern Med*. 2005;165:1022–1027.
17. Kiecolt-Glaser J, Habash DL, Fagundes CP, et al. Daily stressors, past depression, and metabolic responses to high-fat meals: A novel path to obesity. *Biol Psychiatry*. 2015;77(7):653–660.

18. Kiecolt-Glaser J, Jaremeka L, Andridge R, et al. Marital discord, past depression, and metabolic responses to high-fat meals: Interpersonal pathways to obesity. *Psychoneuroendocrinology.* 2015;52:239–250.
19. Epel ES, McEwen B, Seeman T, et al. Stress and body shape: Stress-induced cortisol secretion is consistently greater among women with central fat. *Psychosom Med.* 2000;62(5):623–632.
20. Epel E, Lapidus R, McEwen B, Brownell K. Stress may add bite to appetite in women: A laboratory study of stress-induced cortisol and eating behavior. *Psychoneuroendocrinology.* 2001;26(1):37–49.
21. Newman E, O'Connor DB, Conner M. Daily hassles and eating behaviour: The role of cortisol reactivity status. *Psychoneuroendocrinology.* 2007;32(2):125–132.
22. Adam TC, Epel ES. Stress, eating and the reward system. *Physiology & Behavior.* 2007;91(4):449–458.
23. Lutgendorf SK, Garand L, Buckwalter KC, Reimer TT, Hong SY, Lubaroff DM. Life stress, mood disturbance, and elevated interleukin-6 in healthy older women. *J Gerontol A Biol Sci Med Sci.* 1999;54(9):M434–M439.
24. Maes M, Lin AH, Delmeire L, et al. Elevated serum interleukin-6 (IL-6) and IL-6 receptor concentrations in posttraumatic stress disorder following accidental man-made traumatic events. *Biol Psychiatry.* 1999;45(7):833–839.
25. Glaser R, Robles TF, Sheridan J, Malarkey WB, Kiecolt-Glaser JK. Mild depressive symptoms are associated with amplified and prolonged inflammatory responses after influenza virus vaccination in older adults. *Arch Gen Psychiatry.* 2003;60(10):1009–1014.
26. Knight EL, Majd M, Graham-Engeland JE, Smyth JM, Sliwinski MJ, Engeland CG. Depressive symptoms and other negative psychological states relate to ex vivo inflammatory responses differently for men and women: Cross-sectional and longitudinal evidence. *Physiology & Behavior.* 2022;244:113656.
27. Fagundes CP, Glaser R, Hwang BS, Malarkey WB, Kiecolt-Glaser JK. Depressive symptoms enhance stress-induced inflammatory responses. *Brain Behav Immun.* 2013;31:172–176.
28. Brydon L, Wright CE, O'Donnell K, Zachary I, Wardle J, Steptoe A. Stress-induced cytokine responses and central adiposity in young women. *Int J Obes.* 2008;32(3):443–450.
29. Madison AA, Andridge R, Shrout MR, et al. Frequent interpersonal stress and inflammatory reactivity predict depressive-symptom increases: Two tests of the social-signal-transduction theory of depression. *Psychol Sci.* 2022;33(1):152–164.
30. Mac Giollabhui N, Ng TH, Ellman LM, Alloy LB. The longitudinal associations of inflammatory biomarkers and depression revisited: Systematic review, meta-analysis, and meta-regression. *Mol Psychiatry.* 2021;26(7):3302–3314.
31. Raison CL, Rutherford RE, Woolwine BJ, et al. A randomized controlled trial of the tumor necrosis factor antagonist infliximab for treatment-resistant depression: The role of baseline inflammatory biomarkers. *JAMA Psychiatry.* 2013;70(1):31–41.
32. Bonafede MM, Gandra SR, Watson C, Princic N, Fox KM. Cost per treated patient for etanercept, adalimumab, and infliximab across adult indications: A claims analysis. *Adv Ther.* 2012;29(3):234–248.
33. Berger JS. Aspirin for primary prevention-time to rethink our approach. *JAMA Netw Open.* 2022;5(4):e2210144.
34. Kavyani Z, Musazadeh V, Fathi S, Hossein Faghfouri A, Dehghan P, Sarmadi B. Efficacy of the omega-3 fatty acids supplementation on inflammatory biomarkers: An umbrella meta-analysis. *Int Immunopharmacol.* 2022;111:109104.
35. Gabbs M, Leng S, Devassy JG, Monirujjaman M, Aukema HM. Advances in our understanding of oxylipins derived from dietary PUFAs. *Adv Nutr.* 2015;6:513–540.

36. Pauls SD, Du Y, Clair L, et al. Impact of age, menopause, and obesity on oxylipins linked to vascular health. *Arterioscler Thromb Vasc Biol.* 2021;41(2):883–897.

37. Zampelas A, Panagiotakos DB, Pitsavos C, et al. Fish consumption among healthy adults is associated with decreased levels of inflammatory markers related to cardio-vascular disease: The ATTICA study. *J Am Coll Cardiol.* 2005;46(1):120–124.

38. Pischon T, Hankinson SE, Hotamisligil GS, Rifai N, Willctt WC, Rimm EB. Habitual dietary intake of n-3 and n-6 fatty acids in relation to inflammatory markers among US men and women. *Circulation.* 2003;108(2):155–160.

39. Lopez-Garcia E, Schulze MB, Manson JE, et al. Consumption of (n-3) fatty acids is related to plasma biomarkers of inflammation and endothelial activation in women. *J Nutr.* 2004;134(7):1806–1811.

40. Menoyo D, Izquierdo MS, Robaina L, Gines R, Lopez-Bote CJ, Bautista JM. Adaptation of lipid metabolism, tissue composition and flesh quality in gilthead sea bream (*Sparus aurata*) to the replacement of dietary fish oil by linseed and soyabean oils. *Br J Nutr.* 2004;92(1):41–52.

41. Ferrucci L, Cherubini A, Bandinelli S, et al. Relationship of plasma polyunsaturated fatty acids to circulating inflammatory markers. *J Clin Endocrinol Metab.* 2006;91(2): 439–446.

42. McBurney MI, Tintle NL, Harris WS. Lower omega-3 status associated with higher erythrocyte distribution width and neutrophil-lymphocyte ratio in UK Biobank cohort. *Prostaglandins Leukot Essent Fatty Acids.* 2023;192:102567.

43. Ramos-Campo DJ, Ávila-Gandía V, López-Román FJ, et al. Supplementation of re-esterified docosahexaenoic and eicosapentaenoic acids reduce inflammatory and mus-cle damage markers after exercise in endurance athletes: A randomized, controlled crossover trial. *Nutrients.* 2020;12(3)719.

44. Zhou Q, Zhang Z, Wang P, et al. EPA+DHA, but not ALA, improved lipids and inflam-mation status in hypercholesterolemic adults: A randomized, double-blind, placebo-controlled trial. *Mol Nutr Food Res.* 2019;63(10):e1801157.

45. Limonte CP, Zelnick LR, Ruzinski J, et al. Effects of long-term vitamin D and n-3 fatty acid supplementation on inflammatory and cardiac biomarkers in patients with type 2 diabetes: Secondary analyses from a randomised controlled trial. *Diabetologia.* 2021;64(2):437–447.

46. Abdelhamid AS, Brown TJ, Brainard JS, et al. Omega-3 fatty acids for the primary and secondary prevention of cardiovascular disease. *Cochrane Database Syst Rev.* 2020;3(3):Cd003177.

47. Hibbeln JR. Fish consumption and major depression. *Lancet.* 1998;351(9110):1213.

48. Iribarren C, Markovitz JH, Jacobs DR Jr, Schreiner PJ, Daviglus M, Hibbeln JR. Dietary intake of n-3, n-6 fatty acids and fish: Relationship with hostility in young adults–the CARDIA study. *Eur J Clin Nutr.* 2004;58(1):24–31.

49. Kilkens TOC, Honig A, Maes M, Lousberg R, Brummer RJM. Fatty acid profile and affective dysregulation in irritable bowel syndrome. *Lipids.* 2004;39(5):425–431.

50. Hallahan B, Garland MR. Essential fatty acids and mental health. *Br J Psychiatry.* 2005;186:275–277.

51. Sobczak S, Honig A, Christophe A, et al. Lower high-density lipoprotein cholesterol and increased omega-6 polyunsaturated fatty acids in first-degree relatives of bipolar patients. *Psychol Med.* 2004;34(1):103–112.

52. Kulikova A, Palka JM, Van Enkevort EA, et al. The cross-sectional relationship among omega-3 fatty acid levels, cardiorespiratory fitness, and depressive symptoms from the Cooper Center Longitudinal Study. *J Psychosom Res.* 2023;168:111181.

53. Kiecolt-Glaser JK, Belury MA, Porter K, Beversdorf DQ, Lemeshow S, Glaser R. Depressive symptoms, omega-6:omega-3 fatty acids, and inflammation in older adults. *Psychosom Med.* 2007;69(3):217–224.

54. Maes M, Christophe A, Bosmans E, Lin A, Neels H. In humans, serum polyunsaturated fatty acid levels predict the response of proinflammatory cytokines to psychologic
stress. *Biol Psychiatry.* 2000;47(10):910–920.
55. Kiecolt-Glaser J, Belury MA, Andridge R, Malarkey WB, Glaser R. Omega-3 supplementation lowers inflammation and anxiety in medical students: A randomized controlled trial. *Brain Behav Immun.* 2011;25(8):1725–1734.
56. Kiecolt-Glaser J, Epel ES, Belury MA, et al. Omega-3 fatty acids, oxidative stress, and
leukocyte telomere length: A randomized controlled trial. *Brain Behav Immun.* 2013;
28:16–24.
57. Appleton KM, Voyias PD, Sallis HM, et al. Omega-3 fatty acids for depression in
adults. *Cochrane Database of Syst Rev.* 2021;11(11):Cd004692.
58. Kiecolt-Glaser JK, Derry HM, Fagundes CP. Inflammation: Depression fans the flames
and feasts on the heat. *Am J Psychiatry.* 2015;172(11):1075–1091.
59. Kris-Etherton PM, Harris WS, Appel LJ. Fish consumption, fish oil, omega-3 fatty
acids, and cardiovascular disease. *Circulation.* 2002;106(21):2747–2757.
60. Griel AE, Kris-Etherton PM. Beyond saturated fat: The importance of the dietary fatty
acid profile on cardiovascular disease. *Nutr Rev.* 2006;64(5 Pt 1):257–262.
61. Moshfegh AJ, Goldman JD, Rhodes DG, Friday JE. Usual nutrient intake from food
and beverages, by gender and age, what we eat in America, NHANES 2017-March 2020
Prepandemic. Worldwide Web Site: Food Surveys Research Group; 2023. Available at
https://www.ars.usda.gov/Services/docs.htm?docid=22659.

26 Cancer Prevention and Management

Cramer J. Kallem, MA, Emily K. Tillman, MS, MSW,
Kari R. Campbell, MS, Jennifer Braim, BS, and
Jennifer L. Steel, PhD

KEY POINTS
- Health behaviors potentiate the onset and progression of several cancer types.
- Biological and genetic mediators exist linking health behaviors and the development and progression of cancer.
- Health behavior interventions have been shown to be effective in the prevention of cancer as well as slowing the progression of cancer once diagnosed.

26.1   INTRODUCTION

The pathogenesis of cancer is understood to be a complex multistep process. Hanahan and Weinberg (2011) described eight hallmark functions that are acquired as normal human cells evolve into malignant cells.[1] These hallmarks include sustaining cellular proliferative signaling, evading tumor suppressor mechanisms, evading immune system destruction, resisting cell death, enabling replicative immortality of cells, inducing angiogenesis, reprogramming of energy metabolism, and activating local invasion and metastasis.[1]

Many factors are known to potentiate the onset and progression of cancer, including modifiable health or lifestyle behaviors and environmental factors.[2,3] This chapter will focus on the relationship between health behaviors (e.g., diet, sleep, physical activity, tobacco and alcohol use, UV exposure, sexual behavior) and their biological and genetic mediators in the development and progression of cancers. We will also discuss health behavior interventions to prevent cancer and slow its progression.

26.2   HEALTH BEHAVIORS IN THE DEVELOPMENT
AND PROGRESSION OF CANCER

It is estimated that 52% of cancers are preventable with changes in lifestyle.[4,5] The adoption of a healthy lifestyle (e.g., physical activity, diets rich in fruits and vegetables, no tobacco use) is associated with lower risks of several site-specific cancers.[5] However, to our knowledge, not *all* of these health behaviors contribute to the incidence or progression of *all* types of cancer.[4]

DOI: 10.1201/b22810-30

Tobacco use is the leading preventable risk factor for cancer, accounting for approximately 19% of all cancer cases and 29% of cancer-related deaths.[2,5,6] Studies have demonstrated a dose-response pattern between tobacco use (both intensity and duration) and incidence of lung, larynx, bladder, esophagus, pancreas, kidney, stomach, oral cavity, and pharynx cancer.[7] Moreover, after receiving a tobacco-related cancer diagnosis, continued tobacco use is associated with increased risk of recurrence and cancer-related mortality.[8,9] Even among non-smoking-related cancers, smoking is associated with decreased tolerance and efficacy of radiation and systemic treatments, increased risk of post-surgical complications, greater incidence of second primary tumors, and shorter overall survival.[8]

Physical inactivity is estimated to account for 2.9% of all cancer incidence, with the highest proportion for cancer of the corpus uteri (26.7%), but the largest number of cases was for colon cancer (16.3%) and breast cancer (3.9%).[6] Greater physical activity after being diagnosed with cancer is also associated with lower cancer cell proliferation, cancer cell viability, tumorigenic potential, risk of recurrence, and mortality.[10,11]

Dietary recommendations for cancer prevention vary by cancer type; however, general guidelines include daily consumption of fruits and vegetables, while limiting consumption of alcohol, processed grain products, red meat, and processed meats.[12,13] Alcohol intake is a particularly potent risk factor and was estimated to account for 5.6% of total cancers.[6] Western diets (e.g., high in fat, red meat, and processed foods) tend to increase risk of cancer-related mortality,[14,15] whereas, adherence to a Mediterranean diet and other high-quality dietary patterns are associated with increased quality of life and lower mortality among those diagnosed with cancer.[14,15]

Few studies have demonstrated the role of sleep in the incidence of cancer. Markedly long and short sleep duration, insomnia, parasomnia, night shift work, and obstructive sleep apnea have been associated with a higher cancer incidence.[16–19] Similar to findings in the general population, a U- or J-shape relationship between sleep duration and mortality has been observed in those diagnosed with cancer, wherein markedly short (< 6 hrs.) or long (> 9 hrs.) sleep durations may be associated with increased mortality in certain cancers.[19]

Approximately 95% of skin cancer (e.g., basal cell, squamous cell, and melanoma) cases were attributable to UV radiation (e.g., from indoor tanning and sun exposure).[6] Although only associated with skin cancers, UV radiation contributes to a significant proportion of total cancer cases in both men (5.8%) and women (3.7%).[6] Once diagnosed with skin cancer, ongoing exposure to UV radiation may result in a recurrence or new lesions.[20]

An estimated 3% of cancer cases were attributable to viral infections due to sexual or IV drug risk behaviors.[6] Strategies to prevent infection-related cancers include adherence to screening recommendations, reducing risky behaviors, vaccination for human papillomavirus (HPV) and hepatitis B virus (HBV), using antiviral medications to treat or cure hepatitis C virus (HCV), and using antiretroviral medications to suppress the viral load in patients with human immunodeficiency virus (HIV).[6] Use of these antiretrovirals, once diagnosed with HCV or HIV, can slow the progression to liver failure and/or cancer or AIDS-related cancers, respectively, as well as reduce the risk of infection of others.[6,21]

26.3   BIOLOGICAL MECHANISMS LINKING HEALTH BEHAVIORS AND CANCER

A number of biological mechanisms have been implicated in facilitating health behaviors' influence on cancer development and progression. While a comprehensive review of this topic is beyond the scope of this chapter, this section will provide an overview of possible biological and genetic mechanisms linking health behaviors with the onset and progression of cancer.

More than 60 carcinogens have been detected in cigarette smoke.[4] Tobacco carcinogens react with deoxyribonucleic acid (DNA) to form adducts which can induce gene mutations that promote carcinogenesis in the lungs.[4] There is growing evidence that epigenetic reprogramming appears to play a major role in the association between cigarette smoking and cancer outcomes.[4,22] Smoking causes significant changes to DNA methylation patterns which alter the expression of numerous genes that are implicated in the initiation and progression of cancer.[22] Several studies have demonstrated an inverse association between physical activity and breast cancer risk, even among women at high risk due to tumor suppressor gene mutations (e.g., BRCA1 and BRCA2).[4] A hormonal mechanism is believed to mediate this relationship wherein physical activity lowers estrogen levels, a hormone that stimulates cell proliferation.[4] Physical activity may inhibit the development of colorectal cancer and progression by decreasing bowel transit time, thereby reducing exposure to fecal carcinogens.[4] Physical activity may also attenuate the development and progression of certain cancers by slowing the body's production of insulin-like growth factors, increasing cancer cell growth.[4]

One way in which diet may influence cancer incidence and progression is via the gut microbiota by promoting the growth of bacteria with either oncogenic or tumor-suppressive properties.[12] The beneficial effect of dietary fiber appears to be at least partially mediated by a bacterial fermentation process within the colon that produces butyrate, a fatty acid that suppresses the growth of colorectal cancer cells.[12] Once diagnosed with cancer, diets high in polyphenols (micronutrients found in fruits and vegetables) have the capacity to prevent metastasis and slow tumor progression through epigenetic mechanisms by influencing non-coding ribonucleic acid (RNA) expression, DNA methylation patterns, and histone modifications in cancer cells.[12]

Inflammation has also been proposed as a biological link between diet, including the consumption of alcohol, and cancer, based on evidence that diets categorized as inflammatory (e.g., Western diet) are associated with greater cancer risk compared to anti-inflammatory diets (e.g., Mediterranean diet).[12] Many of the carcinogenic effects of heavy alcohol consumption are attributable to its primary metabolite, acetaldehyde, a mutagenic compound that binds to DNA to form stable adducts.[23] However, alcohol can also directly facilitate the development and progression of certain cancers by causing inflammation and organ/tissue damage, thereby increasing exposure and absorption of other carcinogens.[23]

Immune system dysregulation may explain the link between sleep and cancer development and progression. Short sleep duration has been associated with reduced Natural Killer cell activity, which plays an important role in tumor surveillance and, thereby, plays a vital role in tumor surveillance, putting an individual at risk of developing cancer.[24] Obstructive sleep apnea may also promote tumor onset and growth through its association with increased oxidative stress, induced by intermittent hypoxia.[25] Oxidative stress can cause damage to DNA, RNA, and lipids, which may result in gene mutations that promote tumorigenesis and cancer progression.[25]

26.4   HEALTH BEHAVIOR INTERVENTIONS FOR CANCER PREVENTION AND MANAGEMENT

A multitude of health behavior interventions to prevent cancer exist. Smoking cessation interventions are the most common of health behavior interventions to prevent cancer and have been shown to be effective for decades. Today, tailored smoking cessation interventions are targeted to adolescents and disadvantaged populations who may be at the greatest risk of developing tobacco-related cancers.[26,27] Development of health behavior interventions that focus on diet, exercise, sleep, and alcohol use have been primarily designed to improve overall health and not specifically to reduce cancer risk.[28] With regard to research on using diets to reduce cancer risk, a meta-analysis concluded a vegetarian diet was not associated with lower risk of breast, colorectal, or prostate cancer.[29] However evidence suggests that the Mediterranean diet was related to lower risk of cancer-related mortality.[30] Interventions to increase screening behavior for cancers such as breast, prostate, colorectal, and cervical cancers have also been shown to be effective in reducing cancer-related mortality.[31-34]

Interventions to improve health behaviors after a diagnosis of cancer have also been designed and tested. Schmitz and colleagues (2005), in their meta-analyses of physical activity interventions for those diagnosed with cancer, concluded that the interventions were safe and improved cardiorespiratory fitness, reduced cancer-related symptoms, and decreased fatigue.[35] Physical activity interventions have also been shown to improve all cause and cancer-specific survival.[36] Of note, with interventions targeted toward changing dietary habits after a diagnosis of cancer, a Mediterranean diet was not found to reduce the risk of cancer recurrence or mortality.[30] In a meta-analysis, the greatest efficacy for insomnia exists for cognitive-behavioral therapy for insomnia, but no data regarding the effects of this intervention on cancer-related or overall survival were included in these studies.[37] Interventions to reduce smoking and alcohol use after a diagnosis of cancer have been shown to be effective but have been primarily tested in cancer types in which alcohol or tobacco were the primary contributing factor in the development of the cancer (e.g., lung cancer, head, and neck).[38,39] Smoking cessation after a diagnosis of cancer has been shown to improve all-cause and cancer-related survival.[40]

In the last two decades, technology-assisted interventions have been developed to increase the reach of interventions. However, recent meta-analyses have shown that technology-assisted interventions often have small effect sizes, and at this time, there is not enough evidence to recommend lifestyle interventions delivered using technology (e.g., internet, mobile app).[41,42] Interestingly, couples-focused interventions have been shown to be more effective than individual interventions in changing health behaviors and may be recommended.[43] Mixed findings have been reported with regard to whether targeting multiple health behaviors at one time may be beneficial, and it appears that when smoking cessation is included in these multiple risk behavior interventions, it is not as effective.[28,44] The need for innovative and effective health behavior interventions to prevent cancer as well as to reduce morbidity and mortality once diagnosed with cancer continues to exist despite decades of research.

26.5 CONCLUSION

In summary, health behaviors often play an important role in the onset and progression of several cancer types. These behaviors influence cancer outcomes through a number of biological and genetic processes. Considering that health behavior interventions effectively reduce the incidence and progression of cancer, they represent a promising option to reduce the morbidity and mortality resulting from cancer. Further research is still needed to understand the role of health behaviors in rarer cancer types to maximize the potential for health behavior interventions to reduce cancer morbidity and mortality.

REFERENCES

1. Hanahan D, Weinberg RA. Hallmarks of cancer: The next generation. *Cell.* 2011; 144(5):646–674.
2. Dornelas EA. *Psychological Treatment of Patients with Cancer.* American Psychological Association; 2018.
3. Fisher EB, Fitzgibbon ML, Glasgow RE, et al. Behavior matters. *Am J Prev Med.* 2011;40(5):e15–e30.
4. Coyle YM. Lifestyle, genes, and cancer. *Methods Mol Biol Clifton NJ.* 2009;472:25–56.
5. Zhang YB, Pan XF, Chen J, et al. Combined lifestyle factors, incident cancer, and cancer mortality: A systematic review and meta-analysis of prospective cohort studies. *Br J Cancer.* 2020;122(7):1085–1093.
6. Islami F, Goding Sauer A, Miller KD, et al. Proportion and number of cancer cases and deaths attributable to potentially modifiable risk factors in the United States. *CA Cancer J Clin.* 2018;68(1):31–54.
7. Kuper H, Boffetta P, Adami HO. Tobacco use and cancer causation: Association by tumour type. *J Intern Med.* 2002;252(3):206–224.
8. Jassem J. Tobacco smoking after diagnosis of cancer: Clinical aspects. *Transl Lung Cancer Res.* 2019;8(Suppl 1):S50–S58.
9. Parsons A, Daley A, Begh R, Aveyard P. Influence of smoking cessation after diagnosis of early-stage lung cancer on prognosis: Systematic review of observational studies with meta-analysis. *BMJ.* 2010;340:b5569.
10. Morishita S, Hamaue Y, Fukushima T, Tanaka T, Fu JB, Nakano J. Effect of exercise on mortality and recurrence in patients with cancer: A systematic review and meta-analysis. *Integr Cancer Ther.* 2020;19:1–10.
11. Friedenreich CM, Neilson HK, Farris MS, Courneya KS. Physical activity and cancer outcomes: A precision medicine approach. *Clin Cancer Res.* 2016;22(19):4766–4775.
12. Steck SE, Murphy EA. Dietary patterns and cancer risk. *Nat Rev Cancer.* 2020;20(2): 125–138.
13. Kushi LH, Doyle C, McCullough M, et al. American Cancer Society guidelines on nutrition and physical activity for cancer prevention. *CA Cancer J Clin.* 2012;62(1):30–67.
14. Castro-Espin C, Agudo A. The role of diet in prognosis among cancer survivors: A systematic review and meta-analysis of dietary patterns and diet interventions. *Nutrients.* 2022;14(2):348.

15. Schwedhelm C, Boeing H, Hoffmann G, Aleksandrova K, Schwingshackl L. Effect of diet on mortality and cancer recurrence among cancer survivors: A systematic review and meta-analysis of cohort studies. *Nutr Rev.* 2016;74(12):737–748.

16. Zhao H, Yin JY, Yang WS, et al. Sleep duration and cancer risk: A systematic review and meta-analysis of prospective studies. *Asian Pac J Cancer Prev.* 2013;14(12):7509–7515.

17. Blask DE. Melatonin, sleep disturbance and cancer risk. *Sleep Med Rev.* 2009;13(4): 257–264.

18. Fang HF, Miao NF, Chen CD, Sithole T, Chung MH. Risk of cancer in patients with insomnia, parasomnia, and obstructive sleep apnea: A nationwide nested case-control study. *J Cancer.* 2015;6(11):1140–1147.

19. Collins KP, Geller DA, Antoni M, et al. Sleep duration is associated with survival in advanced cancer patients. *Sleep Med.* 2017;32:208–212.

20. Mahon SM. Skin cancer prevention: Education and public health issues. *Semin Oncol Nurs.* 2003;19(1):52–61.

21. Calvo-Cidoncha E, González-Bueno J, Almeida-González CV, Morillo-Verdugo R. Influence of treatment complexity on adherence and incidence of blips in HIV/HCV coinfected patients. *J Manag Care Spec Pharm.* 2015;21(2):153–157.

22. Ma Y, Li MD. Establishment of a strong link between smoking and cancer pathogenesis through DNA methylation analysis. *Sci Rep.* 2017;7(1):1811.

23. Seitz HK, Cho CH. Contribution of alcohol and tobacco use in gastrointestinal cancer development. In: Verma M, ed. *Cancer Epidemiology: Modifiable Factors.* Humana Press; 2009:217–241.

24. Irwin M, Mascovich A, Gillin JC, Willoughby R, Pike J, Smith TL. Partial sleep deprivation reduced natural killer cell activity in humans. *Psychosom Med.* 1994;56(6): 493–498.

25. Cao J, Feng J, Li L, Chen B. Obstructive sleep apnea promotes cancer development and progression: A concise review. *Sleep Breath Schlaf Atm.* 2015;19(2):453–457.

26. Soneji S, Barrington-Trimis JL, Wills TA, et al. Association between initial use of e-cigarettes and subsequent cigarette smoking among adolescents and young adults: A systematic review and meta-analysis. *JAMA Pediatr.* 2017;171(8):788–797.

27. Myung SK, Yoo KY, Oh SW, et al. Meta-analysis of studies investigating one-year effectiveness of transdermal nicotine patches for smoking cessation. *Am J Health Syst Pharm.* 2007;64(23):2471–2476.

28. Meader N, King K, Wright K, et al. Multiple risk behavior interventions: Meta-analyses of RCTs. *Am J Prev Med.* 2017;53(1):e19–e30.

29. Godos J, Bella F, Sciacca S, Galvano F, Grosso G. Vegetarianism and breast, colorectal and prostate cancer risk: An overview and meta-analysis of cohort studies. *J Hum Nutr Diet.* 2017;30(3):349–359.

30. Schwingshackl L, Schwedhelm C, Galbete C, Hoffmann G. Adherence to mediterranean diet and risk of cancer: An updated systematic review and meta-analysis. *Nutrients.* 2017;9(10):1063.

31. Hewitson P, Glasziou P, Watson E, Towler B, Irwig L. Cochrane systematic review of colorectal cancer screening using the fecal occult blood test (hemoccult): An update. *Am J Gastroenterol.* 2008;103(6):1541–1549.

32. Nelson HD, Tyne K, Naik A, Bougatsos C, Chan BK, Humphrey L. Screening for breast cancer: An update for the U.S. Preventive Services Task Force. *Ann Intern Med.* 2009;151(10):727–737.

33. Peirson L, Fitzpatrick-Lewis D, Ciliska D, Warren R. Screening for cervical cancer: A systematic review and meta-analysis. *Syst Rev.* 2013;2(1):35.

34. Sadate A, Occean BV, Beregi JP, et al. Systematic review and meta-analysis on the impact of lung cancer screening by low dose computed tomography. *Eur J Cancer.* 2020; 134:107–114.

35. Schmitz KH, Holtzman J, Courneya KS, Mâsse LC, Duval S, Kane R. Controlled physical activity trials in cancer survivors: A systematic review and meta-analysis. *Cancer Epidemiol Biomarkers Prev.* 2005;14(7):1588–1595.

36. McTiernan A, Friedenreich CM, Katzmarzyk PT, et al. Physical activity in cancer prevention and survival: A systematic review. *Med Sci Sports Exerc.* 2019;51(6):1252–1261.

37. Ma Y, Hall DL, Ngo LH, Liu Q, Bain PA, Yeh GY. Efficacy of cognitive behavioral therapy for insomnia in breast cancer: A meta-analysis. *Sleep Med Rev.* 2021;55:101376.

38. Lauridsen SV, Thomsen T, Kaldan G, Lydom LN, Tønnesen H. Smoking and alcohol cessation intervention in relation to radical cystectomy: A qualitative study of cancer patients' experiences. *BMC Cancer.* 2017;17(1):793.

39. Shingler E, Robles LA, Perry R, et al. Tobacco and alcohol cessation or reduction interventions in people with oral dysplasia and head and neck cancer: Systematic review protocol. *Syst Rev.* 2017;6(1):161.

40. Walter V, Jansen L, Hoffmeister M, Brenner H. Smoking and survival of colorectal cancer patients: Systematic review and meta-analysis. *Ann Oncol.* 2014;25(8):1517–1525.

41. Kelley MM, Kue J, Brophy L, et al. Mobile Health applications, cancer survivors, and lifestyle modification: An integrative review. *CIN Comput Inform Nurs.* 2021; 39(11):755–763.

42. Furness K, Sarkies MN, Huggins CE, Croagh D, Haines TP. Impact of the method of delivering electronic health behavior change interventions in survivors of cancer on engagement, health behaviors, and health outcomes: Systematic review and meta-analysis. *J Med Internet Res.* 2020;22(6):e16112.

43. Arden-Close E, McGrath N. Health behaviour change interventions for couples: A systematic review. *Br J Health Psychol.* 2017;22(2):215–237.

44. Moug SJ, Bryce A, Mutrie N, Anderson AS. Lifestyle interventions are feasible in patients with colorectal cancer with potential short-term health benefits: A systematic review. *Int J Colorectal Dis.* 2017;32(6):765–775.

27 Depressive and Anxiety Related Conditions

Lydia Wu-Chung, MA and
Christopher P. Fagundes, PhD

KEY POINTS

- Hypothalamic-pituitary-adrenal axis dysregulation and elevated inflammation are implicated in the pathophysiology of depressive and anxiety disorders.
- Biobehavioral interventions successfully reduce relapse rate and symptom severity, although cognitive behavioral therapy is more effective than mind-body interventions.
- Reductionist and transdiagnostic approaches provide a promising perspective for understanding the complex etiology and presentation of depressive and anxiety disorders.

27.1 OVERVIEW

Depressive and anxiety disorders are the most common mental disorders worldwide.[1] They cause significant disruption to daily functioning, enhance the risk of developing cardiovascular illness,[2] increase cardiovascular and all-cause mortality,[3] and worsen disease prognosis and treatment outcomes when present alongside physical illnesses.[4-6] Depressive disorders also increase the risk of cardiovascular multimorbidity, or the presence of multiple cardiometabolic illnesses.[5,7] Moreover, the comorbidity of depressive and anxiety disorders predicts worse psychiatric symptoms and complicates treatment regimens for patients. Indeed, patients with major depressive disorder and comorbid anxiety reported more suicidal ideation, more depressed mood, and greater role impairment compared with patients with only major depressive disorder.[8,9] Identifying pathophysiological mechanisms is crucial for developing individualized treatment plans and improving patient outcomes. However, decades of research underscore the complexity of depressive and anxiety disorders, as their etiology remains elusive and conventional treatment options fail to sufficiently alleviate symptoms for all affected individuals.

The present chapter provides a brief description of depressive and anxiety disorders, their etiology, and current treatment options. In describing the pathophysiology and treatment of depressive and anxiety disorders, we primarily emphasize stress-related mechanisms and interventions, as substantial work implicates stress dysregulation as a pathophysiological mechanism underlying both depressive and anxiety disorders. Throughout the chapter, we occasionally highlight research on patients with comorbid anxiety and depression, as subtle differences in symptom

DOI: 10.1201/b22810-31

presentation and physiology exist between those with "pure" depressive or anxiety disorders and those with both depressive and anxiety disorders. We conclude with a brief discussion about the limitations of a symptom-based diagnostic system, the current research initiative to identify objective biomarkers that quantify risk and symptom severity, and the possibility that stress dysregulation may represent a trans-diagnostic process of depressive and anxiety disorders.

27.2 WHAT ARE DEPRESSIVE DISORDERS?

Depressive disorders are characterized by varying degrees of sad or irritable mood that are accompanied by cognitive and somatic changes.[10] The most common type of depressive disorder is major depressive disorder (MDD). An MDD diagnosis requires a discrete depressive episode lasting at least 2 weeks. A depressive episode is defined as having 5+ of the following symptoms: depressed mood, anhedonia (loss of interest or pleasure in most activities one usually would enjoy), significant weight loss, insomnia or hypersomnia, fatigue, feelings of worthlessness, difficulty concentrating or making decisions, and recurring thoughts of death. At least one of the 5+ symptoms must be depressed mood or anhedonia.[10]

27.3 WHAT ARE ANXIETY DISORDERS?

Excessive and persistent fear, anxiety, and related behavioral disturbances are the hallmark features of anxiety disorders.[10] Fear presents as an emotional response to a real or perceived imminent threat, whereas anxiety often surfaces at the anticipation of future threat. Although similar, fear and anxiety generally manifest differently: While fear often is accompanied by an increase in the fight or flight response, escape behavior, and thoughts of danger, anxiety is associated with muscle tension, hyper-vigilance toward future threats and dangers, and avoidance behaviors. Panic attacks frequently present in anxiety disorders as a type of fear response.

Despite their high comorbidity with each other, anxiety disorders are distin-guished by the types of situations that elicit anxiety symptoms. For example, social anxiety disorder is characterized by extreme fear or anxiety in social situations. Generalized anxiety disorder (GAD) is the presence of core anxiety disorder symp-toms and somatic ailments (e.g., fatigue, sleep disturbance, difficulty concentrating) for 6+ months in various contexts, such as school and work.[10] The most common types of anxiety disorders are specific phobias (intense fear to specific situations or objects) and panic disorder with or without agoraphobia (fear of crowds, leaving home, or in places that are difficult to escape).[11]

27.4 MECHANISMS UNDERLYING DEPRESSIVE AND ANXIETY DISORDERS

27.4.1 GENETICS

Depressive and anxiety disorders are highly heritable with rates ranging between 40-70%[12,13] for depressive disorders and between 24-65% for anxiety disorders,[14] depending on the specific phobia. Clinical features such as duration of longest episode, number of episodes (7-9 episodes), recurrent suicidal ideation, and level of distress and impairment are the strongest predictors of depression risk among co-twins, especially monozygotic twins.[15] The genetic correlation between anxiety disorders and major depressive disorder is high, suggesting that these disorders, which often present together, share common genetic etiology.[16]

27.4.2 PSYCHOLOGICAL STRESS

Stressful life events substantially enhance the risk of MDD[17] and GAD.[18] Depressed individuals have 2.5 to 9.8 times greater risk of experiencing a major life event prior to the onset of a first-time major depressive episode.[19] Similarly, the occurrence of one or more negative life events predicts a threefold risk increase of developing GAD.[18] The highest risk of MDD and GAD occurs within the same month of the negative event.[20] However, there is a progressive decrease in the temporal association between life stress and depressive episodes as the number of previous episodes increases – an observation suggesting that less stress is needed to trigger future episodes.[21]

Certain stressors are more likely to provoke depressive and anxiety episodes more than others.[18,22] Specifically, events characterized by significant loss and humiliation, such as childhood trauma, death of a close relative, job loss, or marital dissolution strongly predict impending depression.[22] Loss events also predict the onset of pure GAD, but the magnitude of the association is weaker than that observed with MDD and MDD with comorbid anxiety.[22] Notably, the specificity of stressful life events for predicting depressive or anxiety episodes is modest, as most events impartially increase the risk of both MDD and GAD.[20]

Research on childhood adversity suggests that increased vulnerability to stress-induced psychopathology is driven by stress sensitization processes occurring across a person's lifetime. Specifically, past life events sensitize individuals to psychopathology following recent major life events by reducing their tolerance to minor stressors. Indeed, one study found that a low amount of stressful life events was associated with an increased risk of a major depressive episode only in individuals reporting a history of adverse childhood events (e.g., parental death, family violence, and divorce).[23] In a sample of 34,653 participants, stressful life events in the past year were associated with an increased risk of MDD and anxiety disorders in individuals reporting three or more negative childhood events (e.g., family violence, emotional and physical abuse).[24] In sum, prior exposure to highly threatening events can shape people's response to life stress years later.

27.4.3 HPA AXIS DYSFUNCTION

The hypothalamic-pituitary-adrenal (HPA) axis regulates the body's response to stress through its main byproduct, the human glucocorticoid cortisol.[25] HPA axis activation involves the sequential release of corticotropin-releasing hormone (CRH) and adrenocorticotropic hormone (ACTH), which stimulate cortisol secretion from the adrenal glands. Cortisol self-regulates itself via a negative feedback system, such that elevated cortisol levels subsequently cause the system to inhibit the production of CRH and ACTH. Cortisol coordinates essential homeostatic functions in the midst of changing environments.[25] These changes include increased blood pressure, heart rate, and temporary suppression of vegetative functions such as inflammation, digestion, and reproduction.[25] To assess HPA axis function, researchers assess levels of CRH, ACTH, or cortisol or evaluate the effectiveness of the negative feedback system through administration of dexamethasone, an exogenous steroid that suppresses ACTH and thereby cortisol production.

Substantial work implicates HPA axis dysregulation as a mechanism linking stress and depressive disorders. Currently depressed subjects, remitted depressed subjects, and non-depressed offspring of depressed subjects, all show increased cortisol levels relative to controls; this suggests that HPA axis dysregulation may represent a vulnerability rather than an indicator of present depressive mood.[26,27] In a meta-analysis of 361 studies, cortisol and ACTH levels, but not CRH, were significantly elevated in depressed individuals relative to non-depressed groups. Notably, cortisol differences between depressed and non-depressed groups are stronger for older samples compared to younger samples.[28,29]

Evidence of HPA axis dysregulation in anxiety disorders is less consistent than that of depressive disorders. Although some studies report less adaptive HPA axis functioning (e.g., higher morning cortisol levels, higher basal cortisol levels, greater non-suppression in the dexamethasone suppression test) in people with anxiety disorders, these relationships are more commonly observed in the context of panic disorder, not generalized anxiety disorder.[26] Instead, there is stronger evidence for a role of HPA axis dysregulation in patients with comorbid anxiety and depression. Whereas those with pure anxiety disorders showed normal ACTH and cortisol responses to a laboratory-induced social stressor, those with comorbid depression and anxiety showed higher levels of ACTH in response to the stressor.[30]

27.4.4 PROINFLAMMATORY ACTIVITY

Inflammatory processes are intimately linked with HPA axis function, making it a biological process sensitive to psychological stress. Although cortisol typically inhibits proinflammatory activity, chronic stress desensitizes immune cells to the anti-inflammatory effects of cortisol.[31] Consequently, psychological stress is associated with elevated proinflammatory activity and less adaptive immune responses to infection and injury.[32] Systemic inflammation contributes to the pathophysiology of many age-related diseases, including cardiovascular disease, Alzheimer's disease, and diabetes.[33]

Observational and experimental studies strongly support elevated proinflammatory activity as a pathophysiological mechanism of depressive disorders.[19] People with inflammatory disorders, such as rheumatoid arthritis, inflammatory bowel diseases, and chronic pain, exhibit increased rates of MDD, relative to the general population.[19] Inflammatory challenges also elicit depressive symptomology. Patients receiving Interferon-alpha (IFN-α) treatment to strengthen their immune system developed clinically significant levels of depression.[34] Specifically, over a 3-month period, a majority of patients developed somatic and neurovegetative symptoms (e.g., fatigue, pain, changes in sleep behavior) while a subset developed depressed mood, cognitive dysfunction, and anxiety. These effects were prevented through treatment of paroxetine, an antidepressant, prior to IFN-α treatment.[35] Even when healthy subjects are given the typhoid vaccination, which is considered the mildest inflammatory challenge, increases in depressed mood and fatigue and decreases in cognitive function are observed; these changes are mediated by the proinflammatory biomarker, Interleukin-6.[36,37]

Elevated levels of proinflammatory biomarkers are also observed in people with anxiety disorder. Meta-analyses of inflammatory biomarkers in people with generalized anxiety disorder[38] and post-traumatic stress disorder[39] demonstrate that there is modest evidence of increased levels of proinflammatory biomarkers. Antidepressants may reduce anxiety symptoms via their effects on proinflammatory pathways. In a sample of 42 subjects, antidepressant medication (e.g., serotonin selective reuptake inhibitors) reduced inflammatory cytokine levels in patients with generalized anxiety disorder, and change in cytokine levels covaried with reduction in anxiety symptoms.[40] However, high study heterogeneity, low sample sizes, and lack of a control group limit the generalizability and strength of the association between anxiety disorders and inflammatory biomarkers.

27.5 TREATMENT FOR DEPRESSIVE AND ANXIETY DISORDERS

27.5.1 STANDARD TREATMENT

Depending on the provider and patient preferences, the initial choice of treatment for MDD usually consists of psychotherapy or pharmacotherapy.[41] There is a 50-50 chance that the first form of treatment is tolerable, successfully reduces symptom severity, and achieves remission.[41] Antidepressants are commonly prescribed for MDD and are effective for depressive disorders of various severity. Serotonin selective reuptake inhibitors (SSRIs) are the first line of antidepressant pharmacotherapy.[41] Continuation of antidepressant treatment for 6-9 months after successful response is crucial for obtaining full remission and preventing relapse. Those at high risk for relapse may be required to take medication indefinitely until more curative treatment is discovered.[41] The combination of antidepressants (e.g., fluoxetine) and antipsychotics (e.g., olanzapine) also yields promising results for people with treatment-resistant depression.[41] Antidepressants and antipsychotics come with several side effects, including nausea, diarrhea, sexual dysfunction, daytime drowsiness, insomnia, weight gain, and increased blood pressure.[41]

Anxiety disorders are relatively undertreated, but treatment typically consists of psychotherapy, pharmacotherapy, or a combination of the two.[42] Selective serotonin norepinephrine reuptake inhibitors (SNRI) and SSRIs are the recommended first line of drugs. Benzodiazepines are sometimes administered, as their effects occur more immediately than SNRIs. However, preference for antidepressants over benzodiazepines is primarily attributed to the side effects associated with benzodiazepines, which include depression, fatigue, dizziness, impaired cognitive functioning, and dependency.[42] Importantly, SNRIs and the combination of SNRIs with benzodiazepines are effective in treating patients with comorbid depression and GAD.[43] While further research is needed to understand how these drugs improve psychological symptoms, there is some evidence suggesting that SSRIs have an anti-inflammatory effect in patients with GAD, which may drive the anxiolytic improvements observed in these patients.[40]

27.5.2 COGNITIVE AND BEHAVIORAL INTERVENTIONS

As one of the most densely researched forms of psychotherapy, cognitive behavioral therapy (CBT), effectively treats depressive disorders, anxiety disorders, and related comorbid illnesses.[44,45] Cognitive behavioral therapy rests on the assumptions that psychological disorders arise from maladaptive cognitive patterns and coping behavior. Thus, CBT aims to modify thinking to subsequently change behavior and emotional responses. Several meta-analytic studies strongly support the use of CBT for improving depressive symptoms, anxiety, sleep quality, and psychosocial functioning and reducing relapse rates among people with depressive and anxiety disorders.[46-48] Indeed, for specific phobia and generalized anxiety disorder, CBT performs more efficaciously compared to control or pill placebo conditions and performs similarly to relaxation therapy and psychopharmacology for generalized anxiety disorder.[48] CBT with antidepressants is also effective for preventing relapse: CBT significantly reduces the rate of recurrent depression and the level of residual depressive symptoms after traditional antidepressant treatment.[49] Although CBT has been found to be effective for patients with both anxiety and depression, higher levels of depression are associated with less effective improvement in anxiety symptoms following CBT.[43] Research on CBT has shifted toward identifying the biological mechanisms of action underlying its effectiveness.

27.5.3 MIND–BODY INTERVENTIONS

Mind–body interventions have been explored as alternative options for reducing stress and depressive symptom severity. Rooted in the understanding that the mind, brain, body, and behavior are intimately connected, mind–body interventions focus on using the mind to promote physical and mental well-being.

Yoga is one of the most commonly studied mind–body interventions. Yoga integrates breathing exercises, physical activity, spiritual practice, and meditation.[50] Across multiple randomized controlled trials, yoga produced short-term improvements in depressive symptom severity, relative to standard treatment.[51] However, the effects of yoga on depression severity are not noticeably different from the effects of other complementary treatments on depression, such as relaxation training and physical activity.[51] Similarly, among people with GAD, yoga improved GAD severity, relative to the stress education attention control condition, but was not as effective as CBT.[52]

Mindfulness-based interventions also improve outcomes for people with psychiatric illness.[53] Mindfulness is purposeful, nonjudgmental attention to the inward and outward experiences of the present moment.[54] Mindfulness-based cognitive therapy (MBCT), which combines components of mindfulness and cognitive therapy to reduce stress and improve psychological health,[55] reduces depressive symptoms from pre- to post-treatment and also prevents depression relapse over a 60-week examination period.[56] Notably, mindfulness-based therapy effectively improves symptoms in people with depressive and anxiety disorders when compared to other active treatments (e.g., psychoeducation, relaxation, art therapy), but it does not out-perform traditional CBT.[53,57]

27.6 TOWARDS A REDUCTIONIST AND TRANSDIAGNOSTIC APPROACH TO UNDERSTANDING DEPRESSIVE AND ANXIETY DISORDERS

Shared biological and psychological vulnerabilities suggest depressive and anxiety disorders may share more similarities than differences. Not only is it common for people with an anxiety disorder to have more than one anxiety diagnosis, significant symptom overlap exists between depressive and anxiety disorders. Indeed, 57% of those with depression present with comorbid anxiety[58] and as much as 67% of patients with GAD have a lifetime history of comorbid MDD.[59] Whether mental disorders are qualitatively different from each other or whether they are better represented as a continuum of psychological functioning remains controversial.

Researchers are increasingly interested in using biobehavioral biomarkers as alternatives to symptom-based diagnosis of mental disorders. Developing an objective, biomarker-based diagnostic system is complicated by the realization that alterations in biological markers exist in more than one mental disorder. To overcome these limitations, researchers are beginning to adopt a reductionist approach toward understanding psychopathology.[60] Rather than defining a mental disorder and subsequently identifying the pathophysiology associated with those symptoms, the aim is to identify relevant systems, understand how they become dysregulated, and relate this dysregulation to symptoms.[60]

Research on etiology and treatment efficacy suggests that stress dysregulation may be a transdiagnostic process of mood and anxiety disorders. Transdiagnostic processes are mechanisms shared across multiple disorders. In addition to considerable evidence linking life stressors and physiological stress dysregulation to depressive or anxiety disorders, treatments that target stress appraisal and stress mediators also prove effective. Indeed, both CBT[47,48] and anti-inflammatory medications improve outcomes in individuals with MDD or GAD.[61,62]

Stress dysregulation as a transdiagnostic process may also explain the co-occurrence of depressive and anxiety disorders with other medical illnesses. Psychological stress, inflammatory cytokines, and HPA axis dysregulation are implicated in the pathophysiology and exacerbation of cardiometabolic disorders, autoimmune disorders, and chronic pain. Transdiagnostic treatments such as CBT also have beneficial, untargeted effects on comorbid mental and physical illness.[63] For example, CBT decreases symptom severity in people with comorbid anxiety and depression and improves depressed mood, quality of life, disability, and pain intensity in patients with chronic pain [64,65] and inflammatory bowel syndrome.[66]

27.7 CONCLUSION

Mood disorders are heterogeneous disorders characterized by complex, yet overlapping etiology. Although genetics play a significant role in the development of depressive and anxiety disorders, exposure to major life stressors, HPA axis dysregulation, and a proinflammatory profile play a prominent role in depressive disorders and, to a lesser extent, anxiety disorders. Interventions that aim to modify stress appraisals, target stress mediators, and reduce perceived stress (e.g., cognitive behavioral therapy, mind–body interventions) have promising effects on depressive and anxiety symptoms; however, whether these effects can be sustained long-term requires further examination. In light of commonalities observed between depressive disorders and affective disorders, researchers are exploring different ways to capture psychopathology outside the conventional symptom-based approach. We considered the possibility that stress dysregulation may represent a transdiagnostic process that explains both the similarities among depressive and anxiety disorders and the comorbidity between these psychological disorders and physical illness.

REFERENCES

1. Harvard Medical School. National Comorbidity Survey (NCS); 2007. https://www.hcp.med.harvard.edu/ncs/index.php.
2. Scott KM. Depression, anxiety and incident cardiometabolic diseases. *Curr Opin Psychiatry.* 2014;27(4):289. doi:10.1097/YCO.0000000000000067
3. Phillips AC, Batty GD, Gale CR, et al. Generalized anxiety disorder, major depressive disorder, and their comorbidity as predictors of all-cause and cardiovascular mortality: The Vietnam experience study. *Psychosom Med.* 2009;71(4):395. doi:10.1097/PSY.0b013e31819e6706
4. Aguglia A, Salvi V, Maina G, Rossetto I, Aguglia E. Fibromyalgia syndrome and depressive symptoms: Comorbidity and clinical correlates. *J Affect Disord.* 2011;128(3):262–266. doi:10.1016/j.jad.2010.07.004
5. Yin J, Ma T, Li J, Zhang G, Cheng X, Bai Y. Association of mood disorder with cardiometabolic multimorbidity trajectory and life expectancy, a prospective cohort study. *J Affect Disord.* 2022;312:1–8. doi:10.1016/j.jad.2022.06.003
6. Tully PJ, Harrison NJ, Cheung P, Cosh S. Anxiety and cardiovascular disease risk: A review. *Curr Cardiol Rep.* 2016;18(12):120. doi:10.1007/s11886-016-0800-3
7. Qiao Y, Ding Y, Li G, Lu Y, Li S, Ke C. Role of depression in the development of cardiometabolic multimorbidity: Findings from the UK Biobank study. *J Affect Disord.* 2022;319:260–266. doi:10.1016/j.jad.2022.09.084
8. Fava M, Alpert JE, Carmin CN, et al. Clinical correlates and symptom patterns of anxious depression among patients with major depressive disorder in STAR*D. *Psychol Med.* 2004;34(7):1299–1308. doi:10.1017/S0033291704002612
9. Kessler RC, Sampson NA, Berglund P, et al. Anxious and non-anxious major depressive disorder in the World Health Organization World Mental Health Surveys. *Epidemiol Psychiatr Sci.* 2015;24(3):210–226. doi:10.1017/S2045796015000189
10. American Psychiatric Association, American Psychiatric Association. DSM-5 task force. *Diagnostic and Statistical Manual of Mental Disorders: DSM-5.* 5th ed. American Psychiatric Association; 2013.
11. Kessler RC, McGonagle KA, Zhao S, et al. Lifetime and 12-month prevalence of DSM-III-R psychiatric disorders in the United States: Results from the national comorbidity survey. *Arch Gen Psychiatry.* 1994;51(1):8–19. doi:10.1001/archpsyc.1994.03950010008002
12. Kendler KS, Neale MC, Kessler RC, Heath AC, Eaves LJ. The lifetime history of major depression in women: Reliability of diagnosis and heritability. *Arch Gen Psychiatry.* 1993;50(11):863–870. doi:10.1001/archpsyc.1993.01820230054003
13. Sullivan PF, Neale MC, Kendler KS. Genetic epidemiology of major depression: Review and meta-analysis. *AJP.* 2000;157(10):1552–1562. doi:10.1176/appi.ajp.157.10.1552

14. Gelernter J, Stein MB. Heritability and genetics of anxiety disorders. In: Antony MM, Stein MB, eds. *Oxford Handbook of Anxiety and Related Disorders*. USA: Oxford University Press; 2009.

15. Kendler KS, Gardner CO, Prescott CA. Clinical characteristics of major depression that predict risk of depression in relatives. *Arch Gen Psychiatry*. 1999;56(4):322–327. doi:10.1001/archpsyc.56.4.322

16. Guffanti G, Gameroff MJ, Warner V, et al. Heritability of major depressive and comorbid anxiety disorders in multi-generational families at high risk for depression. *Am J Med Genet B Neuropsychiatr Genet*. 2016;171(8):1072–1079. doi:10.1002/ajmg.b. 32477

17. Kendler KS, Karkowski LM, Prescott CA. Causal relationship between stressful life events and the onset of major depression. *AJP*. 1999;156(6):837–841. doi:10.1176/ajp. 156.6.837

18. Blazer D, Hughes D, George LK. Stressful life events and the onset of a generalized anxiety syndrome. *Am J Psychiatry*. 1987;144(9):1178–1183. doi:10.1176/ajp.144.9.1178

19. Slavich GM, Irwin MR. From stress to inflammation and major depressive disorder: A social signal transduction theory of depression. *Psychol Bull*. 2014;140(3):774. doi:10.1037/a0035302

20. Kendler KS, Karkowski LM, Prescott CA. Stressful life events and major depression: Risk period, long-term contextual threat, and diagnostic specificity. *J Nerv Ment Dis*. 1998;186(11):661.

21. Kendler KS, Thornton LM, Gardner CO. Genetic risk, number of previous depressive episodes, and stressful life events in predicting onset of major depression. *AJP*. 2001;158(4):582–586. doi:10.1176/appi.ajp.158.4.582

22. Kendler KS, Hettema JM, Butera F, Gardner CO, Prescott, Carol A. Life event dimensions of loss, humiliation, entrapment, and danger in the prediction of onsets of major depression and generalized anxiety. *Arch Gen Psychiatry*. 2003;60(8):789–796.

23. Hammen C, Henry R, Daley SE. Depression and sensitization to stressors among young women as a function of childhood adversity. *J Consult Clin Psychol* . 2000;68(5):782. doi:10.1037/0022-006X.68.5.782

24. McLaughlin KA, Conron KJ, Koenen KC, Gilman SE. Childhood adversity, adult stressful life events, and risk of past-year psychiatric disorder: A test of the stress sensitization hypothesis in a population-based sample of adults. *Psychol Med*. 2010; 40(10):1647–1658. doi:10.1017/S0033291709992121

25. Sapolsky RM, Romero LM, Munck AU. How do glucocorticoids influence stress responses? Integrating permissive, suppressive, stimulatory, and preparative actions. *Endocr Rev*. 2000;21(1):55–89. doi:10.1210/edrv.21.1.0389

26. Vreeburg SA, Hoogendijk WJG, van Pelt J, et al. Major depressive disorder and hypothalamic-pituitary-adrenal axis activity: Results from a large cohort study. *Arch Gen Psychiatry*. 2009;66(6):617–626. doi:10.1001/archgenpsychiatry.2009.50

27. Vreeburg SA, Hartman CA, Hoogendijk WJG, et al. Parental history of depression or anxiety and the cortisol awakening response. *Br J Psychiatry*. 2010;197(3):180–185. doi:10.1192/bjp.bp.109.076869

28. Stetler C, Miller GE. Depression and hypothalamic-pituitary-adrenal activation: A quantitative summary of four decades of research. *Psychosom Med*. 2011;73(2):114. doi:10. 1097/PSY.0b013e31820ad12b

29. Belvederi Murri M, Pariante C, Mondelli V, et al. HPA axis and aging in depression: Systematic review and meta-analysis. *Psychoneuroendocrinology*. 2014;41:46–62. doi:10.1016/j.psyneuen.2013.12.004

30. Young EA, Abelson JL, Cameron OG. Effect of comorbid anxiety disorders on the hypothalamic-pituitary-adrenal axis response to a social stressor in major depression. *Biol Psychiatry*. 2004;56(2):113–120. doi:10.1016/j.biopsych.2004.03.017

31. Miller GE, Cohen S, Ritchey AK. Chronic psychological stress and the regulation of pro-inflammatory cytokines: A glucocorticoid-resistance model. *Health Psychol.* 2002;21(6):531. doi:10.1037/0278-6133.21.6.531
32. Glaser R, Kiecolt-Glaser JK. Stress-induced immune dysfunction: Implications for health. *Nat Rev Immunol.* 2005;5(3):243–251. doi:10.1038/nri1571
33. Franceschi C, Campisi J. Chronic inflammation (Inflammaging) and its potential contribution to age-associated diseases. *J Gerontol A Biol Sci Med Sci.* 2014;69(Suppl_1): S4–S9. doi:10.1093/gerona/glu057
34. Capuron L, Miller AH. Cytokines and psychopathology: Lessons from interferon-α. *Biol Psychiatry.* 2004;56(11):819–824. doi:10.1016/j.biopsych.2004.02.009
35. Musselman DL, Lawson DH, Gumnick JF, et al. Paroxetine for the prevention of depression induced by high-dose interferon alfa. *N Engl J Med.* 2001;344(13):961–966. doi:10.1056/NEJM200103293441303
36. Kuhlman KR, Robles TF, Dooley LN, Boyle CC, Haydon MD, Bower JE. Within-subject associations between inflammation and features of depression: Using the flu vaccine as a mild inflammatory stimulus. *Brain Behav Immun.* 2018;69:540–547. doi:10.1016/j.bbi.2018.02.001
37. Strike PC, Wardle J, Steptoe A. Mild acute inflammatory stimulation induces transient negative mood. *J Psychosom Res.* 2004;57(2):189–194. doi:10.1016/S0022-3999(03)00569-5
38. Costello H, Gould RL, Abrol E, Howard R. Systematic review and meta-analysis of the association between peripheral inflammatory cytokines and generalised anxiety disorder. *BMJ Open.* 2019;9(7):e027925. doi:10.1136/bmjopen-2018-027925
39. Passos IC, Vasconcelos-Moreno MP, Costa LG, et al. Inflammatory markers in post-traumatic stress disorder: A systematic review, meta-analysis, and meta-regression. *Lancet Psychiatry.* 2015;2(11):1002–1012. doi:10.1016/S2215-0366(15)00309-0
40. Hou R, Ye G, Liu Y, et al. Effects of SSRIs on peripheral inflammatory cytokines in patients with Generalized Anxiety Disorder. *Brain Behav Immun.* 2019;81:105–110. doi:10.1016/j.bbi.2019.06.001
41. Thase ME, Denko T. Pharmacotherapy of mood disorders. *Annu Rev Clin Psychol.* 2008;4:53–91. doi:10.1146/annurev.clinpsy.2.022305.095301
42. Bandelow B, Michaelis S, Wedekind D. Treatment of anxiety disorders. *Dialogues Clin Neurosci.* 2017;19(2):93–107.
43. Pollack MH. Comorbid anxiety and depression. *J Clin Psychiatry.* 2005;66(Suppl 8):22–29.
44. Reavell J, Hopkinson M, Clarkesmith D, Lane DA. Effectiveness of cognitive behavioral therapy for depression and anxiety in patients with cardiovascular disease: A systematic review and meta-analysis. *Psychosom Med.* 2018;80(8):742. doi:10.1097/PSY.0000000000000626
45. Otte C. Cognitive behavioral therapy in anxiety disorders: Current state of the evidence. *Dialogues Clin Neurosci.* 2011;13(4):413–421.
46. Butler AC, Chapman JE, Forman EM, Beck AT. The empirical status of cognitive-behavioral therapy: A review of meta-analyses. *Clin Psychol Rev.* 2006;26(1):17–31. doi:10.1016/j.cpr.2005.07.003
47. Stewart RE, Chambless DL. Cognitive-behavioral therapy for adult anxiety disorders in clinical practice: A meta-analysis of effectiveness studies. *J Consult Clin Psychol.* 2009;77(4):595–606. doi:10.1037/a0016032
48. Hofmann SG, Asnaani A, Vonk IJ, Sawyer AT, Fang A. The efficacy of cognitive behavioral therapy: A review of meta-analyses. *Cognit Ther Res.* 2012;36:427–440.
49. Fava GA, Rafanelli C, Grandi S, Conti S, Belluardo P. Prevention of recurrent depression with cognitive behavioral therapy: Preliminary findings. *Arch Gen Psychiatry.* 1998;55(9):816–820. doi:10.1001/archpsyc.55.9.816
50. Feuerstein G. *The Yoga Tradition.* Hohm Press; 1998.

51. Cramer H, Lauche R, Langhorst J, Dobos G. Yoga for depression: A systematic review and meta-analysis. *Depress Anxiety.* 2013;30(11):1068–1083. doi:10.1002/da.22166
52. Simon NM, Hofmann SG, Rosenfield D, et al. Efficacy of yoga vs cognitive behavioral therapy vs stress education for the treatment of generalized anxiety disorder: A randomized clinical trial. *JAMA Psychiatry.* 2021;78(1):13–20. doi:10.1001/jamapsychiatry.2020.2496
53. Khoury B, Lecomte T, Fortin G, et al. Mindfulness-based therapy: A comprehensive meta-analysis. *Clin Psychol Rev.* 2013;33(6):763–771. doi:10.1016/j.cpr.2013.05.005
54. Kabat-Zinn J. *Wherever You Go, There You Are: Mindfulness Meditation in Everyday Life.* 7th ed.; 1994. New York: Hyperion.
55. Teasdale JD, Segal Z, Williams JM. How does cognitive therapy prevent depressive relapse and why should attentional control (mindfulness) training help? *Behav Res Ther.* 1995;33(1):25–39. doi:10.1016/0005-7967(94)e0011-7
56. Kuyken W, Warren FC, Taylor RS, et al. Efficacy of mindfulness-based cognitive therapy in prevention of depressive relapse: An individual patient data meta-analysis from randomized trials. *JAMA Psychiatry.* 2016;73(6):565–574. doi:10.1001/jamapsychiatry.2016.0076
57. Singh SK, Gorey KM. Relative effectiveness of mindfulness and cognitive behavioral interventions for anxiety disorders: Meta-analytic review. *Soc Work Ment Health.* 2018;16(2):238–251. doi:10.1080/15332985.2017.1373266
58. Almeida OP, Draper B, Pirkis J, et al. Anxiety, depression, and comorbid anxiety and depression: Risk factors and outcome over two years. *Int Psychogeriatr.* 2012;24(10):1622–1632. doi:10.1017/S104161021200107X
59. Judd LL, Kessler RC, Paulus MP, Zeller PV, Wittchen HU, Kunovac JL. Comorbidity as a fundamental feature of generalized anxiety disorders: Results from the National Comorbidity Study (NCS). *Acta Psychiatrica Scandinavica.* 1998;98(s393):6–11. doi:10.1111/j.1600-0447.1998.tb05960.x
60. Cuthbert BN. The RDoC framework: Facilitating transition from ICD/DSM to dimensional approaches that integrate neuroscience and psychopathology. *World Psychiatry.* 2014;13(1):28–35. doi:10.1002/wps.20087
61. Köhler O, Benros ME, Nordentoft M, et al. Effect of anti-inflammatory treatment on depression, depressive symptoms, and adverse effects: A systematic review and meta-analysis of randomized clinical trials. *JAMA Psychiatry.* 2014;71(12):1381–1391. doi:10.1001/jamapsychiatry.2014.1611
62. Elnazer HY, Sampson AP, Baldwin DS. Effects of celecoxib augmentation of antidepressant or anxiolytic treatment on affective symptoms and inflammatory markers in patients with anxiety disorders: Exploratory study. *Int Clin Psychopharmacol.* 2021;36(3):126. doi:10.1097/YIC.0000000000000356
63. McEvoy PM, Nathan P, Norton PJ. Efficacy of transdiagnostic treatments: A review of published outcome studies and future research directions. *J Cogn Psychother.* 2009;23(1):20–33.
64. Bernardy K, Füber N, Köllner V, Häuser W. Efficacy of cognitive-behavioral therapies in fibromyalgia syndrome — A systematic review and metaanalysis of randomized controlled trials. *J Rheumatol.* 2010;37(10):1991–2005. doi:10.3899/jrheum.100104
65. Richmond H, Hall AM, Copsey B, et al. The effectiveness of cognitive behavioural treatment for non-specific low back pain: A systematic review and meta-analysis. *PLoS ONE.* 2015;10(8):e0134192. doi:10.1371/journal.pone.0134192
66. Bennebroek Evertsz' F, Sprangers MAG, Sitnikova K, et al. Effectiveness of cognitive–behavioral therapy on quality of life, anxiety, and depressive symptoms among patients with inflammatory bowel disease: A multicenter randomized controlled trial. *J Consult Clin Psychol.* 2017;85:918–925. doi:10.1037/ccp0000227

28 Bipolar Disorders

Steven G Sugden, MD, MPH, MSS,
Gia Merlo, MD, MBA, MEd, and
Gabrielle Bachtel, BS

KEY POINTS

- Bipolar disorder is a chronic mental health disorder that is often associated with poor health outcomes, decreased social connections, reduced quality of life, and increased morbidity and mortality.
- Lifestyle interventions should be initiated in conjunction with psychotropic medication at the onset of mood symptoms to provide patients with the best health outcomes.
- The health consequences of BD are all-pervasive in the lives of those diagnosed with the condition and often necessitate both acute and maintenance therapy.

28.1 INTRODUCTION

Bipolar disorder (BD) is a chronic mental health illness that can cause significant quality of life impairment due to intense and unpredictable shifts in mood, levels of energy, and functional capacity. Descriptions of BD, including the extreme pathological expressions of mood (i.e., severe sadness or extreme mania), date back to Hippocrates,[1] who attributed severe sadness, or "melancholia," to imbalances of black bile; he attributed the observed manic symptoms to imbalances of yellow bile. Bipolar episodes comprise extremes of mood-related symptoms: manic/hypomanic, depressive, or a mixture of both manic and depression, and the subsequent fluctuation or cycling of these symptom clusters. BD exists on a spectrum of disorders based on the severity of these symptoms.[1] The spectrum of BD is now classified within the Diagnostic and Statistical Manual of Mental Disorders, Fifth Edition-Text Revision (DSM 5-TR), as the following: Bipolar I Disorder, Bipolar II Disorder, Cyclothymic Disorder, and Unspecified Bipolar.[2,3] In order to be diagnosed with BD, patients must exhibit distinct episodic cycling between two or more mood episodes (e.g., mania, hypomania, depression). Bipolar I Disorder has the most extreme symptoms with distinct periods of severe mania and major depressive disorder. Bipolar II Disorder has symptoms of major depressive disorder and hypomania. Cyclothymic Disorder has symptoms of hypomania and unresolved major depressive disorder symptoms lasting for at least two years.

The onset of BD symptoms typically develops in adolescents or young adults and persists throughout adulthood. BD is often misdiagnosed or classified as other psychiatric conditions such as personality disorders, major depressive disorder, generalized anxiety disorder, substance use disorders (SUDs), and psychosis, due to the heterogeneous presentation of symptoms.[3] Historically, the first-line treatment for individuals diagnosed with bipolar disorder has been psychotropic medications (i.e. mood stabilizers like lithium or Valproate and/or atypical antipsychotics like olanzapine, risperidone, quetiapine).[4] However, due to the lack of efficacy or the occurrence of side effects associated with antipsychotic medications,[5] individuals with BD are often managed with complex regimens to address both disease-related symptoms and drug-induced side effects. Although there is no cure for BD, therapeutic interventions have been found to attenuate morbidity and mortality associated with the condition. The intent of this chapter is to provide an evidence-based review on the prospective role of lifestyle interventions in the management of BD. Lifestyle interventions are often overlooked by healthcare providers in the setting of psychiatric illnesses. Yet, data suggest that guided lifestyle modifications put into effect by informed professionals can help to improve brain health and decrease mortality and morbidity related to BD.[6] Additionally, lifestyle interventions may be instrumental in reversing common metabolic side effects engendered by psychotropic medications in patients with BD.

28.2   IMPACT OF BIPOLAR DISORDER

The global lifetime prevalence of bipolar spectrum has been estimated at 0.5 to 5.0%.[3,7] Within the United States, the prevalence of BD has been estimated at 1.3 to 2.0%. Nevertheless, BD carries one of the highest disease burdens. The health consequences of BD are all-pervasive in the lives of those diagnosed with the condition and often necessitate both acute and maintenance therapy.[3] The US National Comorbidity Study (NCS) revealed that more than two-thirds of those diagnosed with BD have at least one additional comorbid psychiatric illness, the most common being a SUD. The lifetime prevalence for any SUD and any form of BD is nearly 50%. For individuals with bipolar 1 disorder, the incidence of a SUD is over 60%.[8] The diverse array of symptoms associated with BD puts individuals affected by the condition at high risk for potentially self-harming behaviors. Compared to other mental health disorders, the rate of suicide among those with BD is also higher, and people with BD are 20 to 30 times more likely to commit suicide.[9]

Moreover, the prevalence of significant medical and other psychiatric comorbidities in BD is higher than that of the general population and is currently estimated to be within the range of 60-90%. The variety of potential medical comorbidities in the setting of BD include, but are not limited to, cardiovascular, metabolic, digestive, and respiratory illnesses.[3,10] Thus, the likelihood of patients with BD necessitating increased and more complex healthcare is high. The financial costs associated with living with BD are both direct and indirect. The direct costs of BD include hospitalizations, outpatient treatment, and pharmaceuticals, while indirect costs are correlated with morbidity, premature mortality (i.e., death by suicide), and lack of occupational contribution to society due to functional impairment.[11] There is a paucity of literature calculating the direct costs of bipolar disorder, but in 1990, it was estimated to be $US 12.4-19.2 billion annually. The indirect costs of BD were estimated at $US 45.2 billion in 1991, which was higher than those associated with unipolar depression.[7] Ultimately, BD causes the loss of quality of life and places extreme burden on patients and their social circle. Individuals with BD also have a higher-than-average incarceration rate. It is estimated that nearly 50% of those diagnosed with BD are underperforming in their professional roles.[9] Globally, the disability-adjusted life year, also known as DALY, in patients with BD increased 54.4% from 1990-2017.[12] DALY indicates the overall burden of disease and demonstrates that individuals afflicted by BD are progressively losing more years of healthy life because of premature mortality, spending fewer life years in a state of full health, and experiencing more years of disabled life than those without the disorder.

28.3 NEUROBIOLOGICAL UNDERPINNINGS OF BIPOLAR

Since Emil Kraepelin's observations in 1899, who coined the term "manic-depressive insanity" that would later be referred to as BD,[1] researchers have tried to understand the origins and characteristics of BD.[13] As described above, the latest collective concords of symptoms within the bounds of the BD spectrum are included in the DSM 5-TR. However, due to the frequent enigmatic presentations of BD, there is an expanding body of research on the etiology and nosology of psychiatric illnesses, such as BD, in the effort to attenuate rates of misdiagnosis and lag time between symptom onset and appropriate diagnosis/treatment. As novel technology has continued to evolve, researchers have turned to the field of genetics to gain new insight into the causes of this disorder. Twin studies comparing the concordance of BD between monozygotic and dizygotic twins have reported rates of prevalence between 60 to 90%.[14] Additionally, genetic population studies have expanded their investigational scope beyond that of twins to identify the relative familial risks of BD diagnosis. The largest reported family study examining the hereditary prevalence of BD followed over four million Swedish nuclear families and revealed that the relative risk for first-, second-, and third-degree relatives was as high as 7.9, 3.3, and 1.6, respectively.[14] Cumulatively, current literature suggests that BD is one of the most heritable conditions among all mental health diseases.[15] Despite these findings, researchers have not yet isolated a single candidate gene or candidate region within the human genome responsible for BD.[15]

Recently, neuroimaging has also emerged as a modality to illuminate the etiology and nosology of BD. Thus far, attempts by imaging studies to discern specific foci of injury linked to the origin of a neurotoxic event that could account for clinical BD symptoms have generally been unsuccessful.[16] However, according to a 2020 review article by Kloiber et al., abnormalities in white matter integrity are present in individuals at risk for the development and progression of BD. Postmortem brain biopsies of individuals with BD have also revealed decreased cortical thickness and glial density in the anterior cingulate and reduced neuronal density in the amygdala and prefrontal cortex.[17] Although neuroimaging studies have propounded various homogeneous cerebral features in the setting of BD, the current lack of complete congruence of evidence exemplifies the major challenge of present-day healthcare providers: Patients with BD do not always align with the modern diagnostic framework for psychiatric illnesses.

In addition to their contributions specific to neuroimaging, Kloiber et al. summarized their findings through the identification of potential environmental triggers and formulation of a Neurodevelopmental Model for BD.[17] Key contributory factors within the perinatal period include maternal/neonatal infection, toxin exposure, and poor diet. Significant determinants during the developmental period of adolescence and young adulthood include low vitamin D, lower socioeconomic status, cannabis and tobacco exposure, and early life stress.[17] Poor diet and its role in the development of dysbiosis within the perinatal period is of particular interest, as there is a growing collection of literature suggesting that maternal gut microbiota is unable to provide neuroprotection[18] to the development of the fetal brain and the later onset of mental illness disorders, such as BD, and validates its basis as a predisposing circumstance for the disease.[3,19] Finally, there is a high correlation between childhood trauma and the subsequent development of BP. Garno and colleagues identified that 50% of the population diagnosed with BD experienced childhood trauma.[20]

28.4   LIFESTYLE INTERVENTIONS

As mentioned in the previous sections, the social and financial impacts of bipolar disorder and medical comorbidities are significant. The current recommended treatment for the intense mood symptoms of BD is psychotropic medications. Despite the ongoing exploration and discovery of numerous potential candidate genes and underlying neurodevelopmental pathways for BD, there have not been any significant new treatment advancements. The current pharmacotherapeutic components of BD management have been independently linked to worsening obesity and metabolic syndrome among patients with BP.[21] Of note, individuals diagnosed with BD are already at increased risk for metabolic complications. The long-term use of psychotropic drugs, in conjunction with the persistence of poor lifestyle behaviors, further exacerbates metabolic health circumstances in patients with BD. In spite of these barriers, lifestyle interventions may serve as adjuncts to contemporary therapeutic regimes and may play a vital role in reversing the metabolic consequences induced by psychotropic medications.[3]

28.4.1   IMPROVE SLEEP

Lack of sleep or poor sleep is a common feature of BD. More precisely, sleep disturbances typically escalate in those with BD before, during, and after mood episodes.[22] In the setting of BD, it has been noted that shorter sleep patterns are associated with greater mood fluctuation and intensity during bipolar episodes, earlier age of onset of BD, and a longer duration of manic, hypomanic, and/or depressive symptoms.[23] Importantly, this association has been upheld even in individuals being treated with psychotropic medications.[23] Furthermore, there is growing evidence to support the notion that sleep deprivation during the course of BP episodes has a significant influence on gut microbiota and the development of dysbiosis, as well as a lack of microbiota- and diet-related neuroprotection,[18] which can potentially worsen BD symptoms.[24]

Cognitive behavior therapy for chronic insomnia (CBT-I) has emerged as the first-line therapy for insomnia.[25] Modifications of CBT-I that target BD have been developed and have been found to improve sleep and function outcomes.[22] The RISE-UP routine integrates CBT-I with morning activity and has shown improvement with sleep inertia, the state of compromised cognitive and sensory-motor function during the transition between sleeping to waking state, in individuals with BD.[26] This is significant, as typical CBT-I does not incorporate modifications to address sleep inertia. Sleep inertia can be so severe in patients with BD that it persists for hours and further exacerbates the functional impairments present during bipolar episodes at baseline. The RISE-UP routine has been reported to be associated with high rates of patient compliance and marked improvements in morning activity and operational functioning. Apart from CBT-I, additional lifestyle interventions surrounding sleep in those with BD include the use of light therapy (direct exposure to a bright source of light), which has been demonstrated to treat bipolar depression,[27] and dark therapy (blocking blue wavelength at night), which has been used to treat bipolar mania.[27]

28.4.2 HEALTHIER DIETS

As mentioned, the historical gold standard treatment for BD has been psychotropic medications, typically in the form of a mood stabilizer and/or an antipsychotic. Xu and Zhuang recently reviewed the metabolic sequelae following the use of atypical antipsychotic (AAP) medications in patients with schizophrenia and BD. It was reported that 50% of the patients with schizophrenia and BD undergoing treatment with AAPs experienced weight gain.[28] This study also delineated a relationship between the use of AAPs in individuals with schizophrenia or BD and hyperglycemia, type 2 diabetes mellitus, dyslipidemia, and nonalcoholic fatty liver disease.[28] These findings are consistent with additional reviews on this topic.[21,29] Aside from the metabolic factors associated with long-term AAP administration, individuals with BD had higher-than-average tendencies to consume highly processed foods. A study conducted by Platzer revealed that individuals with BP had greater food cravings for foods with high-fat content and for fast foods. The patient's leptin or ghrelin levels could not explain these tendencies, suggesting the explicit link between AAP use and cravings for unhealthy foodstuffs. Individuals with BD who consumed highly fat-rich and processed foods tended to exhibit worsening depressive symptoms.[30]

With this in mind, Stroup and Gray have recommended the inclusion of diet and exercise in the treatment plan of all patients who are prescribed AAPs.[31] Diets high in whole food plants and low in processed foods have been shown to provide significant cardioprotective implications through the attenuation of metabolic syndrome sequelae (e.g., high blood pressure, high serum triglycerides, compromised fasting blood glucose levels, abdominal obesity, low serum high-density lipoprotein [HDL] levels).[32] Diets high in fruits, vegetables, and unrefined grains, yet low in red meat, have demonstrated neuroprotective effects against depressive symptoms in general, including those in major depressive disorder and other psychiatric illnesses, as well as bipolar symptoms.[33] Overall, the potency of whole foods in improving brain and metabolic health must not be undervalued in developing patient-centered synergistic strategies to manage BD in individuals afflicted with the condition.[34]

28.4.3 EXERCISE MORE

Prior to discussion of the benefits of exercise, there is merit in reviewing the evidence related to immune dysfunction within BD,[35] particularly the increase of pro-inflammatory cytokines that is especially notable throughout the course of manic episodes.[36] Interleukin proteins exhibit unique patterns within the central nervous system,[35] which may provide the basis as to why exercise is beneficial in the management of BD. Consistent and regular exercise has been proven to impart significant anti-inflammatory benefits, including the release of hippocampal brain-derived neurotrophic factor (BDNF), which may mitigate cytokine damage and promote neurogenesis.[37] Sun et al. showed that increased physical activity levels decrease the risk of developing BD. There is scarce literature expounding the benefits of implementing exercise in treatment plans for patients with BD, apart from those describing the role of physical activity in attenuating depressive symptoms and improving overall activity and health.[37,38] Given the higher levels of inactivity reported in patients with hippocampal brain-derived neurotrophic factor (BDNF) BD and the metabolic side effects of psychotropic medications commonly used to treat BD, those diagnosed with BD should be encouraged to exercise to help improve body metabolism, reduce symptoms of bipolar episodes, and improve overall health and quality of life.[39]

28.4.4 AVOID RISKY SUBSTANCES

A common symptom within the BD spectrum is involvement in activities that have a high potential for painful consequences,[2] which include increased use of SUD. As mentioned, the prevalence of SUD in patients with BD is 20-70%, which is a higher prevalence than that of individuals with major depressive disorder (10-30%).[40] Individuals with BD and SUD exhibit worsening cognitive impairment (specifically, executive function) throughout the lifespan, which further complicates the management and burden of the illness.[41] Inversely, a recent review article by Laili et al. has suggested the role of SUD in the development of BD, reporting that those with SUD are 3.7 times as likely to experience the onset of BD than the general population. This study also demonstrated the correlation between cannabis, alcohol, nicotine, and opioids as independent risk factors for the development of BD in individuals who partake in substance use.[42]

Integrated group therapy (IGT), developed by Weiss, Najavits, and Greenfield, has been one of the most studied and effective non-pharmacological treatments for BD and SUD.[43] IGT focuses on identifying triggers preceding substance use, enhancing relationships with friends and family, and processing the pros and cons of recovery while promoting sobriety.[43] This approach has been shown to be successful in community-based settings under the guidance of substance use counselors.[40] It is noteworthy that many of the Lifestyle Medicine pillars are incorporated into the IGT model in several ways (e.g., substance avoidance, healthy social connections).

28.4.5 DECREASE STRESS

Individuals with BD have higher levels of psychosocial comorbidities. A meta analysis from Lex et al. reviewed forty-two studies of over 4200 individuals with BD.

Results from this study revealed that individuals with BD were exposed to significantly more stressful life events preceding acute manic episodes.[44] This correlation suggests that stress management and interventions to improve resiliency among patients with BD may reduce bipolar episode relapses and increase time between acute manic episodes. The formulation of newer treatment recommendations reinforces the importance of including psychological interventions in the treatment of BD.[45] Recent advances in psychotherapeutic modalities include mindfulness-based cognitive therapy (MBCT), which incorporates formal meditation practice (sitting and movement practices), and yoga.[46] Recent review articles by Lovas and Schuman-Olivier, and Xuan et al. have both described the efficacy of MBCT in improving emotional dysregulations, without adverse influences on manic symptoms, in patients with BD.[46,47] Finally, emotionally focused therapy has shown to be effective in emotional balance, and strengthening interpersonal bonds, which can improve feelings of isolation and improve mood symptoms.[48]

28.4.6 HEALTHIER RELATIONSHIPS

Finally, individuals with BD tend to damage social relationships due to the extreme mood states and impaired psychosocial functioning correlated with bipolar episodes. BD leads to the unpredictable loss of social control, social disadvantages, mental health stigmatization, and poor social functioning, thereby constituting the impetus for the development of poor relationships and/or damage to healthy relationships. Kim et al. further related poor relationships with worsening negative symptoms, poor adaptive coping, and less resilience in individuals with BD.[49] Dou et al. have highlighted the importance of including family strategies as part of BD treatment to improve psychosocial functioning, enhance social support, and bolster personal resilience in order to facilitate the development, maintenance, and growth of healthy relationships.[50]

28.5 NEXT STEPS

In alignment with this evidence-based review on the implications of lifestyle interventions in the management of BD, it is essential that healthcare professionals increase their awareness of and familiarity with lifestyle recommendations and treatments. Approaches to treating psychiatric disorders, such as BD, through the lens of lifestyle medicine can provide vital augmentation to the typical psychopharmacology approach through attenuating symptoms, pharmaceutical side effects, and risk factors for comorbid physical and mental/brain illnesses. The extent of this discussion is not limited to mental health care providers. Mental/brain health is a global health crisis that is linked to innumerable public health issues outside of the psychiatric/psychological sphere. Mental health organizations, such as the American Psychiatric Association, must further advocate for lifestyle interventions as first-order interventions in the treatment of psychiatric illnesses in order to provide adequate patient-centered care that fosters health-promoting behaviors, maintenance, patient compliance, and overall health and quality of life in patients impacted by conditions like BD.

REFERENCES

1. Mason BL, Brown ES, Croarkin PE. Historical underpinnings of bipolar disorder diagnostic criteria. *Behav Sci*. 2016;6(3):14. doi:10.3390/bs6030014. PMID: 27429010; PMCID: PMC5039514.
2. American Psychiatric Association. *Diagnostic and Statistical Manual of Mental Disorders, Text Revision (DSM-5-TR (TM))*. American Psychiatric Association Publishing, 2022.
3. Malhi GS, Bell E, Singh AB, et al. The 2020 Royal Australian and New Zealand College of Psychiatrists clinical practice guidelines for mood disorders: Major depression summary. *Bipolar Disord*. 2020;22(8):788–804. doi:10.1111/bdi.13035. PMID: 33320412.
4. Hirschfeld RM, Bowden CL, Gitlin MJ, et al. Practice guideline for the treatment of patients with bipolar disorder (revision). *Focus*. 2003;1(1):64–110.
5. Kessing LV, Vradi E, Andersen PK. Nationwide and population-based prescription patterns in bipolar disorder. *Bipolar Disord*. 2016;18(2):174–182. doi:10.1111/bdi.12371. Epub 2016 Feb 18. PMID: 26890465.
6. Vancampfort D, Firth J, Schuch FB, et al. Sedentary behavior and physical activity levels in people with schizophrenia, bipolar disorder and major depressive disorder: A global systematic review and meta-analysis. *World Psychiatry*. 2017;16(3):308–315. doi:10.1002/wps.20458. PMID: 28941119; PMCID: PMC5608847.
7. Kleinman L, Lowin A, Flood E, Gandhi G, Edgell E, Revicki D. Costs of bipolar disorder. *Pharmacoeconomics*. 2003;21(9):601–622. doi:10.2165/00019053-200321090-00001. PMID: 12807364.
8. Pettinati HM, O'Brien CP, Dundon WD. Current status of co-occurring mood and substance use disorders: A new therapeutic target. *Am J Psychiatry*. 2013;170(1):23–30. doi:10.1176/appi.ajp.2012.12010112. PMID: 23223834; PMCID: PMC3595612.
9. Dong M, Lu L, Zhang L, et al. Prevalence of suicide attempts in bipolar disorder: A systematic review and meta-analysis of observational studies. *Epidemiol Psychiatr Sci*. 2019;29:e63. doi:10.1017/S2045796019000593. PMID: 31648654; PMCID: PMC8061290.
10. Wang Z, Li T, Li S, et al. The prevalence and clinical correlates of medical disorders comorbidities in patients with bipolar disorder. *BMC Psychiatry*. 2022;22(1):176. doi:10.1186/s12888-022-03819-0. Erratum in: BMC Psychiatry. 2022 Apr 1;22(1):232. PMID: 35272642; PMCID: PMC8908627.
11. Marwaha S, Durrani A, Singh S. Employment outcomes in people with bipolar disorder: A systematic review. *Acta Psychiatr Scand*. 2013;128(3):179–193. doi:10.1111/acps.12087. Epub 2013 Feb 4. PMID: 23379960.
12. He H, Hu C, Ren Z, Bai L, Gao F, Lyu J. Trends in the incidence and DALYs of bipolar disorder at global, regional, and national levels: Results from the global burden of disease study 2017. *J Psychiatr Res*. 2020;125:96–105. doi:10.1016/j.jpsychires.2020.03.015. Epub 2020 Mar 27. PMID: 32251918.
13. Surís A, Holliday R, North CS. The evolution of the classification of psychiatric disorders. *Behav Sci*. 2016;6(1):5. doi:10.3390/bs6010005. PMID: 26797641; PMCID: PMC4810039.
14. Song J, Bergen SE, Kuja-Halkola R, Larsson H, Landén M, Lichtenstein P. Bipolar disorder and its relation to major psychiatric disorders: A family-based study in the Swedish population. *Bipolar Disord*. 2015;17(2):184–193. doi:10.1111/bdi.12242. Epub 2014 Aug 13. PMID: 25118125.
15. Bienvenu OJ, Davydow DS, Kendler KS. Psychiatric 'diseases' versus behavioral disorders and degree of genetic influence. *Psychol Med*. 2011;41(1):33–40. doi:10.1017/S003329171000084X. Epub 2010 May 12. PMID: 20459884.
16. Passos IC, Mwangi B, Vieta E, Berk M, Kapczinski F. Areas of controversy in neuroprogression in bipolar disorder. *Acta Psychiatr Scand*. 2016;134(2):91–103. doi:10.1111/acps.12581. Epub 2016 Apr 21. PMID: 27097559.

17. Kloiber S, Rosenblat JD, Husain MI, et al. Neurodevelopmental pathways in bipolar disorder. *Neurosci Biobehav Rev.* 2020;112:213–226. doi:10.1016/j.neubiorev.2020.02.005. Epub 2020 Feb 5. PMID: 32035092.

18. Martínez Leo EE, Segura Campos MR. Effect of ultra-processed diet on gut microbiota and thus its role in neurodegenerative diseases. *Nutrition.* 2020;71:110609. doi:10.1016/j.nut.2019.110609. Epub 2019 Oct 11. PMID: 31837645.

19. Codagnone MG, Spichak S, O'Mahony SM, et al. Programming bugs: Microbiota and the developmental origins of brain health and disease. *Biol Psychiatry.* 2019;85(2): 150–163. doi:10.1016/j.biopsych.2018.06.014. Epub 2018 Jun 27. PMID: 30064690.

20. Garno JL, Goldberg JF, Ramirez PM, Ritzler BA. Impact of childhood abuse on the clinical course of bipolar disorder. *Br J Psychiatry.* 2005;186:121–125. doi:10.1192/bjp.186.2.121. Erratum in: Br J Psychiatry. 2005 Apr;186:357. PMID: 15684234.

21. Mazereel V, Detraux J, Vancampfort D, van Winkel R, De Hert M. Impact of psychotropic medication effects on obesity and the metabolic syndrome in people with serious mental illness. *Front Endocrinol.* 2020;11:573479. doi:10.3389/fendo.2020.573479. PMID: 33162935; PMCID: PMC7581736.

22. Kaplan KA. Sleep and sleep treatments in bipolar disorder. *Curr Opin Psychol.* 2020; 34:117–122. doi:10.1016/j.copsyc.2020.02.001. Epub 2020 Feb 13. PMID: 32203912.

23. Gruber J, Harvey AG, Wang PW, et al. Sleep functioning in relation to mood, function, and quality of life at entry to the Systematic Treatment Enhancement Program for Bipolar Disorder (STEP-BD). *J Affect Disord.* 2009;114(1–3):41–49. doi:10.1016/j.jad.2008.06.028. Epub 2008 Aug 15. PMID: 18707765; PMCID: PMC2677624.

24. Wagner-Skacel J, Dalkner N, Moerkl S, et al. Sleep and microbiome in psychiatric diseases. *Nutrients.* 2020;12(8):2198. doi:10.3390/nu12082198. PMID: 32718072; PMCID: PMC7468877.

25. Qaseem A, Kansagara D, Forciea MA, Cooke M, Denberg TD, Clinical Guidelines Committee of the American College of Physicians. Management of chronic insomnia disorder in adults: A clinical practice guideline from the American College of Physicians. *Ann Intern Med.* 2016;165(2):125–133. doi:10.7326/M15-2175. Epub 2016 May 3. PMID: 27136449.

26. Kaplan KA, Talavera DC, Harvey AG. Rise and shine: A treatment experiment testing a morning routine to decrease subjective sleep inertia in insomnia and bipolar disorder. *Behav Res Ther.* 2018;111:106–112. doi:10.1016/j.brat.2018.10.009. Epub 2018 Oct 27. PMID: 30399503.

27. Benedetti F, Barbini B, Fulgosi MC, et al. Combined total sleep deprivation and light therapy in the treatment of drug-resistant bipolar depression: Acute response and long-term remission rates. *J Clin Psychiatry.* 2005;66(12):1535–1540. doi:10.4088/jcp.v66n1207. PMID: 16401154.

28. Xu H, Zhuang X. Atypical antipsychotics-induced metabolic syndrome and non-alcoholic fatty liver disease: A critical review. *Neuropsychiatr Dis Treat.* 2019;15: 2087–2099. doi:10.2147/NDT.S208061. PMID: 31413575; PMCID: PMC6659786.

29. Barton BB, Zagler A, Engl K, Rihs L, Musil R. Prevalence of obesity, metabolic syndrome, diabetes and risk of cardiovascular disease in a psychiatric inpatient sample: Results of the Metabolism in Psychiatry (MiP) study. *Eur Arch Psychiatry Clin Neurosci.* 2020;270(5):597–609. doi:10.1007/s00406-019-01043-8. Epub 2019 Jul 13. PMID: 31302731.

30. Platzer M, Fellendorf FT, Bengesser SA, et al. The relationship between food craving, appetite-related hormones and clinical parameters in bipolar disorder. *Nutrients.* 2020;13(1):76. doi:10.3390/nu13010076. PMID: 33383670; PMCID: PMC7824587.

31. Stroup TS, Gray N. Management of common adverse effects of antipsychotic medications. *World Psychiatry.* 2018;17(3):341–356. doi:10.1002/wps.20567. PMID: 30192094; PMCID: PMC6127750.

32. Marrone G, Guerriero C, Palazzetti D, et al. Vegan diet health benefits in metabolic syndrome. *Nutrients.* 2021;13(3):817. doi:10.3390/nu13030817. PMID: 33801269; PMCID: PMC7999488.
33. Madani S, Ahmadi A, Shoaei-Jouneghani F, Moazen M, Sasani N. The relationship between the mediterranean diet and axis I disorders: A systematic review of observational studies. *Food Sci Nutr.* 2022;10(10):3241–3258. doi:10.1002/fsn3.2950. PMID: 36249971; PMCID: PMC9548357.
34. Jacobs DR, Tapsell LC. Food synergy: The key to a healthy diet. *Proc Nutr Soc.* 2013; 72(2):200–206. doi:10.1017/S0029665112003011. Epub 2013 Jan 14. PMID: 23312372.
35. Fries GR, Walss-Bass C, Bauer ME, Teixeira AL. Revisiting inflammation in bipolar disorder. *Pharmacol Biochem Behav.* 2019;177:12–19. doi:10.1016/j.pbb.2018.12.006. Epub 2018 Dec 24. PMID: 30586559.
36. Sayana P, Colpo GD, Simões LR, et al. A systematic review of evidence for the role of inflammatory biomarkers in bipolar patients. *J Psychiatr Res.* 2017;92:160–182. doi:10.1016/j.jpsychires.2017.03.018. Epub 2017 Mar 29. PMID: 28458141.
37. Melo MC, Daher Ede F, Albuquerque SG, de Bruin VM. Exercise in bipolar patients: A systematic review. *J Affect Disord.* 2016;198:32–38. doi:10.1016/j.jad.2016.03.004. Epub 2016 Mar 15. PMID: 26998794.
38. Firth J, Solmi M, Wootton RE, et al. A meta-review of "lifestyle psychiatry": The role of exercise, smoking, diet and sleep in the prevention and treatment of mental disorders. *World Psychiatry.* 2020;19(3):360–380. doi:10.1002/wps.20773. PMID: 32931092; PMCID: PMC7491615.
39. Moghetti P, Bacchi E, Brangani C, Donà S, Negri C. Metabolic effects of exercise. *Front Horm Res.* 2016;47:44–57. doi:10.1159/000445156. Epub 2016 Jun 27. PMID: 27348753.
40. Gold AK, Otto MW, Deckersbach T, Sylvia LG, Nierenberg AA, Kinrys G. Substance use comorbidity in bipolar disorder: A qualitative review of treatment strategies and outcomes. *Am J Addict.* 2018;27(3):188–201. doi:10.1111/ajad.12713. PMID: 29596721.
41. Albanese MJ, Pies R. The bipolar patient with comorbid substance use disorder: Recognition and management. *CNS Drugs.* 2004;18(9):585–596. doi:10.2165/00023210-200418090-00004. PMID: 15222775.
42. Lalli M, Brouillette K, Kapczinski F, de Azevedo Cardoso T. Substance use as a risk factor for bipolar disorder: A systematic review. *J Psychiatr Res.* 2021;144:285–295. doi:10.1016/j.jpsychires.2021.10.012. Epub 2021 Oct 20. PMID: 34710665.
43. Weiss RD, Najavits LM, Greenfield SF. A relapse prevention group for patients with bipolar and substance use disorders. *J Subst Abuse Treat.* 1999;16(1):47–54. doi:10.1016/s0740-5472(98)00011-7. PMID: 9888121.
44. Lex C, Bäzner E, Meyer TD. Does stress play a significant role in bipolar disorder? A meta-analysis. *J Affect Disord.* 2017;208:298–308. doi:10.1016/j.jad.2016.08.057. Epub 2016 Oct 11. PMID: 27794254.
45. Kendall T, Morriss R, Mayo-Wilson E, Marcus E, Guideline Development Group of the National Institute for Health and Care Excellence. Assessment and management of bipolar disorder: Summary of updated NICE guidance. *BMJ.* 2014;349:g5673. doi:10.1136/bmj.g5673. PMID: 25258392.
46. Lovas DA, Schuman-Olivier Z. Mindfulness-based cognitive therapy for bipolar disorder: A systematic review. *J Affect Disord.* 2018;240:247–261. doi:10.1016/j.jad.2018.06.017. Epub 2018 Jul 6. PMID: 30086469; PMCID: PMC7448295.
47. Xuan R, Li X, Qiao Y, et al. Mindfulness-based cognitive therapy for bipolar disorder: A systematic review and meta-analysis. *Psychiatry Res.* 2020;290:113116. doi:10.1016/j.psychres.2020.113116. Epub 2020 May 25. PMID: 32480120.

48. Greenman PS, Johnson SM. Emotionally focused therapy: Attachment, connection, and health. *Curr Opin Psychol.* 2022;43:146–150. doi:10.1016/j.copsyc.2021.06.015. Epub 2021 Jun 30. PMID: 34375935.
49. Kim KR, Song YY, Park JY, et al. The relationship between psychosocial functioning and resilience and negative symptoms in individuals at ultra-high risk for psychosis. *Aust N Z J Psychiatry.* 2013;47(8):762–771. doi:10.1177/0004867413488218. Epub 2013 May 9. PMID: 23661784.
50. Dou W, Yu X, Fang H, et al. Family and psychosocial functioning in bipolar disorder: The mediating effects of social support, resilience and suicidal ideation. *Front Psychol.* 2022;12:807546. doi:10.3389/fpsyg.2021.807546. PMID: 35153929; PMCID: PMC8832135.

29 Posttraumatic Stress Disorder

Allison Young, MD and Gia Merlo, MD, MBA, MEd

KEY POINTS

- A growing body of evidence suggests that the pillars of lifestyle medicine, including exercise, nutrition, stress management (i.e., mindfulness), substance use harm reduction, sleep, and social connectedness can help prevent, manage, and sometimes treat PTSD.
- Lifestyle interventions can be used to improve both mental and physical health outcomes of individuals diagnosed with PTSD given the bidirectional relationship between PTSD and poor health outcomes and behaviors.
- It is imperative that more research is conducted in order to formulate effective patient-centered lifestyle treatment recommendations based on the unique comorbidity and mortality rates among those suffering from PTSD.

29.1 INTRODUCTION

Non-clinically, trauma is defined as an emotional response to a disturbing or life-threatening event. An individual may experience or witness a single event or multiple events. These responses are influenced by several factors, including previous history of trauma, the response of the environment to the event(s), availability of treatment, and genetic or other vulnerabilities. There are a number of ways in which trauma can impact a person's psychological, physical, and social well-being, some of which are currently defined as clinical disorders. The current version of DSM (DSM-5TR) lists the trauma- and stress-related disorders as: (1) Reactive Attachment Disorder, (2) Disinhibited Social Engagement Disorder, (3) Posttraumatic Stress Disorder, (4) Acute Stress Disorder, (5) Adjustment Disorders, (6) Prolonged Grief Disorder, (7) Other Specified Trauma- and Stressor-Related Disorder, and (8) Unspecified Trauma- and Stressor-Related Disorder. Although a person can experience dissociative symptoms, such as derealization and depersonalization, as part of certain trauma- and stress-related disorders, there are also discrete dissociative disorders that may intersect with trauma, but are treated and regarded separately due to their differences in presentation.

For the purpose of this chapter, we will be focusing on posttraumatic stress disorder (PTSD). The DSM-5TR defines trauma within the setting of PTSD as exposure to "actual or threatened death, serious injury, or sexual violence." Exposure includes directly experiencing the event, witnessing the event, learning the event occurred to a close family member or friend, or related exposure to details of such

DOI: 10.1201/b22810-33

an event, such as with law enforcement or journalists. The diagnostic criteria for trauma-related PTSD are associated with prolonged traumatic experiences and/or singular or multiple serious life-threatening or distressing events. It is important to note that while other less stressful events (e.g., divorce, job loss) may be traumatic to an individual, they do not meet the criteria regarding trauma in the setting of PTSD. The symptoms of PTSD fall into categories that include intrusion (such as nightmares or flashbacks), avoidance (of thoughts, feelings, or external reminders), negative alterations in cognitions and mood (such as negative thoughts about oneself or the world, exaggerated blame, and decreased interest in activities), and alterations in arousal and reactivity (such as irritability, hypervigilance, and decreased sleep). For a diagnosis of PTSD, symptoms last for more than a month and are significant enough to cause issues in daily functioning.[1]

In addition to this psychological impact, a large body of literature has associated the profound impact of both early life adversity and PTSD with poorer physical health. For example, PTSD severity is associated with increased risk of obesity, diabetes, and cardiovascular disease. Increased severity of symptoms in the setting of PTSD is directly correlated with higher values of body mass index (BMI), leptin, fibrinogen, and blood pressure, and lower values of insulin sensitivity, with early life adversity having an additive effect on these metabolic outcomes.[2] Research suggests a bidirectional relationship between PTSD and poorer health outcomes, with both worsened symptoms impacting health behaviors and poor health behaviors being associated with more severe symptomatology.[3]

Given this bidirectional relationship, there has been increasing interest in the use of lifestyle interventions to improve both the mental and physical health outcomes of those with PTSD. The focuses of these lifestyle interventions include exercise, nutrition, mindfulness (particularly as a stress management tool), substance use, sleep, and social connectedness. This chapter will review each of these topics and explore both the evidence for their relevance in the prevention and management of PTSD, as well as discuss any available evidence for related interventions in improving either physical health outcomes or PTSD symptom severity.

While reading this chapter, it is important to keep two things in mind. One, PTSD is heterogeneous. As mentioned above, the diagnosis of PTSD relies on the presence of a variety of symptoms clustered into categories. Although there are a number of potential symptoms in each category, only 1-2 symptoms are required in each category to have a diagnosis of PTSD. To illustrate, this means that two people can be diagnosed with PTSD, despite presenting with distinct, differing symptoms. Although the current available research on PTSD largely refers to the condition as a singular disorder, it is possible that a certain set of symptoms can be better addressed with specific treatments than other symptom sets. Two, while exposure to trauma can lead to a variety of psychological consequences and health-related sequelae, this chapter is limited to the discussion of PTSD. However, future research endeavors concentrating on lifestyle interventions in the prevention and management of non-PTSD, trauma-related mental distress, as well, may add valuable insight into the fields of both lifestyle medicine and mental & behavioral health.

29.2 EXERCISE

While exercise undoubtedly has physical and psychological benefits, the specific benefits of exercise in the setting of PTSD continue to be researched. It is important to note that different forms of exercise confer different biological and psychological effects. For example, the cardiovascular strain of aerobic exercise varies from that of resistance training. It has also been noted that group fitness or team sports may engender different psychological benefits than those induced by individual training. The current literature on the effects of exercise in the setting of trauma has failed to clearly delineate the impact of various physical activity interventions and exercise modalities on patients with a history of trauma. Studies on exercise as a lifestyle intervention in those with PTSD face a variety of challenges due to the highly variable presentations of the disorder. For example, there are certain types of fitness that may alleviate specific symptoms that may not be present in all diagnosed with PTSD.

A growing body of evidence has indicated that exercise may be a useful adjunct treatment for PTSD. A 2018 review of the literature on this topic found that exercise was an effective adjunct treatment for patients diagnosed with PTSD, particularly in those with subsyndromal symptoms (symptoms similar to those of PTSD, but not severe enough to warrant diagnosis) and those with treatment-resistant PTSD.[4] Further, a 2021 systematic review and meta-analysis studied eleven randomized controlled trials that compared exercise groups to non-exercise groups among participants with symptoms of PTSD. Data from this study demonstrated that exercise benefited those with PTSD, with more voluminous exercise (more than 20 hours in total) being slightly more beneficial than less voluminous (less than 20 hours in total). Subgroup analysis on the various exercise intervention modalities utilized in this study did not exhibit clinical significance. However, the authors noted that the lack of clinical significance with regard to the category of physical activity may be linked to the relatively few studies available on the use of different exercise methodologies in the prevention and management of PTSD among patients.[5] Evidence suggests the prospective therapeutic value of exercise for patients with PTSD. Further research is needed to delineate if specific exercise modalities play a significant role in patient outcomes.

A paucity of data is also apparent regarding the mechanism behind the effect of physical activity on symptoms associated with PTSD. Researchers of a 2021 study of 321 veterans (average age 74, 29.6% of whom had PTSD according to self-report questionnaires) enrolled in a group exercise intervention attempted to identify the mechanism behind clinical improvements in PTSD via physical activity. The study found that self-reported symptoms associated with PTSD, as well as self-reported physical function and social connectedness, significantly improved among those with PTSD subsequent to group exercise intervention Secondary analyses demonstrated that the improvement in social connectedness was significantly associated with improvement in symptoms of PTSD. However, there was no significant association between exercise-induced improvements in physical function and improvements in symptoms of PTSD. Of note, this study was limited by the participation of a specific population of older veterans, the lack of a control group, and the use self-reported data rather than standardized clinical interviews.[6]

The benefits of exercise may extend beyond enhancing social connectedness for those with PTSD and PTSD-related symptoms. Several hypotheses exist for this mechanism including exposure and desensitization to internal hyperarousal cues; increased neuroplasticity; reduced stress response and inflammatory markers; and enhanced cognitive function, behavioral activation, and sense of accomplishment.[7,8]

Positive results have been reported in studies examining the feasibility of exercise as an intervention for patients with PTSD. A randomized controlled study among older veterans with PTSD found that the exercise intervention was well-attended, had high rates of completion, and had high satisfaction ratings, with even higher ratings for group interventions.[9]

The current data collection process still leaves many questions regarding exercise as a treatment for PTSD. It is important to determine whether there is a type of exercise that provides the most benefit for patients with PTSD, if specific symptom clusters of PTSD interact with particular exercise types, how long the benefits of exercise last in patients, and how to create a method for prescribing the appropriate dosage and duration of exercise in the context of PTSD. Exercise may be considered an adjunct treatment for PTSD from the standpoint of its benefits in terms of overall health and physical function, as well as the demonstrated tolerability of interventions. Future research must be conducted to clarify the contemporary gaps in literature on the implications of physical activity in the treatment and management of patients with PTSD.

29.3 NUTRITION

Literature on the link between nutrition and PTSD is scarce, with most studies concentrating on health behaviors, such as diet, in those with the disorder. However, data on this subject are expanding as a result of the relatively new conception and rapid growth of the field of nutritional psychiatry. The practice of nutritional psychiatry aims to treat mental health disorders and improve mental health outcomes through the use of nutrition and supplements.

Research conducted to date has shown that PTSD may be associated with both a poor diet and poor health outcomes, such as an increased risk of obesity and cardiometabolic disease. A secondary analysis conducted in 2021 examined a randomized controlled trial of 54 veterans aged 60 and over to determine the association between diet quality and PTSD. The Dietary Screener Questionnaire (DSQ) was used to assess subjects' daily intake of fiber, calcium, added sugar, whole grains, dairy products, fruits, vegetables, and legumes. Data from this study revealed the prevalence of poor diet among veterans with PTSD. Of note, study participants with PTSD who received exercise intervention improved in some health measures, but diet quality did not improve.[10]

Another study involving United States military veterans similarly found an association between PTSD symptom severity and poor diet quality. An additional correlation between poor diet quality and the suppression of emotions was revealed by mediation models.[11] Unfortunately, a study of the utilization of weight loss programs within Veterans Health Affairs revealed that veterans diagnosed with PTSD used weight loss programs less frequently than those without PTSD. Results from this study demonstrated the positive association between the use of weight loss programs and subsequent improvement in PTSD symptoms.[12]

Furthermore, trauma reactions can have a variety of physical health consequences, including disrupted digestion. A 2022 randomized controlled trial found that 36% of a sample of US veterans with PTSD reported abdominal pain, and 25% met criteria for irritable bowel syndrome (IBS), which is greater than the general US population.[13] Some researchers and physicians have hypothesized that the link between the digestion system and trauma resides in the balance between the sympathetic and parasympathetic nervous systems; however, there is currently little research that has tackled this link. Based on this theoretical link and the increased occurrence of gastrointestinal distress, it has been speculated that anti-inflammatory foods, fermented foods, and probiotics may improve symptoms of PTSD, but research is needed.[14] Ultimately, despite the promise of integrative medicine, which considers nutrition an important factor in PTSD treatment, much of the literature on this topic remains anecdotal. Further long-term studies must be conducted to fully understand the effects of specific foods/diet on PTSD presentation.

Aside from actual diet, eating habits are also an important part of nutrition in PTSD. Multiple small studies have found that PTSD impacts food behaviors, frequently observing skipped meals, decreased general appetite, increased desire for sweetened and processed foods, as well as eating patterns dictated by stress or emotions. This further lends credence to a correlation between PTSD and obesity. It may be beneficial for nutritional treatment plans to focus not just on type of food but also pattern of eating in order to improve both the actual diet of patients and their relationship with food.[15–17]

The link between PTSD and poor diet and higher rates of chronic health conditions, such as cardiometabolic disease and IBS, is well established. Nutritional interventions have not yet been studied among those with PTSD to determine if they improve psychological or physical health. Thus, research suggests that those with PTSD should be screened for chronic conditions and counseled about protective health behaviors, but there is scant scientific literature on specific evidence-based nutritional interventions to recommend in clinical settings.

29.4 MINDFULNESS

Mindfulness is a mental state achieved by focusing one's attention on the present moment while nonjudgmentally acknowledging any thoughts, feelings, and bodily sensations as they arise. There are many different practices through which a state of mindfulness can be achieved. The practice of mindfulness can be as simple as choosing to be fully attentive to the present moment while walking, drinking tea, or even washing dishes. More formal practices, such as meditation or yoga, can also be executed to achieve and promote mindfulness. Research on mindfulness interventions and patients with PTSD is limited, both in terms of quantity and methodology, due to the variety of mindfulness practices available.[18]

A number of trials have used mindfulness-based stress reduction (MBSR), a standardized treatment consisting of 2-2.5-hour long group sessions per week over eight weeks and one full-day retreat, to overcome this methodological challenge in mindfulness research.[19] A recent meta-analysis of 10 randomized controlled trials of MBSR in the setting of PTSD found that MBSR was effective in reducing symptoms of PTSD regardless of trauma type. But, high attrition rates are noted within individual studies.[20] For example, a 2017 feasibility study found MBSR to be effective in reducing symptoms of PTSD as a standalone treatment; however, the high drop-out rate, combined with results from post-study interviews, indicated a need to adapt protocols to incorporate mindfulness exercises targeted at PTSD symptoms with shorter duration of interventions.[21] A multisite randomized controlled trial in 214 United States military veterans compared MBSR to active control (present-centered group therapy). Results from this study demonstrated reductions in PTSD symptoms in both experimental and control groups in accordance with the Clinician-Administered PTSD Scale for DSM-IV (CAPS-IV). Of note, high attrition rates were also observed in this study.[22]

Studies have been conducted on various other forms of mindfulness with mixed results owing in part to the variable nature of the protocols. Pilot studies have shown that metta (loving-kindness) meditation and mantra repetition practice, coupled with traditional treatment methods, showed significant reductions in PTSD symptoms. The low participation numbers of these studies and their concurrent use of other treatments limited their findings.[19,23]

Mindfulness practices have been associated with improvements in PTSD symptoms through various mechanisms. Psychological mechanisms of mindfulness may include increasing self-compassion, improving emotional flexibility, reducing ruminative tendencies, and decreasing hyperarousal. A mindfulness-based approach may facilitate the attenuation of PTSD symptoms by fostering awareness and nonjudgment of one's behaviors, such as in situations where avoidant behaviors are present.[19] PTSD-related emotional reactivity may be regulated by mindfulness on a neurobiological level via top-down modulation of limbic regions.[19] Additional studies have suggested that increased mindfulness can also decrease the likelihood of developing PTSD following a distressing event, perhaps by moderating internalizing symptoms.[19,24]

It is important to consider that those with PTSD who are particularly prone to flashbacks, those who are still developing appropriate distress tolerance skills, and those who are prone to derealization or depersonalization may find mindfulness-based practice to be psychologically challenging.[19] Mindfulness interventions should therefore be administered carefully and as part of a patient-centered approach to care in the setting of PTSD.

Cumulative evidence suggests that mindfulness interventions, such as MBSR, may be effective in the treatment and management of patients with PTSD. The effectiveness of mindfulness-based interventions among those suffering from PTSD should be studied further to determine if any mindfulness-based interventions are superior to others, as well as to determine how to discern individuals who may derive greater benefit or tolerance from mindfulness interventions.

29.5 SUBSTANCE USE

Evidence-based treatments exist for substance use disorders (SUDs) and PTSD as individual conditions, but there is limited data on the treatment of patients in the setting of co-occurring SUD and PTSD. There is extensive research documenting an association between SUDs and PTSD. Approximately 40% of people with PTSD, including military and non-military trauma, have a co-occurring SUD.[25] Individuals with co-occurring PTSD and SUD are at increased risk for other psychiatric problems, such as depression and anxiety, suicidality, neuropsychological impairment, unemployment, and overall increased morbidity and mortality.[25] A 2017 review of randomized controlled trials studying treatments for PTSD found that SUD was an exclusion criteria in three-fourths of the studies, and less than 10% of the studies reported substance use-related outcomes.[26]

The current framework for treatment of patients with PTSD lacks clear guidelines for those with comorbidities due to these limitations in research. Patients with co-occurring PTSD and SUDs are therefore subject to discrepancies in treatment approach and chronology of intervention execution. In some healthcare settings, it is recommended to treat SUDs first, but the US Department of Veterans Affairs recommends that individuals with SUDs receive evidence-based treatments for PTSD regardless of whether they have been diagnosed with an SUD.[27,28] Furthermore, there is evidence linking substance use to severity of PTSD symptoms, suggesting that individual attempts to self-medicate may play a role in the prevalence and development of substance use.[29] This may lead to high drop-out rates in SUD treatments that do not simultaneously address PTSD symptoms as patients may experience an uptick in emotional distress as a self-coping tool is removed without the replacement with other coping mechanisms.[28] Integrated treatments have been developed to address the complex relationship between PTSD and SUD in patients with co-occurring diagnoses.

There are two primary types of integrated treatments: non-trauma (present) focused and trauma (past) focused. The former primarily seeks to improve coping skills and self-compassion, while the latter more actively addresses PTSD symptoms by utilizing evidence-based psychological interventions for PTSD.[29]

A recent meta-analysis examined the available studies on psychological treatments for comorbid SUD and PTSD. This meta-analysis showed that integrated programs and standalone SUD programs similarly reduced substance use. Of note, trauma-focused interventions of the integrated programs more effectively attenuated PTSD symptoms than non-trauma-focused methods.[30] This study was somewhat limited by the lack of quantity and variety of non-trauma-focused and trauma-focused therapies. The majority of studies analyzing the effects of trauma-focused integrated therapies on patients with comorbid SUD and PTSD studied prolonged exposure (PE). Few studies included an evaluation of cognitive processing therapy (CPT) or eye-desensitization movement and reprocessing (EMDR), both of which are evidence-based treatments for PTSD. Notably, there was a high non-completion rate across all of the studies, and treatment effect sizes were relatively modest when comparing integrated programs to traditional treatments.[30]

Ultimately, there is a large body of research that demonstrates the importance of addressing substance use among those with PTSD in order to reduce the psychological, physical, and socioeconomic impact of their symptoms. The procedure by which these efforts may best be addressed remains a subject of research. The number of trials including those with both PTSD and SUD has increased significantly in the past few years, showing potential for future data expansion on the topic.[30]

29.6   SLEEP

A significant portion of those who suffer from PTSD experience sleep disturbances. In fact, sleep disturbances are part of the diagnostic criteria for PTSD.[1] So, it is not surprising that addressing sleep may be a compelling and effective strategy in managing this disorder. Recurrent nightmares, as well as difficulty falling and staying asleep, are the most frequently reported sleep issues among those with PTSD.[31] Other sleep disorders commonly reported among those with PTSD include obstructive sleep apnea and atypical sleep-disruptive behaviors.[31,32] Treatments for PTSD typically improve perceived sleep quality, but sleep disturbances often persist at clinically significant levels in posttreatment stages.[31]

The findings of polysomnographic studies examining sleep abnormalities in PTSD remain inconsistent despite the high prevalence of subjective complaints of sleep disturbances among those with PTSD. A 2020 meta-analysis of 20 polysomnographic studies on individuals with PTSD demonstrated that participants experienced longer duration of stage 1 sleep, less slow wave sleep, and greater rapid eye movement (REM) density compared to individuals without PTSD. The results of this study suggest that variables like depression and other disorders may explain inconsistencies in prior studies.[33]

Meta-analyses of randomized controlled trials have indicated that cognitive behavioral therapy (CBT) for insomnia (CBT-I) is effective in attenuating sleep disturbances in those with PTSD, with low attrition rates. This suggests that the favorable benefit-to-risk ratio conferred by CBT in the general patient population is maintained in patients with PTSD. Therefore, CBT-I may prove an effective and well-tolerated treatment for sleep disturbances in those with PTSD.[32,34] Sleep disturbances, such as nightmares, can also be addressed through psychological approaches with validated protocols, such as imagery rehearsal therapy. Imagery rehearsal therapy offers a therapeutic environment through which patients receive sleep education, rescript aspects of the nightmares, and practice daily imaginal rehearsals of new dream narratives that support healthy sleep.[31,35]

Prazosin can also help reduce the frequency and severity of nightmares, but does not significantly impact other non-sleep-related PTSD symptoms.[36] Of note, other commonly prescribed hypnotics, such as benzodiazepine and non-benzodiazepine receptor agonists (Z drugs), should be approached with extreme caution due to limited positive evidence and the likelihood of adverse side effects (i.e. potential habit formation).[32] It is also important for clinicians to be aware of psychotropic-induced interactions with sleep. For example, selective serotonin reuptake inhibitors (SSRIs) are sometimes used to target PTSD-related mood symptoms or comorbid depressive symptoms. SSRIs can impact sleep architecture, induce hyperarousal, and exacerbate sleep-disruptive behaviors.[37]

There is strong evidence that patients with PTSD should be screened for sleep issues and disorders. A targeted psychological intervention should be undertaken upon the identification of sleep disorders in the setting of PTSD. Future research should consider addressing larger comparisons of PTSD-specific psychological treatments with sleep-specific interventions and include trials comparing the effectiveness of sequential treatments for sleep disturbances and PTSD to approaches incorporating the concurrent treatment of sleep disturbances and PTSD.

29.7 SOCIAL CONNECTEDNESS

Several studies have attempted to explain the relationship between social connectedness and PTSD development and severity. The relationship between social functioning and mental illness can be hard to study because they are often interconnected and coexisting. Mental illnesses, including PTSD, can challenge social relationships. Some PTSD symptoms, including but not limited to irritability, anger, and avoidance, can pose a barrier to the establishment and maintenance of healthy relationships.

One study took a longitudinal approach in its assessment of the relationship between PTSD and two aspects of social connectedness: quality (defined in the study as degree of distress related to interpersonal conflict) and structural social support (defined by the number of days of contact with supportive loved ones). This study consisted of 1491 US military veterans in residential treatment for PTSD at 35 Department of Veterans Affairs facilities who were evaluated at baseline (the 30 days prior to initiating involvement in the study) and 4 months after discharge. Results from this study found that a higher prevalence of irritability/anger at baseline was associated with poorer quality of postdischarge relationships (i.e., more distress related to interpersonal conflict). Additionally, data revealed that more days of contact with loved ones predicted lower severity of avoidance and numbing symptoms in patients with PTSD.[38]

Another longitudinal study used a patient database to study 101 World War II (WWII) veterans, their childhood relationship quality, their relationships with fellow soldiers in WWII, and their severity of PTSD symptoms. This study demonstrated that a higher level of peer relationship quality during deployment was associated with the development of less severe PTSD symptoms. Moreover, it appeared that higher quality early-life relationships were associated with healthier relationships during deployment.[39] Social connection may also moderate other health outcomes in those with PTSD aside from PTSD symptomatology. For example, one study found that social connection moderated the strength of association between poor health outcomes and PTSD symptom severity in a group of older adults with war-related PTSD.[40]

The current studies suggest that social connectedness may be at least one indicator or factor in the development and severity of PTSD symptoms. However, there have not yet been any randomized trials that utilize social connectedness as a specific intervention in the treatment of patients with PTSD. Comparable existing studies using social interventions in patients with PTSD have been conducted in group settings. The findings of these studies are limited by depth of analysis and propose that the group setting itself is responsible for the benefits derived from social interventions in those with PTSD. For example, one of the aforementioned exercise studies examined a group exercise intervention in US military veterans and found that the improvement in PTSD symptoms seen in the intervention group was associated with the social relationships and level of social connectedness facilitated by group exercise programs, rather than individual exercise programs.[6] Further research is needed to elucidate the complex bidirectional relationship between PTSD and social connectedness and to better assess the patient populations affected by PTSD that are most likely to benefit from group intervention.

29.8 CONCLUDING REMARKS

Current research on patients with PTSD has identified lifestyle factors, including exercise, nutrition, mindfulness, substance use, sleep, and social connectedness, as important factors in the prevention, management, and treatment of PTSD. Previous literature on this topic is limited by the isolation of lifestyle factors from other lifestyle variables in data analyses. The entanglement of the benefits and relationships among these interventions must be clarified in order to formulate optimal treatment recommendations in the setting of PTSD and any comorbidities. Future research efforts, particularly within the lifestyle medicine space, should examine the potential of a lifestyle program addressing each of the lifestyle factors in patients with PTSD, as well as the additional conferred benefits of such a regimen plan.

REFERENCES

1. American Psychiatric Association. *Diagnostic and Statistical Manual of Mental Disorders.* 5th ed., Text Revision, American Psychiatric Publishing; 2022, doi:10.1176/appi.books.9780890425787.
2. Farr OM, Ko BJ, Joung KE, et al. Posttraumatic stress disorder, alone or additively with early life adversity, is associated with obesity and cardiometabolic risk. *Nutr Metab Cardiovasc Dis NMCD.* 2015;25(5):479–488. doi:10.1016/j.numecd.2015.01.007
3. Hruby A, Lieberman HR, Smith TJ. Symptoms of depression, anxiety, and posttraumatic stress disorder and their relationship to health-related behaviors in over 12,000 US military personnel: Bi-directional associations. *J Affect Disord.* 2021;283:84–93. doi:10.1016/j.jad.2021.01.029
4. Oppizzi LM, Umberger R. The effect of physical activity on PTSD. *Issues Ment Health Nurs.* 2018;39(2):179–187. doi:10.1080/01612840.2017.1391903
5. Björkman F, Ekblom Ö. Physical exercise as treatment for PTSD: A systematic review and meta-analysis. *Mil Med.* Published online November 26, 2021:usab497. doi:10.1093/milmed/usab497
6. Wilkins SS, Melrose RJ, Hall KS, et al. PTSD improvement associated with social connectedness in Gerofit veterans exercise program. *J Am Geriatr Soc.* 2021;69(4):1045–1050. doi:10.1111/jgs.16973
7. Hegberg NJ, Hayes JP, Hayes SM. Exercise intervention in PTSD: A narrative review and rationale for implementation. *Front Psychiatry.* 2019;10:133. doi:10.3389/fpsyt.2019.00133
8. Fetzner MG, Asmundson GJG. Aerobic exercise reduces symptoms of posttraumatic stress disorder: A randomized controlled trial. *Cogn Behav Ther.* 2015;44(4):301–313. doi:10.1080/16506073.2014.916745
9. Pebole MM, Hall KS. Insights following implementation of an exercise intervention in older veterans with PTSD. *Int J Environ Res Public Health.* 2019;16(14):E2630. doi:10.3390/ijerph16142630
10. Browne J, Morey MC, Beckham JC, et al. Diet quality and exercise in older veterans with PTSD: A pilot study. *Transl Behav Med.* 2021;11(12):2116–2122. doi:10.1093/tbm/ibab116
11. Escarfulleri S, Ellickson-Larew S, Fein-Schaffer D, Mitchell KS, Wolf EJ. Emotion regulation and the association between PTSD, diet, and exercise: A longitudinal evaluation among US military veterans. *Eur J Psychotraumatol.* 2021;12(1):1895515. doi:10.1080/20008198.2021.1895515

12. Scherrer JF, Salas J, Chard KM, et al. PTSD symptom decrease and use of weight loss programs. *J Psychosom Res.* 2019;127:109849. doi:10.1016/j.jpsychores.2019.109849

13. Kearney DJ, Kamp KJ, Storms M, Simpson TL. Prevalence of gastrointestinal symptoms and irritable bowel syndrome among individuals with symptomatic post-traumatic stress disorder. *J Clin Gastroenterol.* 2022;56(7):592–596. doi:10.1097/MCG.0000000000001670

14. Korn LE. Exploring Integrative Medicine and Nutrition for PTSD. *Psychiatric Times*, October 21, 2022, www.psychiatrictimes.com/view/exploring-integrative-medicine-and-nutrition-for-ptsd Accessed September 12, 2023.

15. Roer GE, Solbakken HH, Abebe DS, Aaseth JO, Bolstad I, Lien L. Inpatients experiences about the impact of traumatic stress on eating behaviors: An exploratory focus group study. *J Eat Disord.* 2021;9(1):119. doi:10.1186/s40337-021-00480-y

16. Rijkers C, Schoorl M, van Hoeken D, Hoek HW. Eating disorders and posttraumatic stress disorder. *Curr Opin Psychiatry.* 2019;32(6):510–517. doi:10.1097/YCO.0000000000000545

17. Carmassi C, Antonio Bertelloni C, Massimetti G, et al. Impact of DSM-5 PTSD and gender on impaired eating behaviors in 512 Italian earthquake survivors. *Psychiatry Res.* 2015;225(1–2):64–69. doi:10.1016/j.psychres.2014.10.008

18. Lang AJ. Mindfulness in PTSD treatment. *Curr Opin Psychol.* 2017;14:40–43. doi:10.1016/j.copsyc.2016.10.005

19. Boyd JE, Lanius RA, McKinnon MC. Mindfulness-based treatments for posttraumatic stress disorder: A review of the treatment literature and neurobiological evidence. *J Psychiatry Neurosci JPN.* 2018;43(1):7–25. doi:10.1503/jpn.170021

20. Liu Q, Zhu J, Zhang W. The efficacy of mindfulness-based stress reduction intervention 3 for post-traumatic stress disorder (PTSD) symptoms in patients with PTSD: A meta-analysis of four randomized controlled trials. *Stress Health J Int Soc Investig Stress.* Published online March 6, 2022. doi:10.1002/smi.3138

21. Müller-Engelmann M, Wünsch S, Volk M, Steil R. Mindfulness-based stress reduction (MBSR) as a standalone intervention for posttraumatic stress disorder after mixed traumatic events: A mixed-methods feasibility study. *Front Psychol.* 2017;8:1407. doi:10.3389/fpsyg.2017.01407

22. Davis LL, Whetsell C, Hamner MB, et al. A multisite randomized controlled trial of mindfulness-based stress reduction in the treatment of posttraumatic stress disorder. *Psychiatr Res Clin Pract.* 2019;1(2):39–48. doi:10.1176/appi.prcp.20180002

23. Kearney DJ, Malte CA, McManus C, Martinez ME, Felleman B, Simpson TL. Loving-kindness meditation for posttraumatic stress disorder: A pilot study. *J Trauma Stress.* 2013;26(4):426–434. doi:10.1002/jts.21832

24. Tubbs JD, Savage JE, Adkins AE, Amstadter AB, Dick DM. Mindfulness moderates the relation between trauma and anxiety symptoms in college students. *J Am Coll Health J ACH.* 2019;67(3):235–245. doi:10.1080/07448481.2018.1477782

25. Flanagan JC, Korte KJ, Killeen TK, Back SE. Concurrent treatment of substance use and PTSD. *Curr Psychiatry Rep.* 2016;18(8):70. doi:10.1007/s11920-016-0709-y

26. Leeman RF, Hefner K, Frohe T, et al. Exclusion of participants based on substance use status: Findings from randomized controlled trials of treatments for PTSD. *Behav Res Ther.* 2017;89:33–40. doi:10.1016/j.brat.2016.10.006

27. VA/DOD clinical practice guideline for the management of posttraumatic stress disorder and acute stress disorder: Clinician summary. *Focus J Life Long Learn Psychiatry.* 2018;16(4):430–448. doi:10.1176/appi.focus.16408

28. Forbes D, Bisson JI, Monson CM, Berliner L, eds. *Effective Treatments for PTSD.* Guilford Publications; 2020.

29. Langdon KJ, Fox AB, King LA, King DW, Eisen S, Vogt D. Examination of the dynamic interplay between posttraumatic stress symptoms and alcohol misuse among

combat-exposed Operation Enduring Freedom (OEF)/Operation Iraqi Freedom (OIF) Veterans. *J Affect Disord.* 2016;196:234–242. doi:10.1016/j.jad.2016.02.048

30. Roberts NP, Lotzin A, Schäfer I. A systematic review and meta-analysis of psychological interventions for comorbid post-traumatic stress disorder and substance use disorder. *Eur J Psychotraumatol.* 2022;13(1):2041831. doi:10.1080/20008198.2022.2041831

31. Casement MD, Swanson LM. A meta-analysis of imagery rehearsal for post-trauma nightmares: Effects on nightmare frequency, sleep quality, and posttraumatic stress. *Clin Psychol Rev.* 2012;32(6):566–574. doi:10.1016/j.cpr.2012.06.002

32. Miller KE, Brownlow JA, Gehrman PR. Sleep in PTSD: Treatment approaches and outcomes. *Curr Opin Psychol.* 2020;34:12–17. doi:10.1016/j.copsyc.2019.08.017

33. Kobayashi I, Boarts JM, Delahanty DL. Polysomnographically measured sleep abnormalities in PTSD: A meta-analytic review. *Psychophysiology.* 2007;44(4):660–669. doi:10.1111/j.1469-8986.2007.537.x

34. Ho FYY, Chan CS, Tang KNS. Cognitive-behavioral therapy for sleep disturbances in treating posttraumatic stress disorder symptoms: A meta-analysis of randomized controlled trials. *Clin Psychol Rev.* 2016;43:90–102. doi:10.1016/j.cpr.2015.09.005

35. Hansen K, Höfling V, Kröner-Borowik T, Stangier U, Steil R. Efficacy of psychological interventions aiming to reduce chronic nightmares: A meta-analysis. *Clin Psychol Rev.* 2013;33(1):146–155. doi:10.1016/j.cpr.2012.10.012

36. Zhang Y, Ren R, Sanford LD, et al. The effects of prazosin on sleep disturbances in post-traumatic stress disorder: A systematic review and meta-analysis. *Sleep Med.* 2020; 67:225–231. doi:10.1016/j.sleep.2019.06.010

37. Holshoe JM. Antidepressants and sleep: A review. *Perspect Psychiatr Care.* 2009;45(3): 191–197. doi:10.1111/j.1744-6163.2009.00221.x

38. Sippel LM, Watkins LE, Pietrzak RH, Hoff R, Harpaz-Rotem I. Heterogeneity of posttraumatic stress symptomatology and social connectedness in treatment-seeking military veterans: A longitudinal examination. *Eur J Psychotraumatology.* 2019;10(1): 1646091. doi:10.1080/20008198.2019.1646091

39. Nevarez MD, Yee HM, Waldinger RJ. Friendship in War: Camaraderie and PTSD prevention. *J Trauma Stress.* 2017;30(5):512–520. doi:10.1002/jts.22224

40. Schwartz E, Shrira A. Social connectedness moderates the relationship between warfare exposure, PTSD symptoms and health among older adults. *Psychiatry.* 2019;82(2): 158–172. doi:10.1080/00332747.2018.1534521

30 Eating Disorders

Liana Abascal, PhD, MPH and
Dawn M. Eichen, PhD

KEY POINTS

- Eating disorders are serious mental illnesses that contribute to significant physical and psychological suffering with mortality rates among the highest in mental illnesses.
- Guidelines by both the Academy of Eating Disorders and the Physicians Committee for Responsible Medicine suggest approaches that are specific to and appropriate for patients who follow a vegetarian or vegan diet.
- Collaboration of lifestyle medicine and eating disorder professionals is essential to providing comprehensive mental and physical health to patients with a past or current history of eating disorders.

30.1 INTRODUCTION

Eating disorders (EDs) are serious mental illnesses that contribute to a patient's significant physical and psychological suffering.[1] EDs can present in all ages, races, ethnicities, genders, socioeconomic statuses, and body sizes and types. Lifetime rates of ED diagnosis by age 40 are estimated to be nearly 1 in 7 (14.3%) for men and 1 in 5 for women (19.7%).[2] Given these high rates of prevalence, most clinical settings will encounter a patient with an ED diagnosis (current or by history) or subsyndromal symptoms (disordered eating). While the etiology and symptomology of EDs are complex, overt signs and symptoms observed include specific eating behaviors, exercise behaviors, and medical complications, among others. Notably, eating and exercise behaviors figure prominently in lifestyle medicine (LM) and are two of the six pillars (nutrition, physical activity, sleep, substance use, social connection, stress management). The current chapter will review EDs and discuss the intricacies of treating a patient with a current ED diagnosis, or history of an ED, from a lifestyle medicine perspective.

30.2 EATING DISORDERS

Disturbances of eating or eating-related behaviors that result in altered consumption of food that significantly impacts physical health and/or psychosocial functioning are characteristic of feeding and EDs.[3] The four main EDs, *Anorexia Nervosa (AN)*, *Bulimia Nervosa (BN)*, *Binge-Eating Disorder (BED)*, and *Avoidant/restrictive food intake disorder (ARFID)* are mutually exclusive such that only one diagnosis can be current at any given time, though individuals may cross diagnostic boundaries throughout their lifetime. AN is characterized by persistent restriction of energy

354

DOI: 10.1201/b22810-34

intake resulting in significantly low body weight, fears of being overweight or gaining weight, consistent actions to prevent weight gain, and disturbance in perceived weight or shape.[3] There are two diagnostic subtypes of AN: restricting due to dieting, fasting and/or excessive exercise; or binge-purge, due to recurrent binge eating and/or purging. BN is characterized by recurrent binge eating (i.e. discrete episodes of eating large amounts of food while experiencing a sense of loss of control) and recurrent compensatory behaviors (e.g., purging, misuse of laxatives, diuretics or other medications, excessive exercise, fasting) with self-evaluation unduly influenced by shape and/or weight.

BED is characterized by recurrent binge eating without the presence of compensatory behaviors, occurring on average at least once a week for three months, with marked distress related to binge eating. BED also requires the presence of three of the following criteria related to binge eating: eating much more rapidly; eating until uncomfortably full; eating large amounts when not physically hungry; eating alone due to embarrassment; and feeling disgusted, depressed, or guilty after eating.

The hallmark feature of ARFID is avoidance or restriction of food intake with at least one of the following consequences: significant weight loss (or failure to achieve expected growth in children), significant nutritional deficiency, dependence on enteral feeding or oral nutrition supplements, or significant interference of psychosocial functioning. Although not official subtypes of diagnosis, research suggests that there are three types of presentations (that may not be mutually exclusive) of ARFID related to (1) low interest in food or eating, (2) avoidance based on the sensory characteristics of food, and (3) concern about possible aversive consequences of eating (e.g., choking, vomiting). Presentation of ARFID often appears like "picky eating" where certain categories or textures of foods are avoided.

It is also important to note that a category of *other specified feeding or eating disorder* (OSFED) exists, which represents patients that present with clinical impairments without meeting full criteria for one of the "threshold" EDs (AN, BN, BED, ARFID) or other feeding disorders. Although understudied, many patient presentations fall into this important category, which encompasses subclinical presentations with significant impairment and warrants treatment.[3]

30.3 THE SPECIAL CASE OF ORTHOREXIA

Although not a defined diagnosis in the Diagnostic and Statistical Manual of Mental Disorders, 5th edition, Text Revision (DSM-5-TR) or International Classification of Diseases, 11th Edition (ICD-11),[3,4] Orthorexia Nervosa (ON) is a condition characterized by compulsive behaviors and obsessive thoughts concerning healthy eating to the point of psychological and physical harm. There is considerable disagreement on diagnostic criteria for ON; four sets have been proposed.[5-9] Consistent criteria among the four sets are the following: "(a) obsessive behaviors and preoccupation with healthy nutrition that includes rigidly following a restrictive "healthy" diet (that the individual believes to be health-promoting and pure) with strict avoidance of foods believed to be unhealthy; (b) violations of their restrictive dietary rules resulting in extreme emotional distress with feelings of guilt, shame, and/or anxiety; (c) physical impairments, whereby nutritional deficiencies may lead to significant weight loss,

TABLE 30.1

Prevalence Rates of Anorexia Nervosa (AN), Bulimia Nervosa (BN), and Binge-Eating Disorder (BED)[3,13,14]

	12-month Prevalence Rate			Lifetime Prevalence Rate		
	Total	Women	Men	Total	Women	Men
AN	0.0–0.05%	0–0.08%	0–0.01%	0.60–0.80%	0.9–1.42%	0.12–0.3%
BN	0.14–0.3%	0.22–0.5%	0.05–0.1%	0.28–1.0%	0.46–1.5%	0.05–0.08%
BED	0.44–1.2%	0.6–1.6%	0.26–0.8%	0.85–2.8%	1.25–3.5%	0.42–2%

malnutrition, and/or physical health complications; and (d) psychosocial impairments in social, vocational, and/or academic functioning that may result from the other-diagnostic criteria."[8] Research suggests varying prevalence rates from 6% to nearly 90%, pointing to the need for improved assessment measures.[10] The criteria and assessment of Orthorexia lack clear parameters by which clinicians may distinguish those who enthusiastically adopt a healthy diet from those who develop inflexible beliefs, attitudes, and behaviors related to nutrition and ultimately suffer from related impairments and unhealthy consequences.[11,12] Clinical anecdotes of people with impairments in the setting of ON describe patients as being paralyzed by self-induced pressure to make the "correct" healthy choices due to the abundance of conflicting nutritional information that is pervasive in the media.

30.4 PREVALENCE RATES

The 12-month and lifetime prevalence rates for the three most distinct EDs are presented in Table 30.1.[3,13,14] Women show higher rates across all three diagnoses, with gender differences being smallest in magnitude in BED. A recent simulation suggested that lifetime rates of ED diagnosis by age 40 are nearly 1 in 7 (14.3%) for men and 1 in 5 for women (19.7%) with OSFED being the most common diagnosis.[1] Recent research highlights higher rates of these EDs among sexual and gender minorities.[15] Prevalence rates of ARFID are harder to characterize due to limited research in this area. One study suggests a current prevalence of 0.3% among Australians and another study suggests 0.8% among Germans.[16,17] Also, higher rates of ARFID may be found among individuals with Autism (~21%).

30.5 MEDICAL CONSEQUENCES

EDs are associated with significant medical and psychosocial consequences and can affect nearly every organ system.[18] EDs may result in substantial weight gain, loss, fluctuation, or an otherwise unexplained deviation from growth trajectory in youth. EDs that include restriction or purging (AN, BN, ARFID) can result in malnutrition or nutrient deficiencies. These patients may have cold intolerance or present with hypothermia, weakness, fatigue, dizziness, or fainting. Cardiorespiratory consequences can include heart palpitations or arrhythmias, bradycardia, hypotension, and edema. Endocrine effects may include hypoglycemia, amenorrhea or irregular menses, increased bone fractures due to low bone density, and infertility. Clinicians may observe lanugo hair growth or hair thinning, carotenoderma, and skin that bruises easily. Self-induced vomiting may lead to inflammation and rupture of the esophagus, electrolyte imbalances, pancreatitis, cardiac concerns, GI distress, calluses or sores on the back of the hand, and tooth enamel decay. Health risks of binge-eating behavior include weight gain or obesity, which increases the risk for type 2 diabetes, cancer, hypertension, hypercholesterolemia, sleep apnea, and cardiovascular, gallbladder, and liver disease. EDs are also often comorbid with other psychiatric disorders, including anxiety, depression, obsessive-compulsive disorder, substance use disorders, and suicidality and self-harm. Mortality rates of people with EDs are among the highest in mental illnesses, second only to opioid overdose.[19]

30.6 RISK FACTORS

The complex etiology of EDs involves multiple factors, including genetic, biological, psychosocial, and temperamental vulnerabilities. The risk of developing an ED increases when these risk factors interact with each other and with environmental circumstances.[1,20] Heritability of genetic factors accounts for an estimated 50–83% of the variance in predisposition to and presentation of AN, BN, and BED.[21,22] Additionally, these genetic factors contribute to neurobiological factors inherent in EDs.[22,23] Psychosocial and biological risk factors include weight concerns, dieting, elevated body mass index (BMI), overeating, fasting, drive for thinness, body dissatisfaction, social pressure for thinness, thin-ideal internalization, daily exercise, excessive exercise, low interoceptive awareness, ineffectiveness, alcohol use, negative affect, social support deficits, and early puberty.[24]

30.7 TREATMENT

Family-based therapy (FBT) is the most supported treatment for youth with AN, while cognitive behavioral therapy (CBT) and cognitive behavioral therapy for eating disorders (CBT-E) is the most supported treatment for BN, BED, and adults with AN.[25,26] Antidepressants are also supported for the management of BN and BED, while stimulants are indicated as a therapy for BED.[26] It is recommended that multidisciplinary teams manage patients at all levels of care (outpatient, intensive outpatient, partial hospitalization, inpatient, and residential). Healthcare teams in the management of EDs generally consist of a therapist, dietician, psychiatrist, and primary care provider. Treatment goals specific to nutrition and exercise will be reviewed below, as these are the most relevant to lifestyle medicine.

30.7.1 NUTRITIONAL RECOMMENDATIONS

The consensus among ED professionals is that medical stabilization and fulfillment of basic energy needs are the necessary first steps in treating EDs. This includes weight restoration if the patient is underweight.[27] Once weight is improved by the inclusion of higher energy density foods, the nutritional focus of the healthcare provider should then shift to the improvement of nutrient intake and variety.[27–29] Structured meal plans are used to establish regular patterns of eating. Food plans should emphasize the inclusion of planned exposure to foods that are consumed in binge episodes, as well as "feared and avoided" foods.[27] It is important to note that fewer than 6% of people with EDs are medically diagnosed as "underweight," and approximately 30% of males and 23% of females with EDs have overweight or obesity. For this reason, relatively few patients with EDs will require weight restoration.[30] When patients present with possible dietary-related comorbidities (e.g., elevated cholesterol, triglycerides, glucose, A1C, and blood pressure) the recommendations are to first focus on improving ED behaviors, and then, if comorbidities are not resolved, consultation with the medical provider and the patient is recommended before any dietary restrictions are considered.[27] Patients frequently continue eating patterns they adopted in treatment long after discharge due to familiarity and to maintain structure; these patterns usually have a greater emphasis on food variety than food quality. Additional targeted nutritional counseling may be necessary to shift the focus toward improved nutrient intake.

30.7.2 EXERCISE RECOMMENDATIONS

Excessive or compulsive exercise is present in 30-80% of individuals with EDs.[27,31] Recommendations for exercise are to cease or severely limit activity if the patient has abnormal labs, is underweight, and/or there are signs of bradycardia. Some moderate exercise has been shown to help patients who are restoring weight consistently to accept body changes and decrease their drive to excessively or compulsively exercise, as well as provide enjoyment and improve mood.[27–29] Exercise allowance is often used as an incentive contingent on progress in treatment. Once in recovery, exercise limits include the following: (1) no more than an hour a day of exercise, (2) no more than one exercise session per day, and (3) exercise on no more than five days of a given week.[29]

30.8 PROGNOSIS

Data on the prognosis of EDs vary depending on diagnosis, treatment intensity, and follow-up length.[32] Earlier intervention leads to better outcomes. Relapse rates are high, ranging from 40-50% of patients.[33] For AN, remission rates are between 30-70% of patients and more than 20% of patients continue to have an ED on long-term follow-up. Mortality rates range between 5-15%.[32–34] Remission rates for BN range from 27–70%, with chronicity ranging from 11%-14%, and a mortality rate of 0.5-1%. BED remission rates are 25-80%. OSFED remission rates are reported as 67-69% and do not seem to be affected by treatment intensity or length of follow-up.

30.9 ED AND LM: CONFLICTING RECOMMENDATIONS/ FRAMEWORKS?

Initially, it might appear that LM and EDs specialist recommendations do not align. LM recommends a whole food plant-predominant diet, 150 minutes of moderate or

75 minutes of vigorous activity weekly, and 2 days of strength training. Alternatively, the ED field recommends diets that are not restrictive (i.e., inclusive of all food groups, lack of food rules), and physical activity that is not excessive or compulsive. Although the fields may see these goals as mutually exclusive, we take the position that they are not. When an individual has an ED and it is impacting either their health (e.g., low weight, cardiometabolic issues) or their psychological functioning (e.g., large percent of their day thinking about food or weight, lack of flexibility in food choices or physical activity), primary targets for treatment should be focused on restoring health and psychological functioning. Once the patient progresses, moving toward the pillars of LM can follow. Patients with EDs often tend to be rigid and inflexible and should be monitored closely as they incorporate more LM goals during their healing process. It is expected that improvement will not be linear but can be achieved with the support of knowledgeable and strategic healthcare providers.

To help recognize EDs early, ED professionals recommend evaluating those who present with "sudden changes in eating behaviors (e.g., recent vegetarianism/veganism, gluten-free, lactose free, elimination of certain foods or food groups, eating only 'healthy' foods, uncontrolled binge eating, lack of appetite)."[27] Many ED professionals are suspicious of patients presenting as vegetarian or vegan due to concern that removing complete food groups from one's diet and following strict food rules frequently occur at the onset of EDs. Strict food rules often maintain or can exacerbate ED symptoms. Therefore, it is important that LM professionals thoroughly understand a patient's history, as recommending the removal of entire food groups could precipitate the recurrence of ED symptoms. However, ED treatment guidelines exist for patients who follow a vegetarian or vegan diet.[27,35] While there is evidence of higher rates of vegetarianism among ED samples, the evidence for higher rates of disordered eating symptoms among vegetarians is mixed.[36–38] Some concerns about these data have been posed because many scales that measure ED symptoms do not distinguish between meat-avoiding behaviors characteristic of vegetarians and vegans and food avoidance, which may be more symptomatic of EDs.[35,37] Relatedly, some data indicate that vegetarians and vegans who are motivated for reasons other than weight are more likely to endorse less eating-related pathology than others.[10,39] Interestingly, only one study to date has examined attitudes toward veganism in a sample of health care professionals.[40] In this study, measures asked about attitudes towards veganism in general and not in the clinical context of EDs. Views towards veganism were found to be positive among all professionals; general mental health professionals had more positive attitudes than eating disorder specialists and other healthcare professionals.[40]

30.10   IS THERE SUCH A THING AS A "HEALTHY" RESTRICTION?

As highlighted above, the restriction of food groups in a patient with a history of an ED may raise red flags among ED professionals, as this can be a 'socially acceptable' way to limit total caloric intake or avoid binge-eating trigger foods. The data suggesting that dietary restraint and dieting are causal risk factors for EDs are mixed.[41] Recent publications support the emerging consensus that dietary restraint and actual restriction of dietary intake may be practiced in a healthy manner and are both safe and effective for weight management and the promotion of good physical and mental health in those without significant risks for the development of EDs.[42,43] It is plausible that dietary restraint may activate vulnerability factors (i.e., those who have genetic and neurobiological vulnerabilities), or that dietary restraint may be a correlate or proxy risk factor of ED symptoms.[41,42] Some experimental studies suggest that weight loss and weight maintenance diets actually reduce ED symptoms.[41] In particular, a randomized controlled study, which was effective for inducing a chronic (two-year) reduction in total energy intake that resulted in weight loss, increased dietary restraint, and avoidance of "forbidden foods" (i.e., foods with high dietary fat or added sugar) and decreased binge-eating episodes and concerns about body size; additionally, ED symptoms did not increase.[42] It is also important to note that while most Americans diet and seek to lose weight in culture, relatively few continue to develop EDs.[2,3,10,13,14,21,22] Accordingly, to comprehensively convey public health, it is important to balance the prevention and treatment of obesity and EDs concurrently.[42,44]

30.11 WHERE DOES THIS LEAVE US FROM A LIFESTYLE MEDICINE PERSPECTIVE?

Several questions arise: How do the LM pillars relate to managing people with EDs or history of EDs? What approach can be taken to address any associated sequelae? Is it possible to move a patient towards improved overall health, without any deterioration of ED treatment gains? The following sections will discuss the benefits of targeting each pillar specifically for an individual with ED and provide recommendations for approaches.

30.11.1 NUTRITION

The major mechanisms by which diet affects psychological health include the gastrointestinal (GI) microbiome, inflammation, epigenetics, and the effects of macronutrients and micronutrients.[45] Existing literature also supports a bidirectional relationship between mental health and nutrients. Results of a 2017 meta-analysis indicated that healthier eating patterns may decrease the risk of depression, whereas 'Western' eating patterns may increase the risk of depression.[46] In 2019, another large meta-analysis provided evidence that dietary interventions significantly reduce symptoms of depression; women experienced greater benefits and reduced anxiety.[47] Nutritional choices lead to important improvements in depression and anxiety for ED patients, reducing comorbidity and improving engagement in treatment and recovery.

Recommendations: While approaching nutritional changes in a patient with, or history of, an ED is delicate, it is not necessarily contraindicated. LM principles focus on increasing whole foods, decreasing processed foods, and consuming minimal animal products, if any.[48] There is no specification of caloric limits. Plant-based approaches to nutrition focus on eating until satiation. Recommendations can be made, especially if other health conditions are present, that would improve with dietary changes; however, risks and benefits need to be evaluated. The patient must be interested in making changes with the intention of health improvement in order to engage with and benefit from the process effectively. Major changes to eating patterns may constitute a 'trigger' of eating-disordered thoughts; therefore, it is best to proceed with small changes, particularly with the support of an ED therapist. Recovered individuals often have an ED therapist whom they see periodically for relapse prevention accountability. The patient needs to be willing to see their therapist to evaluate the risks and benefits of dietary changes and to help manage any ED cognitions which may surface.

30.11.2 Physical Activity

The benefits of physical activity (PA) are wide-reaching, including mood and mental health improvements.[49] LM recommends 150 minutes of moderate or 75 minutes of vigorous activity weekly and 2 days of strength training. When appropriate in the context of ED treatment, exercise can be integrated at a safe level, as outlined previously, as long as it is not excessive, compulsive, or compensatory in nature. Improvements in depressive symptoms are important for ED patients not only due to the co-morbid nature of the disorders, but because improvements in depression also lead to increases in self-efficacy, self-esteem, and prosocial behaviors, and these can increase engagement in treatment and contribute to success in recovery.[50,51]

Recommendations: Lifestyle medicine guidelines for physical activity do not conflict with activity guidelines for EDs, as previously discussed, on the condition that the patient is medically stable, weight restored, and did not have previous excessive/compulsive exercise tendencies. In the case of the latter, proceed with caution and only with the support of an ED therapist.

30.11.3 Sleep

EDs and eating issues frequently co-occur with sleep disturbances.[52] This relationship is considered bidirectional, where EDs can negatively affect sleep, and sleep disruptions can contribute to and intensify the symptoms of EDs.[53,54] A large longitudinal study found that an ED diagnosis was predictive of sleeping disturbances over time.[15] Appetite and hunger are regulated by hormone production, which is affected by sleep. Sleeping problems may disrupt the normal production and levels of hormones, resulting in altered eating behavior. Additionally, food intake patterns, and nutrient variety and deficits (malnutrition) may influence both sleep quality and daytime sleepiness.[53,55] Mood or anxiety disorders, which also affect sleep, are highly comorbid with EDs.[56]

Recommendations: Sufficient quantity and good quality of sleep are essential for vital biological processes that maintain physical and mental health symptoms. For adults, at least 7 hours of sleep is recommended.[55,57] Sleep deprivation affects all the pillars of LM and may need to be addressed early to enable the patient to execute their lifestyle changes. Deprivation can lead to reduced energy for exercise, alterations in eating, poor coping with stress, difficulty with interpersonal relationships, and engaging in risky behaviors, all of which interfere with progress in other LM pillars.[58] Sleep improvement has shown a dose-response effect on mental health.[59]

Therefore, increasing sleep duration and quality, even by a modest amount, will benefit the patient.

30.11.4 SOCIAL CONNECTION

Poor social support is a risk factor for the development of EDs.[60,61] Social isolation and feelings of being alone with one's disorder are common for those with EDs. Being diagnosed with and receiving treatment for an ED is disruptive to the patient's social network. Often, family conflict increases and siblings frequently withdraw due to the shift in focus to the patient.[62,63] Friends may disconnect from the patient, rendering the patient with limited social support.

Recommendations: Encouraging patients to focus on building social connection is warranted. Additionally, interpersonal psychotherapy (IPT), which directly focuses on improving relationships/fixing problems with relationships and has been shown to help reduce ED symptoms, may be indicated.[64]

30.11.5 STRESS MANAGEMENT

Stress management is crucial to patients' recovery and relapse prevention with EDs. The comorbidity of anxiety has been reported to be up to 62% of patients.[65] Anxiety and stress are detrimental to one's ability to cope with daily challenges, which hinders the recovery process and may put patients at risk for relapse. Eating patterns change during times of high stress, when diet quality diminishes and there is a tendency to eat foods higher in sugar, salt, and fat, all of which can trigger binge-eating.[66-70]

Recommendations: Therapeutic approaches to EDs generally include a component of mindfulness, where the goal is to manage anxiety responses and increase awareness around emotions, eating, and appetite.[71-73] This has many additional benefits. Incorporating mindfulness practice has been shown to increase cortical thickness in the prefrontal cortex and elevate serotonin levels, both of which can affect mood.[74] Encouraging patients to engage in reasonable physical activity also helps to reduce anxiety and the physiological effects of stress on the body.[49]

30.11.6 SUBSTANCE USE

Any substance use is relevant to mental (and physical) health. In general, the prevalence rates of substance use disorder (SUD) in EDs have been reported as high as 27%.[65] High rates of substance use are seen in those with higher frequencies of binge/purge behavior. Substances are commonly reported as strategies for coping with stress and negative emotions, or general relaxation. However, substance use often leads to negative mental health symptoms; withdrawal from alcohol leads to increases in anxiety, sleep disruption, and risk for major depression.[75-77]

Recommendation: Counseling for reduced substance intake is crucial to managing the ED patient's sleep, mood, and anxiety. Referral for substance use treatment may be indicated. Treatment of ED and SUD is best addressed simultaneously using a multi-disciplinary approach.[78]

30.12 CONCLUSION

This chapter provided an overview of EDs, what might be encountered in clinical practice in the setting of EDs, and how the frameworks of LM and EDs can be used in conjunction to support patients through their recovery process. A review of the LM pillars was given to highlight the benefits of an LM approach to complement recommendations for ED treatment and management. At first glance, treatment recommendations for LM and EDs, particularly for nutrition and exercise, might appear not to align. LM guidelines for physical activity fit well within the activity guidelines for ED patients (stabilized and/or recovered). LM nutrition principles focus on (1) increasing whole foods (2) decreasing processed foods (3) minimizing animal products, and (4) no specification of caloric limits. Existing ED guidelines suggest approaches that are specific to and appropriate for patients who follow a vegetarian or vegan diet. Risks and benefits first need to be explored when any major changes to patterns of eating and exercise are considered. Implementation of changes needs to start with small steps, and with the support of an ED therapist for accountability and relapse prevention. Moving a patient towards improved overall health without any deterioration of ED treatment gains is possible within the LM framework.

REFERENCES

1. Klump KL, Bulik CM, Kaye WH, Treasure J, Tyson E. Academy for eating disorders position paper: Eating disorders are serious mental illnesses. *Int J Eat Disord.* 2009;42(2):97–103. doi:10.1002/eat.20589
2. Ward ZJ, Rodriguez P, Wright DR, Austin SB, Long MW. Estimation of eating disorders prevalence by age and associations with mortality in a simulated nationally representative US cohort. *JAMA Netw Open.* 2019;2(10):e1912925. doi:10.1001/jamanetworkopen.2019.12925
3. American Psychiatric Association, American Psychiatric Association DSM-5 Task Force. *Diagnostic and Statistical Manual of Mental Disorders: DSM-5.* 5th ed. American Psychiatric Association; 2013.
4. *International Classification of Diseases, Eleventh Revision (ICD-11).* World Health Organization (WHO); 2019. https://icd.who.int/browse11
5. Moroze RM, Dunn TM, Craig Holland J, Yager J, Weintraub P. Microthinking about micronutrients: A case of transition from obsessions about healthy eating to near-fatal "orthorexia nervosa" and proposed diagnostic criteria. *Psychosomatics.* 2015;56(4):397–403. doi:10.1016/j.psym.2014.03.003
6. Dunn TM, Bratman S. On orthorexia nervosa: A review of the literature and proposed diagnostic criteria. *Eat Behav.* 2016;21:11–17. doi:10.1016/j.eatbeh.2015.12.006
7. Barthels F, Meyer F, Pietrowsky R. Die Düsseldorfer Orthorexie Skala–Konstruktion und Evaluation eines Fragebogens zur Erfassung ortho-rektischen Ernährungsverhaltens. *Z Für Klin Psychol Psychother.* 2015;44(2):97–105. doi:10.1026/1616-3443/a000310
8. Oberle CD, De Nadai AS, Madrid AL. Orthorexia Nervosa Inventory (ONI): Development and validation of a new measure of orthorexic symptomatology. *Eat Weight Disord EWD.* 2021;26(2):609–622. doi:10.1007/s40519-020-00896-6
9. Setnick J. *The Eating Disorders Clinical Pocket Guide: Quick Reference for Healthcare Providers.* Snack Time Press; 2005: 9780976400240: Amazon.com: Books. https://www.amazon.com/Eating-Disorders-Clinical-Pocket-Guide/dp/0976400243. Accessed September 11, 2022.

10. Dunn TM, Gibbs J, Whitney N, Starosta A. Prevalence of orthorexia nervosa is less than 1%: Data from a US sample. *Eat Weight Disord EWD*. 2017;22(1):185–192. doi:10.1007/s40519-016-0258-8

11. Cena H, Barthels F, Cuzzolaro M, et al. Definition and diagnostic criteria for orthorexia nervosa: A narrative review of the literature. *Eat Weight Disord EWD*. 2019;24(2): 209–246. doi:10.1007/s40519-018-0606-y

12. Bratman S. Orthorexia vs. theories of healthy eating. *Eat Weight Disord EWD*. 2017; 22(3):381–385. doi:10.1007/s40519-017-0417-6

13. Hudson JI, Hiripi E, Pope HG, Kessler RC. The prevalence and correlates of eating disorders in the National Comorbidity Survey Replication. *Biol Psychiatry*. 2007;61(3): 348–358. doi:10.1016/j.biopsych.2006.03.040

14. Udo T, Grilo CM. Prevalence and correlates of DSM-5-defined eating disorders in a nationally representative sample of U.S. Adults. *Biol Psychiatry*. 2018;84(5):345–354. doi:10.1016/j.biopsych.2018.03.014

15. Nagata JM, Ganson KT, Austin SB. Emerging trends in eating disorders among sexual and gender minorities. *Curr Opin Psychiatry*. 2020;33(6):562–567. doi:10.1097/YCO.0000000000000645

16. Hay P, Mitchison D, Collado AEL, González-Chica DA, Stocks N, Touyz S. Burden and health-related quality of life of eating disorders, including Avoidant/Restrictive Food Intake Disorder (ARFID), in the Australian population. *J Eat Disord*. 2017;5:21. doi:10.1186/s40337-017-0149-z

17. Hilbert A, Zenger M, Eichler J, Brähler E. Psychometric evaluation of the Eating Disorders in Youth-Questionnaire when used in adults: Prevalence estimates for symptoms of avoidant/restrictive food intake disorder and population norms. *Int J Eat Disord*. 2021;54(3):399–408. doi:10.1002/eat.23424

18. AED Medical Care Standards Committee. *Eating Disorders: A Guide to Medical Care*. Academy of Eating Disorders. https://www.aedweb.org/publications/medical-care-standards Accessed September 9, 2022.

19. Arcelus J, Mitchell AJ, Wales J, Nielsen S. Mortality rates in patients with anorexia nervosa and other eating disorders: A meta-analysis of 36 studies. *Arch Gen Psychiatry*. 2011;68(7):724–731. doi:10.1001/archgenpsychiatry.2011.74

20. Stice E, Desjardins CD. Interactions between risk factors in the prediction of onset of eating disorders: Exploratory hypothesis generating analyses. *Behav Res Ther*. 2018; 105:52–62. doi:10.1016/j.brat.2018.03.005

21. Bulik CM, Sullivan PF, Tozzi F, Furberg H, Lichtenstein P, Pedersen NL. Prevalence, heritability, and prospective risk factors for anorexia nervosa. *Arch Gen Psychiatry*. 2006;63(3):305–312. doi:10.1001/archpsyc.63.3.305

22. Kaye WH, Wierenga CE, Bailer UF, Simmons AN, Bischoff-Grethe A. Nothing tastes as good as skinny feels: The neurobiology of anorexia nervosa. *Trends Neurosci*. 2013; 36(2). doi:10.1016/j.tins.2013.01.003

23. Kaye WH, Fudge JL, Paulus M. New insights into symptoms and neurocircuit function of anorexia nervosa. *Nat Rev Neurosci*. 2009;10(8):573–584. doi:10.1038/nrn2682

24. Stice E, Gau JM, Rohde P, Shaw H. risk factors that predict future onset of each DSM-5 eating disorder: predictive specificity in high-risk adolescent females. *J Abnorm Psychol*. 2017;126(1):38–51. doi:10.1037/abn0000219

25. Hay P. A systematic review of evidence for psychological treatments in eating disorders: 2005–2012. *Int J Eat Disord*. 2013;46(5):462–469. doi:10.1002/eat.22103

26. Monteleone AM, Pellegrino F, Croatto G, et al. Treatment of eating disorders: A systematic meta-review of meta-analyses and network meta-analyses. *Neurosci Biobehav Rev*. Published online September 6, 2022:104857. doi:10.1016/j.neubiorev.2022.104857

27. Academy for Eating Disorders Nutrition Working Group. *Guidebook for Nutrition Treatment of Eating Disorders*. Academy of Eating Disorders; 2020. https://www.aedweb.org/publications

28. Cook BJ, Wonderlich SA, Mitchell JE, Thompson R, Sherman R, McCallum K. Exercise in eating disorders treatment: Systematic review and proposal of guidelines. *Med Sci Sports Exerc.* 2016;48(7):1408–1414. doi:10.1249/MSS.0000000000000912

29. Herrin M, Larkin M. *Nutrition Counseling in the Treatment of Eating Disorders.* 2nd ed. Routledge; 2012. doi:10.4324/9780203870600

30. Flament MF, Henderson K, Buchholz A, et al. Weight status and DSM-5 diagnoses of eating disorders in adolescents from the community. *J Am Acad Child Adolesc Psychiatry.* 2015;54(5):403–411.e2. doi:10.1016/j.jaac.2015.01.020

31. Quesnel DA, Libben M, D Oelke N, I Clark M, Willis-Stewart S, Caperchione CM. Is abstinence really the best option? Exploring the role of exercise in the treatment and management of eating disorders. *Eat Disord.* 2018;26(3):290–310. doi:10.1080/10640266.2017.1397421

32. Keel PK, Brown TA. Update on course and outcome in eating disorders. *Int J Eat Disord.* 2010;43(3):195–204. doi:10.1002/eat.20810

33. Miller CA, Golden NH. An introduction to eating disorders. *Nutr Clin Pract.* 2010;25(2):110–115. doi:10.1177/0884533609357566

34. Steinhausen HC. Outcome of eating disorders. *Child Adolesc Psychiatr Clin N Am.* 2009;18(1):225–242. doi:10.1016/j.chc.2008.07.013

35. Physicians Committee for Responsible Medicine. Eating Disorders | Nutrition Guide for Clinicians. https://nutritionguide.pcrm.org/nutritionguide/view/Nutrition_Guide_for_Clinicians/1342074/all/Eating_Disorders?refer=true. Accessed September 9, 2022.

36. Zickgraf HF, Hazzard VM, O'Connor SM, et al. Examining vegetarianism, weight motivations, and eating disorder psychopathology among college students. *Int J Eat Disord.* 2020;53(9):1506–1514. doi:10.1002/eat.23335

37. McLean CP, Kulkarni J, Sharp G. Disordered eating and the meat-avoidance spectrum: A systematic review and clinical implications. *Eat Weight Disord EWD.* Published online June 21, 2022. doi:10.1007/s40519-022-01428-0

38. Bardone-Cone AM, Fitzsimmons-Craft EE, Harney MB, et al. The inter-relationships between vegetarianism and eating disorders among females. *J Acad Nutr Diet.* 2012;112(8):1247–1252. doi:10.1016/j.jand.2012.05.007

39. Forestell CA, Spaeth AM, Kane SA. To eat or not to eat red meat. A closer look at the relationship between restrained eating and vegetarianism in college females. *Appetite.* 2012;58(1):319–325. doi:10.1016/j.appet.2011.10.015

40. Fuller SJ, Hill KM. Attitudes toward veganism in eating disorder professionals. *BJPsych Bull.* 2022;46(2):95–99. doi:10.1192/bjb.2021.57

41. Stice E, Presnell K. Dieting and the eating disorders. In: Agras WS, ed. *The Oxford Handbook of Eating Disorders.* Oxford University Press; 2010:148–179.

42. Stewart TM, Martin CK, Williamson DA. The complicated relationship between dieting, dietary restraint, caloric restriction, and eating disorders: Is a shift in public health messaging warranted? *Int J Environ Res Public Health.* 2022;19(1):491. doi:10.3390/ijerph19010491

43. Chen JY, Singh S, Lowe MR. The food restriction wars: Proposed resolution of a primary battle. *Physiol Behav.* 2021;240:113530. doi:10.1016/j.physbeh.2021.113530

44. Stewart TM. Why thinking we're fat won't help us improve our health: Finding the middle ground. *Obesity.* 2018;26(7):1115–1116. doi:10.1002/oby.22241

45. Merlo G, Vela A. Mental health in lifestyle medicine: A call to action. *Am J Lifestyle Med.* Published online May 21, 2021:15598276211013312. doi:10.1177/15598276211013313

46. Li Y, Lv MR, Wei YJ, et al. Dietary patterns and depression risk: A meta-analysis. *Psychiatry Res.* 2017;253:373–382. doi:10.1016/j.psychres.2017.04.020

47. Firth J, Marx W, Dash S, et al. The effects of dietary improvement on symptoms of depression and anxiety: A meta-analysis of randomized controlled trials. *Psychosom Med.* 2019;81(3):265–280. doi:10.1097/PSY.0000000000000673

48. Overview | American College of Lifestyle Medicine. https://lifestylemedicine.org/overview/. Accessed September 13, 2022.

49. Noordsy DL. *Lifestyle Psychiatry*. 1st ed. Amer Psychiatric Pub Inc.; 2019.

50. Kandola A, Ashdown-Franks G, Hendrikse J, Sabiston CM, Stubbs B. Physical activity and depression: Towards understanding the antidepressant mechanisms of physical activity. *Neurosci Biobehav Rev.* 2019;107:525–539. doi:10.1016/j.neubiorev.2019.09.040

51. McAuley E, Morris KS. State of the art review: Advances in physical activity and mental health: Quality of life. *Am J Lifestyle Med.* 2007;1(5):389–396. doi:10.1177/1559827607303243

52. Aspen V, Weisman H, Vannucci A, et al. Psychiatric comorbidity in women presenting across the continuum of disordered eating. *Eat Behav.* 2014;15(4):686–693. doi:10.1016/j.eatbeh.2014.08.023

53. Allison KC, Spaeth A, Hopkins CM. Sleep and eating disorders. *Curr Psychiatry Rep.* 2016;18(10):92. doi:10.1007/s11920-016-0728-8

54. Kim KR, Jung YC, Shin MY, Namkoong K, Kim JK, Lee JH. Sleep disturbance in women with eating disorder: Prevalence and clinical characteristics. *Psychiatry Res.* 2010;176(1):88–90. doi:10.1016/j.psychres.2009.03.021

55. The Impact of an Eating Disorder on Sleep. Sleep Foundation; 2021. https://www.sleepfoundation.org/mental-health/eating-disorders-and-sleep

56. Goel NJ, Sadeh-Sharvit S, Trockel M, et al. Depression and anxiety mediate the relationship between insomnia and eating disorders in college women. *J Am Coll Health J ACH.* 2021;69(8):976–981. doi:10.1080/07448481.2019.1710152

57. Consensus Conference Panel. Recommended amount of sleep for a healthy adult: A joint consensus statement of the American academy of sleep medicine and sleep research society. *Sleep.* 2015;38(6):843–844. doi:10.5665/sleep.4716

58. McEwen BS, Karatsoreos IN. Sleep deprivation and circadian disruption: Stress, allostasis, and allostatic load. *Sleep Med Clin.* 2015;10(1):1–10. doi:10.1016/j.jsmc.2014.11.007

59. Scott AJ, Webb TL, Martyn-St James M, Rowse G, Weich S. Improving sleep quality leads to better mental health: A meta-analysis of randomised controlled trials. *Sleep Med Rev.* 2021;60:101556. doi:10.1016/j.smrv.2021.101556

60. Limbert C. Perceptions of social support and eating disorder characteristics. *Health Care Women Int.* 2010;31(2):170–178. doi:10.1080/07399330902893846

61. Leonidas C, dos Santos MA. Social support networks and eating disorders: An integrative review of the literature. *Neuropsychiatr Dis Treat.* 2014;10:915–927. doi:10.2147/NDT.S60735

62. Hutchison S, House J, McDermott B, Simic M, Baudinet J, Eisler I. Silent witnesses: The experience of having a sibling with anorexia nervosa. *J Eat Disord.* 2022;10(1):134. doi:10.1186/s40337-022-00655-1

63. Maon I, Horesh D, Gvion Y. Siblings of individuals with eating disorders: A review of the literature. *Front Psychiatry.* 2020;11.https://www.frontiersin.org/articles/10.3389/fpsyt.2020.00604. Accessed September 12, 2022.

64. Miniati M, Callari A, Maglio A, Calugi S. Interpersonal psychotherapy for eating disorders: Current perspectives. *Psychol Res Behav Manag.* 2018;11:353–369. doi:10.2147/PRBM.S120584

65. Hambleton A, Pepin G, Le A, et al. Psychiatric and medical comorbidities of eating disorders: Findings from a rapid review of the literature. *J Eat Disord.* 2022;10(1):132. doi:10.1186/s40337-022-00654-2

66. Kazmierski KFM, Gillespie ML, Kuo S, Zurita T, Felix D, Rao U. Stress-induced eating among Racial/Ethnic groups in the United States: A systematic review. *J Racial Ethn Health Disparities.* 2021;8(4):912–926. doi:10.1007/s40615-020-00849-w

67. Kandiah J, Yake M, Jones J, Meyer M. Stress influences appetite and comfort food preferences in college women. *Nutr Res.* 2006;26(3):118–123. doi:10.1016/j.nutres.2005.11.010

68. Greeno CG, Wing RR. Stress-induced eating. *Psychol Bull.* 1994;115:444–464. doi:10.1037/0033-2909.115.3.444

69. Ling J, Zahry NR. Relationships among perceived stress, emotional eating, and dietary intake in college students: Eating self-regulation as a mediator. *Appetite.* 2021; 163:105215. doi:10.1016/j.appet.2021.105215

70. Khaled K, Tsofliou F, Hundley V, Helmreich R, Almilaji O. Perceived stress and diet quality in women of reproductive age: A systematic review and meta-analysis. *Nutr J.* 2020;19(1):92. doi:10.1186/s12937-020-00609-w

71. Godsey J. The role of mindfulness based interventions in the treatment of obesity and eating disorders: An integrative review. *Complement Ther Med.* 2013;21(4):430–439. doi:10.1016/j.ctim.2013.06.003

72. Wanden-Berghe RG, Sanz-Valero J, Wanden-Berghe C. The application of mindfulness to eating disorders treatment: A systematic review. *Eat Disord.* 2010;19(1):34–48. doi:10.1080/10640266.2011.533604

73. Yu J, Song P, Zhang Y, Wei Z. Effects of mindfulness-based intervention on the treatment of problematic eating behaviors: A systematic review. *J Altern Complement Med.* 2020;26(8):666–679. doi:10.1089/acm.2019.0163

74. Sarris J, O'Neil A, Coulson CE, Schweitzer I, Berk M. Lifestyle medicine for depression. *BMC Psychiatry.* 2014;14:107. doi:10.1186/1471-244X-14-107

75. Bayard M, Mcintyre J, Hill KR, Jack Woodside JR. Alcohol withdrawal syndrome. *Am Fam Physician.* 2004;69(6):1443–1450.

76. Bowen MT, George O, Muskiewicz DE, Hall FS. Factors contributing to the escalation of alcohol consumption. *Neurosci Biobehav Rev.* 2022;132:730–756. doi:10.1016/j.neubiorev.2021.11.017

77. Boden JM, Fergusson DM. Alcohol and depression. *Addict Abingdon Engl.* 2011;106(5): 906–914. doi:10.1111/j.1360-0443.2010.03351.x

78. Gregorowski C, Seedat S, Jordaan GP. A clinical approach to the assessment and management of co-morbid eating disorders and substance use disorders. *BMC Psychiatry.* 2013;13:289. doi:10.1186/1471-244X-13-289

31 | Psychotic Disorders

Vanika Chawla, MD, FRCPC,
Maryam S. Makowski, PhD,
Heather Freeman, PsyD, E-RYT 500,
and Douglas L. Noordsy, MD

KEY POINTS

- Lifestyle psychiatry goes beyond the biopsychosocial model to include evidence-based recommendations such as exercise, diet, and sleep to prevent and address mental illness.
- Schizophrenia spectrum disorders (SSD) are characterized by mental health symptoms such as positive symptoms, negative symptoms and neurocognitive deficits, impairments in quality of life and function, and poor physical health outcomes including reduced life expectancy of up to ten to twenty years compared to the general population.
- There is a bidirectional relationship between lifestyle factors such as diet, physical activity, and mental and physical health outcomes of the illness.
- There is evidence for the benefits of lifestyle interventions such as yoga, exercise, and nutrition in improving positive, negative, and cognitive symptoms as well as quality of life and function and physical health parameters.
- Lifestyle interventions are feasible, relatively low-risk, can complement existing treatments for SSD, and should be integrated into routine mental health care.

31.1 INTRODUCTION

Lifestyle psychiatry is a subspeciality of lifestyle medicine that focuses on the management of psychiatric disorders through an integrated and holistic approach that may complement medication and psychotherapy. Lifestyle psychiatry goes beyond the biopsychosocial model to include evidence-based recommendations such as exercise, diet, and sleep to prevent and address mental illness.[1]

Schizophrenia spectrum disorders (SSD) are characterized by positive symptoms (such as hallucinations and delusions as well as disorganized behaviors and thoughts), negative symptoms (such as amotivation and social withdrawal) as well as neurocognitive deficits. These symptoms have a significant impact on quality of life and functional outcomes. The lifetime prevalence of schizophrenia is approximately one percent worldwide. The onset is typically in adulthood with many individuals having a chronic and relapsing course, with persistent symptoms in two-thirds of individuals despite optimal treatment. The etiology of schizophrenia is yet to be fully understood but involves a combination of genetics, biological, and social

DOI: 10.1201/b22810-35

factors. Neurodegeneration related to excess synaptic pruning has been implicated as an element in the underlying pathophysiology.

Conventional treatment of schizophrenia involves medical interventions with the mainstay being treatment with antipsychotics as well as psychosocial interventions such as cognitive behavioral therapy for psychosis (CBTp), supportive employment, and family education. Antipsychotics have less efficacy for negative and cognitive symptoms, which generates a greater symptom burden on the functional status of people with SSD.

There is a need for low-cost, accessible, and patient-centered treatments that reduce negative symptoms and cognitive deficits, increase quality of life, promote functional recovery, and improve the physical health of people with SSD to reduce morbidity and mortality.

31.2 RISK FACTORS ASSOCIATED WITH THE ILLNESS THAT IMPACT HEALTH

Individuals with schizophrenia have high rates of cardiometabolic disease leading to a reduced life expectancy of up to ten to twenty years compared to the general population. A meta-analysis found that individuals with schizophrenia spectrum disorders (SSD) were 4 times more likely to have abdominal obesity, 2.4 times more likely to have metabolic syndrome, and twice as likely to have diabetes.[1]

The causes of increased cardiometabolic risk factors are complex and include genetics of the disease; side effects of antipsychotic medications including the negative impact of antipsychotic drugs on lipid and glucose metabolism, appetite, weight, and increased risk of metabolic syndrome;[2] illness factors that impact engagement in care and social determinants of health; as well as lifestyle factors such as unhealthy diet, smoking, and sedentary behaviors. The shortest life expectancy is among those who do not take antipsychotic medication, suggesting that cardiovascular mortality in schizophrenia is attributable to factors other than antipsychotic treatment;[3] thus illness factors and lifestyle factors are the dominant drivers of mortality Furthermore, individuals with serious mental illness have difficulty accessing health care and typically receive poorer quality health care services,[4] and socioeconomic disparities are also contributory to these health inequities.

People with schizophrenia are less physically active than the general population, with research showing that only one-quarter of individuals with schizophrenia adhere to guideline-recommended levels of physical activity. Research shows that individuals with SSD have higher levels of sedentary behavior, engage in less physical activity, and have low cardiorespiratory fitness (CRF) levels compared to age and gender-matched controls[5,6]

Unhealthy dietary habits, such as high intake of fat and sugar and low intake of fruits and vegetables, are also common.[7] Research suggests that individuals with schizophrenia tend to have diets that are higher in caloric intake,[8] energy, fat, and lower in fruits and vegetables, fiber, vitamin C, and beta carotene compared to the general population.[8,9] Some studies have noted that individuals with SSD have a higher propensity for metabolic abnormalities at the onset of illness even prior to medication initiation.[1,8] Furthermore, epidemiological studies that examined the role of prenatal nutrition relative to mental health conditions have found that prenatal caloric malnutrition, low birth weight, and prematurity increase the risk for disorders such as schizophrenia.[10] In 2004, Malcolm Peet completed an ecological study that evaluated outcomes of people with schizophrenia in relation to diet. The consumption of the "Western" diet such as red meat, dairy, and refined sugar significantly worsened 2-year mental health outcomes (such as hospitalization and social impairment) of patients with schizophrenia, whereas consumption of foods such as legumes significantly improved outcomes. Peet postulated that dietary patterns that were causal in physical diseases, such as diabetes and coronary artery disease, may also contribute to psychiatric disorders such as schizophrenia, making a seminal link between diet and mental health.[11,12]

People with schizophrenia show a high incidence of metabolic syndrome, which is associated with greater mortality from cardiovascular disease. The prevalence of metabolic syndrome in a large sample clinical trial was 44%. The etiology of the metabolic syndrome in schizophrenia is multifactorial and may involve antipsychotic treatment, high levels of stress, and an unhealthy lifestyle, such as poor diet and sedentary behavior. Illness factors are also contributory, and some studies indicate a risk for elevated cortisol levels and cardiometabolic abnormalities in those with schizophrenia prior to antipsychotic initiation.

Sleep disturbances occur at high rates in people with schizophrenia spectrum disorder. Sleep disturbances can precede the onset of schizophrenia, can be a warning sign or predictor of an acute exacerbation of psychotic symptoms, and can be related to symptom severity. Psychotic symptoms can also directly lead to sleep disturbances, including insomnia, due to the intrusion of unwanted thoughts and hallucinations when trying to sleep. Schizophrenia is associated with various sleep disturbances including circadian dysregulation. difficulty with sleep onset and maintenance, decreased total sleep time, and reduced rapid eye movement (REM) sleep. Obstructive sleep apnea is observed in a greater proportion of people with schizophrenia compared to the general population.

Approximately 50% of patients with schizophrenia develop a substance use disorder in their lifetime, and 60 to 90% endorse cigarette smoking. People with schizophrenia smoke tobacco at a rate of three to four times greater than the general population. The mechanistic underpinnings may include a shared genetic vulnerability or blunted brain reward responsiveness. Substance use both increases the risk of developing psychotic symptoms and negatively affects the course of SSD resulting in more positive symptoms; higher rates of treatment non-adherence, relapse, and hospitalization; worsened mood; as well as psychosocial, legal, and medical issues.

There is a bi-directional relationship between the risk factors associated with the illness and physical health outcomes. These factors impact the quality of life, function, and mental and physical health outcomes for those with schizophrenia spectrum disorders.

31.3 LIFESTYLE INTERVENTIONS

Lifestyle interventions are a first-line approach for decreasing cardiovascular disease risk for individuals with schizophrenia. There is also emerging evidence for the benefits of lifestyle interventions such as exercise and diet in improving positive, negative, and cognitive symptoms as well as quality of life and function.[2–4,13]

Interventions as part of the field of lifestyle psychiatry include yoga, diet and nutrition, exercise, mindfulness and meditation, and sleep management. This chapter will focus specifically on yoga, diet and nutrition, exercise, and the evidence for the use and recommended guidelines in people with schizophrenia, given both the strength of evidence and the expertise of the authors.

31.4 BARRIERS

There are several barriers that need to be considered and addressed when implementing lifestyle interventions in people with schizophrenia spectrum disorders. Persistent negative symptoms, including amotivation, can prevent patients from engaging in behavioral change. Strategies such as group formats, rewards, and engaging support networks can be helpful to address barriers related to negative symptoms. Cognitive symptoms can also impact engagement in lifestyle change, and necessary modifications such as delivering information in simple, engaging, and approachable ways can be helpful. Antipsychotic treatment can cause side effects such as sedation and further cognitive and negative symptoms, and modifications as indicated should be considered to minimize such side effects. Social determinants of health such as homelessness, financial difficulties, transportation difficulties, childcare and family duties, as well as social isolation and medical comorbidity, are other considerations that should be explored and addressed.

31.5 INTERVENTIONS

31.5.1 YOGA

Yoga is an ancient practice, originating in India, that integrates psychology with spirituality. The word yoga in Sanskrit means to "unite." Yoga is a science and philosophy that involves disciplined physical and contemplative practices that unite the body, mind, and spirit. In its most comprehensive form, yoga embodies the raja or eight-limbed path, including ethical practices (yamas), inner disciplines (niyamas), physical postures (asana), breathing (pranayama), inner-focused sense awareness (pratyahara), concentration (dharana), meditation (dhyana), and absorption (samadhi).

Physiologically, yoga has a role in regulating the autonomic nervous system, and is theorized to evoke the relaxation response and reduce the fight-flight stress response through creating changes in hypothalamic-pituitary-adrenal axis activity and sympathetic/parasympathetic balance.[14–16] Studies have demonstrated reductions of physiological markers of stress following yoga including blood pressure, heart rate, inflammatory cytokines, and cortisol[17] and increases in neurotransmitters implicated in various psychiatric disorders including mood and anxiety disorders such as gamma-aminobutyric acid (GABA) and oxytocin.[18,19]

Yoga as an intervention is known for its generalizability and adaptability with varied practices of the eight limbs meeting the needs of the individual and the group that the intervention is designed for. Patients with schizophrenia each carry unique presentations of the disorder while all need support with creating physiological, physical, and psychological change for their own healing and resilience.

A systematic review of randomized controlled trials indicated that yoga reduced both positive and negative symptoms of schizophrenia and improved the health-related quality of life of people with schizophrenia, although evidence was limited, as the review included only three trials. None of the randomized controlled trials (RCTs) encountered adverse events. Another systematic review and meta-analysis found moderate evidence for short-term improvements in quality of life in schizophrenia patients after yoga interventions. This review included 5 RCTs with a total of 337 patients. Moderate evidence was found for short-term effects of yoga on quality of life compared to usual care; no evidence was found for positive symptoms, negative symptoms, or social function. There was only one RCT that reported adverse effects; none were identified.[20] A review of 29 studies on exercise in patients with schizophrenia spectrum disorder found that yoga improved cognitive domains of long-term memory, attention, and executive function, and these results were not seen in other forms of exercise in this review[21]

There were 3 Cochrane reviews conducted on yoga among people with schizophrenia; one compared yoga versus non-standard care (another exercise comparator), one compared yoga versus standard care, and one compared yoga as part of a package of care versus standard care. The first review found minimal difference between yoga and non-standard care.[22] The next review comparing yoga and standard of care found that the outcomes were in favor of the yoga group with a positive impact of yoga on mental state, social functioning, and quality of life.[23] Lastly, comparing yoga as part of a package of care for schizophrenia versus standard of care found that of the three studies included, there was some evidence in favor of the yoga package for quality of life endpoint scores.[24] Issues with the reviews included many outcomes not reported and missing key outcomes, limited sample sizes and short-term follow-up, and low to moderate quality of RCTs; and thus the results must be interpreted with caution but can be seen as promising.

Yoga can also have several positive impacts on physical health for individuals with schizophrenia spectrum disorders. A systematic review of seven trials with 794 participants showed that yoga had beneficial effects on systolic blood pressure and waist circumference in adults with metabolic syndrome.[25] A Cochrane review with 800 participants at high risk of developing cardiovascular disease showed that yoga led to a reduction in diastolic blood pressure and triglycerides as well as an increase in HDL cholesterol; however, the studies were small, short-term, and low-quality.[26] The proposed mechanism for the impact of yoga on cardiometabolic health, in addition to being a form of physical activity, includes effects on stress reduction, which can lead to positive impacts on neuroendocrine status and metabolic and cardiac-vagal function and related inflammatory responses.[27]

Yoga can also create physiological changes that impact emotional and social functioning, key components in schizophrenia recovery. A randomized controlled trial showed an increase in plasma oxytocin levels, as well as social functioning, after 1 month of yoga practice. Oxytocin dysregulation is theorized to be involved in social cognitive deficits in schizophrenia; thus yoga may impact this domain possibly through the mediation of the vagus nerve, which is proposed to modulate neural circuits associated with social functioning.[28]

With respect to safety, a systematic review and meta-analysis of 94 RCTs of yoga found no significant differences in terms of safety risk between yoga versus comparative exercise in participants of all ages.[29]

There are several limitations to the current research landscape including a small number of total randomized controlled trials (RCTs), high risk of bias, limited reporting on long-term effects, insufficient reporting of safety data, and significant heterogeneity in yoga techniques, duration, and frequency. Future research endeavors should focus on high-quality RCTs and standardization of yoga protocols. Nonetheless, the current research is promising and overall shows positive benefits for various symptom domains with no significant adverse effects.

Barriers to yoga practice for people with schizophrenia include accessibility and financial cost.[30] Financial barriers can be addressed within healthcare settings by creating low-cost yoga programs or enlisting insurance companies to fund minimally invasive and promising therapeutic yoga offered by trained health care professionals that teach yoga specifically to those with psychotic disorders. For patients with schizophrenia, healthcare professionals cannot just refer them to "yoga" in the community. Community setting yoga classes have limitations, and general yoga practitioners may lack knowledge of the mental health needs of the patient. Yoga therapists should be certified and have mental healthcare experience. Education and training specific to yoga practitioners in health care settings should be widely disseminated.

31.5.2 Diet and Nutrition

A scoping review examined dietary patterns associated with psychosis and diets that can serve as an intervention for psychopathology. Oxidative stress, methylation cycle, inflammation, food sensitivity, essential amino acid and fatty acid deficiency, gut microbiome, blood sugar dysregulation, and vitamin and mineral insufficiency are all possible mechanisms linking diet and psychosis.[31]

Observational studies indicate an association of higher levels of carbohydrate intake among people with psychosis, which may be mediated by reactive hypoglycemia. Theoretically, ketogenic diets (low carbohydrate and high fat) may exert effects by impacting abnormalities in glucose tolerance and insulin resistance that have been associated with the pathogenesis of psychosis, leading to improvement in psychiatric symptoms.[32] However, currently, there are no published randomized control trials on the efficacy and safety of ketogenic diets on schizophrenia outcomes.

There is increasing recognition that a bidirectional communication exists between the brain and the gut through neural, hormonal, and immunological routes. Preliminary data suggest that people with schizophrenia may have differences in gut microbiome composition,[31] as well as alterations in gut immune system function.[33] Prebiotics, probiotics, and avoidance of foods that contribute to dysbiosis may have therapeutic relevance.[31] Patients with schizophrenia are three to four times more likely to have celiac disease and also have higher levels of antigliadin antibody levels, indicative of gluten sensitivity, compared to the general population.[8,9] There are some studies demonstrating the benefits of a gluten-free diet in patients with SSD. A systematic review examined nine studies evaluating outcomes in SSD after the implementation of a gluten-free diet, and six of the nine studies showed beneficial effects.[11] There may be a specific subset of patients with schizophrenia with gluten sensitivity who may benefit most from gluten-free diets.[17]

Increasing the intake of fruits and vegetables can have a positive impact on mental health through the provision of nutrients such as fiber, vitamins, minerals, and phytonutrients. Fiber may exert an effect by decreasing reactive hypoglycemia and modifying gut microbiome. Higher vegetable intake is also associated with reduced cardiovascular risk and all-cause mortality.[31]

Several specific nutraceuticals have been studied. Randomized trials have examined the impact of N-Acetyl Cysteine (NAC) compared to placebo, and found that NAC (1 gram orally twice daily) improved clinical global impression, Positive and Negative Syndrome Scale (PANSS), negative symptoms with moderate effect sizes over 24 weeks, and after 4 weeks of discontinuation, symptoms returned to baseline levels.[12] Similar findings were reported by Farokhnia et al., 2013 and Breier et al., 2018, who evaluated the effects of NAC (3600 mg/day) in a 52-week, double-blind placebo-controlled trial in early phase SSD and found improvement in PANSS total, negative and disorganized thought but not in positive and cognitive symptoms, and preliminary analysis showed an increase in cortical thickness.[34]

Omega-3 fatty acids have also been studied extensively due to their potential neuroprotective effects. There are three main omega-3 fatty acids: alpha-linolenic acid (ALA) which is found mainly in plant oils and the long-chain omega-3 fatty acids, eicosapentaenoic acid (EPA), and docosahexaenoic acid (DHA). EPA and DHA are found in seaweed and seafood; since EPA and DHA cannot be synthesized de novo by humans, supplementation is required. Essential polyunsaturated fatty acids are important components of the phospholipids that comprise specialized cell membranes which play a central role in the physiology and function of the brain.[9] Abnormal polyunsaturated fatty acid metabolism may be one of many factors involved in the development of schizophrenia.[21] Studies have shown that omega-3 polyunsaturated fatty acid supplementation (700 mg EPA and 480 mg DHA) reduced the conversion rate to psychosis and improved both positive and negative symptoms and global functions in adolescents at ultra-high risk for psychosis.[35,36] Another study also showed improvement in general psychopathology, depressive symptoms, level of functioning, and clinical global impression in first-episode psychosis patients after 6 months of supplementation with 2.2 g per day of EPA and DHA (compared to olive oil placebo in a randomized double-blind trial).[37] Supplementation with omega-3 fatty acids may demonstrate greater efficacy in clinical high-risk or first-episode psychosis populations,[38] in those with lower baseline levels of polyunsaturated fatty acids,[21] or those who have more severe symptomatology.[39]

A systematic review showed that omega-3 fatty acids did not induce serious adverse effects and that supplementation with EPA and DHA up to 5g/day is not dangerous for the general population.[40] Another systematic review showed that the ratio of EPA to DHA did not influence treatment outcomes.[39] Only supplements containing EPA at a dosage of more than 1g/day had significant beneficial effects on the psychopathology of schizophrenia.[39] There is also evidence that omega-3 fatty acids can reduce markers of metabolic syndrome.[38] Firth et al., 2017 conducted a meta-analysis and found that high dose B vitamins have evidence in reducing residual symptoms in people with schizophrenia; however, they noted significant heterogeneity among study findings.[3] There is also preliminary interest in nutraceuticals such as vitamin C for symptomatic improvement, and vitamin D deficiency as a risk factor for schizophrenia;[9,42] however, further research is needed. Furthermore, dietary supplements are not regulated in many countries and lack data on safety, efficacy, and effective dose and interactions, and are administered in heterogenous forms, and thus must be administered under a medical professional's supervision.

Evidence-informed dietary recommendations for individuals with psychotic disorders include: (1) reduction of refined carbohydrates and processed/packaged foods, (2) increased consumption of fruits and vegetables, (3) adequate dietary sources of fiber and omega-3 fatty acids, and (4) sufficient intake of vitamin B12, vitamin B6, folate, zinc, and protein. Dietary patterns to consider include whole foods diets such as the Mediterranean diet, or a therapeutic trial of a gluten-free or ketogenic diet.[31]

Though routine metabolic screening is part of the standard of care for patients with schizophrenia; few receive appropriate screening and care. Collaborations must occur among psychiatrists, primary care physicians, dieticians, and other multidisciplinary team members. Antipsychotics are also associated with weight gain, increasing appetite via antagonism of histamine H1 and serotonin 2C, and metabolic symptoms. Providers should consider strategies such as utilizing medications with lower risk for metabolic derangement first line, treating hyperlipidemia with lipid-lowering agents, offering metformin preventive therapy when indicated, and providing tailored nutrition counseling.

Integrating nutrition-focused professions into the multidisciplinary team can provide opportunities to deliver dietary interventions to this population. If food insecurity is present, educate about local food programs, emergency food relief programs, and capacity building.

31.5.3 EXERCISE

Several recent meta-analyses have shown that physical activity can significantly improve positive symptoms, negative symptoms, and social functioning, as well as cardiorespiratory fitness and metabolic health in patients with schizophrenia.[14,43,44] The proposed mechanisms of action of exercise include biochemical changes such as an increase in endorphins, changes in stress reactivity via the hypothalamus-pituitary-adrenal (HPA) axis, physiological changes such as improved cardiovascular function, and psychological changes such as increased sense of autonomy, self-efficacy, and coping. Exercise-induced neurogenesis and synaptic proliferation may be another mechanism by which exercise is helpful for people with schizophrenia. The hippocampus is a primary site of neurogenesis and a region with structural and functional abnormalities in psychosis.[45] Studies have shown that exercise increases hippocampal volume[46,47] and metabolism in both people with schizophrenia as well as healthy controls. Further, exercise increases gray matter volume and cortical thickness, [48] and white matter integrity.[49] Physical exercise upregulates brain neurotrophic factors that stimulate neoneurogenesis and synaptic plasticity which results in a partial reversal of regional volume loss in critical areas of the brain impacted by schizophrenia.[50] The onset of psychosis is associated with progressive neurodegeneration, and exercise may potentially reverse neurodegeneration and has the potential for neuroprotection and prevention of progression of the illness.

Furthermore, exercise may target negative and cognitive symptoms; both of which are not adequately treated by antipsychotic medication and for which there are limited other available treatment options, yet significant symptom burden. Firth et al., 2016 found that exercise was particularly beneficial in improving social cognition, working memory, and attention in a dose-dependent manner.[50] It has been theorized that this may be mediated through upregulation of brain-derived neurotrophic factor (BDNF), a family of proteins that promote growth and differentiation and maintenance of neurons, leading to increased neurogenesis and cognitive performance. Another systematic review showed that aerobic exercise had a small but statistically significant beneficial effect on negative symptoms.[51] A 12-week study involving 17 patients with SSD delivering moderate-intensity aerobic and weight-bearing exercise showed a decrease in symptom severity, improvement in social functioning, improvement in depression scores, and an increase in hippocampal volume.[46] A recent systematic review examining 22 studies showed that all exercise training modalities (including aerobic training, resistance training, and combined aerobic and resistance training) revealed significant effects on body mass index, maximal/peak oxygen consumption, body weight, PANSS negative scores, and Scale for the Assessment of Negative Symptoms (SANS) total scores.[52]

In people with schizophrenia, the presence of metabolic syndrome and metabolic risk factors is associated with significantly reduced aerobic fitness.[5] Exercise is capable of improving cardiorespiratory fitness (CRF) and thereby reducing risk factors for cardiovascular disease (CVD) and associated mortality.[6] A systematic review by Firth et al., 2015 noted that exercise interventions did not yield consistent reductions in body weight and body mass index (BMI); however, waist circumference reduction was noted, which may be a more valuable measure of metabolic health.[29] Of 11 studies measuring cardiovascular fitness and/or exercise capacity, 10 reported significant improvement from exercise.[29] There is evidence that the addition of a dietary intervention in conjunction with exercise may improve weight-related outcomes in people with schizophrenia.[45]

In one study, participants with schizophrenia spectrum disorder were most commonly motivated to exercise for "self-image." These individuals reported improved global well-being, depression, anxiety, energy, motivation, and cognition after individual exercise sessions.[44]

Exercise has clear neurotrophic effects and benefits for mental and physical health. It is an intervention with few risks, requires no equipment, and is low-cost. Additionally, it can be made available to individuals who are apprehensive about medications, or as an adjunct to minimize other modes of therapy, or it can work to address side effects related to medications such as weight gain. There is an urgent need to better integrate physical activity interventions into mental health settings.

Physical activity may be challenging for those with SSD due to barriers such as negative symptoms including lack of motivation, cognitive symptoms, cardiometabolic comorbidities, medication side effects, lack of support, lack of knowledge about the benefits of physical activity, and low self-efficacy.[44] Socioeconomic factors such as limited finances, poor transport and access to resources, and social isolation are also potential barriers.

For exercise recommendations, consider factors such as the patient's interests, goals, and current capacity. Guidelines suggest 150 minutes of moderate or 75 minutes of vigorous aerobic exercise + 2 strength training sessions/week for healthy adults. Allowing individuals to choose their type of physical activity may help with both the initiation and continuation of exercise for individuals over time, and the optimal modality is simply the type of activity that the individual will engage in regularly. Both aerobic and resistance exercises act together on the brain through independent yet complementary neural mechanisms.[17] Research shows that the dose of physical activity is more important than the modality and noted that benefits were prominent in those who were engaged in approximately 90 minutes or more per week of moderate to vigorous physical activity.[29] Tailoring exercise programs based on the individual's physical fitness, physical activity history, goals, level of motivation, and specific needs increases adherence and engagement in the program. Follow-up assessments should focus on adherence to the plan, highlighting changes in core symptoms, as well as sleep, appetite, energy, well-being, and general health effects. Further, goals should be modified and refined as needed, and triggers to lapse should be identified and addressed.

One of the most important predictors of dropping out from exercise was the qualifications of the person providing the physical activity intervention, and interventions that were being supervised by qualified professionals such as exercise physiologists, physical therapists, and yoga instructors had a much better outcome. Exercise professionals are ideally positioned to provide safe, evidence-based exercise interventions.[53] Other factors that reduced dropout rate of exercise programs included supervision, motivation components, rewards, incorporation of motivational interviewing techniques, and incorporation of video games.[53] Utilizing technology including mobile apps may also be a helpful avenue to increase engagement and sustainability of exercise programs. Intervention at the earliest stages of psychosis can help prevent weight gain and other metabolic dysregulation typically seen at the commencement of antipsychotic medication. Collaboration between mental health and allied health team members is important; family and carers may be valuable to provide holistic interventions. Importantly, all interventions should apply recovery-oriented practices and incorporate stakeholder feedback for sustainability. Programs should work to optimize long-term effectiveness and cost-effectiveness. Principles of behavior-change strategies can be helpful, including motivational interviewing and behavior-change counseling.[17] The Society of Behavioral Medicine and the American College of Sports Medicine advocate for more funding to train qualified professionals to deliver physical activity, embedding these services within mental health programs, more reimbursement strategies for providers, and adequate length and face-to-face contact of programs.[17] In addition to more comprehensive clinical services, additional research is needed to provide further evidence regarding the most effective treatment approaches, including further data on modality, frequency, and duration, including longer-term follow-up, and the efficacy of exercise at different stages of disease progression.[54] Efforts should also be made to engage hard-to-reach populations such as older individuals and racial minorities in clinical programming and research endeavors[17] and to continue to address barriers to engaging in exercise including both disease-related factors as well as socio-economic factors and issues related to health care delivery models.

31.5.4 OTHER INTERVENTIONS

Jon Kabat Zinn is credited with introducing mindfulness to Western cultures and has conceptualized it as "paying attention in a particular way: on purpose, in the present moment, and non-judgmentally." A systematic review and meta-analysis including 10 studies with 1094 participants showed that mindfulness-based interventions combined with treatment as usual are effective when compared to treatment as usual control groups and active treatment control groups. There were moderate to large effects in reducing overall symptomatology and small to moderate effects in reducing both positive and negative symptoms; some studies showed benefit for improving functioning level and awareness of the illness, and there were no harmful effects noted in this analysis.[55]Another systematic review and meta-analysis showed that mindfulness-based interventions decreased psychotic symptoms immediately post-intervention and also had an effect on negative symptoms both immediately post-intervention as well as at 3- to 6-month follow-up.[56]

Regular sleep-wake cycles, regular meals, and physical and social activity can help with sleep. A modified CBT insomnia protocol has been developed for people with schizophrenia.[57] Some antipsychotic medications can improve sleep by reducing the time to fall asleep and increasing total sleep time. However, some medications like clozapine may prolong sleep duration significantly (12-14 hours). Antipsychotics can also induce restless leg syndrome and periodic limb movement disorder as well as parasomnias such as sleepwalking. Obstructive sleep apnea (OSA) is observed in a greater proportion of people with schizophrenia compared to the general population. Weight gain is the strongest link to OSA, and addressing contributing lifestyle factors and medications can be helpful, as well as following the standard of care to treat OSA and implementing screening for OSA and sleep disorders more widely.[58]

Approximately 50% of patients with schizophrenia develop a substance use disorder in their lifetime,[59] and 60 to 90% endorse cigarette smoking.[60] Cigarette smoking contributes to cardiovascular morbidity and mortality and is a modifiable risk factor. People who use cannabis appear to develop psychosis 2.7 years earlier on average than those who do not.[60] Programs that coordinate pharmacotherapy, psychosocial treatment, and substance abuse counseling into a single package with consideration of motivation for change, comprehensive services, and a long term perspective are more likely to achieve good treatment outcomes.[59]

31.6 CONCLUSION

Schizophrenia spectrum disorders (SSD) are characterized by positive symptoms, negative symptoms, as well as neurocognitive deficits. Individuals with schizophrenia have high rates of cardiometabolic disease leading to a reduced life expectancy of up to ten to twenty years compared to the general population. There is a need for low-cost, accessible, and patient-centered treatments that reduce negative symptoms and cognitive deficits, increase quality of life, promote functional recovery, and improve the physical health of people with SSD to reduce morbidity and mortality. Interventions as part of the field of lifestyle psychiatry include yoga, diet and nutrition, exercise, mindfulness and meditation, sleep management, and addressing substance use. These interventions have evidence for reducing cardiometabolic risk factors, improving quality of life and functional outcomes, and addressing positive, negative, and cognitive symptoms in people with schizophrenia spectrum disorders, with relatively low risk of adverse effects. Clinicians should consider integrating these interventions into routine clinical practice as well as broader health policy and work to address barriers.

REFERENCES

1. Noordsy D. *Lifestyle Psychiatry*. American Psychiatric Association Publishing; 2019.
2. Dauwan M, Begemann MJH, Heringa SM, Sommer IE. Exercise improves clinical symptoms, quality of life, global functioning, and depression in schizophrenia: A systematic review and meta-analysis. *Schizophr Bull.* 2016;42(3):588–599. doi:10.1093/schbul/sbv164
3. Firth J, Stubbs B, Sarris J, et al. The effects of vitamin and mineral supplementation on symptoms of schizophrenia: A systematic review and meta-analysis. *Psychol Med.* 2017;47(9):1515–1527. doi:10.1017/S0033291717000022
4. Ward PB, Firth J, Rosenbaum S, Samaras K, Stubbs B, Curtis J. Lifestyle interventions to reduce premature mortality in schizophrenia. *Lancet Psychiatry.* 2017;4(7):e14. doi:10.1016/S2215-0366(17)30235-3
5. Vancampfort D, Guelinkcx H, Probst M, et al. Associations between metabolic and aerobic fitness parameters in patients with schizophrenia. *J Nerv Ment Dis.* 2015; 203(1):23–27. doi:10.1097/NMD.0000000000000229
6. Schmitt A, Maurus I, Rossner MJ, et al. Effects of aerobic exercise on metabolic syndrome, cardiorespiratory fitness, and symptoms in schizophrenia include decreased mortality. *Front Psychiatry.* 2018;9. doi:10.3389/fpsyt.2018.00690
7. Brems C. *Ancient Wisdoms and Science of Yoga: A Companion for 200-Hour Yoga Teacher Training for Healthcare and Allied Healthcare Settings.* Santa Barbara, CA: Self Published. 2021
8. Porcelli B, Verdino V, Bossini L, Terzuoli L, Fagiolini A. Celiac and non-celiac gluten sensitivity: A review on the association with schizophrenia and mood disorders. *Auto Immun Highlights.* 2014;5(2):55–61. doi:10.1007/s13317-014-0064-0
9. Arroll MA, Wilder L, Neil J. Nutritional interventions for the adjunctive treatment of schizophrenia: A brief review. *Nutr J.* 2014;13(1):91. doi:10.1186/1475-2891-13-91
10. Davison KM, Ng E, Chandrasekera U, et al. Role of Nutrition in Mental Health Promotion and Prevention. Dietitians of Canada. 2012
11. Levinta A, Mukovozov I, Tsoutsoulas C. Use of a gluten-free diet in schizophrenia: A systematic review. *Adv Nutr.* 2018;9(6):824–832. doi:10.1093/advances/nmy056
12. Berk M, Copolov D, Dean O, et al. N-acetyl cysteine as a glutathione precursor for schizophrenia—A double-blind, randomized, placebo-controlled trial. *Biol Psychiatry.* 2008;64(5):361–368. doi:10.1016/j.biopsych.2008.03.004
13. Firth J, Cotter J, Elliott R, French P, Yung AR. A systematic review and meta-analysis of exercise interventions in schizophrenia patients. *Psychol Med.* 2015;45(7): 1343–1361. doi:10.1017/S0033291714003110
14. Balasubramaniam M, Telles S, Doraiswamy PM. Yoga on our minds: A systematic review of yoga for neuropsychiatric disorders. *Frontiers in Psychiatry.* 2012;3:117. doi:10.3389/fpsyt.2012.00117
15. Hatha Yoga for Depression_ Critical Review of the Evidence for Efficacy, Plausible Mechanisms of Action, and Directions for Future Research. 2010
16. Muehsam D, Lutgendorf S, Mills PJ, et al. The embodied mind: A review on functional genomic and neurological correlates of mind-body therapies. *Neuroscience and Biobehavioral Reviews.* 2017;73:165–181. doi:10.1016/j.neubiorev.2016.12.027

17. Pascoe MC, Bauer IE. A systematic review of randomised control trials on the effects of yoga on stress measures and mood. *Journal of Psychiatric Research*. 2015;68: 270–282. doi:10.1016/j.jpsychires.2015.07.013

18. Mehta UM, Gangadhar BN. Yoga: Balancing the excitation-inhibition equilibrium in psychiatric disorders. *Progress in Brain Research*. 2019;244:387–413. doi:10.1016/bs. pbr.2018.10.024

19. Govindaraj R, Naik SS, Mehta UM, Sharma M, Varambally S, Gangadhar BN. Yoga therapy for social cognition in schizophrenia: An experimental medicine-based randomized controlled trial. *Asian Journal of Psychiatry*. 2021;62:102731. doi:10.1016/j. ajp.2021.102731

20. Cramer H, Lauche R, Klose P, Langhorst J, Dobos G. Yoga for schizophrenia: A systematic review and meta-analysis. *BMC Psychiatry*. 2013;13(1):32. doi:10.1186/1471-244X-13-32

21. Hsu M, Huang Y, Ouyang W. Beneficial effects of omega-3 fatty acid supplementation in schizophrenia: Possible mechanisms. *Lipids Health Dis*. 2020;19(1). doi:10.1186/s12944-020-01337-0

22. Broderick J, Crumlish N, Waugh A, Vancampfort D. Yoga versus non-standard care for schizophrenia. *Cochrane Database Syst Rev*. 2017;9(9). doi:10.1002/14651858.CD012052.pub2

23. Broderick J, Knowles A, Chadwick J, Vancampfort D, Broderick J. Yoga versus standard care for schizophrenia. *Cochrane Database Syst Rev*. 2015;2015(10):CD010554. doi:10.1002/14651858.CD010554.pub2

24. Broderick J, Vancampfort D. Yoga as part of a package of care versus standard care for schizophrenia. *Cochrane Database Syst Rev*. 2017;9(9). doi:10.1002/14651858.CD012145.pub2

25. Cramer H, Langhorst J, Dobos G, Lauche R. Yoga for metabolic syndrome: A systematic review and meta-analysis. *Eur J Prev Cardiol*. 2016;23(18):1982–1993. doi:10.1177/2047487316665729

26. Hartley L, Dyakova M, Holmes J, et al. Yoga for the primary prevention of cardiovascular disease. *Cochrane Library*. 2014;2014(6):CD010072. doi:10.1002/14651858.CD010072.pub2

27. Chu P, Gotink RA, Yeh GY, Goldie SJ, Hunink MM. The effectiveness of yoga in modifying risk factors for cardiovascular disease and metabolic syndrome: A systematic review and meta-analysis of randomized controlled trials. *Eur J Prev Cardiol*. 2016;23(3):291–307. doi:10.1177/2047487314562741

28. Jayaram N, Varambally S, Behere RV, et al. Effect of yoga therapy on plasma oxytocin and facial emotion recognition deficits in patients of schizophrenia. *Indian J Psychiatry*. 2013;55(Suppl 3):409. doi:10.4103/0019-5545.116318

29. Cramer H, Ward L, Saper R, Fishbein D, Dobos G, Lauche R. The safety of yoga: A systematic review and meta-analysis of randomized controlled trials. *American Journal of Epidemiology*. 2015;182(4):281–293. doi:10.1093/aje/kwv071

30. Broderick J, Vancampfort D, Mockler D, et al. Yoga for schizophrenia. *Cochrane Database Syst Rev*. 2018;2018(12). doi:10.1002/14651858.CD013213

31. Aucoin M, LaChance L, Cooley K, Kidd S. Diet and psychosis: A scoping review. *Neuropsychobiology*. 2020;79(1):20–42. doi:10.1159/000493399

32. Sarnyai Z, Kraeuter AK, Palmer CM. Ketogenic diet for schizophrenia: Clinical implication. *Curr Opin Psychiatry*. 2019;32(5):394–401. doi:10.1097/YCO.0000000000000535

33. Patrono E, Svoboda J, Stuchlík A. Schizophrenia, the gut microbiota, and new opportunities from optogenetic manipulations of the gut-brain axis. *Behav Brain Funct*. 2021;17(1):7. doi:10.1186/s12993-021-00180-2

34. Breier A, Liffick E, Hummer TA, et al. Effects of 12-month, double-blind N-acetyl cysteine on symptoms, cognition and brain morphology in early phase schizophrenia spectrum disorders. *Schizophr Res*. 2018;199:395–402. doi:10.1016/j.schres.2018.03.012

35. Amminger GP, Schäfer MR, Papageorgiou K, et al. Long-chain omega-3 fatty acids for indicated prevention of psychotic disorders: A randomized, placebo-controlled trial. *Arch Gen Psychiatry.* 2010;67(2):146–154. doi:10.1001/archgenpsychiatry.2009.192

36. Amminger GP, Schäfer MR, Schlögelhofer M, Klier CM, McGorry PD. Longer-term outcome in the prevention of psychotic disorders by the Vienna omega-3 study. *Nature Communications.* 2015;6(1):7934. doi:10.1038/ncomms8934

37. Pawełczyk T, Grancow-Grabka M, Kotlicka-Antczak M, Trafalska E, Pawełczyk A. A randomized controlled study of the efficacy of six-month supplementation with concentrated fish oil rich in omega-3 polyunsaturated fatty acids in first episode schizophrenia. *J Psychiatr Res.* 2015;73:34–44. doi:10.1016/j.jpsychires.2015.11.013

38. Pawelczyk T, Grancow-Grabka M, Zurner N, Pawelczyk A. Omega-3 fatty acids reduce cardiometabolic risk in first-episode schizophrenia patients treated with antipsychotics: Findings from the OFFER randomized controlled study. *Schizophr Res.* 2021;230:61–68. doi:10.1016/j.schres.2021.02.012

39. Goh K, Chen C, Chen C-H, Lu M-L. Effects of omega-3 polyunsaturated fatty acids supplements on psychopathology and metabolic parameters in schizophrenia: A meta-analysis of randomized controlled trials. *J Psychopharmacol.* 2021;35(3):221–235.

40. Bozzatello P, Brignolo E, De Grandi E, Bellino S. Supplementation with omega-3 fatty acids in psychiatric disorders: A review of literature data. *J Clin Med.* 2016;5(8):67. doi:10.3390/jcm5080067

41. Firth J, Stubbs B, Sarris J, et al. The effects of vitamin and mineral supplementation on symptoms of schizophrenia: A systematic review and meta-analysis. *Psychological Medicine.* 2017;47(9):1515–1527. doi:10.1017/S0033291717000022

42. Brown HE, Roffman JL. Vitamin supplementation in the treatment of schizophrenia. *CNS Drugs.* 2014;28(7):611–622. doi:10.1007/s40263-014-0172-4

43. Vancampfort D, Vansteelandt K, Scheewe T, et al. Yoga in schizophrenia: A systematic review of randomised controlled trials. *Acta Psychiatrica Scandinavica.* 2012;126(1):12–20. doi:10.1111/j.1600-0447.2012.01865.x

44. Ho PA, Dahle DN, Noordsy DL. Why do people with schizophrenia exercise? A mixed methods analysis among community dwelling regular exercisers. *Front Psychiatry.* 2018;9:596. doi:10.3389/fpsyt.2018.00596

45. Mittal VA, Vargas T, Juston Osborne K, et al. Exercise treatments for psychosis: A review. *Curr Treat Options Psych.* 2017;4(2):152–166. doi:10.1007/s40501-017-0112-2

46. Woodward ML, Gicas KM, Warburton DE, et al. Hippocampal volume and vasculature before and after exercise in treatment-resistant schizophrenia. *Schizophr Res.* 2018;202:158–165. doi:10.1016/j.schres.2018.06.054

47. Pajonk F, Wobrock T, Gruber O, et al. Hippocampal plasticity in response to exercise in schizophrenia. *Arch Gen Psychiatry.* 2010;67(2):133–143. doi:10.1001/archgenpsychiatry.2009.193

48. Scheewe TW, Backx FJG, Takken T, et al. Exercise therapy improves mental and physical health in schizophrenia: A randomised controlled trial. *Acta Psychiatr Scand.* 2013;127(6):464–473. doi:10.1111/acps.12029

49. Firth J, Cotter J, Elliott R, French P, Yung AR. A systematic review and meta-analysis of exercise interventions in schizophrenia patients. *Psychological Medicine.* 2015;45(7):1343–1361. doi:10.1017/S0033291714003110

50. Firth J, Stubbs B, Rosenbaum S, et al. Aerobic exercise improves cognitive functioning in people with schizophrenia: A systematic review and meta-analysis. *Schizophr Bull.* 2017;43(3). doi:10.1093/schbul/sbw115

51. Sabe M, Kaiser S, Sentissi O. Physical exercise for negative symptoms of schizophrenia: Systematic review of randomized controlled trials and meta-analysis. *Gen Hosp Psychiatry.* 2020;62:13–20. doi:10.1016/j.genhosppsych.2019.11.002

52. Bredin SSD, Kaufman KL, Chow MI, et al. Effects of aerobic, resistance, and combined exercise training on psychiatric symptom severity and related health measures

in adults living with schizophrenia: A systematic review and meta-analysis. *Front Cardiovasc Med.* 2022;8. doi:10.3389/fcvm.2021.753117

53. Vancampfort D, Rosenbaum S, Schuch FB, Ward PB, Probst M, Stubbs B. Prevalence and predictors of treatment dropout from physical activity interventions in schizophrenia: a meta-analysis. *Gen Hosp Psychiatry.* 2016;39:15. doi:10.1016/j.genhosppsych.2015.11.008

54. Girdler SJ, Confino JE, Woesner ME. Exercise as a treatment for schizophrenia: A review. *Psychopharmacol Bull.* 2019;49(1):56–69.

55. Hodann-Caudevilla RM, Díaz-Silveira C, Burgos-Julián FA, Santed MA. Mindfulness-based interventions for people with schizophrenia: A systematic review and meta-analysis. *Int J Environ Res Public Health.* 2020;17(13):4690. doi:10.3390/ijerph17134690

56. Liu Y, Li I, Hsiao F. Effectiveness of mindfulness-based intervention on psychotic symptoms for patients with schizophrenia: A meta-analysis of randomized controlled trials. *J Adv Nurs.* 2021;77(6):2565. doi:10.1111/jan.14750

57. Freeman D, Waite F, Startup H, et al. Efficacy of cognitive behavioural therapy for sleep improvement in patients with persistent delusions and hallucinations (BEST): a prospective, assessor-blind, randomised controlled pilot trial. Lancet Psychiatry. 2015;2(11):975-983. doi:10.1016/S2215-0366(15)00314-4

58. Kaskie RE, Graziano B, Ferrarelli F. Schizophrenia and sleep disorders: Links, risks, and management challenges. *Nat Sci Sleep.* 2017;9:227–239. doi:10.2147/NSS.S121076

59. Green AI, Drake RE, Brunette MF, Noordsy DL. Schizophrenia and co-occurring substance use disorder. *Am J Psychiatry.* 2007;164(3):402–408. doi:10.1176/ajp.2007.164.3.402

60. Crockford D, Addington D. Canadian Schizophrenia guidelines: Schizophrenia and other psychotic disorders with coexisting substance use disorders. *Can J Psychiatry.* 2017;62(9):624–634. doi:10.1177/0706743717720196

Section V

Specific Populations

32 Pediatric Mental and Physical Health

Wendi Waits, MD and Megan Marumoto, MD

KEY POINTS

- Environmental and societal factors have contributed to the emergence of chronic diseases at younger and younger ages.
- By 2021, the rates of depression and anxiety symptoms in youth had doubled compared to pre-pandemic levels, triggering the United States Surgeon General to release a 53-page advisory on the state of Youth Mental Health in America.
- Declining physical and mental health in pediatric populations is deepening our national healthcare crisis and threatening our national security.

Lifestyle Medicine is the practice of applying evidence-based interventions proven to prevent, treat, and reverse chronic disease. These interventions are critically important in young people, who – for the most part – have yet to develop the chronic, disabling mental and physical illnesses that afflict many adults and strain the healthcare system. Children have traditionally been the most healthy subset of our population, bringing happy, playful, and active energy to their families and communities. However, over the past few decades, environmental and societal factors have contributed to the emergence of chronic diseases at younger and younger ages. We have seen a rise in the rates of physical ailments in young people that were previously only seen in older populations, including obesity, type 2 diabetes, hypertension, fatty liver, and colorectal cancers.[1–5] As of 2018, nearly 60% of young people were ineligible to join the military due to health reasons, obesity being the primary reason in 31% of them.[6] This was an increase from 28% in 2013, and is expected to be even higher in today's post-pandemic era.[7] Unfortunately, obesity and its related health conditions are not the only problems increasing among children. In 2011, the Center for Disease Control reported that 1 in 5 American youth were also experiencing anxiety or depression.[8] By 2021, the rates of depression and anxiety symptoms in youth had doubled compared to pre-pandemic levels,[9] triggering the United States Surgeon General to release a 53-page advisory on the state of Youth Mental Health in America in December 2021.[10] We are facing a clear physical and mental health crisis in our pediatric population and cannot afford to forget about kids when it comes to Lifestyle Medicine.

Poor physical health in children contributes to poor mental health. This can happen physiologically, such as when low-nutrient, additive-heavy diets starve the body of beneficial nutrients and contribute to inflammation, concentration problems, and mood symptoms. Or it can happen indirectly, such as when lack of sleep, exercise, and good nutrition contribute to conditions such as acne, weight gain, and other

DOI: 10.1201/b22810-37

undesirable physical issues that can upset the child and contribute to peer ridicule. Nutrients in food become the building blocks of nerves, brain tissue, and glands. When nutrients are in low supply, kids' bodies cannot create a sufficient supply of the neurochemicals that keep them happy and mentally well-adjusted. Happiness, confidence, and resilience may give way to anxiety, loneliness, sadness, and despair, reducing overall quality of life. And children are less able than adults to control their diet and daily routines. They cannot make healthy choices 100% of the time, and their caregivers may be prevented from doing so by financial and logistical limitations.

Additionally, unlike adults, children rarely experience immediate consequences when they make poor health choices. Symptoms like gastric distress, bloating, and lethargy, which serve as negative reinforcers to adults who have overindulged, occur uncommonly in children, who can feel perfectly fine after a lunch of pizza, cake, and soda. Developmentally, children often feel immortal and their bodies recover easily from injury and illness. Incentivizing a child to eat healthy, be physically active, and socialize can be difficult unless you make it fun.

So while adults–motivated by the discomfort of their ailments and their fear of death–may be able to muscle through a complete reboot of their lifestyle, children will naturally be less motivated to make healthy lifestyle choices. The primary goal with children may look more like a subtle shift than a dramatic change. We should aspire to keep moving their lifestyle dial in the right direction by helping their parents and teachers create an environment and daily routine that support children's overall health and reduce their risk for chronic disease down the road.

The following vignettes are based on actual cases in which lifestyle interventions improved behavioral symptoms in children and adolescents.

32.1   CASE 1

An adolescent girl presented with significant depressive symptoms and suicidal ideation. After a thorough evaluation, including education on the benefits of diet and lifestyle interventions, she agreed to try a Mediterranean Diet. Over the next two weeks, she shifted her diet to include more vegetables, whole grains, fish, and healthy fats. She reported that her depressive symptoms were significantly improved and her suicidal thoughts had resolved.

32.2   CASE 2

A young boy presented with generalized anxiety, as well as separation anxiety and intermittent panic attacks. He scored in the severe range on the Screen for Child Anxiety Related Disorders (SCARED). On evaluation, he was consuming an extreme amount of apple juice, as well as many whole apples each day. His psychiatrist recommended that he stop drinking apple juice in order to decrease the level of sugar in his diet. With the assistance of his parents, the boy completely eliminated apple juice from his diet, leading to a dramatic reduction in his overall anxiety.

32.3 CASE 3

An adolescent girl presented with profound depression, suicidal thinking, panic attacks, fatigue, and severe nausea that had contributed to a 30-pound weight loss. She had been seeing a therapist regularly and had tried several antidepressants without benefit. Upon evaluation, she admitted to binge drinking at large social events and smoking marijuana daily for three to four months. Motivational interviewing and supportive psychotherapy inspired the patient to abstain from all substances. Within two months, her depression, anxiety, and nausea had all improved to the point that she no longer needed medications or psychiatric treatment.

32.4 PHYSICAL ACTIVITY

Physical activity has been strongly correlated with improving mood, improving anxiety, and decreasing suicidal ideation in adults as well as adolescents, and vigorous physical activity has been shown to be particularly beneficial.[11-17] Increased physical activity in children has also been shown to improve attention, cognitive flexibility (i.e., multi-tasking), decision-making, and processing speed.[18-20] Children and adolescents who are active are therefore more likely to be attentive, resilient, successful, and happy than those who are sedentary. The US Physical Activity Guidelines for Americans (see Table 32.1) provides specific guidance regarding the duration and types of activities most likely to benefit youth mental health.

32.5 NUTRITION

Perhaps more than any other lifestyle factor, children's nutrition is regulated almost entirely by their caregivers, who buy groceries, prepare food, and pay for meals outside the home. It is therefore paramount for caregivers to not only understand why it is important for children to eat healthy (ideally a whole-food, plant-based diet[23]),

---

TABLE 32.1

US Physical Activity Guidance for Children

Age	Guidance[21,22]	Examples
3–5 years	Should be physically active throughout the day, ideally for 3 hours daily. Adult caregivers should encourage active play that includes a variety of activity types.	Going to the playground, walking the dog, throwing/kicking balls, riding a tricycle or bicycle, hopping, skipping, jumping, dance party, tumbling, playing "clean-up," etc.
6–17 years	Moderate to vigorous activity for 60 minutes or more per day. This should include vigorous activity 3 days/week, muscle-strengthening activity 3 days/week, and bone-strengthening activity 3 days/week.	Outdoor games, dancing, hiking, running, biking, swimming, gymnastics, sports, exercise classes, weights (in older kids), etc.

TABLE 32.2

Nutrition Guidance for Children

Age	Guidance[29,30]	Notes
4–6 months	Consider introducing solids if child's healthcare provider agrees. Start with bitter greens (expect gagging and faces!), then add a rainbow of fruits, vegetables, and iron-fortified, whole-grain baby cereal.	Avoid honey, sugared beverages (including fruit juice), nuts, grapes, and other choking hazards
1–2 years	As child starts to eat solid foods, ensure their diet includes plenty of vegetables, fruits, and healthy grains.	Keep prepped finger foods handy to simplify meal creation. Ideas include oatmeal, rice, steamed broccoli, chickpeas, kidney beans, pitted dates, and raspberries.
3–5 years	Identify plant-based foods your kids enjoy and serve them more often. Make meal menus and stick to them. Apple slices, grapes, celery with peanut butter, bean burritos, soups, and chia pudding are some ideas.	Children will want to eat what they see adults eating, so adopt healthy eating habits, including fresh, non-processed snacks low in fat and sugar.
6–12 years	Introduce kids to the Lifestyle Medicine plate, create games to challenge their knowledge and spark creativity, and have them help with food prep and cooking.	These years are absolutely critical to establish good habits for adolescence and early adulthood.
13–18 years	Prepare as many meals at home as possible and aim for a colorful plate of predominately plant-based foods. Use herbs and spices generously and introduce ethnic meals.	Healthy eating habits will give teens more energy, better skin, a more stable mood, and faster healing from injuries.

but also how to serve up the best food possible (see Table 32.2). It also appears to be important for parents to make the same dietary changes themselves that they desire for their children.[24] While many recent studies about the cognitive and psychological benefits of healthy eating have focused on adult populations, several studies in adolescents from around the world have also demonstrated a clear relationship between healthy diets, fewer depressive symptoms, and better mental health.[25–28]

32.6 SLEEP

Better sleep health in children and teens has been associated with fewer depressive and anxiety symptoms, cognitive problems, physical complaints, and social problems related to friends and family,[31] as well as better academic performance [32,33] and fewer attention-deficit/hyperactivity disorder (ADHD) symptoms in children with ADHD.[34] Insufficient sleep has also been recently found to contribute to suicidal ideation in high-risk adolescents.[35] For these reasons, maximizing sleep should be a key priority for pediatric clinicians (see Table 32.3).

TABLE 32.3
Sleep Guidance for Children

Age	Guidance[36,37]	Notes
4–12 months	Should sleep 12–16 hours per 24 hours (including naps)	Child should sleep in nearly empty crib with minimal blankets, pillows, etc. Keep room dark and temperature comfortable. Use low, warm lights during feeding times.
1–2 years	Should sleep 11-14 hours per 24 hours (including naps)	Child should sleep in own crib/bed. Put child to sleep as soon as they appear tired. Do not respond immediately to crying as it will often stop within a few minutes.
3–5 years	Should sleep 10–13 hours per 24 hours (including naps)	Child should sleep in own bed. Avoid screen devices. Establish bedtime routine (e.g. brush, book, bed) and consistent sleep/wake times.
6–12 years	Should sleep 9–12 hours per 24 hours	Too little sleep can contribute to problems with attention, behavior, learning, and emotional regulation. Too much sleep can contribute to mental health problems.
13–18 years	Should sleep 8–10 hours per 24 hours	Insufficient sleep is associated with increased risk of self-harm and suicide attempts.

32.7   SOCIAL CONNECTEDNESS

The term connectedness has different meanings depending on the age of the child in question. In infants and toddlers, connectedness refers to the strength of the bond between the child and their caregiver(s). As children enter elementary school and beyond, connectedness refers to their sense of belonging, within their family, their peer group, and their community. Prominent twentieth-century researchers demonstrated that children's connections to others are critical for normal growth and development, particularly their connection to a primary caregiver from 6-24 months of age.[38] Failure of a child to securely attach with a caregiver during this time period can lead to anxiety disorders and other problems later in childhood.[39] Similarly, adolescents with low levels of social and family connectedness are more likely to experience emotional distress and suicidal ideation as adults.[40] In adulthood, loneliness has been associated with a 26% increase in the risk of premature mortality.[41] Conversely, adults with strong social connections have been found to have a 50% greater likelihood of survival.[42] Equipping children with the self-confidence and social skills that will become necessary for them to effectively connect with others as adults is therefore a paramount task for caregivers (see Table 32.4).

32.8   STRESS MANAGEMENT

Life in the 21st century is busy. Children, teens, and adults are exposed to more sources of stress now than ever before. The stress management suggestions in Table 32.5 are intended primarily for caregivers. However, there is a lot that young people, especially teens, can learn to do on their own to decrease stress. Staying connected to positive peers and limiting exposure to negativity, such as

TABLE 32.4
Social Guidance for Children

Age	Guidance	Notes
Infancy	Cuddle, hold, and otherwise maximize physical closeness and skin-to-skin contact with the child. Attend to their cries to ensure feeding and toileting needs are met.	Responding quickly to distressed infants will reassure them of their safety and improve their ability to self-soothe over time.
Pre-school	Provide reassurance and connect with them through play. Bath and bedtime games are important. Encourage social connections by scheduling play dates.	Preschoolers are still developing their sense of security, so family support remains important as children begin to meet other children.
Elem. School	Create fun family memories whenever possible. Support and encourage the child's participation in school events, parties, sleepovers, sports, scouts, Sunday school, etc. Take reports of bullying or ostracization seriously.	Allow child to socialize with different groups in different venues. Gentle encouragement may be necessary, but children should not be forced to participate in activities they don't enjoy.
Middle School	Expect shifting friendships and alliances. Permit children to define their preferred social activities, but be attuned to signs of peer rejection, depression, or severe anxiety. Remain available in case child wants to talk.	Puberty heightens social insecurities in both genders. Successful development requires children to learn how to eventually navigate peer interactions on their own.
High School	Support the child's choice of friends and activities as long as they are safe and supportive. Negotiate ground rules with child that will permit them to attend social events with increasing degrees of autonomy.	Adolescents should be seeking out ways to connect with peers. Failure to connect to peers in meaningful ways could be a concerning sign necessitating mental health evaluation.

abusive peers, bullies, and social media, will go a long way to decreasing stress and improving emotional resilience. There is significant evidence that using social media, especially if extensive, obsessional, or passive (i.e., observing and not posting), can contribute to low self-esteem, depression, and suicidal ideation.[43] Youth identifying as female, as well as lesbian, gay, bisexual, transexual, and questioning (LGBTQ) youth are particularly susceptible to negative outcomes.[44]

32.9 SUBSTANCE USE

Experimentation with substances is common among youth, especially among adolescents,[46] and addressing this problem clinically can be difficult since young people have a limited appreciation of their own mortality and often engage in impulsive and risky behaviors. Substance use in children and adolescents has been associated with low grades, higher rates of school absence, social problems, legal problems, physical illnesses, unprotected and/or non-consensual sexual activity,

TABLE 32.5

Stress Management Guidance for Children

Age	Guidance[45]	Notes
Pre-school	Establish routines to help children learn self-regulation. Give them resources to reset themselves when they get overwhelmed. Think A-B-C (emotional Awareness, Breathing, and Calming).	Helpful tools may include emotion identification charts, breathing apps/sites (e.g., xhalr.com, Calm, Headspace), stuffed animals, blankies, calm corner, etc.
Elem. School	Emphasize physical play and social connectedness. Ensure downtime is a part of every day. Teach kids how to breathe when they're stressed and don't overload them with activities. Address any bullying with school staff.	Show kids it's okay to make mistakes and that you love them no matter what. Use outdoor games and toys to keep them active and playful.
Middle School	Consider providing a simple phone with basic texting/calling capability. Limit non-academic screen time to 2 hours/day and monitor content. Encourage social activities but don't pry, monitor for social withdrawal and intense anxiety.	Learn to ride the child's wave of emotions. Provide a listening ear or a hug when they seem to need it, but don't be offended if they back away or respond with hostility.
High School	Stay involved in your teen's life, at a distance if needed. Don't take hostility personally and show them you still care. Applaud successes, discipline without judgment, and catch them if they fall instead of criticizing their decision-making.	If necessary, consider negotiating a written contract with teen that sets expectations and consequences. Get involved at any sign of drug use, severe depression, or violence.

stunted physical development, physical and sexual violence, motor vehicle accidents, accidental injuries and death, concentration difficulties, suicide, homicide, and permanent changes in brain development.[47–50] Motivating children and teens to avoid using substances is challenging, but possible. Caregivers should try to minimize children's early exposure to substances and related paraphernalia. Institutions, such as schools, sports teams, and medical clinics, should provide children with continuous, age-appropriate education about the potential dangers of substance use (see Table 32.6).

32.10 CAFFEINE

It bears mentioning that caffeine is an often overlooked substance to which children can be especially sensitive. Several research studies on caffeine use in youth have found evidence of side effects such as hypertension, tachycardia, arrhythmias, chest pain, tremor, abdominal pain, headaches, hyperactivity, inattentiveness, anxiety, insomnia, increased stress, depression, and suicidal ideation.[51] Energy drinks have been cited as being particularly problematic since they are often marketed to young people, contain unregulated levels of caffeine, and can include high levels of sugar, vitamins, and energizing herbs, which collectively may contribute to additional problems such as obesity, tooth decay, seizures, and death.[52–54] For these reasons, Canada recommends limiting overall daily caffeine consumption to 45 mg in children ages 4-6, 62.5 mg in children ages 7-9, 85 mg in children ages 10-14,

TABLE 32.6
Risky Substance Use Guidance for Children

Age	Guidance	Notes
Pre-school	Avoid exposing children to second-hand smoke and remove substance-related paraphernalia from their environment. Abstain from substances or use them out of children's view.	Young children are highly curious about their environment and often explore it using their hands and mouth.
Elem. School	Same as above. Additionally, education about the dangers of substance use should begin in elementary school, using age-appropriate tools such as memorable testimonials, videos, activities, toys, etc.	The goal in elementary school is to deter children from experimenting with substances until they are cognitively able to appreciate the risks of doing so.
Middle School	Continue to educate children about the dangers of substance use. Engage your child in dialogue and remain inquisitive about their life even as they start to become more independent (and sometimes aloof).	Experimentation may begin in these years when children are able to access substances easily, i.e. drugs from older siblings, inhalants from the garage, etc.
High School	Establish a relationship with your teen that promotes disclosure and honesty. Be observant for changes in their appearance, performance, and mood. Give them the chance to self-report before looking through their room and personal effects.	Drug use can be a sign of underlying mental illness and a form of self-medication; don't forget to evaluate the reason behind the use. Some addictions will require regular urine drug testing and inspections.

and 2.5 mg per kg in older adolescents, and the American Academy of Pediatrics has stated that "caffeine and other stimulant substances contained in energy drinks have no place in the diet of children and adolescents."[45,55]

32.11 SUMMARY

Although children and adolescents do not typically share the same motivation and resources that compel adults to make health-promoting lifestyle changes, attending to important lifestyle factors early in children's development will equip them both emotionally and physically to successfully navigate adulthood. Caregivers, teachers, coaches, clinicians, and others have important roles in optimizing children's physical activity, nutrition, sleep, social connectedness, stress management, and use of substances. Staying healthy in today's world is not getting any easier; we owe it to our kids to give them the best chance possible at avoiding the chronic health conditions afflicting their parents and grandparents.

REFERENCES

1. Centers for Disease Control and Prevention National Center for Health Statistics. National Health and Nutrition Examination Survey 2017–March 2020 prepandemic data files—development of files and prevalence estimates for selected health outcomes. *Natl Health Stat Report.* 2021;158:1–14. https://stacks.cdc.gov/view/cdc/106273.

2. Divers J, Mayer-Davis EJ, Lawrence JM, et al. Trends in incidence of type 1 and type 2 diabetes among youths — selected counties and Indian reservations, United States, 2002–2015, *MMWR Morb Mortal Wkly Rep.* 2020;69(6):161–164.

3. Jackson SL, Zhang Z, Wiltz JL, et al. Hypertension among youths—United States, 2001–2016. *MMWR Morb Mortal Wkly Rep.* 2018;67:758–762.

4. Shaunak M, Byrne CD, Davis N, Afolabi P, Faust SN, Davies JH. Non-alcoholic fatty liver disease and childhood obesity. *Arch Dis Child.* 2021;106(1):3–8.

5. Siegel RL, Fedewa SA, Anderson WF, et al. Colorectal cancer incidence patterns in the United States, 1974–2013. *JNCI J Natl Cancer Inst.* 2017;109(8):djw322. https://www. ncbi.nlm.nih.gov/pmc/articles/PMC6059239/pdf/djw322.pdf.

6. Mission: Readiness. Ready, Willing, and Unable to Serve, 2017;2018 https://strongnation. s3.amazonaws.com/documents/484/389765e0-2500-49a2-9a67-5c4a090a215b. pdf?1539616379&inline;%20filename=%22Unhealthy%20and%20Unprepared% 20report.pdf%22.

7. Defense Advisory Committee on Women in the Services. The Target Population for Military Recruitment: Youth Eligible to Enlist Without a Waiver; 2016. https://dacowits. defense.gov/Portals/48/Documents/General%20Documents/RFI%20Docs/Sept2016/ JAMRS%20RFI%2014.pdf.

8. Centers for Disease Control and Prevention. Mental health surveillance among children— United States, 2005–2011. *MMWR Morb Mortal Wkly Rep.* 2013;62(Suppl 2);1–35. https://www.cdc.gov/mmwr/pdf/other/su6202.pdf.

9. Racine N, McArthur BA, Cooke JE, Eirich R, Zhu J, Madigan S. Global prevalence of depressive and anxiety symptoms in children and adolescents during COVID-19: A meta-analysis. *JAMA Pediatrics.* 2021;175(11):1142–1150.

10. U.S. Department of Health and Human Services. Protecting Youth Mental Health: The U.S. Surgeon General's Advisory; 2021. https://www.hhs.gov/sites/default/files/ surgeon-general-youth-mental-health-advisory.pdf

11. Chekroud SR, Gueorguieva R, Zheutlin AB, et al. Association between physical exercise and mental health in 1·2 million individuals in the USA between 2011 and 2015: A cross-sectional study. *Lancet Psychiatry.* 2018;5(9):739–746.

12. Grasdalsmoen M, Eriksen HR, Lonning KJ, Sivertsen B. Physical exercise, mental health problems, and suicide attempts in university students. *BMC Psychiatry.* 2020; 20(1):175–186.

13. Kandola AA, del Pozo Cruz B, Osborn DPJ, Stubbs B, Choi KW, Hayes JF. Impact of replacing sedentary behaviour with other movement behaviours on depression and anxiety symptoms: A prospective cohort study in the UK Biobank. *BMC Med.* 2021;19:133.

14. Oberste M, Medele M, Javelle F, et al. Physical activity for the treatment of adolescent depression: A systematic review and meta-analysis. *Front Physiol.* 2020;11:185.

15. Cecchini JA, Fernandez-Rio J, Mendez-Gimenes A, Sanchez-Martinez B. Connections among physical activity, motivation, and depressive symptoms in adolescent girls. *Eur Phy Educ Rev.* 2020;26:682–694.

16. Kandola A, Lewis G, Osborn DPJ, et al. Depressive symptoms and objectively measured physical activity and sedentary behaviour throughout adolescence: A prospective co-hort study. *Lancet Psychiatry.* 2020;7:262–271.

17. Hughes CW, Barnes S, Barnes C, et al. Depressed adolescents treated with exercise (DATE): A pilot randomized controlled trial to test feasibility and establish preliminary effect sizes. *Ment Health Phys Act.* 2013;6(2):10.

18. Hillman CH, Pontifex MB, Castelli DM, et al. Effects of the FIT Kids randomized controlled trial on executive control and brain function. *Pediatrics.* 2014;134(4):e1063–e1071.

19. Hillman CH, Buck SM, Themanson JR, Pontifex MB, Castelli DM. Aerobic fitness and cognitive development: Event-related brain potential and task performance indices of executive control in preadolescent children. *Dev Psychol.* 2009;45(1):114–129.

20. Pontifex MB, Raine LB, Johnson CR, et al. Cardiorespiratory fitness and the flexible modulation of cognitive control in preadolescent children. *J Cogn Neurosci*. 2011;23(6): 1332–1345.
21. U.S. Department of Health and Human Services. Physical Activity Guidelines, 2nd edition; 2018. https://health.gov/sites/default/files/2019-09/Physical_Activity_Guidelines_2nd_edition.pdf.
22. American College of Lifestyle Medicine handout on Promoting Physical Activity in Young Children. https://connect.lifestylemedicine.org/resources. Accessed December 18, 2022.
23. American College of Lifestyle Medicine. ACLM Plate Graphic for Child Tween Teen 2019. https://connect.lifestylemedicine.org/resources. Accessed December 18, 2022.
24. Mahmood L, Flores-Barrantes P, Moreno LA, Manios Yannis, Gonzalez-Gil EM. The influence of parental dietary behaviors and practices on children's eating habits. *Nutrients*. 2021;13(4):1138.
25. Jacka FN, Kremer PJ, Berk M, et al. A prospective study of diet quality and mental health in adolescents. *PLoS ONE*. 2011;6(9):e24805.
26. Jacka FN, Rothon C, Taylor S, Berk M, Stansfeld SA. Diet quality and mental health problems in adolescents from East London: A prospective study. *Soc Psychiatry Psychiatr Epidemiol*. 2013;48(8):1297–1306.
27. Kulkarni AA, Swinburn BA, Utter J. Associations between diet quality and mental health in socially disadvantaged New Zealand adolescents. *Eur J Clin Nutr*. 2015; 69(1):79–83.
28. Sinclair R, Millar L, Allender S, et al. The cross-sectional association between diet quality and depressive symptomology amongst Fijian adolescents. *PLoS ONE*. 2016; 11(8):e0161709.
29. American College of Lifestyle Medicine. Infant Food Introduction handout. https://connect.lifestylemedicine.org/resources. Accessed December 18, 2022.
30. American College of Lifestyle Medicine. Lifestyle Medicine Adolescent Mental Health Toolkit. https://connect.lifestylemedicine.org/resources. Accessed December 18, 2022.
31. Dong L, Martinez AJ, Buysse DJ, Harvey AG. A composite measure of sleep health predicts concurrent mental and physical health outcomes in adolescents prone to eveningness. *Sleep Health*. 2019;5(2):166–174.
32. Gruber R, Somerville G, Bergmame L, Fontil L, Paquin S. School-based sleep education program improves sleep and academic performance of school-age children. *Sleep Med*. 2016;21:93–100.
33. Gruber R, Somerville G, Enros P, Paquin S, Kestler M, Gillies-Poitras E. Sleep efficiency (but not sleep duration) of healthy school-age children is associated with grades in math and languages. *Sleep Med*. 2014;15(12):1517–1525.
34. Sciberras E, Mulraney M, Mensah F, Oberklaid F, Efron D, Hiscock H. Sustained impact of a sleep intervention and moderators of treatment outcome for children with ADHD: A randomised controlled trial. *Psychol Med*. 2020;50(2):210–219.
35. Hamilton JL, Tsypes A, Zelazny J, et al. Sleep influences daily suicidal ideation through affective reactivity to interpersonal events among high-risk adolescents and young adults. *J Child Psychology and Psychiatry*. 2022 July; issued ahead of print. https://acamh.onlinelibrary.wiley.com/doi/epdf/10.1111/jcpp.13651. Accessed July 17, 2022.
36. Paruthi S, Brooks LJ, D'Ambrosio C, et al. Recommended amount of sleep for pediatric populations: A consensus statement of the American Academy of Sleep Medicine. *J Clin Sleep Med*. 2016;12(6):785–786.
37. American College of Lifestyle Medicine. Sleep in Children handout. https://connect.lifestylemedicine.org/resources. Accessed December 18, 2022.
38. Cherry K. What is attachment theory? The importance of early emotional bonds. https://www.verywellmind.com/what-is-attachment-theory-2795337. Accessed December 18, 2022.

39. Warren SL, Huston L, Egeland B, Sroufe LA. Child and adolescent anxiety disorders and early attachment. *J Am Acad Child Adolesc Psychiatry.* 1997;36(5):637–644.

40. Steiner R, Sheremenko G, Lesesne C, et al. Adolescent connectedness and adult health outcomes. *Pediatrics.* 2019;144(1):1–22.

41. Cacciopo JT, Cacciopo S. The growing problem of loneliness. *Lancet.* 2018;391(10119): 426–427.

42. Holt-Lunstad J, Smith TB, Layton JB. Social relationships and mortality risk: A meta-analytic review. *PLoS Medicine.* 2010;7(7):1–20.

43. Keles B, McCrae N, Grealish A. A systematic review: The influence of social media on depression, anxiety and psychological distress in adolescents. *Int J Adol and Youth.* 2020;25(1):79–93.

44. Vidal C, Lhaksampa T, Miller L, Platt R. Social media use and depression in adolescents: A scoping review. *Int Rev Psychiatry.* 2020;32(3):235–253.

45. American College of Lifestyle Medicine. Managing Stress in Early Childhood Years handout. https://connect.lifestylemedicine.org/resources. Accessed December 18, 2022

46. Centers for Disease Control. Youth Risk Behavioral Surveillance System (YRBSS). https://www.cdc.gov/healthyyouth/data/yrbs/reports_factsheet_publications.htm. Accessed December 18, 2022.

47. Jones CM, Clayton HB, Deputy NP, et al. Prescription opioid misuse and use of alcohol and other substances among high school students—Youth Risk Behavior Survey, United States, 2019. *MMWR Suppl.* 2020;69(Suppl-1):38–46.

48. U.S. Department of Health and Human Services (HHS), Office of the Surgeon General. *Facing Addiction in America: The Surgeon General's Report on Alcohol, Drugs, and Health.* Washington, DC: HHS; 2016.

49. Miller JW, Naimi TS, Brewer RD, Jones SE. Binge drinking and associated health risk behaviors among high school students. *Pediatrics.* 2007;119:76–85.

50. Esser MB, Guy GP, Zhang K, Brewer RD. Binge drinking and prescription opioid misuse in the U.S., 2012-2014. *Am J Prev Med.* 2019;57:197–208.

51. Soós R, Gyebrovszki Á, Tóth Á, Jeges S, Wilhelm M. Effects of caffeine and caffeinated beverages in children, adolescents and young adults: Short review. *Int. J. Environ. Res. Public Health.* 2021;18(12389)1–20.

52. De Sanctis V, Soliman N, Soliman AT, et al. Caffeinated energy drink consumption among adolescents and potential health consequences associated with their use: A significant public health hazard. *Acta Biomed.* 2017;88(2):222–231.

53. American Academy of Pediatrics, Committee on Nutrition and the Council on Sports Medicine and Fitness. Clinical report–sports drinks and energy drinks for children and adolescents: Are they appropriate? *Pediatrics.* 2011;127(6):1182–1189.

54. Institute of Medicine. *Nutrition Standards for Foods in Schools: Leading the Way Toward Healthier Youth.* Washington, DC: The National Academies Press; 2007. https://nap.nationalacademies.org/catalog/11899/nutrition-standards-for-foods-in-schools-leading-the-way-toward. Accessed December 18, 2022.

55. Health Canada Information Update RA-34021. https://recalls-rappels.canada.ca/en/alert-recall/health-canada-reminds-canadians-manage-their-caffeine-consumption. Accessed December 18, 2022.

33 Healthy Aging
A Lifestyle Approach to Cognitive Health

Emma Dotson, DNP, AGPCNP-BC and
Nancy Isenberg, MD, MPH, FAAN

KEY POINTS
- Dementia is a leading cause of morbidity, mortality, and financial burden.
- Forty percent of all-cause dementia is preventable.
- The seven pillars of cognitive health can both prevent dementia and slow dementia progression.

33.1 INTRODUCTION

Dementia is defined as a decline in cognition across multiple domains (more recently across one domain to include aphasias) that is severe enough to impact function.[1] Dementia is an umbrella term whereas Alzheimer's disease (AD), vascular dementia, and Lewy body dementia are examples of various types of dementias. Neurodegeneration due to AD accounts for the majority of dementia cases, with cerebrovascular disease (CVD) as the second most common cause. However, increasing evidence from neuroimaging and neuropathological studies demonstrates that mixed etiologies (with neurodegenerative and vascular features) account for many cases of dementia, especially in people older than 80 years.[2] Stroke doubles the risk of developing dementia and shares many of the same risk factors.[3,4]

Dementia is characterized by a long pre-clinical phase without cognitive symptoms, followed by mild cognitive challenges with preserved overall functioning (mild cognitive impairment stage) that can progress to clinical dementia. Cognitive impairment is currently recognized as a spectrum, as reflected in the latest edition of the *Diagnostic and Statistical Manual of Mental Disorders* fifth edition (DSM-5), with its syndromes of mild and major neurocognitive disorders (the latter replacing the term dementia).[5] In addition to the pre-clinical phase, mild cognitive impairment (MCI) is also a critical period in dementia prevention.

Approximately 15% of those with MCI will go on to develop AD after 2 years and one-third will within 5 years.[6,7] However, some individuals will revert to normal, or the clinician will identify a reversible cause for cognitive decline such as sleep apnea, hearing loss, micronutrient deficiencies, medications and/or polypharmacy, and mood disturbances which, when treated, may improve or resolve cognitive challenges.

DOI: 10.1201/b22810-38

Age is the single greatest risk factor for dementia, and as the United States (US) aging population continues to grow, so will the prevalence of dementia. The population of Americans aged 65 and older is expected to grow from 58 million in 2021 to 88 million by 2050. In 2011, the largest ever American demographic cohort, the baby boomer generation, began reaching age 65. By 2030, 74 million older adults will compose over 20% of our US population.[8]

An estimated 6.5 million Americans aged 65 and older are affected by AD in 2022 with 73% of those aged 75 or older. Alternatively, about 1 in 9 people aged 65 and older has AD in the US.[9] The incidence rate of AD appears to be declining, which is speculated to be related to improvements in hypertension management and level of education advancements. However, although the incidence rate is declining, the number of people affected by AD, or the prevalence rate, is still increasing due to the growth in aging adults.[10]

AD remains the fifth leading cause of death in adults aged 65 and older, which is likely underestimated.[11] AD is also a leading cause of morbidity due to the often-numerous years of living with the illness. The financial burden of AD is astonishing. In 2022, the total national cost of caring for people living with AD and other dementias is projected to reach $321 billion.[10] Evidently, dementia is one of the most costly and burdensome diseases that plague our humanity. This chapter will highlight and summarize the important research findings in both the risk and protective factors for dementia through the lens of lifestyle medicine.

33.2   RISK FACTORS

Early recognition of individuals at risk of dementia provides a critical window to intervene along the lifespan through holistic, multimodal interventions that delay or prevent the onset of this disabling neurocognitive disorder. Estimates suggest that delay of onset of just one year could prevent more than 9 million cases of dementia by 2050, and if the onset is delayed by 5 years, then the prevalence of dementia could be halved globally.[12]

Non-modifiable risk factors for dementia are age, family history, and genetics. Apolipoprotein 4 (APOE 4) is considered a risk factor gene for late-onset AD and is carried by approximately 25% of the population.[13] Yet, fewer than half of those who carry this susceptibility gene will develop dementia, and lifestyle factors such as cognitive and social stimulation, a positive outlook on aging, higher level of education, and minimizing cardiometabolic risk factors can mitigate this risk.[14,15] Interestingly, APOE 4 expression is influenced by ancestry, and individuals with European ancestry have a stronger risk of AD, whereas no association has been found in individuals of African and Native American ancestry.[16,17] In a large population-based study, having a parent with dementia was associated with an independent risk.[18]

Modifiable risk factors are key in dementia prevention and account for 40% of dementia prevention across the lifespan. The 2020 *Lancet* Commission on dementia prevention, intervention, and care lists twelve modifiable risk factors: less education in early life, hypertension, hearing loss, smoking, obesity, depression, physical inactivity, diabetes, social isolation, excessive alcohol consumption, traumatic brain injury, and air pollution (Figure 33.1).[19] Furthermore, a recent study in the US found

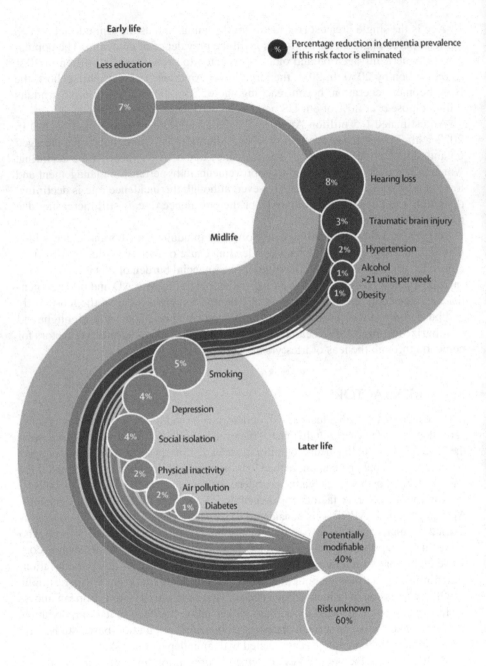

FIGURE 33.1 Population attributable fraction of potentially modifiable risk factors for dementia. Used with permission. Livingston G, Huntley J, Sommerlad A, et al. Dementia prevention, intervention, and care: 2020 report of the Lancet Commission. Lancet. 2020;396 (10248):413–446.

that preventable dementia is more common in people of color.[20] Social determinants of health such as gender and racial discrimination, socioeconomic status, education level, health literacy, and exposure to environmental pollutants all influence cognitive health. Policy and public health efforts addressing structural factors and underlying risk factor differences, as well as those targeting midlife obesity, hypertension, and physical inactivity, are necessary to achieve cognitive health equity and population-level dementia prevention.

33.3 SEVEN PILLARS OF COGNITIVE HEALTH: SLEEP, DIET, EXERCISE, SOCIALIZATION, STRESS MANAGEMENT, COGNITIVE ENGAGEMENT, TEAM/SUPPORT CARE

The seven pillars of cognitive health are crucial lifestyle approaches that can shape one's cognitive trajectory. They are all important health behaviors for both dementia prevention and slowing the progression of existing dementia. Furthermore, given our lack of clinically effective, safe, and affordable disease-modifying therapies for dementia, the importance of implementing lifestyle medicine interventions across the lifespan is not only timely but also imperative.

Pillar 1: Sleep is the first of the seven pillars, one that is often dysregulated in the elderly population. Sleep is crucial for removal of toxins and waste from the brain that can interfere with neuronal, synaptic, and overall brain function. Specifically, sleep is needed for the clearance of beta-amyloid and tau, neuropathological toxins of AD.[21] Sleep is also important for the consolidation of memories as well as supporting emotional well-being.

Additionally, untreated sleep apnea is associated with increased stroke risk, cognitive deficits, as well as an increased incidence of dementia.[22,23] According to a meta-analysis, insomnia is associated with a 27% increase in cognitive decline. Six types of self-reported sleep conditions were found to be a risk for cognitive disorders in non-demented adults with moderate to high level evidence: insomnia, sleep fragmentation, daytime dysfunction, prolonged latency, rapid eye movement sleep behavior disorder, and an extended period of time in bed.[24] Sleep hygiene, behavioral interventions, and cognitive behavioral therapy for insomnia (CBT-I) continue to be the most evidence-based approaches to psychophysiological insomnia.[25]

Pillar 2: Diet has been shown to have complex interactions on cognition that include behavioral, genetic, systemic and brain factors (Figure 33.2).[26] The MIND diet is the most evidence-based diet to prevent dementia.[27–29] The MIND diet incorporates leafy greens, berries, fish and poultry, healthy fats, nuts, beans, whole grains, eating the rainbow, and minimizing red meat and processed foods. Adherence to the MIND diet has been shown to improve cognitive performance, prevent cognitive decline, and slow progression of dementia.[28–33]

Ultra-processed foods are defined as foods changed from their natural state with additives, preservatives, and artificial colors and flavors. A recent cohort study found a higher consumption of ultra-processed foods was associated with a higher risk of dementia, whereas unprocessed or minimally processed foods were associated with a lower risk.[34] Helping patients focus on whole foods and purchasing grocery items

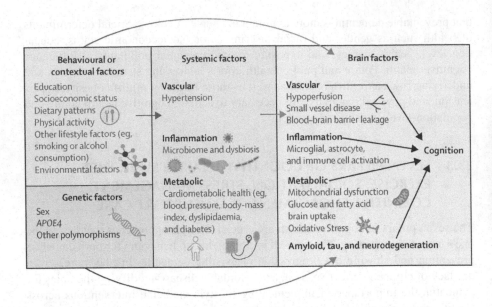

FIGURE 33.2 Biological pathways mediating the relationship of the diet with cognition. The effect of the diet on cognition involves complex interactions that include behavioral, genetic, systemic, and brain factors. The diet can affect the brain directly or indirectly through chronic diseases (dementia risk factors). The blood-brain barrier has pleiotropic functions that include nutrient brain delivery, and a leaky blood-brain barrier in Alzheimer's disease is associated with brain glucose hypometabolism. Used with permission. Yassine HN, Samieri C, Livingston G, et al. Nutrition state of science and dementia prevention: recommendations of the Nutrition for Dementia Prevention Working Group. Lancet Healthy Longev. 2022;3(7):e501–e512.

with minimal ingredients that are easy to understand is key to simplifying nutritional recommendations. In a recent mixed-methods study, shared medical appointments in a resourced-challenged community where participants were educated about sleep, physical activity, and MIND diet were effective in increasing fruit and vegetable intake and improving confidence in preparing healthy meals.[35] Innovative lifestyle medicine programs in resource-challenged community settings further support positive health behaviors including dietary changes to improve physical and cognitive health.

Additionally, excessive alcohol, greater than 21 units per week, increases risk for dementia.[19] A U-shaped curve with alcohol is demonstrated in multiple studies. There is an increased risk of dementia in those who abstained from alcohol in midlife or consumed greater than 14 units per week.[36,37] However, personalized provider recommendations are required given the heterogeneity in each individual's risk profile. Heavy chronic alcohol use can also lead to a thiamine deficiency and subsequent Wernicke-Korsakoff syndrome which causes memory impairment and dementia.

In addition to approaches to nutrition, substances such as methamphetamine and cocaine increase susceptibility to cerebral vascular disease, significantly increasing dementia risk. Smoking tobacco and opioid use are also associated with increased dementia risk. Polypharmacy, especially medications that are on the American Geriatrics Society Beers® criteria list of potentially harmful medications in elderly individuals, also increases risk of cognitive decline, clouds thinking, and can cause falls and adverse events in the geriatric population.[38] Anti-cholinergic medications such as diphenhydramine, oxybutynin, and amitriptyline are some examples of medications that can cause confusion, cognitive dysfunction, and other adverse effects in the elderly.

Pillar 3: We have substantial evidence to support the positive role of exercise in cognition.[39-46] A meta-analysis found that a duration of 45-60 minutes per session and at least moderate-intensity exercise with aerobics and resistance training was associated with benefits in cognition in adults over 50 regardless of the cognitive status of participants.[39] Both aerobic and strength-training exercise have been associated with both dementia prevention and slowing progression of dementia. The American Heart Association recommends 150 minutes of moderate-intensity exercise per week or 75 minutes of high intensity exercise per week for maintaining cardiovascular health, and heart health is brain health. Aerobic exercise promotes angiogenesis, boosts brain-derived neurotrophic factor (BDNF) which supports the formation of new neurons, releases neurotransmitters and endorphins involved in improving cognition and mood, and has an anti-inflammatory, neuroprotective effect. In individuals with established AD, both aerobic and strength exercise are associated with lower mortality risk, lower degree of brain atrophy in early stages, and can improve cognitive functioning, behavior, and functional mobility.[40-42] Strength training is particularly important in aging because it improves bone density and mobility. The hippocampus is a key structure of the brain affected by AD. The hippocampus is thought to be predominantly involved in both spatial and declarative memory. Numerous studies have shown that aerobic and strength training can increase the size of the hippocampus to both protect against AD and improve cognition in individuals who are affected.[43,44] Specifically, an exerkine called irisin, that is released during exercise, has been shown to increase hippocampal neurons, release BDNF, and decrease amyloid beta plaque formation.[45] New research on exerkines, a signaling moiety released with exercise, demonstrates effects on endocrine, autocrine and/or paracrine pathways. Nervous system effects from exerkines include an increase in BDNF and neurogenesis as well as enhanced mood, cognition, and synaptic plasticity. Exerkines enhance resilience, healthspan, and longevity.[46]

Pillar 4: Social connection is neuroprotective and associated with longevity and reduced dementia risk; conversely, social isolation is an important risk factor for dementia.[19] Loneliness is correlated with increased mortality in older adults. Cognitive processes are also impacted by loneliness, for example, impairment in executive functioning and promotion of an inflammatory stress response.[47] Even in midlife, socialization is key to dementia prevention and is associated with a 26% reduction in dementia onset.[48] In individuals with established AD, increased social interaction has been shown to be of benefit by minimizing sense of loneliness, isolation, stress, and vascular factors that contribute to cognitive decline.[49]

Pillar 5: Cognitive Engagement plays an important role in neurogenesis and building cognitive reserve. Early life education and cognitive stimulation across the lifespan contribute to cognitive reserve and play a key role in the brain's capacity to compensate for neurodegenerative and cerebrovascular burden. The higher the educational attainment and job complexity, the greater the cognitive reserve. Early life educational attainment is inversely associated with dementia incidence.[19] In a meta-analysis of 15 randomized control trials (RCTs), there was consistent evidence that cognitive stimulation benefits people with mild to moderate dementia by decreasing severity of behavioral symptoms while increasing memory performance, abstraction, planning, and visuospatial ability.[50] Senior centers, joining groups and organizations, volunteering, group exercise classes, and learning novel and challenging activities are ways adults in mid and late life can not only prevent dementia occurrence but also vastly slow progression of neurodegenerative disease. Many of these activities can combine three or even four of the pillars: socialization, cognitive engagement, stress management, and exercise. The Finnish Geriatric Intervention Study to Prevent Cognitive Impairment and Disability (FINGER), targeting lifestyle and vascular risk factors, is the first RCT demonstrating that multidomain lifestyle interventions can prevent cognitive decline in at-risk individuals with high cardio-metabolic burden. The intervention group received nutritional counseling, exercise, cognitive stimulation, and socialization while managing cardiovascular risk factors. This two-year study demonstrated a 25% improvement in cognitive function in the intervention group compared to control group, specifically improved speed of processing and executive function, both key factors to support independent functioning, as well as larger brain volumes, and greater functional connectivity. In addition to the cognitive benefits, quality of life and physical functioning were better maintained in the intervention group, with fewer new chronic diseases.[51-53]

Pillar 6: Stress management is the sixth pillar of dementia prevention and management. Chronic stress equates to chronically elevated levels of cortisol, and over time, causes increased levels of circulating cytokines, promoting systemic and neuroinflammation. Chronic inflammation can lead to stroke, cancers, diabetes, anxiety and depression, and neurodegeneration, which are all risk factors for dementia.[19] Cognitively, chronic stress causes neurotoxic effects on the brain such as hippocampal, prefrontal cortical atrophy, and amygdala hypertrophy.[54]

Neuroplasticity and epigenetics support the potential to rewire our brains, creating new neurons in regions vital for memory and learning, new connections in brain systems, and improving blood flow as well as cognitive reserve. Mind-body practices such as mindfulness, yoga, and tai chi are lifestyle medicine approaches to manage stress and promote stress resilience, improving cognition and brain health. Meditation slows the rate of hippocampal volume atrophy in those with mild cognitive impairment when compared to a randomized control group.[55] At age fifty, brains of meditators were estimated to be 7.5 years younger than those of controls on magnetic resonance imaging (MRI) scans.[56] Mindset medicine matters: having a positive outlook on aging has an astounding impact on dementia prevention. For example, among individuals with the APOE4 allele and an increased susceptibility risk, those with positive aging beliefs were almost 50% less likely to develop dementia than those with negative aging beliefs.[15]

In addition to chronic stress, depression is associated with reduced white matter integrity in the brain.[57] Depression can also cause cognitive impairment and mimic dementia. Hence it is imperative for clinicians to assess for mood changes in patients reporting cognitive dysfunction, as treating mood disorders can improve cognition.

Pillar 7: Lastly, team and supportive care impact both the person affected by dementia and the care partner(s). Having a timely and comprehensive approach to cognitive changes over time; targeting modifiable risks along the lifespan; performing a careful medication review; and assessing for perceptual disturbance (such as hearing loss), micronutrient or endocrine abnormalities, sleep disturbance, and mood disorders are all critical in providing person and family/care partner-centered cognitive care. Support groups show significant positive effects on caregivers' psychological well-being.[58] According to a review that examined seven meta-analyses and 17 systematic reviews of RCTs, the following were prominent characteristics that deemed caregiver interventions effective: caregivers are actively involved in the intervention, the intervention is tailored and personalized to the changing needs of the individual with dementia and his or her caregivers, and the intervention meets the needs of all parties involved.[59]

Lifestyle medicine offers a comprehensive approach to support both the person with dementia and his or her care partner(s) by promoting longer healthspan and quality of life along the cognitive health continuum.

33.4 DISPARITIES

Sex, gender, racial, and socioeconomic inequities exist in persons with dementia and in those caring for them. Older Blacks and Hispanic Americans are twice to 1.5 times more likely than older Whites to have AD or other dementias, respectively.[60,61] Both Hispanic and African American populations will see the greatest increase in AD and related dementias between 2015 and 2060. By 2060, the number of AD cases is expected to grow to 14 million people, with historically marginalized communities affected the most.[62] Evidence supports that these disparities are greatly affected by marginalization of people of color and structural racism.[63] Residential segregation is a consequence of structural racism and is associated with cognitive dysfunction and increased dementia risk.[64] Additionally, Black caregivers are more likely to provide more than 40 hours of caregiving per week, much more than White caregivers, and are also more likely than White caregivers to be caring for someone with dementia. Black caregivers were also 69% less likely to have access to respite services.[65]

Moreover, women are disproportionately affected by AD. Almost two-thirds of Americans with AD are women, and two-thirds of dementia caregivers are also women. Initial research in prevalence rates had suggested these sex differences are attributable to the increased longevity of women compared to men. However, emerging research identifies a number of factors including the menopause transition, stress, neuroinflammation, mood disorders, and dementia risk. In a large prospective cohort study, less estradiol exposure associated with later menarche, early menopause, shorter reproductive span, and hysterectomies was associated with a higher risk of dementia.[66]

Current studies examining menopause hormone therapy (HT) for dementia prevention in women are mixed.[67] Currently, HT is not recommended for AD prevention or cognition preservation in women of menopausal age; rather, a personalized approach with consideration of key factors including age, menopausal stage, comorbidities, and symptoms is warranted. Longitudinal studies are needed to further explore the association between cumulative estrogen exposure and cognitive function in later life.

Recognizably, there is a large gap in including historically marginalized groups in dementia research. More studies that focus on diverse sex, ethnic, and racial backgrounds are needed to draw conclusions about disparity gaps within dementia care to direct policy and public health efforts. Providing culturally competent care and removing barriers to timely access and treatment of cognitive decline and dementia in disproportionately affected groups is paramount to population health. Lifestyle medicine is well suited to promote cognitive health equity through scalable community partnerships and innovative systems of care such as shared medicine appointments.

33.5 CONCLUSION

In conclusion, dementia prevalence is on the rise with our aging population and is a public health priority.[8–12] Cognitive impairment is a spectrum that necessitates our focus on preventative and lifestyle interventions. There are numerous, modifiable risk and protective factors to target our efforts in reducing dementia and slowing progression of cognitive impairment with the seven pillars of cognitive health.[21–59] A lifestyle medicine approach to cognitive health is essential for prevention of cognitive impairment, slowing progression of dementia, increasing healthspan, and promoting quality of life.

REFERENCES

1. Arvanitakis Z, Shah RC, Bennett DA. Diagnosis and management of dementia: Review. *JAMA*. 2019;322(16):1589–1599. doi:10.1001/jama.2019.4782
2. Hachinski V, Ganten D, Lackland D, et al. Implementing the proclamation of stroke and potentially preventable dementias. *J Clin Hypertens*. 2018;20(10):1354–1359. doi:10.1111/jch.13382
3. Azarpazhooh MR, Avan A, Cipriano LE, et al. Concomitant vascular and neurodegenerative pathologies double the risk of dementia. *Alzheimers Dement*. 2018;14(2):148–156.
4. Solomon A, Mangialasche F, Richard E, et al. Advances in the prevention of Alzheimer's disease and dementia. *J Intern Med*. 2014;275(3):229–250.
5. American Psychiatric Association., American psychiatric association. DSM-5 task force. *Diagnostic and Statistical Manual of Mental Disorders: DSM-5*, 5th ed. Washington, D.C.: American Psychiatric Association; 2013.
6. Petersen RC, Lopez O, Armstrong MJ, et al. Practice guideline update summary: Mild cognitive impairment: Report of the guideline development, dissemination, and implementation subcommittee of the American academy of neurology. *Neurology*. 2018;90(3):126–135. doi:10.1212/WNL.0000000000004826.
7. Ward A, Tardiff S, Dye C, et al. Rate of conversion from prodromal Alzheimer's disease to Alzheimer's dementia: A systematic review of the literature. *Dement Geriatr Cogn Dis Extra*. 2013;3(1):320–332. doi:10.1159/000354370
8. He W, Goodkind D, Kowal P. *U.S. Census Bureau, International Population Reports, P95/16-1, An Aging World: 2015*. Washington, D.C.: U.S. Government Publishing Office; 2016. Available at http://www.census.gov/content/dam/Census/library/publications/2016/demo/p95-16-1.pdf.
9. Rajan KB, Weuve J, Barnes LL, McAninch EA, Wilson RS, Evans DA. Population estimate of people with clinical Alzheimer's disease and mild cognitive impairment in the United States (2020-2060). *Alzheimers Dement*. 2021;17(12):1966–1975. doi:10.1002/alz.12362
10. Alzheimer's Association. 2022 Alzheimer's disease facts and figures. *Alzheimers Dement*. 2022;18(4):700–789. doi:10.1002/alz.12638
11. Xu JQ, Murphy SL, Kochanek KD, et al. Mortality in the United States, 2018. NCHS Data Brief; No. 355. Hyattsville, MD: National Center for Health Statistics; 2020.
12. Jorm AF, Dear KB, Burgess NM. Projections of future numbers of dementia cases in Australia with and without prevention. *Aust N Z J Psychiatry*. 2005;39(11–12):959–963.
13. Beydoun MA, Boueiz A, Abougergi MS, et al. Sex differences in the association of the apolipoprotein e epsilon 4 allele with incidence of dementia, cognitive impairment, and decline. *Neurobiol Aging*. 2012;33(4):720–731.e724.

14. Liu CC, Kanekiyo T, Xu H, et al. Apolipoprotein E and Alzheimer disease: Risk, mechanisms and therapy. *Nat Rev Neurol.* 2013;9(2):106–118.
15. Levy BR, Slade MD, Pietrzak RH, et al. Positive age beliefs protect against dementia even among elders with high-risk gene. *PLoS ONE.* 2018;13(2):e0191004. doi:10.1371/journal.pone.0191004
16. Suchy-Dicey A, Howard B, Longstreth WT Jr, et al. APOE genotype, hippocampus, and cognitive markers of Alzheimer's disease in American Indians: Data from the strong heart study [published online ahead of print, 2022 Feb 10]. *Alzheimers Dement.* 2022. doi:10.1002/alz.12573.
17. Griswold AJ, Celis K, Bussies PL, et al. Increased APOE ε4 expression is associated with the difference in Alzheimer's disease risk from diverse ancestral backgrounds. *Alzheimers Dement.* 2021;17(7):1179–1188. doi:10.1002/alz.12287
18. Wolters FJ, van der Lee SJ, Koudstaal PJ, et al. Parental family history of dementia in relation to subclinical brain disease and dementia risk. *Neurology.* 2017;88(17):1642–1649. doi:10.1212/WNL.0000000000003871
19. Livingston G, Huntley J, Sommerlad A, et al. Dementia prevention, intervention, and care:2020 report of the Lancet Commission. *Lancet.* 2020;396(10248):413–446.
20. Lee M, Whitsel E, Avery C, et al. Variation in population attributable fraction of dementia associated with potentially modifiable risk factors by race and ethnicity in the US. *JAMA Netw Open.* 2022;5(7):e2219672. doi:10.1001/jamanetworkopen.2022.19672
21. Winer JR, Mander BA, Kumar S, et al. Sleep disturbance forecasts β-amyloid accumulation across subsequent years. *Curr Biol.* 2020;30(21):4291–4298.e3. doi:0.1016/j.cub.2020.08.017
22. Dunietz GL, Chervin RD, Burke JF, Conceicao AS, Braley TJ. Obstructive sleep apnea treatment and dementia risk in older adults. *Sleep.* 2021;44(9):zsab076. doi:10.1093/sleep/zsab076
23. Spira AP, Chen-Edinboro LP, Wu MN, Yaffe K. Impact of sleep on the risk of cognitive decline and dementia. *Curr Opin Psychiatry.* 2014;27(6):478–483. doi:10.1097/YCO.0000000000000106
24. Xu W, Tan C, Zou J, et al. Sleep problems and risk of all-cause cognitive decline or dementia: An updated systematic review and meta-Analysis. *Journal of Neurology, Neurosurgery & Psychiatry.* 2020;91:236–244.
25. Sharma MP, Andrade C. Behavioral interventions for insomnia: Theory and practice. *Indian J Psychiatry.* 2012;54(4):359–366. doi:10.4103/0019-5545.104825
26. Yassine HN, Samieri C, Livingston G, et al. nutrition state of science and dementia prevention: Recommendations of the nutrition for dementia prevention working group. *Lancet Healthy Longev.* 2022;3(7):e501–e512. doi:10.1016/s2666-7568(22)00120-9
27. Hosking DE, Eramudugolla R, Cherbuin N, et al. MIND not mediterranean diet related to 12-year incidence of cognitive impairment in an Australian longitudinal cohort study. *Alzheimers Dement.* 2019;15(4):581–589.
28. Morris MC, Tangney CC, Wang Y, et al. MIND diet associated with reduced incidence of Alzheimer's disease. *Alzheimers Dement.* 2015;11(9):1007–1014.
29. Dhana K, James BD, Agarwal P, et al. MIND diet, common brain pathologies, and cognition in community-dwelling older adults. *J Alzheimers Dis.* 2021;83(2):683–692. doi:10.3233/JAD-210107
30. Berendsen AM, Kang JH, Feskens EJM, et al. Association of long-term adherence to the MIND diet with cognitive function and cognitive decline in American women. *J Nutr Health Aging.* 2018;22(2):222–229.
31. Melo van Lent D, O'Donnell A, Beiser AS, et al. Mind diet adherence and cognitive performance in the Framingham Heart Study. *J Alzheimers Dis.* 2021;82(2):827–839. doi:10.3233/JAD-201238

32. Munoz-Garcia MI, Toledo E, Razquin C, et al. "A priori" dietary patterns and cognitive function in the SUN project. *Neuroepidemiology*. 2020;54(1):45–57.
33. Solfrizzi V, Frisardi V, Seripa D, et al. Mediterranean diet in predementia and dementia syndromes. *Curr Alzheimer Res*. 2011;8(5):520–542. doi:10.2174/156720511796391809
34. Li H, Li S, Yang H, et al. Association of ultraprocessed food consumption with risk of dementia: A prospective cohort [published online ahead of print, 2022 Jul 27]. *Neurology*. 2022. doi:10.1212/WNL.0000000000200871
35. Bharmal N, Beidelschies M, Alejandro-Rodriguez M, et al. A nutrition and lifestyle-focused shared medical appointment in a resource-challenged community setting: A mixed-methods study. *BMC Public Health*. 2022;22(447). doi:10.1186/s12889-022-12833-6
36. Sabia S, Fayosse A, Dumurgier J, et al. Alcohol consumption and risk of dementia: 23 year follow-up of Whitehall II cohort study. *BMJ*. 2018;362:k2927. doi:10.1136/bmj.k2927
37. Koch M, Fitzpatrick AL, Rapp SR, et al. Alcohol consumption and risk of dementia and cognitive decline among older adults with or without mild cognitive impairment. *JAMA Netw Open*. 2019;2(9):e1910319. doi: 10.1001/jamanetworkopen.2019.10319
38. 2019 American Geriatrics Society Beers Criteria® Update Expert Panel. American geriatrics society 2019 updated AGS beers criteria® for potentially inappropriate medication use in older adults. *J Am Geriatr Soc*. 2019;67(4):674–694. doi:10.1111/jgs.15767
39. Northey JM, Cherbuin N, Pumpa KL, et al. Exercise interventions for cognitive function in adults older than 50: A systematic review with meta-analysis. *Br J Sports Med*. 2018;52(3):154–160. doi:10.1136/bjsports-2016-096587
40. Scarmeas N, Luchsinger JA, Brickman AM, et al. Physical activity and Alzheimer disease course. *Am J Geriatr Psychiatry*. 2011;19(5):471–481. doi:10.1097/JGP.0b013e3181eb00a9
41. Burns JM, Cronk BB, Anderson HS, et al. Cardiorespiratory fitness and brain atrophy in early Alzheimer disease. *Neurology*. 2008;71(3):210–216. doi:10.1212/01.wnl.0000317094.86209.cb
42. Cancela JM, Ayán C, Varela S, et al. Effects of a long-term aerobic exercise intervention on institutionalized patients with dementia. *J Sci Med Sport*. 2016;19(4):293–298. doi:10.1016/j.jsams.2015.05.007
43. Erickson KI, Voss MW, Prakash RS, et al. Exercise training increases size of hippocampus and improves memory. *Proc Natl Acad Sci USA*. 2011;108(7):3017–3022.
44. Kim YS, Shin SK, Hong SB, et al. The effects of strength exercise on hippocampus volume and functional fitness of older women. *Exp Gerontol*. 2017;97:22–28. doi:10.1016/j.exger.2017.07.007
45. Jin Y, Sumsuzzman DM, Choi J, et al. Molecular and functional interaction of the myokine irisin with physical exercise and Alzheimer's disease. *Molecules*. 2018;23(12):3229. doi:10.3390/molecules23123229
46. Chow LS, Gerszten RE, Taylor JM, et al. Exerkines in health, resilience and disease. *Nat Rev Endocrinol*. 2022;18(5):273–289. doi:10.1038/s41574-022-00641-2
47. Ong AD, Uchino BN, Wethington E. Loneliness and health in older adults: A mini-review and synthesis. *Gerontology*. 2016;62(4):443–449. doi:10.1159/000441651
48. Crooks VC, Lubben J, Petitti DB, et al. Social network, cognitive function, and dementia incidence among elderly women. *Am J Public Health*. 2008;98(7):1221–1227. doi:10.2105/AJPH.2007.115923
49. Ruthirakuhan M, Luedke AC, Tam A, et al. Use of physical and intellectual activities and socialization in the management of cognitive decline of aging and in dementia: A review. *J Aging Res*. 2012;2012:384875. doi:10.1155/2012/384875
50. Woods B, Aguirre E, Spector AE, et al. Cognitive stimulation to improve cognitive functioning in people with dementia. *Cochrane Database Syst Rev*. 2012;(2):CD005562. doi:10.1002/14651858.CD005562.pub2

51. Marengoni A, Rizzuto D, Fratiglioni L, et al. The effect of a 2-year intervention consisting of diet, physical exercise, cognitive training, and monitoring of vascular risk on chronic morbidity-the FINGER randomized controlled trial. *J Am Med Dir Assoc.* 2018;19(4):355–360.e1. doi:10.1016/j.jamda.2017.09.020

52. Rosenberg A, Ngandu T, Rusanen M, et al. Multidomain lifestyle intervention benefits a large elderly population at risk for cognitive decline and dementia regardless of baseline characteristics: The FINGER trial. *Alzheimers Dement.* 2018;14(3):263–270. doi:10.1016/j.jalz.2017.09.006

53. Ngandu T, Lehtisalo J, Korkki S, et al. The effect of adherence on cognition in a multidomain lifestyle intervention (FINGER). *Alzheimers Dement.* 2022;18(7):1325–1334. doi:10.1002/alz.12492

54. Lupien SJ, Juster RP, Raymond C, et al. The effects of chronic stress on the human brain: From neurotoxicity, to vulnerability, to opportunity. *Front Neuroendocrinol.* 2018;49:91–105. doi:10.1016/j.yfrne.2018.02.001

55. Wells RE, Yeh GY, Kerr CE, et al. Meditation's impact on default mode network and hippocampus in mild cognitive impairment: A pilot study. *Neurosci Lett.* 2013;556: 15–19. doi:10.1016/j.neulet.2013.10.001

56. Luders E, Toga AW, Lepore N, et al. The underlying anatomical correlates of long-term meditation: Larger hippocampal and frontal volumes of gray matter. *Neuroimage.* 2009;45(3):672–678. doi:10.1016/j.neuroimage.2008.12.061

57. Harris MA, Cox SR, de Nooij L, et al. Structural neuroimaging measures and lifetime depression across levels of phenotyping in UK biobank. *Transl Psychiatry.* 2022; 12(1):157. doi:10.1038/s41398-022-01926-w

58. Chien LY, Chu H, Guo JL, et al. Caregiver support groups in patients with dementia: A meta-analysis. *Int J Geriatr Psychiatry.* 2011;26(10):1089–1098. doi:10.1002/gps.2660

59. Gitlin LN, Hodgson N. Caregivers as therapeutic agents in dementia care: The evidence-base for interventions supporting their role. In: Gaugler JE, Kane RL, eds. *Family Caregiving in the New Normal.* Philadelphia, PA: Elsevier, Inc.; 2015:305–356.

60. Dilworth-Anderson P, Hendrie HC, Manly JJ, et al. Diagnosis and assessment of Alzheimer's disease in diverse populations. *Alzheimers Dement.* 2008;4(4):305–9.

61. Steenland K, Goldstein FC, Levey A, et al. A meta-analysis of Alzheimer's disease incidence and prevalence comparing African-Americans and Caucasians. *J Alzheimers Dis.* 2016;50(1):71–76. doi:10.3233/JAD-150778

62. Matthews KA, Xu W, Gaglioti AH, et al. Racial and ethnic estimates of Alzheimer's disease and related dementias in the United States (2015-2060) in adults aged ≥65 years. *Alzheimers Dement.* 2019;15(1):17–24.

63. Glymour MM, Manly JJ. Lifecourse social conditions and racial and ethnic patterns of cognitive aging. *Neuropsychol Rev.* 2008;18(3):223–254.

64. Pohl DJ, Seblova D, Avila JF, et al. Relationship between residential segregation, later-life cognition, and incident dementia across race/ethnicity. *Int J Environ Res Public Health.* 2021;18(21):11233. doi:10.3390/ijerph182111233

65. Parker LJ, Fabius CD. Racial differences in respite use among black and white caregivers for people living with dementia. *J Aging Health.* 2020;32(10):1667–1675.

66. Gilsanz P, Lee C, Corrada MM, et al. Reproductive period and risk of dementia in a diverse cohort of health care members. *Neurology.* 2019;92(17):e2005–e2014. doi:10. 1212/WNL.0000000000007326

67. Jett S, Malviya N, Schelbaum E, et al. Endogenous and exogenous estrogen exposures: How women's reproductive health can drive brain aging and inform Alzheimer's prevention. *Front Aging Neurosci.* 2022;14:831807. doi:10.3389/fnagi.2022.831807

34 Women's Mental and Physical Health

Ryan Linn Brown, PhD

KEY POINTS

- Sex-specific, reproductive-related experiences of menarche, pregnancy, and menopause contribute to women's mental and physical health across the lifespan.
- Early menarche, adverse pregnancy outcomes, and early menopause each uniquely contribute to women's health.
- Lifestyle interventions can reduce the number of women adversely affected by elements of these experiences and may disrupt their association with women's psychological and physical (ill) health.

34.1 INTRODUCTION

Despite women's longevity advantage compared to men, women tend to experience worse health and a greater disease burden in older adulthood (i.e., male-female, health-survival paradox).[1-3] Women are disproportionately impacted by age-related diseases[4] and experience elevated morbidity from acute and chronic physical and psychiatric diseases.[5]

Accumulating evidence points to the contribution of sex-specific, reproductive-related experiences of menarche, pregnancy, and menopause to women's mental and physical health. Sex-specific reproductive aging factors promote individual differences in women's experiences of these developmental stages that contribute uniquely to women's mental health and cardiometabolic risk.[6,7] This chapter primarily focuses on physical health outcomes related to cardiometabolic health because cardiovascular disease is the leading cause of death for women in the United States and women are less likely than men to be diagnosed appropriately or receive preventive care. There is strong evidence that there are certain reproductive events in a woman's medical history that may serve as risk factors for poor cardiovascular health.[8] In this chapter, I consider how these factors may contribute to women's health across the lifespan while acknowledging that for any individual woman, these reproductive factors vary concerning whether and how they occur. Related topics, such as the health of transgender individuals and the influence of abortion access for women's mental and physical health, are beyond the scope of this review but represent critical areas of ongoing and future research.

DOI: 10.1201/b22810-39

34.2 MENARCHE

Sex differences in many forms of psychopathology begin to emerge during the pubertal transition.[9,10] In childhood, boys and girls experience similar rates of depression and anxiety until around age 13 when sex differences in internalizing symptoms and disorders widen throughout adolescence.[11-14] Adolescent girls experience substantial emotional shifts (e.g., greater sensitivity to affective facial expressions[15,16]) and stressful negative psychological and social consequences of puberty (e.g., body dissatisfaction, peer stressors).[17-19]

The average age of menarche (i.e., central event of female puberty) is approximately 12 years in the United States. Early menarche is associated with increased risk for internalizing psychopathology,[20,21] eating disorders,[22,23] substance use disorders,[20] as well as increased cardiometabolic risk,[7,24-29] and all-cause mortality.[30] The cardiovascular disease risk appears to be U-shaped as there may also be an increased cardiovascular risk associated with late menarche (after age 17).[26-28] The timing of menarche is influenced by genetic factors and potentially modifiable factors such as lower birthweight and higher childhood body mass index.[31] Exposure to early life adversity, particularly threat of harm, is also associated with earlier menarche.[32-34] Early menarche confers a 15 to 30% higher risk of future cardiovascular disease separate from sociodemographic factors.[24,26,27]

While the physical health risks associated with early menarche may be somewhat attributable to physiology (e.g., metabolic dysregulation),[7,35,36] there is less evidence for the increased risk for internalizing psychopathology to be attributable to physiological changes. Instead, researchers theorize that the psychosocial experience of developing secondary sexual characteristics before most of one's peers may drive an increased vulnerability to depression and anxiety through maladaptive emotion regulatory strategies.[21] For example, one prospective study found that early pubertal timing predicted increased rumination for adolescent girls (but not boys) and that rumination mediated the association between pubertal timing and increased depressive symptoms for adolescent girls.[37] Accordingly, early menarche may be a critical transdiagnostic mechanism that contributes to the association between early life adversity and emergent adolescent psychopathology.[33]

34.2.1 Interventions for Early Menarche: Targeting Substance Use and Close Relationships

Given the evidence for puberty as a developmentally sensitive period of psychological vulnerability, there is an opportunity for lifestyle interventions to influence girls' mental and physical health trajectories. Although puberty timing effects remain small and are not the sole predictor of psychopathology or cardiovascular health, sex-specific reproductive factors like early menarche should also be assessed in clinical practice and discussed to increase girls' and women's awareness of their existing risk factors.

Since puberty begins outside of girls' control, stress-management interventions may be appropriate to navigate the feeling of uncontrollability stemming from early menarche. Broadly, interventions that promote adaptive emotion regulation strategies may help girls adjust to the sheer number and magnitude of social, psychological, and physiological changes experienced through puberty. Emotion regulation interventions here may also be targeted to the family system given the importance of parental involvement and the impact of parental regulation.[38] Further, girls who experience early puberty are at high-risk for early use of both alcohol and cigarettes, with evidence accumulating that this risk may depend on one's household risk (e.g., parental monitoring, parental substance use, fewer resources, more conflict).[39-41] Accordingly, the family system may be an appropriate target to reduce the risk for early substance use among girls who experience early menarche. By targeting substance use for those at high-risk of early alcohol or cigarette use *before consistent drug use behaviors or drug dependence are established*,[42] these interventions may be health-promoting across developmental stages addressed throughout the rest of this chapter. However, more work is needed to tailor many of these interventions to be applicable for young people.[42]

34.3 PREGNANCY

Pregnancy is a vulnerable period for maternal mental and physical health. The transition to parenthood also presents challenges across psychological, biological, familial, and social domains. In addition to the impact of prenatal stress on the developing fetus, maternal stress in pregnancy contributes to maternal mental and physical health conditions. Women's nutritional status during pregnancy affects the growth and development of the fetus,[43-45] as well as their own health. Food insecurity in pregnancy is a potent source of stress that affects eating behaviors (e.g., diet quality,[46,47] food addiction[48]) and the stress conferred by food insecurity may additionally influence metabolic processes.[49-51] Further, several sex-specific risk factors related to one's pregnancy history are increasingly recognized by cardiovascular and obstetric society guidelines, such as adverse pregnancy outcomes, to increase risk for cardiovascular diseases and dementias (including Alzheimer's disease).

Hypertensive disorders of pregnancy include chronic hypertension, gestational hypertension, and preeclampsia (either alone or superimposed on preexisting chronic hypertension).[52]

Preeclampsia is a pregnancy-specific multisystem hypertensive disorder (mediated by the placenta) that affects 2-8% of pregnancies,[53] has a robust genetic component,[54,55] and is characterized by increased oxidative stress, vascular damage, systemic inflammation, and global endothelial damage.[56] Women who experience preeclampsia or gestational hypertension during pregnancy have a 2-fold risk of cardiovascular disease (CVD)[57-59] with the highest risk among those who developed preeclampsia early in pregnancy (before 34 weeks), who had preeclampsia with severe features, or who have had recurrent hypertensive disorders of pregnancy in more than one pregnancy.[59,60] Strikingly, early-onset preeclampsia is associated with more than a 9-fold increased risk of cardiovascular death.[61]

Hypertensive disorders of pregnancy are associated with developing future chronic hypertension and cardiovascular conditions in both the short and long term.[7] In the weeks immediately following delivery, women with a history of hypertensive disorders of pregnancy have increased odds of stroke, cardiomyopathy, myocardial infarction, and spontaneous coronary artery dissection.[62–64] The cardiovascular risk persists into later life as hypertensive disorders of pregnancy and vascular aging (the hallmark of cardiovascular disease) share common mechanisms that may lead to the development of both preeclampsia and cardiovascular disease in a woman's life course[65]; however, it is unknown if preeclampsia simply identifies who may be at later risk or if preeclampsia causally induces changes that increase overall risk for cardiovascular disease later in life. Separate from hypertensive disorders of pregnancy, gestational diabetes mellitus increases one's risk of developing type 2 diabetes mellitus by 7-fold[66] and is associated with a significant increase in cardiovascular disease risk (independent from the development of type 2 diabetes mellitus).[67]

Although less well defined, preeclampsia is also associated with long-term cognitive effects[68–70] (e.g., vascular dementia[71,72]), which may be due to the increased risk of chronic hypertension as there is a robust positive association between blood pressure and cognitive change.[73,74] There is also evidence that preeclampsia and Alzheimer's disease share direct pathophysiological pathways (e.g., protein misfolding and defective amyloid processing).[75]

Pregnancy is also a unique moment in women's lives where weight gain is both essential for fetal development and stigmatized for women who gain excess weight. Women's body image is a relevant factor when considering perinatal depression: prospective cohort studies identify that body image dissatisfaction predicted incident prenatal and postpartum depression.[76,77] Pregnancy and weight gained during pregnancy may also permanently alter women's bodies. Accordingly, weight stigma may shape physical and psychological (ill) health from pregnancy to postpartum.[76,78–80] For example, pregnant and postpartum women who reported facing weight stigma from more sources experienced more depressive symptoms, maladaptive dieting behavior, and perceived stress.[79] This area of research highlights a more complex relationship between weight gain in pregnancy and women's mental and physical health as weight stigma can affect women's relationships with their bodies, food, and trust in healthcare providers.[81,82]

34.3.1 INTERVENTIONS IN PREGNANCY: HEALTHY EATING, PHYSICAL ACTIVITY, AND STRESS MANAGEMENT

This section focuses on interventions aiming to promote cardiometabolic health in pregnancy that also address the stress of one's transition to parenthood. Smoking cessation interventions are also established to promote better cardiometabolic health in pregnancy and lower preterm birth rates, especially the earlier in pregnancy one quits smoking.[83] However, the sensitive period of pregnancy makes it an ideal timepoint for key lifestyle interventions that promote cardiometabolic health while also supporting a lower stress transition to parenthood with critical implications for maternal mental health and offspring development. Accordingly, this section primarily focuses on interventions that target stress-reduction mechanisms.

Excess gestational weight gain is a common target of interventions in pregnancy, particularly for higher weight women, as excessive gestational weight gain is a risk factor for various pregnancy complications (e.g., gestational diabetes) that affect women's risk for age-related diseases later in life. However, there is wide variability in the efficacy of diet and exercise interventions for limiting gestational weight gain,[84] which is likely due to the multifactorial nature of obesity and weight gain, heterogeneity in sample characteristics and access to resources, experiences of weight stigma, and a lack of tailored interventions for racially and ethnically diverse populations. Chronic stress may promote weight gain or weight loss, but regardless of the direction of weight change, chronic stressors often alter metabolic control (e.g., insulin resistance, reward value of food); accordingly, behavioral change interventions are increasingly focusing on stress management and aiming to address the limited success of diet- and exercise-focused interventions by affecting dysregulated eating behaviors and metabolic parameters.[84,85]

One promising intervention involves teaching mindfulness techniques throughout an 8-week intervention targeting eating behavior and reducing stress for pregnant women. Although this quasi-experimental trial did not significantly reduce the number of women gaining excessive weight, it did increase physical activity and reduced the likelihood of impaired glucose tolerance for those in the intervention group.[85] Participants also experienced significantly greater improvements in perceived stress and depression and greater increases in attitudes of acceptance (versus avoidance) about stressful experiences.[85] By 18 months postpartum, those in the mindfulness intervention had lower odds of being in the highest depressive symptom severity group in this sample compared to treatment as usual[86]; critically, the benefits of this intervention persisted eight years later as those in the intervention group had significantly reduced odds of experiencing moderate or high depressive symptoms, compared to those receiving treatment as usual.[87] Lastly, 42% of the participants in this study were food insecure, which points to greater systemic barriers that interventions likely need to address (e.g., by providing food or additional financial resources) since food insecurity is associated with food addiction symptoms in pregnant individuals and caregivers, as well as gestational weight gain, and pregnancy complications.[48,88–91] These results broadly emphasize the immense difficulty of affecting weight gain during pregnancy even when successfully affecting metabolic markers, particularly for those at the most significant risk for adverse pregnancy outcomes, and highlight the exciting potential for mental health effects from a lifestyle intervention to persist nearly a decade after this critical period in a woman's life.

34.4   MENOPAUSE

The menopausal transition marks the end of women's fertility, a critical event of reproductive aging where one's risk for cardiovascular disease can accelerate.[92] Menopause typically occurs around age 50 (median age),[93] and one's age at menopause is well-recognized as a marker of somatic aging and general health.[94] Experiencing menopause at earlier ages is associated with elevated risk of cardiovascular conditions, cardiovascular disease mortality, and all-cause mortality.[29,95–97] Early menopause is considered to occur between ages 40 to 45, whereas premature menopause indicates menopause before age 40. Genetic effects may explain approximately half of the variability in the timing of menopause, and the strongest additional influences are age at menarche, nulliparity, being underweight, and cigarette smoking.[98]

The exact mechanisms underlying the relationship between age at menopause with cardiovascular health are not clear; however, there is some evidence that the association may be bidirectional. Menopause may occur spontaneously or following use of certain medications or surgeries; these differences affect one's level of risk for developing cardiovascular diseases. For example, in a large study of nearly 12000 women in the UK, surgical premature menopause was associated with an 87% increased risk of a composite of cardiovascular diseases compared to only a 36% increased risk for natural premature menopause.[95] In another key study, early menopause had the strongest association with cardiovascular disease risk among women who were current or former smokers, had higher body weight, and those with lower socioeconomic status.[99]

Other characteristics of the menopausal transition, such as vasomotor symptoms, are also related to a greater risk of cardiovascular disease and brain aging. Over 70% of women experience vasomotor symptoms (i.e., hot flashes, night sweats – the cardinal symptoms of menopausal transition) at some point in midlife.[100,101] Meta-analytic evidence highlights a 28% increased risk of cardiovascular disease associated with vasomotor symptoms (beyond traditional risk factors),[97] and there is additional evidence of a dose-dependent relationship between the frequency of vasomotor symptoms and cardiovascular disease risk factors.[102] The severity of vasomotor symptoms is also associated with an increased risk of cardiovascular disease.[103] There is burgeoning evidence that vasomotor symptoms are important for understanding women's risk of memory decline at midlife.[104] Most excitingly, early pilot randomized control trial evidence shows that the effects of vasomotor symptoms on cognition may be able to be reversed if vasomotor symptoms are treated.[105]

34.4.1 INTERVENTIONS FOR MENOPAUSAL TRANSITION: SMOKING CESSATION

There is very limited research surrounding the ideal timing of lifestyle interventions for the menopausal transition; accordingly, randomized clinical trials of lifestyle interventions do not adequately represent this high-risk population.[92] Of the traditional cardiovascular disease risk factors, cigarette smoking is the most clear-cut to address both to reduce the likelihood of early menopause and potentially to ameliorate the risk of early menopause on cardiovascular health. There is some evidence for the potential reversibility of cigarette smoking effects on menopausal timing based on a large prospective cohort study comparing current smokers to those who quit smoking[106]; however, additional research with more precise measurement is necessary to determine the impact of smoking cessation around the menopausal transition.[106–108] Smoking cessation interventions may be targeted for women who are already at heightened risk of early menopause (e.g., due to early menarche or based on family histories).

34.5 CONCLUSION

Considering characteristics of women's reproductive experiences (i.e., menarche, pregnancy, and menopause) provides the opportunity to influence trajectories of health through developmentally sensitive and/or vulnerable periods, incorporate additional

TABLE 34.1

Clinical Applications for Practitioners

1	Clinicians should consider assessing female patients' reproductive history.
2	Reducing stress and cigarette smoking are promising lifestyle interventions to prevent early menarche, adverse pregnancy outcomes, and early menopause.
3	Diet and exercise interventions should be delivered in a manner that does not amplify weight-based stigmatization.

sex-specific risk factors into risk algorithms, and provide women of all ages with the knowledge of their own reproductive-related risk. Because there is also evidence for interactions between aspects of women's reproductive history and traditional cardiovascular disease risk factors, there is ample opportunity for researchers and clinicians to target the six pillars of lifestyle medicine to promote women's mental and physical health across the lifespan. Table 34.1 summarizes a few clinical applications for practitioners.

REFERENCES

1. Archer CR, Recker M, Duffy E, Hosken DJ. Intralocus sexual conflict can resolve the male-female health-survival paradox. *Nat Commun.* 2018;9(1):5048. doi:10.1038/s41467-018-07541-y
2. Oksuzyan A, Juel K, Vaupel JW, Christensen K. Men: Good health and high mortality. Sex differences in health and aging. *Aging Clin Exp Res.* 2008;20(2):91–102. doi:10.1007/BF03324754
3. Gordon EH, Peel NM, Samanta M, Theou O, Howlett SE, Hubbard RE. Sex differences in frailty: A systematic review and meta-analysis. *Exp Gerontol.* 2017;89:30–40. doi:10.1016/j.exger.2016.12.021
4. Austad SN, Fischer KE. Sex differences in lifespan. *Cell Metab.* 2016;23(6):1022–1033. doi:10.1016/j.cmet.2016.05.019
5. Almagro P, Ponce A, Komal S, et al. Multimorbidity gender patterns in hospitalized elderly patients. *PLoS ONE.* 2020;15(1):e0227252. doi:10.1371/journal.pone.0227252
6. Miller EC, Wilczek A, Bello NA, Tom S, Wapner R, Suh Y. Pregnancy, preeclampsia and maternal aging: From epidemiology to functional genomics. *Ageing Res Rev.* 2022;73:101535. doi:10.1016/j.arr.2021.101535
7. O'Kelly AC, Michos ED, Shufelt CL, et al. Pregnancy and reproductive risk factors for cardiovascular disease in women. *Circ Res.* 2022;130(4):652–672. doi:10.1161/CIRCRESAHA.121.319895
8. Vogel B, Acevedo M, Appelman Y, et al. The Lancet women and cardiovascular disease Commission: Reducing the global burden by 2030. *The Lancet.* 2021;397(10292):2385–2438. doi:10.1016/S0140-6736(21)00684-X
9. Mendle J. Why puberty matters for psychopathology. *Child Dev Perspect.* 2014;8(4):218–222. doi:10.1111/cdep.12092
10. Hayward C, Sanborn K. Puberty and the emergence of gender differences in psychopathology. *J Adolesc Health Off Publ Soc Adolesc Med.* 2002;30(4 Suppl):49–58. doi:10.1016/s1054-139x(02)00336-1

11. Jane Costello E, Erkanli A, Angold A. Is there an epidemic of child or adolescent depression? *J Child Psychol Psychiatry*. 2006;47(12):1263–1271. doi:10.1111/j.1469-7610.2006.01682.x

12. Hankin BL, Abramson LY, Moffitt TE, Silva PA, McGee R, Angell KE. Development of depression from preadolescence to young adulthood: Emerging gender differences in a 10-year longitudinal study. *J Abnorm Psychol*. 1998;107(1):128–140. doi:10.1037//0021-843x.107.1.128

13. Letcher P, Sanson A, Smart D, Toumbourou JW. Precursors and correlates of anxiety trajectories from late childhood to late adolescence. *J Clin Child Adolesc Psychol Off J Soc Clin Child Adolesc Psychol Am Psychol Assoc Div 53*. 2012;41(4):417–432. doi:10.1080/15374416.2012.680189

14. Merikangas KR, Zhang H, Avenevoli S, et al. Longitudinal trajectories of depression and anxiety in a prospective community study: The Zurich Cohort Study. *Arch Gen Psychiatry*. 2003;60(10):993–1000. doi:10.1001/archpsyc.60.9.993

15. Goddings AL, Burnett Heyes S, Bird G, Viner RM, Blakemore SJ. The relationship between puberty and social emotion processing. *Dev Sci*. 2012;15(6):801–811. doi:10.1111/j.1467-7687.2012.01174.x

16. Moore WE, Pfeifer JH, Masten CL, Mazziotta JC, Iacoboni M, Dapretto M. Facing puberty: Associations between pubertal development and neural responses to affective facial displays. *Soc Cogn Affect Neurosci*. 2012;7(1):35–43. doi:10.1093/scan/nsr066

17. Hamlat EJ, Stange JP, Alloy LB, Abramson LY. Early pubertal timing as a vulnerability to depression symptoms: Differential effects of race and sex. *J Abnorm Child Psychol*. 2014;42(4):527–538. doi:10.1007/s10802-013-9798-9

18. Ge X, Conger RD, Elder GH. Pubertal transition, stressful life events, and the emergence of gender differences in adolescent depressive symptoms. *Dev Psychol*. 2001;37(3):404–417. doi:10.1037//0012-1649.37.3.404

19. Hamilton JL, Stange JP, Kleiman EM, Hamlat EJ, Abramson LY, Alloy LB. Cognitive vulnerabilities amplify the effect of early pubertal timing on interpersonal stress generation during adolescence. *J Youth Adolesc*. 2014;43(5):824–833. doi:10.1007/s10964-013-0015-5

20. Stice E, Presnell K, Bearman SK. Relation of early menarche to depression, eating disorders, substance abuse, and comorbid psychopathology among adolescent girls. *Dev Psychol*. 2001;37(5):608–619. doi:10.1037//0012-1649.37.5.608

21. Graber JA. Pubertal timing and the development of psychopathology in adolescence and beyond. *Horm Behav*. 2013;64(2):262–269. doi:10.1016/j.yhbeh.2013.04.003

22. Zehr JL, Culbert KM, Sisk CL, Klump KL. An association of early puberty with disordered eating and anxiety in a population of undergraduate women and men. *Horm Behav*. 2007;52(4):427–435. doi:10.1016/j.yhbeh.2007.06.005

23. Klump KL. Puberty as a critical risk period for eating disorders: A review of human and animal studies. *Horm Behav*. 2013;64(2):399–410. doi:10.1016/j.yhbeh.2013.02.019

24. Lakshman R, Forouhi NG, Sharp SJ, et al. Early age at menarche associated with cardiovascular disease and mortality. *J Clin Endocrinol Metab*. 2009;94(12):4953–4960. doi:10.1210/jc.2009-1789

25. Bubach S, De Mola CL, Hardy R, Dreyfus J, Santos AC, Horta BL. Early menarche and blood pressure in adulthood: Systematic review and meta-analysis. *J Public Health*. 2018;40(3):476–484. doi:10.1093/pubmed/fdx118

26. Peters SA, Woodward M. Women's reproductive factors and incident cardiovascular disease in the UK biobank. *Heart*. 2018;104(13):1069–1075. doi:10.1136/heartjnl-2017-312289

27. Canoy D, Beral V, Balkwill A, et al. Age at menarche and risks of coronary heart and other vascular diseases in a large UK cohort. *Circulation*. 2015;131(3):237–244. doi:10.1161/CIRCULATIONAHA.114.010070

28. Lee JJ, Cook-Wiens G, Johnson BD, et al. Age at menarche and risk of cardiovascular disease outcomes: Findings from the national heart lung and blood institute-sponsored Women's ischemia syndrome evaluation. *J Am Heart Assoc.* 2019;8(12):e012406. doi:10.1161/JAHA.119.012406

29. Ley SH, Li Y, Tobias DK, et al. Duration of reproductive life span, age at menarche, and age at menopause are associated with risk of cardiovascular disease in women. *J Am Heart Assoc.* 2017;6(11):e006713. doi:10.1161/JAHA.117.006713

30. Charalampopoulos D, McLoughlin A, Elks CE, Ong KK. Age at menarche and risks of all-cause and cardiovascular death: A systematic review and meta-analysis. *Am J Epidemiol.* 2014;180(1):29–40. doi:10.1093/aje/kwu113

31. Juul F, Chang VW, Brar P, Parekh N. Birth weight, early life weight gain and age at menarche: A systematic review of longitudinal studies. *Obes Rev.* 2017;18(11): 1272–1288. doi:10.1111/obr.12587

32. Colich NL, Rosen ML, Williams ES, McLaughlin KA. Biological aging in childhood and adolescence following experiences of threat and deprivation: A systematic review and meta-analysis. *Psychol Bull.* 2020;146(9):721–764. doi:10.1037/bul0000270

33. Colich NL, Platt JM, Keyes KM, Sumner JA, Allen NB, McLaughlin KA. Earlier age at menarche as a transdiagnostic mechanism linking childhood trauma with multiple forms of psychopathology in adolescent girls. *Psychol Med.* 2020;50(7):1090–1098. doi:10.1017/S0033291719000953

34. Lei MK, Beach SRH, Simons RL. Childhood trauma, pubertal timing, and cardiovascular risk in adulthood. *Health Psychol Off J Div Health Psychol Am Psychol Assoc.* 2018;37(7):613–617. doi:10.1037/hea0000609

35. Matkovic V, Ilich JZ, Skugor M, et al. Leptin is inversely related to age at menarche in human females. *J Clin Endocrinol Metab.* 1997;82(10):3239–3245. doi:10.1210/jcem. 82.10.4280

36. Remsberg KE, Demerath EW, Schubert CM, Chumlea WC, Sun SS, Siervogel RM. Early menarche and the development of cardiovascular disease risk factors in adolescent girls: The Fels Longitudinal Study. *J Clin Endocrinol Metab.* 2005;90(5): 2718–2724. doi:10.1210/jc.2004-1991

37. Alloy LB, Hamilton JL, Hamlat EJ, Abramson LY. Pubertal development, emotion regulatory styles, and the emergence of sex differences in internalizing disorders and symptoms in adolescence. *Clin Psychol Sci.* 2016;4(5):867–881. doi:10.1177/ 2167702616643008

38. Hajal NJ, Paley B. Parental emotion and emotion regulation: A critical target of study for research and intervention to promote child emotion socialization. *Dev Psychol.* 2020;56:403–417. doi:10.1037/dev0000864

39. Andrews JA, Hops H, Duncan SC. Adolescent modeling of parent substance use: The moderating effect of the relationship with the parent. *J Fam Psychol.* 1997;11:259–270. doi:10.1037/0893-3200.11.3.259

40. Westling E, Andrews JA, Hampson SE, Peterson M. Pubertal timing and substance use: The effects of gender, parental monitoring and deviant peers. *J Adolesc Health Off Publ Soc Adolesc Med.* 2008;42(6):555–563. doi:10.1016/j.jadohealth.2007.11.002

41. Dick DM, Rose RJ, Viken RJ, Kaprio J. Pubertal timing and substance use: Associations between and within families across late adolescence. *Dev Psychol.* 2000;36(2):180–189.

42. Stockings E, Hall WD, Lynskey M, et al. Prevention, early intervention, harm reduction, and treatment of substance use in young people. *Lancet Psychiatry.* 2016;3(3):280–296. doi:10.1016/S2215-0366(16)00002-X

43. Fall CHD, Yajnik CS, Rao S, Davies AA, Brown N, Farrant HJW. Micronutrients and fetal growth. *J Nutr.* 2003;133(5):1747S–1756S. doi:10.1093/jn/133.5.1747S

44. Siega-Riz AM, Herrmann TS, Savitz DA, Thorp JM. Frequency of eating during pregnancy and its effect on preterm delivery. *Am J Epidemiol.* 2001;153(7):647–652. doi:10.1093/aje/153.7.647

45. Belkacemi L, Nelson DM, Desai M, Ross MG. Maternal undernutrition influences placental-fetal development. *Biol Reprod*. 2010;83(3):325–331. doi:10.1095/biolreprod.110.084517

46. Laraia BA, Siega-Riz AM, Kaufman JS, Jones SJ. Proximity of supermarkets is positively associated with diet quality index for pregnancy. *Prev Med*. 2004;39(5):869–875. doi:10.1016/j.ypmed.2004.03.018

47. Leung CW, Fulay AP, Parnarouskis L, Martinez-Steele E, Gearhardt AN, Wolfson JA. Food insecurity and ultra-processed food consumption: The modifying role of participation in The Supplemental Nutrition Assistance Program (SNAP). *Am J Clin Nutr*. 2022;116(1):197–205. doi:10.1093/ajcn/nqac049

48. Parnarouskis L, Gearhardt AN, Mason AE, et al. Association of food insecurity and food addiction symptoms: A secondary analysis of two samples of low-income female adults. *J Acad Nutr Diet*. 2022;122(10):1885–1892. doi:10.1016/j.jand.2022.04.015

49. Epel E, Lapidus R, McEwen B, Brownell K. Stress may add bite to appetite in women: A laboratory study of stress-induced cortisol and eating behavior. *Psychoneuroendocrinology*. 2001;26(1):37–49. doi:10.1016/S0306-4530(00)00035-4

50. Epel E, Jimenez S, Brownell K, Stroud L, Stoney C, Niaura R. Are stress eaters at risk for the metabolic syndrome? *Ann N Y Acad Sci*. 2004;1032:208–210. doi:10.1196/annals.1314.022

51. Bermúdez-Millán A, Wagner JA, Feinn RS, et al. Inflammation and stress biomarkers mediate the association between household food insecurity and insulin resistance among latinos with type 2 diabetes. *J Nutr*. 2019;149(6):982–988. doi:10.1093/jn/nxz021

52. Task Force on Hypertension in Pregnancy. Hypertension in pregnancy: Executive summary. *Obstet Gynecol*. 2013;122(5):1122–1131. doi:10.1097/01.AOG.0000437382.03963.88

53. Abalos E, Cuesta C, Grosso AL, Chou D, Say L. Global and regional estimates of preeclampsia and eclampsia: A systematic review. *Eur J Obstet Gynecol Reprod Biol*. 2013;170(1):1–7. doi:10.1016/j.ejogrb.2013.05.005

54. Skjærven R, Vatten LJ, Wilcox AJ, Rønning T, Irgens LM, Lie RT. Recurrence of preeclampsia across generations: Exploring fetal and maternal genetic components in a population based cohort. *BMJ*. 2005;331(7521):877. doi:10.1136/bmj.38555.462685.8F

55. Serrano NC, Quintero-Lesmes DC, Dudbridge F, et al. Family history of pre-eclampsia and cardiovascular disease as risk factors for pre-eclampsia: The GenPE case-control study. *Hypertens Pregnancy*. 2020;39(1):56–63. doi:10.1080/10641955.2019.1704003

56. Burton GJ, Redman CW, Roberts JM, Moffett A. Pre-eclampsia: Pathophysiology and clinical implications. *BMJ*. 2019:l2381. doi:10.1136/bmj.l2381

57. Haug EB, Horn J, Markovitz AR, et al. Association of conventional cardiovascular risk factors with cardiovascular disease after hypertensive disorders of pregnancy: Analysis of the Nord-Trøndelag Health Study. *JAMA Cardiol*. 2019;4(7):628. doi:10.1001/jamacardio.2019.1746

58. Leon LJ, McCarthy FP, Direk K, et al. Preeclampsia and cardiovascular disease in a large UK pregnancy cohort of linked electronic health records: A CALIBER Study. *Circulation*. 2019;140(13):1050–1060. doi:10.1161/CIRCULATIONAHA.118.038080

59. Grandi SM, Filion KB, Yoon S, et al. Cardiovascular disease-related morbidity and mortality in women with a history of pregnancy complications. *Circulation*. 2019;139(8):1069–1079. doi:10.1161/CIRCULATIONAHA.118.036748

60. Riise HKR, Sulo G, Tell GS, et al. Association between gestational hypertension and risk of cardiovascular disease among 617 589 Norwegian women. *J Am Heart Assoc*. 2018;7(10):e008337. doi:10.1161/JAHA.117.008337

61. Mongraw-Chaffin ML, Cirillo PM, Cohn BA. Preeclampsia and cardiovascular disease death: Prospective evidence from the child health and development studies cohort. *Hypertens Dallas Tex 1979*. 2010;56(1):166–171. doi:10.1161/HYPERTENSIONAHA.110.150078

62. Wu P, Chew-Graham CA, Maas AH, et al. Temporal changes in hypertensive disorders of pregnancy and impact on cardiovascular and obstetric outcomes. *Am J Cardiol.* 2020;125(10):1508–1516. doi:10.1016/j.amjcard.2020.02.029

63. Afana M, Brinjikji W, Kao D, et al. Characteristics and in-hospital outcomes of peripartum cardiomyopathy diagnosed during delivery in the United States from the nationwide inpatient sample (NIS) database. *J Card Fail.* 2016;22(7):512–519. doi:10.1016/j.cardfail.2016.02.008

64. Tweet MS, Hayes SN, Codsi E, Gulati R, Rose CH, Best PJM. Spontaneous coronary artery dissection associated with pregnancy. *J Am Coll Cardiol.* 2017;70(4):426–435. doi:10.1016/j.jacc.2017.05.055

65. Berends AL, de Groot CJM, Sijbrands EJ, et al. Shared constitutional risks for maternal vascular-related pregnancy complications and future cardiovascular disease. *Hypertens Dallas Tex 1979.* 2008;51(4):1034–1041. doi:10.1161/HYPERTENSIONAHA.107.101873

66. Bellamy L, Casas JP, Hingorani AD, Williams D. Type 2 diabetes mellitus after gestational diabetes: A systematic review and meta-analysis. *The Lancet.* 2009;373(9677): 1773–1779. doi:10.1016/S0140-6736(09)60731-5

67. Vrachnis N, Augoulea A, Iliodromiti Z, Lambrinoudaki I, Sifakis S, Creatsas G. Previous gestational diabetes mellitus and markers of cardiovascular risk. *Int J Endocrinol.* 2012;2012:458610. doi:10.1155/2012/458610

68. Adank MC, Hussainali RF, Oosterveer LC, et al. Hypertensive disorders of pregnancy and cognitive impairment: A prospective cohort study. *Neurology.* 2021;96(5):e709–e718. doi:10.1212/WNL.0000000000011363

69. Postma IR, Bouma A, de Groot JC, Aukes AM, Aarnoudse JG, Zeeman GG. Cerebral white matter lesions, subjective cognitive failures, and objective neurocognitive functioning: A follow-up study in women after hypertensive disorders of pregnancy. *J Clin Exp Neuropsychol.* 2016;38(5):585–598. doi:10.1080/13803395.2016.1143453

70. Elharram M, Dayan N, Kaur A, Landry T, Pilote L. Long-term cognitive impairment after preeclampsia: A systematic review and meta-analysis. *Obstet Gynecol.* 2018;132(2):355–364. doi:10.1097/AOG.0000000000002686

71. Basit S, Wohlfahrt J, Boyd HA. Pre-eclampsia and risk of dementia later in life: Nationwide cohort study. *BMJ.* 2018;363:k4109. doi:10.1136/bmj.k4109

72. Andolf E, Bladh M, Möller L, Sydsjö G. Prior placental bed disorders and later dementia: A retrospective Swedish register-based cohort study. *BJOG Int J Obstet Gynaecol.* 2020;127(9):1090–1099. doi:10.1111/1471-0528.16201

73. Gottesman RF, Schneider ALC, Albert M, et al. Midlife hypertension and 20-year cognitive change: The atherosclerosis risk in communities neurocognitive study. *JAMA Neurol.* 2014;71(10):1218–1227. doi:10.1001/jamaneurol.2014.1646

74. Muela HCS, Costa-Hong VA, Yassuda MS, et al. Hypertension severity is associated with impaired cognitive performance. *J Am Heart Assoc.* 2017;6(1):e004579. doi:10.1161/JAHA.116.004579

75. Buhimschi IA, Nayeri UA, Zhao G, et al. Protein misfolding, congophilia, oligomerization, and defective amyloid processing in preeclampsia. *Sci Transl Med.* 2014; 6(245):245ra92. doi:10.1126/scitranslmed.3008808

76. Silveira ML, Ertel KA, Dole N, Chasan-Taber L. The role of body image in prenatal and postpartum depression: A critical review of the literature. *Arch Womens Ment Health.* 2015;18(3):409–421. doi:10.1007/s00737-015-0525-0

77. Singh Solorzano C, Porciello G, Violani C, Grano C. Body image dissatisfaction and interoceptive sensibility significantly predict postpartum depressive symptoms. *J Affect Disord.* 2022;311:239–246. doi:10.1016/j.jad.2022.05.109

78. Rode L, Kjærgaard H, Ottesen B, Damm P, Hegaard HK. Association between gestational weight gain according to body mass index and postpartum weight in a large cohort of Danish women. *Matern Child Health J.* 2012;16(2):406–413. doi:10.1007/s10995-011-0775-z

79. Incollingo Rodriguez AC, Dunkel Schetter C, Brewis A, Tomiyama AJ. The psychological burden of baby weight: Pregnancy, weight stigma, and maternal health. *Soc Sci Med.* 2019;235:112401. doi:10.1016/j.socscimed.2019.112401

80. Incollingo Rodriguez AC, Tomiyama AJ, Guardino CM, Dunkel Schetter C. Association of weight discrimination during pregnancy and postpartum with maternal postpartum health. *Health Psychol.* 2019;38:226–237. doi:10.1037/hea0000711

81. Rubino F, Puhl RM, Cummings DE, et al. Joint international consensus statement for ending stigma of obesity. *Nat Med.* 2020;26(4):485–497. doi:10.1038/s41591-020-0803-x

82. Brown A, Flint SW, Batterham RL. Pervasiveness, impact and implications of weight stigma. *EClinicalMedicine.* 2022;47:101408. doi:10.1016/j.eclinm.2022.101408

83. Soneji S, Beltrán-Sánchez H. Association of maternal cigarette smoking and smoking cessation with preterm birth. *JAMA Netw Open.* 2019;2(4):e192514. doi:10.1001/jamanetworkopen.2019.2514

84. Bahri Khomami M, Teede HJ, Enticott J, O'Reilly S, Bailey C, Harrison CL. Implementation of antenatal lifestyle interventions into routine care: Secondary analysis of a systematic review. *JAMA Netw Open.* 2022;5(10):e2234870. doi:10.1001/jamanetworkopen.2022.34870

85. Epel E, Laraia B, Coleman-Phox K, et al. Effects of a mindfulness-based intervention on distress, weight gain, and glucose control for pregnant low-income women: A quasi-experimental trial using the ORBIT model. *Int J Behav Med.* 2019;26(5):461–473. doi:10.1007/s12529-019-09779-2

86. Felder JN, Roubinov D, Bush NR, et al. Effect of prenatal mindfulness training on depressive symptom severity through 18-months postpartum: A latent profile analysis. *J Clin Psychol.* 2018;74(7):1117–1125. doi:10.1002/jclp.22592

87. Roubinov DS, Epel ES, Coccia M, et al. Long-term effects of a prenatal mindfulness intervention on depressive symptoms in a diverse sample of women. *J Consult Clin Psychol.* 2022: doi:10.1037/ccp0000776

88. Troller-Renfree SV, Brito NH, Desai PM, et al. Infants of mothers with higher physiological stress show alterations in brain function. *Dev Sci.* 2020;23(6). doi:10.1111/desc.12976

89. Troller-Renfree SV, Costanzo MA, Duncan GJ, et al. The impact of a poverty reduction intervention on infant brain activity. *Proc Natl Acad Sci.* 2022;119(5):e2115649119. doi:10.1073/pnas.2115649119

90. Arteaga S. The Abundant Birth Project: Community-driven methods to design and evaluate a guaranteed income program for Black and Pacific Islander pregnant women and birthing people. In: APHA; 2022. https://apha.confex.com/apha/2022/meetingapp.cgi/Paper/517947. Accessed December 21, 2022

91. Laraia BA, Siega-Riz AM, Gundersen C. Household food insecurity is associated with self-reported pregravid weight status, gestational weight gain, and pregnancy complications. *J Am Diet Assoc.* 2010;110(5):692–701. doi:10.1016/j.jada.2010.02.014

92. El Khoudary SR, Aggarwal B, Beckie TM, et al. Menopause transition and cardiovascular disease risk: Implications for timing of early prevention: A scientific statement from the American Heart Association. *Circulation.* 2020;142(25). doi:10.1161/CIR.0000000000000912

93. Zhu D, Chung HF, Pandeya N, et al. Relationships between intensity, duration, cumulative dose, and timing of smoking with age at menopause: A pooled analysis of individual data from 17 observational studies. *PLoS Med.* 2018;15(11):e1002704. doi:10.1371/journal.pmed.1002704

94. El Khoudary SR. Age at menopause onset and risk of cardiovascular disease around the world. *Maturitas.* 2020;141:33–38. doi:10.1016/j.maturitas.2020.06.007

95. Honigberg MC, Zekavat SM, Aragam K, et al. Association of premature natural and surgical menopause with incident cardiovascular disease. *JAMA.* 2019;322(24):2411. doi:10.1001/jama.2019.19191

96. Muka T, Oliver-Williams C, Kunutsor S, et al. Association of age at onset of menopause and time since onset of menopause with cardiovascular outcomes, intermediate vascular traits, and all-cause mortality: A systematic review and meta-analysis. *JAMA Cardiol.* 2016;1(7):767–776. doi:10.1001/jamacardio.2016.2415

97. Muka T, Oliver-Williams C, Colpani V, et al. Association of vasomotor and other menopausal symptoms with risk of cardiovascular disease: A systematic review and meta-analysis. *PLoS ONE.* 2016;11(6):e0157417. doi:10.1371/journal.pone.0157417

98. Mishra GD, Chung HF, Cano A, et al. EMAS position statement: Predictors of premature and early natural menopause. *Maturitas.* 2019;123:82–88. doi:10.1016/j.maturitas.2019.03.008

99. Zhu D, Chung HF, Dobson AJ, et al. Age at natural menopause and risk of incident cardiovascular disease: A pooled analysis of individual patient data. *Lancet Public Health.* 2019;4(11):e553–e564. doi:10.1016/S2468-2667(19)30155-0

100. Avis NE, Crawford SL, Greendale G, et al. Duration of menopausal vasomotor symptoms over the menopause transition. *JAMA Intern Med.* 2015;175(4):531. doi:10.1001/jamainternmed.2014.8063

101. Gold EB, Colvin A, Avis N, et al. Longitudinal analysis of the association between vasomotor symptoms and race/ethnicity across the menopausal transition: Study of Women's Health Across the Nation. *Am J Public Health.* 2006;96(7):1226–1235. doi:10.2105/AJPH.2005.066936

102. Franco OH, Muka T, Colpani V, et al. Vasomotor symptoms in women and cardiovascular risk markers: Systematic review and meta-analysis. *Maturitas.* 2015;81(3):353–361. doi:10.1016/j.maturitas.2015.04.016

103. Zhu D, Chung HF, Dobson AJ, et al. Vasomotor menopausal symptoms and risk of cardiovascular disease: A pooled analysis of six prospective studies. *Am J Obstet Gynecol.* 2020;223(6):898.e1–898.e16. doi:10.1016/j.ajog.2020.06.039

104. Maki PM, Thurston RC. Menopause and brain health: Hormonal changes are only part of the story. *Front Neurol.* 2020;11. doi:10.3389/fneur.2020.562275. Accessed March 24, 2023

105. Maki PM, Rubin LH, Savarese A, et al. Stellate ganglion blockade and verbal memory in midlife women: Evidence from a randomized trial. *Maturitas.* 2016;92:123–129. doi:10.1016/j.maturitas.2016.07.009

106. Hayatbakhsh MR, Clavarino A, Williams GM, Sina M, Najman JM. Cigarette smoking and age of menopause: A large prospective study. *Maturitas.* 2012;72(4):346–352. doi:10.1016/j.maturitas.2012.05.004

107. Parente RC, Faerstein E, Celeste RK, Werneck GL. The relationship between smoking and age at the menopause: A systematic review. *Maturitas.* 2008;61(4):287–298. doi:10.1016/j.maturitas.2008.09.021

108. Sun L, Tan L, Yang F, et al. Meta-analysis suggests that smoking is associated with an increased risk of early natural menopause. *Menopause N Y N.* 2012;19(2):126–132. doi:10.1097/gme.0b013e318224f9ac

35 Physical and Mental Health at Work

Jensine Paoletti, PhD, Joanne Angosta, PhD,
and Leo Alexander III, PhD

KEY POINTS

- Work stress and downstream health outcomes have profound effects on employees' quality of life.
- Positive experiences at work may affect employees' health behaviors (e.g., physical activity) as well as their psychological well-being.
- Organizational leaders have many interventional levers at their disposal to benefit their employees' mental and physical health.

For most adults between the ages of 25 and 64, the workplace is one of the most important social contexts in people's lives, as employees spend one-third of their lives at work.[1,2] Work can be a source of favorable health outcomes, including life satisfaction and meaningfulness, but it can also be a source of stress, burnout, and other adverse health outcomes. This chapter aims to summarize some of the research on work and health, especially from occupational health psychology (OHP). OHP is an interdisciplinary field that applies psychology to protecting and promoting workers' health, safety, and well-being. The field of OHP primarily focuses on a healthy, adult workforce; therefore, many of the studies examine subclinical effects on employee health. A detailed review of the field is beyond the scope of this chapter, but further readings are listed in Table 35.1.

35.1 HEALTH PROBLEMS AT WORK

Healthy workplaces function to protect the employees from experiencing chronic stress and burnout (two of the most studied OHP outcomes) and other related adverse health outcomes. According to theory, work experiences can impair health via multiple mechanisms. Job demands are the aspects of jobs that require mental or physical effort (e.g., time demands); job resources are the aspects of a job that help an employee achieve his or her goals (e.g., social support).[3,4] When job demands exceed job resources, employees are more likely to experience strain, fatigue, burnout, and other health problems.[3,4] Over time, these effects result in higher healthcare costs, disease diagnoses, and mortality. Many everyday work-related stressors, including shiftwork, long work hours, low job security, high work-family conflict, high job demands, and low social support at work, were related to increased American healthcare costs, conservatively estimated at an increase of $125 billion annually.[5]

DOI: 10.1201/b22810-40

TABLE 35.1
Suggested Review Articles for Further Reading

Topic	Citation
Health problems at work	
Emotional labor	Zapf D, Kern M, Tschan F, Holman D, Semmer NK. Emotion work: A work psychology perspective. *Annu Rev Organ Psychol Organ Behav.* 2021;8(1):139–172. doi:10.1146/annurev-orgpsych-012420-062451
Work stress and inflammation	Wright BJ, Eddy PJ, Kent S. Work Stress, immune, and inflammatory markers. In: Theorell T, ed. *Handbook of Socioeconomic Determinants of Occupational Health: From Macro-Level to Micro-Level Evidence.* Handbook Series in Occupational Health Sciences. Springer International Publishing; 2020:1–19. doi:10.1007/978-3-030-05031-3_28-1
Economic costs of work stress	Hassard J, Teoh KRH, Visockaite G, Dewe P, Cox T. The cost of work-related stress to society: A systematic review. *Journal of Occupational Health Psychology.* 2017;23(1):1–17. doi:10.1037/ocp0000069
Health benefits from work	
Employee life satisfaction	Erdogan B, Bauer TN, Truxillo DM, Mansfield LR. Whistle while you work: A review of the life satisfaction literature. *Journal of Management.* 2012;38(4):1038–1083. doi:10.1177/0149206311429379
Opportunities for improving employee health	
Safety climate interventions	Lee J, Huang YH, Cheung JH, Chen Z, Shaw WS. A systematic review of the safety climate intervention literature: Past trends and future directions. *Journal of Occupational Health Psychology.* 2019;24(1):66–91. doi:10.1037/ocp0000113
Family-supportive supervisor behaviors	Crain TL, Stevens SC. Family-supportive supervisor behaviors: A review and recommendations for research and practice. *Journal of Organizational Behavior.* 2018;39(7):869–888.
Workplace mindfulness trainings	Bartlett L, Martin A, Neil AL, et al. A systematic review and meta-analysis of workplace mindfulness training randomized controlled trials. *Journal of Occupational Health Psychology.* 2019;24(1):108. doi:10.1037/ocp0000146

Conservative estimates indicate that 127,000 annual deaths may be attributed to work-related stressors.[5]

35.1.1 WORK STRESS AND BURNOUT

At work, employees experience a myriad of stressors with disparate outcomes. The challenge-hindrance framework is often used to distinguish between challenge stressors, which may cause eustress in moderate amounts, and hindrance stressors, which interfere with one's goal and often cause distress.[6,7] One significant stressor is emotional labor, an affective process that involves the suppression of genuine emotions and manufacturing inauthentic emotions as required by one's job.[8] Researchers have found that a form of response-focused emotion regulation at work has a stronger relationship with psychosomatic complaints when compared to a form of antecedent-focused emotion regulation.[9] Much of the research on emotional labor focuses on customer service roles, although it also occurs in collaborative work.[10] In a recent profile analysis, people high in emotional labor reported significantly greater sleeping problems and burnout than those in other profiles.[11]

35.1.2 BURNOUT

Job burnout is a psychological syndrome resulting from chronic stress, especially interpersonal stress, in the workplace. Burnout is especially relevant for occupations that require frequent contact with coworkers or clients.[12] The conceptualization of job burnout that has emerged from the vast body of research on human services occupations and other professions comprises three components: (1) emotional exhaustion, (2) depersonalization, and (3) reduced personal accomplishment. Emotional exhaustion is marked by a feeling of mental fatigue and depletion of emotional resources.[13] Emotional exhaustion results from chronic stress on the job and a lack of emotional resources to deal with those stressors. Depersonalization can be described as treating others in the workplace as objects rather than people. In these cases, workers may develop a cynical attitude toward the organization and their coworkers to cognitively distance themselves from the stress and discouragement that accompanies overwhelming, emotionally exhausting work. Lastly, reduced personal accomplishment refers to a feeling of inefficacy at work. Those suffering from reduced personal accomplishment (or reduced professional efficacy as it is known outside of the human services context) tend to hold negative evaluations of their competence, effectiveness, and work achievements.

35.2 HOW WORK STRESS AND BURNOUT TRANSLATE TO OTHER NEGATIVE HEALTH OUTCOMES

Findings from psychoneuroimmunology demonstrate the relationship between chronic stress and an overactive inflammatory network.[14,15] Inflammation is associated with a large spectrum of conditions, including cardiovascular disease, type 2 diabetes, cancers, osteoporosis, fatigue, frailty, Alzheimer's disease and related dementias, premature aging, and all-cause mortality.[16–18] As expected, work-related stress is related to adverse health outcomes, presumably via overactive inflammation. The Whitehall Studies demonstrated that job demands were related to coronary heart disease (CHD), as British civil servants at lower levels were more likely to have CHD[19]; these results are attributable to elevated, chronic inflammation. More recent meta-analytic findings align with the results of the Whitehall Studies, as low levels of job control were related to 31,000 annual deaths.[5]

Beyond these direct effects of work stressors and health, there are many mediated pathways between work stress and negative health outcomes. For instance, the interactions between burnout and depression may synergistically increase the risk of inflammation-related conditions. Burnout is a direct predictor of all-cause mortality.[20] According to one study, burnout is predictive of depressive symptoms, especially among employees who engage in lower levels of physical activity.[21] Depression can prime the inflammatory response to subsequent stressors, increasing the risk of negative health conditions.[22] Work-related stressors may also affect employees' health directly. One study found that shift work, long work hours, high job demands, and low social support at work were related to higher cases of physician-diagnosed major diseases.[5] Specifically, these stressors increased employees' likelihood of being diagnosed with heart disease, angina, myocardial infarction, stroke, emphysema, asthma, high cholesterol, diabetes, and arthritis.[5] Finally, organizational leaders should understand the emerging evidence of crossover effects from a family member's work experiences to his or her family's health. In one recent example of a crossover effect, fathers' work-family conflict was related to their children's chronic inflammation through depressive symptoms and worry symptoms.[23] Future research should continue to delve into the various pathways and boundary conditions between work stress and negative health outcomes.

35.3 HEALTH BENEFITS FROM WORK

Under some circumstances, positive experiences at work may buffer stress.[24] Positive experiences at work increase an individual's work-related satisfaction, which buffers stress.[25] Employment may satisfy financial needs from pay, interpersonal needs through interactions with coworkers, and status-oriented needs from an organizational position of power.[26] Likewise, positive work experiences include a sense of challenge, growth, and meaningfulness associated with work (i.e., feeling as though your work makes a difference in the world or allows you to be a part of something larger than yourself promotes a sense of meaningfulness).[26] These positive experiences often encourage feelings of competence, self-esteem, and life satisfaction, which also buffer feelings of stress.[25] Work experiences affect the employee's quality of life through a process called spillover; work experiences may affect one's family's quality of life through a process crossover.[27-29] Altogether, fulfilling psychological employment experiences serve to enrich life by serving as an additional domain in which employees may garner psychosocial resources. Finally, there may also be direct physical health benefits due to work experiences, as one study found that seeing coworkers eating fruits and vegetables was positively related to respondents' vegetable consumption; similarly, seeing coworkers exercising was positively associated with respondents' physical activity levels.[30]

35.3.1 MEANINGFUL WORK

Meaningful work is work that an individual finds particularly significant and holds positive meaning.[31] In their review, Rosso and colleagues propose four main categories that describe the sources of meaning in work: the self, other persons, the work context, and spirituality. As these categories suggest, finding meaning in one's work is not limited to interpersonal contexts. Research has previously shown that a sense of meaningful work can reduce emotional exhaustion.[32] Evidence also suggests that employees who spend more time on meaningful work tasks have a lower risk of burnout.[33] Tei and colleagues concluded that medical professionals' sense of meaning in their work reduced their stress by increasing their feelings of purpose and making work feel less distressing. Relatedly, providing support to another coworker was positively correlated with one's feeling of meaningfulness in work.[34] Meaningful work motivates people to rally their character strengths to cope with the demands of stressful work tasks, staving off emotional exhaustion. The same mechanism likely allows meaningful work to mediate the relationship between other traits that influence perceptions of work that lead to emotional exhaustion.

35.3.2 OPPORTUNITIES FOR PROMOTING EMPLOYEES' HEALTH

Organizational leaders have many opportunities to make changes that may promote employee health. Goh and colleagues found that many changeable workplace stressors were related to self-reported physical and mental health, physician-diagnosed health conditions, and mortality. In one study, work-family conflict and family-supportive supervisor behaviors (i.e., supervisors providing empathy and flexibility with work-family management) were significantly related to sleep quality and quantity.[35] In another study, the availability of flexible work hours was related to fewer health-related work limitations among older workers with chronic health conditions.[36] Employee health promotion interventions may also benefit organizations. When employees feel undervalued or mistreated, they may engage in unethical behavior at work.[37] Results from one study suggest that interventions focused on increasing employees' sleep quality and quantity may reduce unethical behavior at work.[37] Below, we delve into two specific opportunities to improve employee health.

35.3.3 BREAKS AND RECOVERY

Work is effortful and depletes psychological resources; to replenish those resources, employees engage in work recovery experiences, which allow employees to return to pre-work levels of energy or exhaustion.[38] Recovery experiences include (1) detachment from work, (2) control of one's time, (3) relaxation, and (4) feelings of mastery due to challenging experiences.[39] According to meta-analytic evidence, after-work relaxation, mastery, and control are positively related to vigor and negatively associated with fatigue.[40] Research on lunch breaks suggests that mid-day recovery experiences, especially lunch breaks that allow employees to experience a sense of control and relaxation, can reduce end-of-day exhaustion.[41,42] In one 10-day lunchtime intervention, employees were sorted into a park walk group, a relaxation exercise group, or a control group. Those in the relaxation group experienced lower strain and fatigue from their pre-intervention levels; they also had higher levels of afternoon concentration caused by their lunchtime experiences of detachment from work.[43] Extant findings suggest that mid-day breaks and after-work recovery experiences can promote employee health. Primordial prevention like these interventions may decrease the risk factors for burnout prior to the onset of burnout.[44]

35.3.4 SUPPORT FROM COLLEAGUES

In many modern workplaces, individuals must rely on giving and receiving instrumental support or task assistance from their coworkers and collaborators to perform their jobs. Exchanging support creates dependencies between the relationship partners such that a relationship will become more interdependent in the future through the dependencies created by support behavior.[45] Early findings indicate that giving support can reduce one's stress from emotional labor.[46] Likewise, receiving high levels of workplace social support is negatively related to the prevalence of cardiovascular disease.[47]

Workplace social support is not universally beneficial. Giving support to others may hurt the support giver, particularly in cases where it takes too much of the support giver's energy.[48,49] One study of service industry workers suggested that support must be appropriate for the recipient's needs.[50] The recipient interprets social support and the provider; therefore, providing or receiving support from individuals who are unresponsive to others' needs may not be accompanied by health benefits.[51] Together, the evidence indicates there may be understudied moderators, mediators, and boundary conditions in the relationship between social support and employee well-being. Interventions that increase supervisors' emotional and instrumental support of their employees' nonwork lives have improved employee's marital relationship quality and reduced stress among employees who provide eldercare in and/ or outside of work.[52,53] Scientists and practitioners should consider utilizing interventions to enhance social support as a method of targeting enhancing employee well-being.

35.4 CONCLUSION

Work experiences have profound effects on the mental and physical health of employees. Positive work experiences can promote human flourishing, while negative experiences are related to higher rates of illness and mortality. For instance, healthy workplaces can contribute to employees' own healthy eating and regular physical activity. Healthy workplaces allow for positive social connection and may promote employees' healthy aging. Emerging research suggests that workplace experiences may also impact employees' families and their health. Despite decades of progress, opportunities abound for more research and practical application of prior findings.

REFERENCES

1. *Household Data: Annual Averages.* Bureau of Labor Statistics; 2021. https://www.bls.gov/cps/cpsaat03.pdf
2. Stewart N. *Winning Friends at Work.* Ballantine Books; 1985.
3. Bakker AB, Demerouti E. The Job demands-resources model: State of the art. *Journal of Managerial Psychology.* 2007;22(3):309–328. doi:10.1108/02683940710733115
4. Kinnunen U, Feldt T, Siltaloppi M, Sonnentag S. Job demands–resources model in the context of recovery: Testing recovery experiences as mediators. *Eur J Work Organ Psychol.* 2011;20(6):805–832. doi:10.1080/1359432X.2010.524411
5. Goh J, Pfeffer J, Zenios SA. The relationship between workplace stressors and mortality and health costs in the United States. *Manage Sci.* 2016;62(2):608–628. doi:10.1287/mnsc.2014.2115
6. Cavanaugh MA, Boswell WR, Roehling MV, Boudreau JW. An empirical examination of self-reported work stress among U.S. managers. *J Appl Psychol.* 2000;85(1):65–74. doi:10.1037/0021-9010.85.1.65

7. O'Brien KE, Beehr TA. So far, so good: Up to now, the challenge–hindrance framework describes a practical and accurate distinction. *J Organ Behav.* 2019;40(8):962–972. doi:10.1002/job.2405

8. Grandey AA. Emotional regulation in the workplace: A new way to conceptualize emotional labor. *J Occup Health Psychol.* 2000;5(1):95–110.

9. Hülsheger UR, Schewe AF. On the costs and benefits of emotional labor: A meta-analysis of three decades of research. *J Occup Health Psychol.* 2011;16(3):361–389. doi:10.1037/a0022876

10. Ozcelik H. An empirical analysis of surface acting in intra-organizational relationships. *J Organ Behav.* 2013;34(3):291–309. doi:10.1002/job.1798

11. Fouquereau E, Morin AJS, Lapointe É, Mokounkolo R, Gillet N. Emotional labour profiles: Associations with key predictors and outcomes. *Work & Stress.* 2019;33(3): 268–294. doi:10.1080/02678373.2018.1502835

12. Maslach C, Schaufeli WB, Leiter MP. Job burnout. *Annu Rev Psychol.* 2001;52(1): 397–422. doi:10.1146/annurev.psych.52.1.397

13. Cordes CL, Dougherty TW. A review and an integration of research on job burnout. *AMR.* 1993;18(4):621–656. doi:10.5465/amr.1993.9402210153

14. Gouin JP, Glaser R, Malarkey WB, Beversdorf D, Kiecolt-Glaser J. Chronic stress, daily stressors, and circulating inflammatory markers. *Health Psychol.* 2012;31(2):264.

15. Wright BJ, Eddy PJ, Kent S. Work stress, immune, and inflammatory markers. In: Theorell T, ed. *Handbook of Socioeconomic Determinants of Occupational Health: From Macro-Level to Micro-Level Evidence.* Handbook Series in Occupational Health Sciences. Springer International Publishing; 2020:1–19. doi:10.1007/978-3-030-05031-3_28-1

16. Akiyama H, Barger S, Barnum S, et al. Inflammation and Alzheimer's disease. *Neurobiol Aging.* 2000;21(3):383–421. doi:10.1016/S0197-4580(00)00124-X

17. Fagundes CP, Way B. Early-life stress and adult inflammation. *Curr Dir Psychol Sci.* 2014;23(4):277–283. doi:10.1177/0963721414535603

18. Willerson JT, Ridker PM. Inflammation as a cardiovascular risk factor. *Circulation.* 2004;109(21 Suppl 1):II2–II10. doi:10.1161/01.CIR.0000129535.04194.38

19. Marmot M, Bosma H, Hemingway H, Brunner E, Stansfeld S. Contribution of job control and other risk factors to social variations in coronary heart disease incidence. *Lancet.* 1997;350(9073):235–239. doi:10.1016/S0140-6736(97)04244-X

20. Ahola K, Väänänen A, Koskinen A, Kouvonen A, Shirom A. Burnout as a predictor of all-cause mortality among industrial employees: A 10-year prospective register-linkage study. *J Psychosom Res.* 2010;69(1):51–57. doi:10.1016/j.jpsychores.2010.01.002

21. Toker S, Biron M. Job burnout and depression: Unraveling their temporal relationship and considering the role of physical activity. *J Appl Psychol.* 2012;97(3):699–710.

22. Kiecolt-Glaser JK, Wilson SJ. Caregiver vulnerability and brain structural markers: Compounding risk. *Am J Geriatr Psychiatry.* 2017;25(6):592–594. doi:10.1016/j.jagp.2017.02.019

23. Ganguli A, Jones EJ, Feinberg ME, Schreier HMC. Association between parent work-family conflict and offspring inflammation. *Psychoneuroendocrinology.* 2021;131: 105473. doi:10.1016/j.psyneuen.2021.105473

24. Martire LM, Stephens MAP, Atienza AA. The interplay of work and caregiving: Relationships between role satisfaction, role involvement, and caregivers' well-being. *J Gerontol B Psychol Sci Soc Sci.* 1997;52(5):S279–S289.

25. Lee RT, Ashforth BE. A meta-analytic examination of the correlates of the three dimensions of job burnout. *J Appl Psychol.* 1996;81(2):123–133. doi:10.1037/0021-9010.81.2.123

26. Erdogan B, Bauer TN, Truxillo DM, Mansfield LR. Whistle while you work: A review of the life satisfaction literature. *J Manage.* 2012;38(4):1038–1083. doi:10.1177/0149206311429379

27. Adams GA, King LA, King DW. Relationships of job and family involvement, family social support, and work–family conflict with job and life satisfaction. *J Appl Psychol.* 1996;81(4):411–420. doi:10.1037/0021-9010.81.4.411

28. Bakker AB, Demerouti E, Burke R. Workaholism and relationship quality: A spillover-crossover perspective. *J Occup Health Psychol.* 2009;14(1):23. doi:10.1037/a0013290

29. Bakker AB, Xanthopoulou D. The crossover of daily work engagement: Test of an actor–partner interdependence model. *J Appl Psychol.* 2009;94(6):1562. doi:10.1037/a0017525

30. Tabak RG, Hipp JA, Marx CM, Brownson RC. Workplace social and organizational environments and healthy-weight behaviors. *PLoS ONE.* 2015;10(4):e0125424. doi:10.1371/journal.pone.0125424

31. Rosso BD, Dekas KH, Wrzesniewski A. On the meaning of work: A theoretical integration and review. *Res Organ Behav.* 2010;30:91–127. doi:10.1016/j.riob.2010.09.001

32. Allan BA, Owens RL, Douglass RP. Character strengths in counselors: Relations with meaningful work and burnout. *J Career Assess.* 2019;27(1):151–166. doi:10.1177/1069072717748666

33. Shanafelt TD, West CP, Sloan JA, et al. Career fit and burnout among academic faculty. *Arch Intern Med.* 2009;169(10):990–995. doi:10.1001/archinternmed.2009.70

34. Colbert AE, Bono JE, Purvanova RK. Flourishing via workplace relationships: Moving beyond instrumental support. *AMJ.* 2016;59(4):1199–1223. doi:10.5465/amj.2014.0506

35. Crain TL, Hammer LB, Bodner T, et al. Work–family conflict, family-supportive supervisor behaviors (FSSB), and sleep outcomes. *J Occup Health Psychol.* 2014;19(2):155–167. doi:10.1037/a0036010

36. Vanajan A, Bültmann U, Henkens K. Health-related work limitations among older workers—the role of flexible work arrangements and organizational climate. *Gerontologist.* 2020;60(3):450–459. doi:10.1093/geront/gnz073

37. Barnes CM, Schaubroeck J, Huth M, Ghumman S. Lack of sleep and unethical conduct. *Organ Behav Hum Decis Process.* 2011;115(2):169–180. doi:10.1016/j.obhdp.2011.01.009

38. Sonnentag S, Venz L, Casper A. Advances in recovery research: What have we learned? What should be done next? *J Occup Health Psychol.* 2017;22(3):365–380. doi:10.1037/ocp0000079

39. Sonnentag S, Fritz C. The recovery experience questionnaire: Development and validation of a measure for assessing recuperation and unwinding from work. *J Occup Health Psychol.* 2007;12(3):204–221.

40. Bennett AA, Bakker AB, Field JG. Recovery from work-related effort: A meta-analysis. *J Organ Behav.* 2018;39(3):262–275. doi:10.1002/job.2217

41. Bosch C, Sonnentag S, Pinck AS. What makes for a good break? A diary study on recovery experiences during lunch break. *J Occup Organ Psychol.* 2018;91(1):134–157. doi:10.1111/joop.12195

42. Trougakos JP, Hideg I, Cheng BH, Beal DJ. Lunch breaks unpacked: The role of autonomy as a moderator of recovery during lunch. *AMJ.* 2014;57(2):405–421. doi:10.5465/amj.2011.1072

43. Sianoja M, Syrek CJ, de Bloom J, Korpela K, Kinnunen U. Enhancing daily well-being at work through lunchtime park walks and relaxation exercises: Recovery experiences as mediators. *J Occup Health Psychol.* 2018;23(3):428–442. doi:10.1037/ocp0000083

44. Merlo G, Rippe J. Physician burnout: A lifestyle medicine perspective. *Am J Lifestyle Med.* 2021;15(2):148–157.

45. Hillman AJ, Withers MC, Collins BJ. Resource dependence theory: A review. *J Manage.* 2009;35(6):1404–1427. doi:10.1177/0149206309343469

46. Uy MA, Jia Lin K, Ilies R. Is it better to give or receive? The role of help in buffering the depleting effects of surface acting. *Acad Manage J.* 2017;60(4):1442–1461. doi:10.5465/amj.2015.0611

47. Johnson JV, Hall EM. Job strain, work place social support, and cardiovascular disease: A cross-sectional study of a random sample of the Swedish working population. *Am J Public Health*. 1988;78(10):1336–1342. doi:10.2105/AJPH.78.10.1336

48. Koopman J, Lanaj K, Scott BA. Integrating the bright and dark sides of OCB: A daily investigation of the benefits and costs of helping others. *AMJ*. 2015;59(2):414–435. doi:10.5465/amj.2014.0262

49. Lanaj K, Johnson RE, Wang M. When lending a hand depletes the will: The daily costs and benefits of helping. *J Appl Psychol*. 2016;101(8):1097. doi:10.1037/apl0000118

50. Tews MJ, Michel JW, Stafford K. Social support and turnover among entry-level service employees: Differentiating type, source, and basis of attachment. *Hum Resour Manage*. 2020;59(3):1–14. doi:10.1002/hrm.21989

51. Holt-Lunstad J, Smith TW, Uchino BN. Can hostility interfere with the health benefits of giving and receiving social support? The impact of cynical hostility on cardiovascular reactivity during social support interactions among friends. *Ann Behav Med*. 2008;35(3):319–330. doi:10.1007/s12160-008-9041-z

52. Brady JM, Hammer LB, Mohr CD, Bodner TE. Supportive supervisor training improves family relationships among employee and spouse dyads. *J Occup Health Psychol*. 2021;26(1):31–48. doi:10.1037/ocp0000264

53. Kossek EE, Thompson RJ, Lawson KM, et al. Caring for the elderly at work and home: Can a randomized organizational intervention improve psychological health? *J Occup Health Psychol*. 2019;24(1):36–54. doi:10.1037/ocp0000104

36 The Health of Sexually-Diverse and Gender-Diverse Populations

Lisa M. Diamond, PhD

KEY POINTS

- The stigma facing sexually- and gender- diverse individuals has consequences on their mental and physical health.
- Social threat can contribute to chronic stress that has negative, long-term effects on health.
- Interventions can aim at social safety to promote well-being and protect sexually- and gender-diverse individuals from negative health consequences.

36.1 INTRODUCTION

Over the past several decades, a growing body of research has focused on the unique mental and physical health needs of sexually-diverse individuals (i.e., those who identify as lesbian, gay, bisexual, pansexual, queer, or asexual, or who engage in sexual or romantic relationships with the same gender) and gender-diverse individuals (i.e., those who identify as transgender, non-binary, gender non-conforming, or gender fluid). Such individuals are commonly described in the scientific and medical literature as *sexual and gender minorities,* but we describe them here as *sexually- and gender-diverse* (SGD) to underscore that it is their *differentness* from mainstream sexual/gender norms that renders them a distinct population, rather than their statistical prevalence. Importantly, sexually-diverse individuals and gender-diverse individuals have unique life experiences and stigma-related challenges, and they are by no means interchangeable populations. We group them together in the present discussion because of their shared experience of stigma and social marginalization, which is the primary driver of their well-documented health disparities. Most SGD individuals grow up exposed to consistent and pervasive social denigration over their lifespans, from multiple sources, and many face explicit discrimination and interpersonal violence as well. In this chapter, we review the processes by which these experiences feed forward to affect mental and physical health of SGD individuals, and we conclude by discussing research on intervention strategies aimed at mitigating the immediate and long-term health risks associated with sexual/gender stigma.

DOI: 10.1201/b22810-41

36.2 HEALTH DISPARITIES

SGD individuals show notable disparities in both physical and mental health over the lifespan, and health psychologists have called for targeted research on their underlying mechanisms and potential strategies for intervention.[1,2] Regarding mental health, numerous population studies and meta-analyses find that SGD adolescents and adults show disproportionate levels of depression, generalized anxiety, obsessive compulsive disorder, suicidal ideation, and suicidal behavior.[3–7] In light of such findings, some scholars have argued that major depression poses a greater threat to the health of gay and bisexual men than HIV.[8]

Physical health disparities in SGD populations have shown more variation from study to study, often depending on the method of categorizing respondents and the specific covariates included (race/ethnicity, age, income, health insurance status, substance use, etc.). Diamond et al.[9] reviewed 22 population studies published in the last decade that assessed disparities in SGD adults' physical health outcomes, relative to cisgender and heterosexual adults. They found substantial variation across studies, depending on the specific health conditions assessed (cardiovascular disease, cardiovascular risk factors, asthma, cancer, etc.) and whether demographic and health-relevant covariates were accounted for. The most consistent disparities were found for self-reported functional disabilities, self-reported global assessments of physical wellness, cardiovascular disease, asthma, and arthritis. Yet the specific SGD subgroups showing elevated health risks differed from study to study: Some studies found moderating effects of gender, race/ethnicity, age, or specific identity subgroupings (for example, bisexual versus lesbian/gay). These findings show that health disparities in SGD populations have no single, all-purpose, easy-to-grasp cause. Rather, they are driven by multiple biobehavioral mechanisms that interact dynamically with individuals' genetic predispositions and environmental contexts.

One of the most well-researched mechanisms is stress reactivity. Meyer's influential "minority stress" theory[10] postulated that the elevated mental health problems of sexually-diverse individuals were attributable to the "pile up" of stigma-related stressors that they commonly experience, including discrimination, bullying, internalized shame, physical victimization, and closeting. Numerous measures have been designed to assess these phenomena in the lives of sexually-diverse and gender-diverse individuals, across a range of time scales, developmental periods, and situational contexts, for example.[11–13] Although self-reports of the frequency of stigma-related stressors tend to correlate with self-report measures of anxiety and depression in SGD populations,[14,15] stress exposure does not reliably predict biological indices of stress reactivity (such as secretion of cortisol) or physical health outcomes.[9] Notably, this is also the case for measures of racial/ethnic stigmatization. Like SGD populations, ethnically-marginalized populations show pronounced health disparities, but individual-level exposures to racial/ethnic stigma do not reliably predict individual-level health outcomes.[16] For these reasons, health psychologists have begun expanding their theoretical models of the links between social stigma and health outcomes in order to capture a broader range of biobehavioral mechanisms, such as *threat-related hypervigilance*.

36.3   SAFETY, UNCERTAINTY, AND HYPERVIGILANCE

In recent years, scholars have noted that our common-sense notions of "stress reactivity" – in which individuals occupy a default state of calm until we encounter an activating stressor – are inaccurate. As argued by Brosschot and colleagues, the human nervous system evolved to *presume* a certain degree of danger in the immediate environment, and hence to maintain a default state of chronic threat-vigilance in order to facilitate rapid and efficient responsiveness to unpredictable threats.[17–19] Chronic threat-vigilance involves a coordinated set of biobehavioral processes, such as perseverative cognition, heightened attention to threat cues, chronic self- and other-monitoring, and social withdrawal.[20–22] Although these strategies are adaptive in providing self-protection within uncertain environments, they are energetically demanding, and over time may deplete the attentional resources necessary for goal-directed, social, and restorative activity.[23,24]

If chronic threat vigilance is the default state of the human nervous system, then what *interrupts* this vigilance sufficiently for individuals to maintain adaptive patterns of emotional, cognitive, behavioral, and immunological functioning? The answer is s*ocial safety*, defined as social connection, social inclusion, social protection, social recognition, and social acceptance.[17,25] Because humans have lived in small social groups throughout our evolutionary history, social belonging is a fundamental and primary human need.[25–27] When we feel sufficiently protected and included by those around us, our prefrontal cortex suppresses the neural systems responsible for threat vigilance, freeing up our attention and energy for exploration, goal-directed activity, and social engagement.[20,28] When individuals do not have sufficient and consistent access to social safety, their threat vigilance remains engaged, eating up their attention and energy even in the absence of direct threat.

This is precisely what may be happening in the minds and bodies of SGD individuals and other marginalized populations: Stigma, by definition, excludes individuals from the broader social fabric by marking them as "other" and "lesser."[29] Stigmatized individuals do not need to experience direct physical threats or discrete instances of discrimination to *know* that they cannot count on the unconditional protection of their neighbors, colleagues, and political leaders. For example, studies have found that routine cues of social safety and belonging (respectful treatment, offers of assistance, friendly eye contact, explicit signs of social inclusion) are often withdrawn from SGD individuals once their identities are known,[30,31] and hence many SGD individuals learn to fend for themselves by closely monitoring their surroundings for signs of disapproval and altering their speech and behavior in order to avoid danger.[32] Concealment, isolation, and chronic wariness may prove adaptive in the short term, by helping individuals to avoid direct exposure to discrimination or harassment, but when sustained over time these processes exact a psychological and biological toll that may be just as health-consequential as heightened stress exposure.

36.4   THE RELEVANCE OF THE IMMUNE SYSTEM

The biological mechanisms through which stigma (and other stressors) influence long-term health have been the topic of extensive study over the past several decades, and an increasing body of work suggests a primary role for *immunological inflammation*. Inflammation is the immune system's response to threat or injury and is mediated by the release of "communication" molecules called pro-inflammatory cytokines, such as interleukin-1β (IL-1β), interleukin-6 (IL-6), and tumor necrosis factor-alpha, or TNF-α. Acute inflammatory responses promote healing, but chronic, low-grade inflammation can increase individuals' long-term susceptibility to infections, reduce the effectiveness of vaccines, and directly damage tissues and organs throughout the body.[33] These processes have been shown to make unique contributions to a broad range of disease processes and health outcomes, including fatigue, frailty, disability, type 2 diabetes, cardiovascular disease, Alzheimer's disease, asthma, osteoporosis, rheumatoid arthritis, periodontal disease, some forms of cancer, and all-cause mortality.[33,34]

Systemic inflammation poses a particular health risk for SGD individuals because it is known to be triggered by *social threat* – i.e., experiences of rejection, isolation, denigration, exclusion, ostracization, and shame.[35,36] For example, observational studies have found that individuals show significant elevations in inflammation after experiencing social rejection, the loss of close social ties, or negative/conflictual interactions with social partners.[37–40] Additionally, studies have found that *perceived* threats are just as influential on threat-related inflammation as actual threats,[41] which indicates *fearing* social rejection may be just as health consequential as experiencing rejection. These studies suggest that because SGD typically face disproportionate risks for social rejection, shame, denigration, and exclusion, they face disproportionate risks for systemic inflammation and its downstream health consequences, and a growing number of studies support this view.[42–49] Nonetheless, the magnitude of associations between sexual/gender stigmatization and inflammation has varied from study to study, and researchers have called for greater attention to moderating factors, such as race/ethnicity, age, or health behaviors.[47–49]

Early life adversity may be among the most important of these moderators, and scholars have increasingly investigated whether some of the long-term health effects of sexual/gender stigma are traceable to SGD individuals' disproportionate exposure to neglect, abuse, economic insecurity, and household dysfunction during childhood and adolescence. Approximately one-third of SGD adults report having such experiences prior to age 18, which is nearly double the rates observed among cisgender heterosexuals reviewed in ref. 9. The reasons for disproportionate exposure to childhood adversity among SGD populations are unknown: Some of this effect is likely due to differential reporting: SGD individuals may be more aware/open about childhood adversity because the process of questioning one's gender or sexuality often involves extended reflection and interrogation about childhood and adolescent feelings and experiences.[50] Additionally, evidence suggests that children who appear "different" from other children (because of gender-atypicality or other domains) face higher rates of maltreatment by the adults and age-mates in their life reviewed in ref. 51. Early life adversity has well-documented implications for long-term mental and physical health reviewed in ref. 52, and studies suggest that it may enhance stigma-related health vulnerabilities among SGD individuals. For example, studies have found that SGD individuals with histories of childhood sexual abuse have significantly greater rates of substance problems, perceived stress, depressive symptoms,

PTSD, and suicidal ideation and behavior than those without such histories.[53-55] Such findings indicate that in order to successfully mitigate the long-term health consequences of stigma among SGD populations, we must devote as much attention to their childhood histories of psychological threat and social safety as to their current experiences.

36.5 INTERVENTION APPROACHES

If SGD health disparities are partly attributable to insufficient social safety and chronic threat-vigilance, then how can we mitigate these effects? Several recent reviews provide evidence-based guidance on the most effective strategies for interrupting the cognitive, behavioral, emotional, and biological sequelae of sexual/gender stigma.[56,57] Some interventions have focused on enhancing SGD individuals' psychological coping resources, for example, by creating educational interventions that counteract negative stereotypes, teach strategies for reframing stigma-related challenges, and enhance individuals' ability to identity and modulate their emotional responses.[58,59] To some degree, such interventions are designed to address the immediate psychological processes that unfold in the wake of stigma, such as rumination, isolation, and self-blame,[60] given that stigma itself may prove difficult and slow to change, especially in certain communities.

Other interventions tackle stigma directly, attempting to reduce SGD individuals' vulnerability to stigma-related health problems by altering local attitudes and expectations about SGD individuals within a particular social environment. For example, numerous school districts have established Gender-Sexuality Alliances (sometimes called "Gay-Straight Alliances") to foster a sense of belonging and protection for SGD youth within their school settings.[61,62] Other interventions disseminate educational trainings and materials aimed at reducing homophobia, promoting contact with SGD individuals, and increasing community knowledge and empathy about their experiences.[63] These interventions have generally proven successful in creating "safe spaces" for SGD individuals within specific settings and social relationships, for example, within the family,[64] although it remains unclear whether such localized approaches are sufficient to counteract the broad and pervasive nature of structural and institutional stigma, as it remains manifested in social practices, laws, and policies.[65]

Of course, social structures and institutions are made up of individual people, and hence interventions that seek to decrease stigma and enhance social safety at the immediate, interpersonal level may, over time, "trickle up" to shape broader social norms and policies. The opposite may take place, as well: Several studies have found that when states and municipalities pass laws and policies that protect the well-being of SGD citizens (for example, laws prohibiting sexual orientation discrimination in housing, employment, or public accommodations), SGD individuals often show subsequent *improvements* in mental and physical health, regardless of whether they are directly affected by the legislation of interest.[66-69] These broad-based effects are thought to reflect the symbolic nature of laws and policies.[70] Laws punishing anti-gay discrimination and harassment serve to affirm the basic dignity and self-worth of SGD individuals, which may explain why SGD individuals who live in regions of the US with anti-discrimination laws are viewed as more "hirable" by local managers and report less organizational discrimination.[71-73]

Intervention initiatives are likely to be most successful when implemented across multiple levels and domains (for example, affirmative laws and policies at the state and municipal level, ability of SGD individuals to access local community support, affirmative school and workplace environments, etc.). The Centers for Disease Control (CDC) advocates a social-ecological approach to health promotion which integrates prevention efforts across four different levels: societal, community, relational, and individual.[74] This strategy has proven successful in the domain of suicide prevention,[75] and it offers a promising framework for addressing stigma-related health problems in SGD populations, by creating a *consistent, multilevel safety net* across multiple social domains.

36.6 CONCLUSION

The human brain's sensitivity to social threat and social belonging is a legacy of our ancestral, group-living nature. Quite simply, our brains evolved to explore and thrive when protected and nurtured by those around us. Hence, we cannot promote health and well-being in stigmatized populations simply by reducing their exposure to stress and hardship: we must also amplify their experiences of reliable social connection, validation, and affirmation, at all stages of life. Accordingly, health promotion efforts should adopt a "safety first" approach which begins by identifying whether individuals have sufficient and reliable access to affirmative and protective social ties that foster feelings of belonging and protection, and that are capable of down-regulating chronic threat-vigilance, rumination, and self-blame. Devoting just as much attention to SGD individuals' access to social safety as we have historically devoted to their stress exposure may be one of the most important intervention strategies available for reducing stigma-related health disparities in sexually-diverse and gender-diverse populations.

REFERENCES

1. Institute of Medicine. *The Health of Lesbian, Gay, Bisexual, and Transgender People: Building a Foundation for Better Understanding.* Washington, D.C.: The National Academies Press; 2011.
2. Sexual and gender minorities formally designated as a health disparity population for research purposes [press release]. October 6 2016.
3. Cicero EC, Reisner SL, Merwin EI, Humphreys JC, Silva SG. The health status of transgender and gender nonbinary adults in the United States. *PLoS ONE.* 2020;15(2): e0228765.
4. Newcomb ME, Mustanski B. Internalized homophobia and internalizing mental health problems: A meta-analytic review. *Clin Psychol Rev.* 2010;30(8):1019–1029.
5. Krueger EA, Upchurch DM. Are sociodemographic, lifestyle, and psychosocial characteristics associated with sexual orientation group differences in mental health disparities? Results from a national population-based study. *Soc Psychiatry Psychiatr Epidemiol.* 2019;54(6):755–770.
6. Raifman J, Charlton BM, Arrington-Sanders R, et al. Sexual orientation and suicide attempt disparities among US adolescents: 2009-2017. *Pediatrics.* 2020;145(3).

7. McCabe SE, Hughes TL, West BT, et al. Sexual orientation, adverse childhood experiences, and comorbid dsm-5 substance use and mental health disorders. *J Clin Psychiatry.* 2020;81(6):20m13291.

8. Bromberg DJ, Paltiel AD, Busch SH, Pachankis JE. Has depression surpassed HIV as a burden to gay and bisexual men's health in the United States? A comparative modeling study. *Soc Psychiatry Psychiatr Epidemiol.* 2021;56(2):273–282.

9. Diamond LM, Dehlin AJ, Alley J. Systemic inflammation as a driver of health disparities among sexually-diverse and gender-diverse individuals. *Psychoneuroendocrinology.* 2021;129:105215.

10. Meyer IH. Prejudice, social stress, and mental health in lesbian, gay, and bisexual populations: Conceptual issues and research evidence. *Psychol Bull.* 2003;129(5):674–697.

11. Eldahan AI, Pachankis JE, Rendina HJ, Ventuneac A, Grov C, Parsons JT. Daily minority stress and affect among gay and bisexual men: A 30-day diary study. *Journal of Affective Disorders.* 2016;190:828–835.

12. Szymanski DM, Kashubeck-West S, Meyer J. Internalized heterosexism: Measurement, psychosocial correlates, and research directions. *Couns Psychol.* 2008;36(4):525–574.

13. Hidalgo MA, Petras H, Chen D, Chodzen G. The gender minority stress and resilience measure: Psychometric validity of an adolescent extension. *Clin Pract Pediatr Psychol.* 2019;7(3):278–290.

14. Plöderl M, Tremblay P. Mental health of sexual minorities. A systematic review. *Int Rev Psychiatry.* 2015;27(5):367–385.

15. Semlyen J, King M, Varney J, Hagger-Johnson G. Sexual orientation and symptoms of common mental disorder or low wellbeing: Combined meta-analysis of 12 UK population health surveys. *BMC Psychiatry.* 2016;16:67.

16. Diamond LM, Alley J. Rethinking minority stress: A social safety perspective on the health effects of stigma in sexually-diverse and gender-diverse population. *Neurosci Biobehav Rev.* 2022;138:104720.

17. Brosschot JF, Verkuil B, Thayer JF. Generalized unsafety theory of stress: Unsafe environments and conditions, and the default stress response. *Int J Environ Res Public Health.* 2018;15(3):1–27.

18. Brosschot JF, Verkuil B, Thayer JF. Exposed to events that never happen: Generalized unsafety, the default stress response, and prolonged autonomic activity. *Neurosci Biobehav Rev.* 2017;74(Pt B):287–296.

19. Brosschot JF, Verkuil B, Thayer JF. The default response to uncertainty and the importance of perceived safety in anxiety and stress: An evolution-theoretical perspective. *J Anxiety Disord.* 2016;41:22–34.

20. Richards HJ, Benson V, Donnelly N, Hadwin JA. Exploring the function of selective attention and hypervigilance for threat in anxiety. *Clin Psychol Rev.* 2014;34(1):1–13.

21. Wieser MJ, Reicherts P, Juravle G, von Leupoldt A. Attention mechanisms during predictable and unpredictable threat—A steady-state visual evoked potential approach. *NeuroImage.* 2016;139:167–175.

22. Cornwell BR, Garrido MI, Overstreet C, Pine DS, Grillon C. The unpredictive brain under threat: A neurocomputational account of anxious hypervigilance. *Biol Psychiatry.* 2017;82(6):447–454.

23. Martin JT, Whittaker AH, Johnston SJ. Pupillometry and the vigilance decrement: Task-evoked but not baseline pupil measures reflect declining performance in visual vigilance tasks. *Eur J Neurosci.* 2022;55(3):778–799.

24. Rivera-Rodriguez A, Sherwood M, Fitzroy AB, Sanders LD, Dasgupta N. Anger, race, and the neurocognition of threat: Attention, inhibition, and error processing during a weapon identification task. *Cogn Res Princ Implic.* 2021;6:74.

25. Slavich GM. Social safety theory: A biologically based evolutionary perspective on life stress, health, and behavior. *Annu Rev Clin Psychol.* 2020;16:265–295.

26. Bowlby J. The nature of the child's tie to his mother. *Int J Psychoanal.* 1958;39:350–373.

27. Baumeister RF, Leary MR. The need to belong: Desire for interpersonal attachments as a fundamental human motivation. *Psychol Bull.* 1995;117(3):497–529.

28. Gomes N, Semin GR. Mapping human vigilance: The influence of conspecifics. *Evol Hum Behav.* 2020;41(1):69–75.

29. Pachankis JE, Hatzenbuehler ML, Wang K, et al. The burden of stigma on health and well-being: A taxonomy of concealment, course, disruptiveness, aesthetics, origin, and peril across 93 stigmas. *Pers Soc Psychol Bull.* 2018;44(4):451–474.

30. Ellis J, Fox P. The effect of self-identified sexual orientation on helping behavior in a British sample: Are lesbians and gay men treated differently? *J Appl Soc Psychol.* 2001;31(6):1238–1247.

31. Gabriel U, Banse R. Helping behavior as a subtle measure of discrimination against lesbians and gay men: German data and a comparison across countries. *J Appl Soc Psychol.* 2006;36(3):690–707.

32. Sloss M. Queer folks are sharing the unwritten rules they follow that most straight people are clueless about, and it's eye-opening. BuzzFeed. March 21, 2022.

33. Furman D, Campisi J, Verdin E, et al. Chronic inflammation in the etiology of disease across the life span. *Nat Med.* 2019;25(12):1822–1832.

34. Couzin-Frankel J. Inflammation bares a dark side. *Science.* 2010;330(6011):1621.

35. Slavich GM, O'Donovan A, Epel ES, Kemeny ME. Black sheep get the blues: A psychobiological model of social rejection and depression. *Neurosci Biobehav Rev.* 2010;35(1):39–45.

36. Kemeny ME. Psychobiological responses to social threat: Evolution of a psychological model in psychoneuroimmunology. *Brain Behav Immun.* 2009;23(1):1–9.

37. Murphy MLM, Slavich GM, Rohleder N, Miller GE. Targeted rejection triggers differential pro- and anti-inflammatory gene expression in adolescents as a function of social status. *Clin Psychol Sci.* 2013;1(1):30–40.

38. Schultze-Florey CR, Martínez-Maza O, Magpantay L, et al. When grief makes you sick: Bereavement induced systemic inflammation is a question of genotype. *Brain Behav Immun.* 2012;26(7):1066–1071.

39. Chiang JJ, Eisenberger NI, Seeman TE, Taylor SE. Negative and competitive social interactions are related to heightened proinflammatory cytokine activity. *Proc Natl Acad Sci USA.* 2012;109(6):1878–1882.

40. Marin TJ, Chen E, Munch JA, Miller GE. Double-exposure to acute stress and chronic family stress is associated with immune changes in children with asthma. *Psychosom Med.* 2009;71(4):378–384.

41. Slavich GM, Irwin MR. From stress to inflammation and major depressive disorder: A social signal transduction theory of depression. *Psychol Bull.* 2014;140(3):774–815.

42. Wardecker BM, Graham-Engeland JE, Almeida DM. Perceived discrimination predicts elevated biological markers of inflammation among sexual minority adults. *J Behav Med.* 2021;44:53–65. doi:10.1007/s10865-020-00180-z

43. Mays VM, Juster R-P, Williamson TJ, Seeman TE, Cochran SD. Chronic physiologic effects of stress among lesbian, gay, and bisexual adults: Results from the National Health and Nutrition Examination Survey. *Psychosom Med.* 2018;80(6):551–563.

44. Everett BG, Rosario M, McLaughlin KA, Austin SB. Sexual orientation and gender differences in markers of inflammation and immune functioning. *Ann Behav Med.* 2014;47(1):57–70.

45. Hatzenbuehler ML, McLaughlin KA, Slopen N. Sexual orientation disparities in cardiovascular biomarkers among young adults. *Am J Prev Med.* 2013;44(6):612–621.

46. Simenson AJ, Corey S, Markovic N, Kinsky S. Disparities in chronic health outcomes and health behaviors between lesbian and heterosexual adult women in Pittsburgh: A longitudinal study. *J Womens Health (Larchmt).* 2020;29(8):1059–1067.

47. Wood EP, Cook SH. Father support is protective against the negative effects of perceived discrimination on CRP among sexual minorities but not heterosexuals. *Psychoneuroendocrinology*. 2019;110.

48. Morgan E, D'Aquila R, Carnethon MR, Mustanski B. Cardiovascular disease risk factors are elevated among a cohort of young sexual and gender minorities in Chicago. *J Behav Med*. 2019;42(6):1073–1081.

49. Doyle DM, Molix L. Minority stress and inflammatory mediators: Covering moderates associations between perceived discrimination and salivary interleukin-6 in gay men. *J Behav Med*. 2016;39(5):782–792.

50. Savin-Williams RC. *"... And Then I Became Gay": Young Men's Stories*. New York: Routledge; 1998.

51. Corliss HL, Cochran SD, Mays VM. Reports of parental maltreatment during childhood in a United States population-based survey of homosexual, bisexual, and heterosexual adults. *Child Abuse & Neglect*. 2002;26(11):1165–1178.

52. Ellis BJ, Sheridan MA, Belsky J, McLaughlin KA. Why and how does adversity influence development? Toward an integrated model of dimensions of environmental experience. *Dev Psychopathol*. 2022;34:447–471.

53. Mattera B, Levine EC, Martinez O, et al. Long-term health outcomes of childhood sexual abuse and peer sexual contact among an urban sample of behaviourally bisexual Latino men. *Cult Health Sex*. 2018;20(6):607–624.

54. Boroughs MS, Valentine SE, Ironson GH, et al. Complexity of childhood sexual abuse: Predictors of current post-traumatic stress disorder, mood disorders, substance use, and sexual risk behavior among adult men who have sex with men. *Arch Sex Behav*. 2015;44(7):1891–1902.

55. Schneeberger AR, Dietl MF, Muenzenmaier KH, Huber CG, Lang UE. Stressful childhood experiences and health outcomes in sexual minority populations: A systematic review. *Soc Psychiatry Psychiatr Epidemiol*. 2014;49(9):1427–1445.

56. Chaudoir SR, Wang K, Pachankis JE. What reduces sexual minority stress? A review of the intervention "toolkit". *J Soc Issues*. 2017;73(3):586–617.

57. Layland EK, Carter JA, Perry NS, et al. A systematic review of stigma in sexual and gender minority health interventions. *Transl Behav Med*. 2020;10(5):1200–1210.

58. Pachankis JE, Hatzenbuehler ML, Rendina HJ, Safren SA, Parsons JT. LGB-affirmative cognitive-behavioral therapy for young adult gay and bisexual men: A randomized controlled trial of a transdiagnostic minority stress approach. *J Consult Clin Psychol*. 2015;83(5):875–889.

59. Lucassen MFG, Merry SN, Hatcher S, Frampton CMA. Rainbow SPARX: A novel approach to addressing depression in sexual minority youth. *Cogn Behav Pract*. 2015;22(2):203–216.

60. Hatzenbuehler ML. How does sexual minority stigma "get under the skin"? A psychological mediation framework. *Psychol Bull*. 2009;135(5):707–730.

61. Lessard LM, Puhl RM, Watson RJ. Gay-straight alliances: A mechanism of health risk reduction among lesbian, gay, bisexual, transgender, and questioning adolescents. *Am J Prev Med*. 2020;59(2):196–203.

62. Wheeler Black W, Fedewa A, Gonzalez K. Effects of "safe school" programs and policies on the social climate for sexual-minority youth: A review of the literature. *J LGBT Youth*. 2012;9:321–339.

63. Tucker EW, Potocky-Tripodi M. Changing heterosexuals' attitudes toward homosexuals: A systematic review of the empirical literature. *Res Soc Work Pract*. 2006;16(2):176–190.

64. Huebner DM, Rullo JE, Thoma BC, McGarrity LA, Mackenzie J. Piloting Lead with Love: A film-based intervention to improve parents' responses to their lesbian, gay, and bisexual children. *J Prim Prev*. 2013;34(5):359–369.

65. Hatzenbuehler ML. Structural stigma and the health of lesbian, gay, and bisexual populations. *Curr Dir Psychol.* 2014;23(2):127–132.
66. Hatzenbuehler ML, McKetta S, Goldberg N, et al. Trends in state policy support for sexual minorities and HIV-related outcomes among men who have sex with men in the united states, 2008-2014. *J Acquir Immune Defic Syndr.* 2020;85(1):39–45.
67. Du Bois SN, Yoder W, Guy AA, Manser K, Ramos S. Examining associations between state-level transgender policies and transgender health. *Transgend Health.* 2018;3(1):220–224.
68. Raifman J, Moscoe E, Austin SB, Hatzenbuehler ML, Galea S. Association of state laws permitting denial of services to same-sex couples with mental distress in sexual minority adults: A difference-in-difference-in-differences analysis. *JAMA Psychiatry.* 2018;75(7):671–677.
69. van der Star A, Pachankis JE, Bränström R. Country-level structural stigma, school-based and adulthood victimization, and life satisfaction among sexual minority adults: A life course approach. *J Youth Adolesc.* 2021;50(1):189–201.
70. Barron LG, Hebl M. Reducing 'acceptable' stigmatization through legislation. *Soc Issues Policy Rev.* 2010;4(1):1–30.
71. Griffith KH, Hebl MR. The disclosure dilemma for gay men and lesbians: 'Coming out' at work. *J Appl Psychol.* 2002;87(6):1191–1199.
72. Barron LG, Hebl M. The force of law: The effects of sexual orientation antidiscrimination legislation on interpersonal discrimination in employment. *Psychol Public Policy, Law.* 2013;19(2):191–205.
73. Barron LG. Promoting the underlying principle of acceptance: The effectiveness of sexual orientation employment antidiscrimination legislation. *J Workplace Rights.* 2009; 14:251–268.
74. Centers for Disease Control and Prevention. *The Social-Ecological Model: A Framework for Prevention* 2017. https://www.cdc.gov/violenceprevention/about/social-ecologicalmodel. html
75. Cramer RJ, Kapusta ND. A social-ecological framework of theory, assessment, and prevention of suicide. *Front Psychol.* 2017;8:1756–1756.

37 Historically Marginalized Ethnic and Racial Communities

Luz M. Garcini, PhD, MPH,
Ivanova Veras-de Jesús, BA,
Kaivalya Gudooru, BS, and
Michelle T. Garza, MS

KEY POINTS

- The use of lifestyle medicine is an effective approach to address the mental health needs of historically marginalized ethnic/racial communities.
- Cultural factors, such as practices, values, social networks, and interpersonal dynamics, are important to address in the development and implementation of lifestyle interventions aimed at addressing the mental health of diverse populations.
- Contextual considerations, including attending to the role of intersectionality, the effect of the social environment, barriers and facilitators to health services and resources, and fostering conditions that facilitate resilience, are important considerations needed to inform mental health interventions for diverse populations.
- As we strive towards health equity, attending to and addressing the mental health of historically marginalized ethnic/racial communities requires innovation and commitment, as well as interdisciplinary efforts.

37.1 INTRODUCTION

Historically marginalized ethnic/racial communities exist on the edges of dominant society with scarce access to opportunities, resources, and vital services, including medical and mental healthcare.[1] Marginalized communities impacted by social disadvantage, life adversity, and economic hardship have experienced disparities and inequities across a range of health outcomes, including mental health.[2] In the face of the 2019 Coronavirus (COVID-19) pandemic, marginalized ethnic/racial communities have endured a significant burden from widening mental health gaps. Indeed, when compared to White individuals, people of African American, Latino, Asian, and Indigenous backgrounds have experienced a more pronounced decline in mental health outcomes throughout the pandemic.[3] Although suicide rates declined in 2019 and 2020 when compared to 2018 for most populations, suicide rates among

DOI: 10.1201/b22810-42

Latino men and non-Latino multiracial women increased in 2020.[4] In the face of added stressors, such as widespread uncertainty, mistrust, economic losses, reduced access to healthcare, social isolation, and limited access to digital technologies, the mental health of individuals from ethnic/racial marginalized communities has been neglected.[5] Amidst increasing mental health disparities, attending to the mental health of marginalized ethnic/racial communities is more relevant than ever.

People from marginalized backgrounds face complex chronic stressors that are toxic to their mental health. Poverty, limited health information, difficulties navigating healthcare systems, racism, discrimination, isolation, mental health stigma, and inadequate social support are some of the many compounded stressors at the root of psychological distress and mental disorders that marginalized individuals face.[6–12] The aforementioned stressors often interfere with individuals' ability to access health resources and obtain timely services that address the complex interplay of systemic, environmental, cultural, and individual factors affecting their mental health. Indeed, individuals from underserved and under-resourced communities, such as people from lower socioeconomic backgrounds and underrepresented racial and ethnic groups (e.g., Black individuals and African Americans, Asian Americans, Indigenous Peoples, Latino or Hispanic, Pacific Islander, Middle Eastern and North African populations) are less likely to seek mental health treatment and to receive quality mental healthcare.[13] Limited or lack of health insurance and the inability to pay out of pocket for mental health services are additional barriers that prevent individuals from marginalized backgrounds from receiving mental healthcare.[14] Addressing deeply entrenched mental health disparities requires devising innovative, more efficient, effective ways to address the current mental health crises.[15]

Lifestyle medicine may offer a valuable opportunity to address mental health among marginalized ethnic/racial communities by overcoming salient barriers to traditional approaches to mental healthcare. With its focus on the promotion and maintenance of health behaviors that are incorporated into everyday life, lifestyle medicine and its focus on improved nutrition, regular physical activity, restorative sleep, stress management, the building of supportive social networks, and avoidance of risky substances may provide a more appealing, non-stigmatizing, and holistic approach to self-care and mental health promotion. Although stigma toward psychological treatment exists in many communities, it is more pronounced among communities of color, given the added stress that underrepresented individuals face from segregation, stereotyping, and discrimination.[16] By emphasizing self-care as needed to reduce stress, lifestyle medicine may open avenues to address mental health in non-stigmatizing ways. For instance, research shows that a high-quality diet and engagement in relaxing physical activities are helpful to improve mood and effective in reducing stress-related fatigue. Similarly, restful sleep and spending time with loved ones improve motivation to pursue meaningful life goals. Moreover, lifestyle medicine for mental health can set the stage for mental health conversations rooted in self-care, which can be useful to demystify mental illnesses. Given the complex and chronic stressors marginalized ethnic/racial communities face, lifestyle medicine could help buffer the effects of toxic stress, build resilience, and provide empowerment and hope in the face of adversity, disadvantage, and marginalization. In the next section of this chapter and summarized in Table 37.1, we highlight cultural and

TABLE 37.1

Cultural and Contextual Considerations for Lifestyle Medicine Interventions with Historically Marginalized Ethnic/Racial Communities.

Cultural Considerations[a]	
Domain	**Examples**
Cultural Humility	• Intentionally engage in self-critique and reflexivity to recognize and accept biases and assumptions. Use these questions to engage in self-reflection: What is it like to be a member of the community? What do I know about this person's experience? Am I centering my own culture and perspective when interacting with this person? What is it about this person that makes them culturally unique? What aspects of this person's culture impact their reasons for engaging/not engaging? How may this person's culture be a strength in working towards a particular goal? How may this person's and my own culture impact our interaction and our ability to connect and work together?
	• Engage in active listening and be genuine in your interpersonal interactions with the community.
	• Ask open-ended questions respectfully and with an honest desire to learn and communicate with the community.
	• Ask for guidance and feedback while conversing, including being accountable for micro and macro aggressions that may happen. Apply the feedback you are given by the community.
	• Ask for permission to share your knowledge about a topic, such as when discussing mental health.
	• Avoid giving unsolicited advice, but rather provide the tools and knowledge for people to make their decisions.
Cultural Competence	• Acquire a robust knowledge about the culture and history of the community, including knowledge of past circumstances that have contributed to a community's current economic, social, and political status within the broader culture.
	• Build liaisons and consult periodically with experts or members of the community to identify gaps in your knowledge and to increase your competence. This includes using consultation, literature, and training to understand culturally specific behaviors that demonstrate respect for the community.
	• Explore, acknowledge, and validate the worldviews of members of the community.
	• Provide training and resources to educate staff and other members of your team about the community.
	• Select or build culturally appropriate screenings and assessment tools with feedback from key experts and/or members of the community.
	• Conduct periodic evaluation of your engagement and communication efforts, and adapt as needed. This includes assessing progress toward desired goals established by the community.
	• Use a collaborative approach when interacting with members of the community.
Values	• Ask and consider what is important and needed by the community, and frame interventions accordingly.
	• Engage in efforts to build trust and establish credibility with guidance, advice and feedback from the community. Periodically assess your efforts at building trust and credibility.

(Continued)

TABLE 37.1 (*Continued*)

Cultural Considerations[a]	
Domain	**Examples**
	• Use verbal and nonverbal responses, approaches, or styles to convey respect for the community and its values.
	• Learn about the history and past experiences associated with the development of norms and values in the community.
	• Learn about the community's views of the past and future, as well as the community's perception of its place within the broader culture, society, and the world.
	• Use values that are important to the community to frame or formulate messages, including health messages. Examples of important values among non-western communities are collectivism, *familism,* religiosity and spirituality, tenacity, respect, and gratitude, among many others. Identify and learn about important values in the community.
Practices	• Recognize and respect help-seeking practices and collaborate with trusted health providers in the community.
	• If appropriate and preferred by the community, incorporate religiosity and spirituality in interventions with guidance and collaboration from the community and its faith-based leaders.
	• Learn preferred cognitive and learning styles of the community (e.g., placing more attention on reflecting and processing than on content; being task-oriented; use of roleplay), and incorporate its preferences in the intervention.
	• Learn and be respectful of rituals, ceremonies, celebrations, and traditions.
	• Abstain from appropriating or exploiting practices, rituals, and traditions.
Social Networks	• Acquire knowledge about the structure of social networks.
	• Learn about the role of the family as a support system and different family structures and systems that exist.
	• Learn about informal sources of emotional and affective support outside the family structure, as well as primary sources of instrumental and informational help to canalize the delivery of health information and resources.
	• Leverage support networks and be mindful of norms that guide interpersonal interactions.
	• Acquire knowledge and be mindful of rules and norms of interpersonal dynamics, including those that may facilitate or hinder the implementation of healthy living (e.g., gender roles, intergenerational differences).
	• Learn about preferred styles of verbal and non-verbal communication. Consider, for instance, the use of direct versus indirect communication, appropriate personal space, social parameters for displays of physical contact, use of silence, preferred ways of moving, meaning of gestures, degree to which arguments and verbal confrontations are acceptable, degree of formality expected in communication, and amount of eye contact expected.
	• Learn about preferred strategies for mediating conflict and how to respectfully engage in problem solving. This includes learning about reward and sanction concepts and how these influence decision making and goal achievement.
	• Learn how prejudice, stereotypes, and expectations from others influence interpersonal dynamics in the community and keep in mind such knowledge when interacting with the community.

(*Continued*)

TABLE 37.1 *(Continued)*

Contextual Considerations[a]

Domain	Examples
Intersectionality	• Become aware and be respectful of intersectional identities that may be prevalent in the community and invite reflection about intersectionality in your conversations. Aspects to consider in addition to ethnicity and race include age, disability, gender identity, religion, education, socioeconomic status, sexual orientation, among many others. • Understand how a person's multiple identities may be barriers and/or resources to opportunities and services, as well as how intersectionality may influence a person's mental health, health behaviors, and lifestyle choices. • Be mindful of the ways in which the community has been harmed by different systems of oppression and of your engagement with said systems.
Social Context	• Identify and become aware of systemic and structural barriers (e.g., racism, discrimination) that increase stress and interfere/undermine an individual's access to opportunities, services, and resources. • Assist, support, and provide resources for the community to help overcome barriers imposed by social disadvantage. • Raise awareness and join advocacy efforts to reduce the harmful effects of social disadvantage on the community. This can be done by writing policy briefs, engaging in media campaigns, or collaborating with local grassroots community organizations that advocate for social justice and health equity.
Resilience	• Learn and incorporate preferred coping strategies used by the community to cope with social disadvantage and adversity. For instance, among some historically marginalized communities, some effective strategies include cognitive reframing, behavioral adaptability, acceptance (i.e., gratefulness, contentment), sociability, courage, and ancestral or cultural pride. • Adopt a strength-based approach that focuses on building upon people's strengths, skills, and qualities over a deficits approach. This includes facilitating strengths-based discussions and exercises, which can be done through testimonials and story-telling. • Incorporating the use of folk and local art (e.g., dance, music, acting, writing, painting, sculpture) in the delivery of health messages that can help foster cultural identity and pride.
Access	• Ask about and address accessibility needs in the community. • Be strategic about delivering health interventions in the communities where people live, work, learn, and play (e.g., engage in home or work visits). • Collaborate and prioritize the use of non-traditional sources of service delivery (e.g., community health workers (CHWs), pastors, priests) for the effective dissemination of lifestyle medicine interventions to the communities. This includes collaborating with members of the community as part of your team. • Utilize peer-support groups and strategies in collaboration with trusted members in the community (e.g., CHWs, pastors, priests) to implement and disseminate interventions to the community. • Disseminate health information and resources using clear, consistent, and easy to understand messages in the preferred language of the community.

(Continued)

TABLE 37.1 (Continued)

Contextual Considerations[a]	
Domain	**Examples**
	• Use patient navigators that can assist community members in accessing and navigating complex healthcare systems and informational resources.
	• Develop local outreach and educational programs. Become knowledgeable about and use available local goods and services (e.g., health, social, legal, educational) and make this knowledge accessible to the community. This could be done for instance through toolkits or resource sheets that can be delivered at local community events, via social media or through a website.
	• Periodically analyze community demographic trends and populations served to ensure representation and inclusion in your work.

[a] Some of the considerations in Table 37.1 have been adapted from SAMHSA.[17]

contextual considerations in developing, implementing, and disseminating lifestyle medicine approaches to address mental health among historically marginalized ethnic/racial communities.

37.2 CULTURAL CONSIDERATIONS OF LIFESTYLE MEDICINE FOR MENTAL HEALTH AMONG MARGINALIZED ETHNIC/RACIAL COMMUNITIES

37.2.1 CULTURAL HUMILITY AND CULTURAL COMPETENCE

The successful use of lifestyle medicine to improve the mental health of marginalized communities requires cultural humility and cultural competence. Cultural humility requires acknowledging one's inability to know everything about another person's culture and contextual experience and requires an awareness of one's biases and limitations.[18] When working with historically marginalized communities, it is important to engage in constant self-reflection and to commit to building robust knowledge based on the targeted community. Similarly, cultural competence requires developing an ability to understand, appreciate, and interact effectively with people of different backgrounds.[19] The best way to increase cultural competence for working with marginalized communities is to build ongoing collaborative alliances with community members, which can facilitate accomplishing practical goals such as building support networks that can assist in the implementation of lifestyle changes.[20] Also essential to cultural competence is the building of knowledge about beliefs, preferences, practices, and values that motivate and guide behaviors in the community of focus. For instance, becoming familiar with perceptions, myths, and taboos surrounding mental illnesses and mental health treatments, as well as knowledge of preferred terms or ways of thinking and talking about mental health, can help create safe environments to talk about mental health in non-stigmatizing ways.

37.2.2 Cultural Values

Value-based approaches to lifestyle medicine can be particularly beneficial to address mental health among marginalized ethnic/racial communities. Cultural values are important beliefs that can guide and motivate individuals' choices in pursuing their well-being. For instance, in a recent study of marginalized Latino communities in South Texas, we found that collectivistic thinking, which is having the ability to focus on how an individual's behaviors or actions have an impact on others, is important to foster an increased sense of responsibility, strength, and unity while reducing symptoms of anxiety and depression.[18] From a collectivistic perspective, framing or formulating health messages that approach engagement in health behaviors as acts of love towards others can help to motivate and sustain engagement in lifestyle changes and recommendations. Similarly, we found that having self-compassion and gratitude are important values that can help discover the silver linings of gloomy situations.[21] Inviting community members to reflect upon important cultural values as the driving force to engage in and maintain a healthy lifestyle can motivate individuals to change and persevere in the face of challenges, strengthen cultural pride, and reaffirm one's cultural identity. Living in agreement with one's cultural values promotes health and well-being, whereas losing sight of one's important values can lead to stress, anxiety, and increased risk for mental illnesses, substance use, and unhealthy lifestyles.[22] Failure to incorporate cultural values in health interventions for marginalized ethnic/racial communities increases attrition rates and reduces treatment efficacy.[23]

37.2.3 Cultural Practices

Cultural practices are equally important to consider in lifestyle medicine for mental health among marginalized communities. Building collaborative networks with local providers who are knowledgeable of the target population conveys respect for the community and is more likely to lead to desired change. An important cultural practice to bear in mind is the role of religious and/or spiritual practices in preserving well-being. Religiosity and spirituality are at the center of the lives of many marginalized individuals, given that they provide a sense of mastery and control over one's actions, enhance self-esteem, give a sense of intrinsic moral self-worth, and provide life purpose and meaning, particularly amid hardship, uncertainty, and adversity.[24] Lifestyle medicine interventions that have a spiritual or religious focus have been shown to be useful in building hope, increasing social support, promoting dietary behaviors, improving sleep quality, and modifying harmful lifestyles, such as reducing the use of harmful substances.[25-28] For many marginalized ethnic/racial communities, religion and spirituality represent a mechanism helpful to organize thoughts and actions to assist in the development and maintenance of healthy living.

37.2.4 Social Networks and Interpersonal Dynamics

The effectiveness of lifestyle medicine interventions for marginalized ethnic/racial communities requires in-depth knowledge of structured social networks and customary interpersonal dynamics. Although social networks vary considerably across cultures and contexts, the stability of nuclear and extended family systems is often essential to preserve good physical and mental health.[22] Unfortunately, family separation and loss of social support systems are common among marginalized communities (e.g., undocumented immigrants, refugees, asylum seekers), thus forcing individuals to build new social networks within churches, advocacy groups, and work settings.[29] The aforesaid social networks often become informal sources of emotional and affective support, as well as primary sources of instrumental and informational help to canalize the delivery of health information and resources, including providing assistance navigating complex systems of care and the building of skills to facilitate adjustment to challenging situations.[30] In addition to attending to the structure of social networks, it is imperative to gain knowledge about rules related to interpersonal dynamics and their possible effects on health, including those that may facilitate or hinder the implementation of healthy living. For instance, internalized gender roles, which are determined by sociocultural expectations and vary widely across cultures, may influence individuals' preferences or engagement in specific health behaviors.[31] Gender roles and gender inequality interact with social and economic factors, such as opportunities and resources, to promote different lifestyle patterns.[32,33] In a study exploring binary gender differences in the engagement of health behaviors among various communities of color, results showed that women and men have important, but different, influences on household health practices (e.g., women are responsible for instilling healthy eating habits in the home, while men dictate habits related to physical activity).[33] Additionally, due to increased discrimination and stigma, transgender and gender-nonconforming people are less often involved in consistent physical activity and experience higher rates of substance use than their cisgender counterparts.[32] Leveraging support networks and being mindful of norms that guide interpersonal interactions can be powerful determinants of success in implementing and maintaining healthy lifestyles and their associated mental health benefits.

37.3 CONTEXTUAL CONSIDERATIONS OF LIFESTYLE MEDICINE FOR MENTAL HEALTH AMONG MARGINALIZED ETHNIC/RACIAL COMMUNITIES

37.3.1 INTERSECTIONALITY

Historically marginalized ethnic/racial communities are highly heterogeneous. While these communities share the experience of being marginalized and stigmatized, their experiences are shaped by the intersectionality of multiple aspects of their identity, including race, ethnicity, age, disability, religion, education, socioeconomic status, sexual orientation, gender identity, and more.[34,35] When considering the implementation of lifestyle interventions, the intersectional experiences of each marginalized individual must be considered in the context of how such experiences shape his or her sense of self, lifestyle choices, and ability to implement health behavior changes. Differences in experiences of hardship and opportunity can contribute to different motivational factors, emotional reactions, and abilities that influence how individuals engage and sustain health behaviors. Studies have shown that holding multiple marginalized identities (e.g., being Black, disabled, and transgender) is associated with a variety of detrimental physical and mental health outcomes and behaviors (e.g., depression, suicide, substance abuse).[36,37] The greater number of marginalized identities an individual endorses, the greater the challenges the person may face to maintain a healthy lifestyle or make lifestyle changes. Understanding the complexities of different aspects of an individual's identity and how this influences his or her mental health, health behaviors, and ability to engage in lifestyle changes is important to increase empathy and can facilitate validating, healing, and fulfilling interactions that are more conducive to change.[38–40]

37.3.2 SOCIAL CONTEXT

Social disadvantage has detrimental effects on the physical and mental health of marginalized ethnic/racial individuals, including restricting their ability to engage and sustain favorable health behaviors.[36] Racism, discrimination, exploitation, isolation, financial hardship, demanding work and family schedules, challenging living arrangements (e.g., crowded housing or reduced spaces), unsafe neighborhoods, insufficient health information, and limited access to technological advances, healthcare, and resources are some of the many barriers leading to chronic toxic stress among marginalized individuals. The aforesaid challenges are damaging to their health and make it difficult to adopt and sustain healthy lifestyles.[13,36,39] For instance, it may be difficult for marginalized individuals to maintain a regular sleep schedule or a consistent physical activity routine in the face of competing economic stressors, multiple demanding jobs, and challenging family caregiving duties. To better understand health among marginalized communities, it is important to consider the context that shapes a person's viewpoints, social norms, and behaviors, rather than adopting an individual lens.[41] Awareness of systemic and structural barriers that interfere or undermine an individual's healthy lifestyle (e.g., racism, discrimination), along with understanding how such barriers influence an individual's behaviors, cognitions, and emotional responses, is vital to developing effective lifestyle medicine interventions. Assisting, supporting, and providing resources for marginalized individuals to succeed in implementing lifestyle changes despite social disadvantage, although challenging, can be validating, empowering, and reassuring. Also, raising awareness of how social disadvantage interferes with healthy lifestyles is needed to reduce harmful stereotypes, given that marginalized individuals often have limited or no control over contextual influences that restrict their lifestyle choices.

37.3.3 RESILIENCE

It is important to emphasize that people from marginalized ethnic/racial communities are extremely resilient. For instance, in a recent study with undocumented Latinx immigrants in the US, we identified numerous strategies used by these immigrants to cope with adversity, marginalization, and trauma.[21] Among the strategies they used were cognitive reframing, behavioral adaptability, acceptance (i.e., gratefulness, contentment), sociability, courage, and ancestral or cultural pride.[21] The aforesaid strategies were associated with positive mental health effects including fostering a sense of meaning and purpose, building hope and self-confidence, increasing self-reliance and sense of identity, maintaining motivation, increasing positive affect, and facilitating connections with other people.[21] Given the racism and social disadvantage faced by marginalized ethnic/racial communities, strength-based approaches that focus on building upon people's strengths, skills, and qualities should be prioritized over intervention approaches that focus on weaknesses and deficits.[15] Prior studies support the effectiveness of strength-based approaches to improve mental health, including increasing positive feelings (i.e., happiness) and diminishing negative affect (i.e., depression).[42] When trying to implement lifestyle changes, strengths-based discussions can promote empowerment, which is healing for marginalized individuals who have been victimized, oppressed, and abused.[43] Building pride and a robust sense of identity can be restorative, energizing, and motivating.[44] Guiding marginalized individuals to use their strengths, talents, and skills to build healthy lifestyle routines promotes their overall well-being and boosts their mental health. An important way to build pride and increase a sense of identity is through the use of testimonials and story-telling. In reflecting upon one's life journey, individuals can increase their self-awareness and sense of resilience despite the adversity they have faced, which fosters identity formation and cognitive reframing.[45] By thinking about the lessons learned from past challenges, people can see things in a new light and often find renewed meaning, purpose, and hope even amid adversity.

37.3.4 ACCESS TO HEALTHCARE

Limited or lack of access to health services, including mental healthcare, is prevalent among marginalized ethnic/racial communities. When access to traditional health services is limited or lacking, it is important to be strategic about delivering health interventions in the communities where people live, work, learn, and play. The use of non-traditional sources of service delivery is vital for effectively disseminating lifestyle medicine interventions to marginalized communities. Non-traditional health providers play a vital role given their already trusted roles, reliance on cultural similarity, and established networks across different marginalized communities.[46,47] For instance, the effective use of Community Health Workers (CHWs) or *promotoras/es* who work in tandem with local healthcare, community agencies, and local governments in the provision of health services to marginalized communities, has been well documented.[48] CHWs and *promotora/es* perform a variety of roles in education and healthcare delivery, including acting as liaisons with their communities, assisting with navigation of current healthcare services and case management, counseling, combating misinformation and rumors, delivering health education and resources, and collecting data for disease surveillance, among many other important activities.[48,49] Furthermore, peer-support groups led by CHWs have been described as effective approaches to health promotion and disease prevention when working with marginalized ethnic/racial communities.[50,51] There is growing evidence that when CHWs utilize peer group strategies, social support can be reinforced.[52] The Community Health Club (CHC) model is one strategy recently adopted in the US, where trained CHWs form voluntary peer groups who meet regularly to co-create health knowledge, build consensus, and take action to foster healthy living that takes culture and context into account.[53,54] To maximize success, collaborations between public health authorities and non-traditional sources of service delivery have to be carefully and respectfully established, adequately funded, and provided with ongoing training, support, and resources. Importantly, resources and health information need to be disseminated in a clear, consistent, and easy to understand format in the preferred language of the targeted community.

37.4 CONCLUSION

Consistent with trends in healthcare innovation and a focus on personalized approaches to health, the use of lifestyle medicine is vital and can open avenues to address the mental health needs of historically marginalized ethnic/racial communities. Yet, the development and implementation of lifestyle interventions must occur through a culturally sensitive and contextually appropriate lens that facilitates an understanding of structural barriers and communities' strengths. As we strive towards achieving health equity, attending to and addressing the mental health of historically marginalized ethnic/racial communities require innovation and commitment, as well as a focus on interdisciplinary collaborations to ensure that no community is left behind.

REFERENCES

1. Cho S, Crenshaw KW, McCall L. Toward a field of intersectionality studies: Theory, applications, and praxis. *Signs.* 2013;38(4):785–810. doi:10.1086/669608
2. Thakur N, Lovinsky-Desir S, Bime C, Wisnivesky JP, Celedón JC. The structural and social determinants of the racial/ethnic disparities in the US COVID-19 pandemic. What's our role? *Am J Respir Crit Care Med.* 2020;202(7):943–949. doi:10.1164/rccm. 202005-1523PP
3. Thomeer MB, Moody MD, Yahirun J. Racial and ethnic disparities in mental health and mental health care during the CoViD-19 pandemic. *J Racial Ethn Health Disparities.* 2022:1–6. doi:10.1007/s40615-022-01284-9
4. Ehlman DC. Changes in suicide rates—United States, 2019 and 2020. *MMWR. Morbidity and Mortality Weekly Report.* 2022;71. doi:10.15585/mmwr.mm7108a5
5. Mongelli F, Georgakopoulos P, Pato MT. Challenges and opportunities to meet the mental health needs of underserved and disenfranchised populations in the United States. *Focus.* 2020;18(1):16–24. doi:10.1176/appi.focus.20190028
6. Benoit C, Jansson SM, Smith M, Flagg J. Prostitution stigma and its effect on the working conditions, personal lives, and health of sex workers. *J Sex Res.* 2018;55(4–5): 457–471. doi:10.1080/00224499.2017.1393652
7. Bowen S, Elliott S, Hardison-Moody A. The structural roots of food insecurity: How racism is a fundamental cause of food insecurity. *Sociol Compass.* 2021;15(7):e12846. doi:10.1111/soc4.12846
8. Cano MÁ, Schwartz SJ, MacKinnon DP, et al. Exposure to ethnic discrimination in social media and symptoms of anxiety and depression among Hispanic emerging adults: Examining the moderating role of gender. *J Clin Psychol.* 2021;77(3):571–586. doi:10.1002/jclp.23050

9. Garcini LM, Chen MA, Brown RL, et al. Kicks hurt less: Discrimination predicts distress beyond trauma among undocumented Mexican immigrants. *Psychol Violence.* 2018;8(6):692. doi:10.1037/vio0000205

10. Glick JL, Lopez A, Pollock M, Theall KP. Housing insecurity and intersecting social determinants of health among transgender people in the USA: A targeted ethnography. *Int J Transgend Health.* 2020;21(3):337–349. doi:10.1080/26895269.2020.1780661

11. Nadal KL. *Microaggressions and Traumatic Stress: Theory, Research, and Clinical Treatment.* American Psychological Association; 2018. doi:10.1037/0000073-000

12. Ramirez JL, Paz Galupo M. Multiple minority stress: The role of proximal and distal stress on mental health outcomes among lesbian, gay, and bisexual people of color. *J Gay Lesbian Ment Health.* 2019;23(2):145–167. doi:10.1080/19359705.2019.1568946

13. Alang SM. Mental health care among blacks in America: Confronting racism and constructing solutions. *Health Serv Res.* 2019;54(2):346–355. doi:10.1111/1475-6773.13115

14. Berkowitz SA, Basu S. Unemployment insurance, health-related social needs, health care access, and mental health during the COVID-19 pandemic. *JAMA Intern Med.* 2021;181(5):699–702. doi:10.1001/jamainternmed.2020.7048

15. Garcini LM, Rosenfeld J, Kneese G, Bondurant RG, Kanzler KE. Dealing with distress from the COVID-19 pandemic: Mental health stressors and coping strategies in vulnerable latinx communities. *Health Soc Care Community.* 2022;30(1):284–294. doi:10.1111/hsc.13402

16. Eylem O, De Wit L, Van Straten A, et al. Stigma for common mental disorders in racial minorities and majorities a systematic review and meta-analysis. *BMC Public Health.* 2020;20(1):1–20. doi:10.1186/s12889-020-08964-3

17. Substance Abuse and Mental Health Services Administration. Improving Cultural Competence. Treatment Improvement Protocol (TIP) Series No. 59. HHS Publication No. (SMA) 14–4849. Rockville, MD: Substance Abuse and Mental Health Services Administration, 2014.

18. Mosher DK, Hook JN, Captari LE, Davis DE, DeBlaere C, Owen J. Cultural humility: A therapeutic framework for engaging diverse clients. *Practice Innovations.* 2017; 2(4):221. doi:10.1037/pri0000055

19. DeAngelis T. In search of cultural competence. *Monit Psychol,* 2015;46(3). https://www.apa.org/monitor/2015/03/cultural-competence

20. Berryman M, SooHoo S, Nevin A, et al. Culturally responsive methodologies at work in education settings. *Int J Res Dev.* 2013;4(2):102–116. doi:10.1108/IJRD-08-2013-0014

21. Garcini LM, Cadenas G, Domenech Rodríguez MM, et al. Lessons learned from undocumented Latinx immigrants: How to build resilience and overcome distress in the face of adversity. *Psychol Serv.* 2021;19(Suppl 1):62–71. doi:10.1037/ser0000603

22. Krishnaswami J, del C. Colon-Gonzalez M. Reforming women's health care: A call to action for lifestyle medicine practitioners to save lives of mothers and infants. *Am J Lifestyle Med.* 2019;13(5):495–504. doi:10.1177/1559827619838461

23. Miranda J, Siddique J, Der-Martirosian C, Belin TR. Depression among Latina immigrant mothers separated from their children. *Psychiatr Serv.* 2005;56(6):717–720. doi:10.1176/appi.ps.56.6.717

24. Koh KB. The role of religion and spirituality in health and illness. *InStress and Somatic Symptoms.* Cham: Springer; 2018:305–313. doi:10.1007/978-3-030-02783-4_26

25. Hou SI, Cao X. A systematic review of promising strategies of faith-based cancer education and lifestyle interventions among racial/ethnic minority groups. *J Cancer Educ.* 2018;33(6):1161–1175. doi:10.1007/s13187-017-1277-5

26. Le D, Holt CL, Hosack DP, Huang J, Clark EM. Religious participation is associated with increases in religious social support in a national longitudinal study of African Americans. *J Relig Health.* 2016;55(4):1449–1460. doi:10.1007/s10943-015-0143-1

27. Litalien M, Atari DO, Obasi I. The influence of religiosity and spirituality on health in Canada: A systematic literature review. *J Relig Health*. 2021;6:1–42. doi:10.1007/s10943-020-01148-8

28. Nguyen AW, Taylor HO, Lincoln KD, Wang F, Hamler T, Mitchell UA. Religious involvement and sleep among older African Americans. *J Aging Health*. 2022;34(3):413–423. doi:10.1177/08982643221085408

29. Galvan T, Rusch D, Domenech Rodríguez MM, Garcini LM. Familias divididas [divided families]: Transnational family separation and undocumented Latinx immigrant health. *J Fam Psychol*. 2022;36(4):513–522. doi:10.1037/fam0000975

30. Ley D. The immigrant church as an urban service hub. *Urban Studies*. 2008;45(10):2057–2074. doi:10.1177/0042098008094873

31. Varì R, Scazzocchio B, D'Amore A, Giovannini C, Gessani S, Masella R. Gender-related differences in lifestyle may affect health status. *Annali dell'Istituto Superiore Di Sanita*. 2016;52(2):158–166. doi:10.4415/ANN_16_02_06

32. Aparicio-García ME, Díaz-Ramiro EM, Rubio-Valdehita S, López-Núñez MI, García-Nieto I. Health and well-being of cisgender, transgender and non-binary young people. *Int J Environ Res*. 2018;15(10):2133. doi:10.3390/ijerph15102133

33. Simonsen SE, Digre KB, Ralls B, et al. A gender-based approach to developing a healthy lifestyle and healthy weight intervention for diverse Utah women. *Eval Program Plann*. 2015;51:8–16. doi:10.1016/j.evalprogplan.2014.12.003.

34. American Psychological Association. Multicultural Guidelines: An Ecological Approach to Context, Identity, and Intersectionality. 2017. Retrieved from: http://www.apa.org/about/policy/multicultural-guidelines.pdf

35. Crenshaw K. Demarginalizing the intersection of race and sex: A black feminist critique of antidiscrimination doctrine, feminist theory and antiracist politics. University of Chicago Legal Forum. 1989(1):Article 8. http://chicagounbound.uchicago.edu/uclf/vol1989/iss1/8

36. Gattamorta KA, Salerno JP, Castro AJ. Intersectionality and health behaviors among U.S. high school students: Examining race/ethnicity, sexual identity, and sex. *J Sch Health*. 2019;89(10):800–808. doi:10.1111/josh.12817

37. Lefevor GT, Janis RA, Franklin A, Stone WM. Distress and therapeutic outcomes among transgender and gender nonconforming people of color. *Couns Psychol*. 2019;47(1):34–58. doi:10.1177/0011000019827210

38. Alizaga NM, Aguayo-Romero RA, Glickman CP. Experiences of health care discrimination among transgender and gender nonconforming people of color: A latent class analysis. *Psychol Sex Orientat Gend Divers*. 2021;9(2):141–151. doi:10.1037/sgd0000479

39. Gkiouleka A, Huijts T, Beckfield J, Bambra C. Understanding the micro and macro politics of health: Inequalities, intersectionality & institutions-a research agenda. *Soc Sci Med*. 2018;200:92–98. doi:10.1016/j.socscimed.2018.01.025

40. Rai SS, Peters RM, Syurina EV, Irwanto I, Naniche D, Zweekhorst M. Intersectionality and health-related stigma: Insights from experiences of people living with stigmatized health conditions in Indonesia. *Int J Equity Health*. 2020;19(1):1–5. doi:10.1186/s12939-020-01318-w

41. Teuscher D, Bukman AJ, van Baak MA, Feskens EJ, Renes RJ, Meershoek A. Challenges of a healthy lifestyle for socially disadvantaged people of Dutch, Moroccan and Turkish origin in the Netherlands: A focus group study. *Crit Public Health*. 2015;25(5):615–626. doi:10.1080/09581596.2014.962013

42. Rashid T. Positive psychotherapy: A strength-based approach. *J Posit Psychol*. 2015;10(1):25–40. doi:10.1080/17439760.2014.920411

43. Lambrinou E, Hansen TB, Beulens JW. Lifestyle factors, self-management and patient empowerment in diabetes care. *Eur J Prev Cardiol*. 2019;26(2):55–63. doi:10.1177/2047487319885455

44. Yip T. Ethnic/racial identity—A double-edged sword? Associations with discrimination and psychological outcomes. *Curr Dir Psychol Sci.* 2018;27(3):170–175. doi:10.1177/0963721417739348

45. Cadenas GA, Campos L, Minero LP, Aguilar C. A guide for providing mental health services to immigrants impacted by changes to DACA and the COVID-19 pandemic. 2020. https://www.informedimmigrant.com/guides/daca-mental-health-providers/

46. Weaver A, Lapidos A. Mental health interventions with community health workers in the United States: A systematic review. *J Health Care Poor Underserved.* 2018;29(1):159–180. doi:10.1353/hpu.2018.0011.

47. Barnett ML, Gonzalez A, Miranda J, Chavira DA, Lau AS. Mobilizing community health workers to address mental health disparities for underserved populations: A systematic review. *Adm Policy Ment Health.* 2018;45(2):195–211. doi:10.1007/s10488-017-0815-0

48. Landers SJ, Stover GN. Community health workers—practice and promise. *Am J Public Health.* 2011;101(12):2198–2198. doi:10.2105/AJPH.2011.300371

49. Peretz PJ, Islam N, Matiz LA. Community health workers and Covid-19—addressing social determinants of health in times of crisis and beyond. *N Engl J Med.* 2020;383(19):e108. doi:10.1056/NEJMp2022641

50. Mosavel M, Simon C, Van Stade D, Buchbinder M. Community-based participatory research (CBPR) in South Africa: Engaging multiple constituents to shape the research question. *Soc Sci Med.* 2005;61(12):2577–2587. doi:10.1016/j.socscimed.2005.04.041

51. Scarinci IC, Garces-Palacio IC, Partridge EE. An examination of acceptability of HPV vaccination among African American women and Latina immigrants. *J Women's Health.* 2007;16(8):1224–1233. doi:10.1089/jwh.2006.0175

52. Wallerstein N, Duran B, Oetzel JG, Minkler M, eds. *Community-Based Participatory Research for Health: Advancing Social and Health Equity.* John Wiley & Sons; 2017.

53. Meza C, Ruiz M, McMaster J, Chung M, Escareño J, Ibarra E, Rosenfeld J. Cooking up Convivencia in the Lower Rio Grande Valley: A peer-group health promotion model that improves physical, social and mental well-being. Oral presentation at: Texas Public Health Association Annual Education Conference; Irving, TX; 2020.

54. Waterkeyn J, Cairncross S. Creating demand for sanitation and hygiene through Community Health Clubs: A cost-effective intervention in two districts in Zimbabwe. *Soc Sci Med.* 2005;61(9):1958–1970. doi:10.1016/j.socscimed.2005.04.012

Index

Printed in the United States
by Baker & Taylor Publisher Services